Advanced Abnormal Psychology

Second Edition

Advanced Abnormal Psychology
Second Edition

Edited by

MICHEL HERSEN

Pacific University
Forest Grove, Oregon

and

VINCENT B. VAN HASSELT

Nova Southeastern University
Fort Lauderdale, Florida

KLUWER ACADEMIC/PLENUM PUBLISHERS
NEW YORK, BOSTON, DORDRECHT, LONDON, MOSCOW

Library of Congress Cataloging-in-Publication Data

Advanced abnormal psychology/edited by Michel Hersen and Vincent B. Van
Hasselt.—2nd ed.
    p. cm.
  Includes bibliographical references and index.
  ISBN 0-306-46381-4
    1. Psychology, Pathological.   2. Mental illness—Treatment.   I. Hersen, Michel.   II. Van
Hasselt, Vincent B.

RC454 .A325 2000
616.89—dc21

                                                00-046624

ISBN 0-306-46381-4

©2001 Kluwer Academic/Plenum Publishers, New York
233 Spring Street, New York, N.Y. 10013

http://www.wkap.nl/

10 9 8 7 6 5 4 3 2 1

A C.I.P. record for this book is available from the Library of Congress

Printed in the United States of America

To

Irene Papadopolous for Her Inspiration

Alexandra and Melanie

Contributors

MARC S. ATKINS, Department of Psychiatry, University of Illinois at Chicago, Chicago, Illinois 60612

KRISTINE L. BRADY, California School of Professional Psychology, San Diego, California 92121

JAMES E. BRYAN, Oregon Health Sciences University, Portland, Oregon 97201

DEVIN A. BYRD, Department of Psychology, Virginia Polytechnic Institute and State University, Blacksburg, Virginia 24061

KEITH CHENG, Child and Adolescent Treatment Program, Emanuel Hospital, Portland, Oregon 97227

FREDERICK L. COOLIDGE, Department of Psychology, University of Colorado at Colorado Springs, Colorado Springs, Colorado 80933-7150

LISA W. COYNE, Department of Psychology, University of Mississippi, University, Mississippi 38677

BRITTA D. DINSMORE, Pacific University Student Counseling Center, Forest Grove, Oregon 97116

CARRIE L. DODRILL, Department of Psychology, University of Houston, Houston, Texas 77204-5341

JAMIE A. DYCE, Department of Psychology, Concordia University College of Alberta, Edmonton, Alberta, Canada T5B 4E4

MORRIS EAGLE, Derner Institute, Adelphi University, Garden City, New York 11530

JOSHUA EHRLICH, Department of Psychiatry, University of Michigan, Ann Arbor, Michigan 48104

PAUL M. G. EMMELKAMP, Department of Clinical Psychology, University of Amsterdam, 1018 WB Amsterdam, The Netherlands

KARYN EWART, California School of Professional Psychology, Fresno, California 93727

PATRICIA L. FIERO, Medical University of South Carolina, Charleston, South Carolina 29425-0742

CHANDRA M. GRABILL, Sexton Woods Psychoeducational Center, DeKalb County School System, Chamblee, Georgia 30341

GERALD GOLDSTEIN, VA Pittsburgh Healthcare System, Pittsburgh, Pennsylvania, 15206

JEANA R. GRIFFITH, Department of Psychiatry and Behavioral Sciences, Emory University School of Medicine at Grady Memorial Hospital, Atlanta, Georgia 30335

ALAN M. GROSS, Department of Psychology, University of Mississippi, University, Mississippi 38677

ANN MARIE HAMER, Oregon State University College of Pharmacy, Portland, Oregon 97201

DANIEL M. HARRIS, Oregon Health Sciences University, Portland, Oregon 97201

JOSHUA K. HARROWER, University of California at Santa Barbara, Santa Barbara, California 93106

NADINE J. KASLOW, Department of Psychiatry and Behavioral Sciences, Emory University School of Medicine at Grady Memorial Hospital, Atlanta, Georgia 30335

LYNN KERN KOEGEL, University of California at Santa Barbara, Santa Barbara, California 93106

ROBERT L. KOEGEL, University of California at Santa Barbara, Santa Barbara, California 93106

KEVIN T. LARKIN, Department of Psychology, West Virginia University, Morgantown, West Virginia 26506-6040

HOWARD D. LERNER, Department of Psychiatry, University of Michigan, Ann Arbor, Michigan 48104; *Current address*: Ann Arbor, Michigan 48104

LESTER LUBORSKY, Department of Psychiatry, University of Pennsylvania, Philadelphia, Pennsylvania 19104

F. DUDLEY MCGLYNN, Department of Psychology, Auburn University, Auburn, Alabama 36849-5214

MARY M. MCKAY, Columbia University School of Social Work, New York, New York 10025

PARAS MEHTA, Department of Psychology, University of Houston, Houston, Texas 77204-5341

CYNTHIA L. MILLER-LONCAR, Department of Pediatrics, Infant Development Center, Women & Infant's Hospital, Providence, Rhode Island 02903

DOIL D. MONTGOMERY, Center for Psychological Studies, Nova Southeastern University, Fort Lauderdale, Florida, 33314

ERIN A. MUELLER, Oregon Health Sciences University, Portland, Oregon 97201

KIM T. MUESER, Department of Psychiatry and Community and Family Medicine, Dartmouth Medical School, Dartmouth College, Concord, New Hampshire 03301-3852

KATHLEEN MYERS, Outpatient Child and Adolescent Psychiatry, Department of Psychiatry, Oregon Health Sciences University, Portland, Oregon 97201

BRIAN P. O'CONNOR, Department of Psychology, Lakehead University, Thunder Bay, Ontario, Canada P7B SE1

KEVIN J. O'CONNOR, California School of Professional Psychology, Fresno, California 93727

WILLIAM O'DONOHUE, Department of Psychology, University of Nevada-Reno, Reno, Nevada 89557-0062

TIMOTHY J. O'FARRELL, Department of Psychiatry, Harvard Medical School, Boston, Massachusetts; and Veterans Affairs Medical Center, Brockton, Massachusetts 02301

THOMAS H. OLLENDICK, Department of Psychology, Virginia Polytechnic Institute and State University, Blacksburg, Virginia 24061

PAMELA M. PLANTHARA, Center for Psychological Studies, Nova Southeastern University, Fort Lauderdale, Florida 33314

TAMARA PENIX, Department of Psychology, University of Nevada-Reno, Reno, Nevada 89557-0062

LINDA KRUG PORZELIUS, School of Professional Psychology, Pacific University, Forest Grove, Oregon 97116

MARK D. RAPPORT, Department of Psychology, University of Central Florida, Orlando, Florida 32816

LISA REGEV, Department of Psychology, University of Nevada-Reno, Reno, Nevada 89557-0062

LYNN P. REHM, Department of Psychology, University of Houston, Houston, Texas 77204-5341

MICHELLE P. SALYERS, Department of Psychology, Indiana University-Purdue University Indianapolis, Indianapolis, Indiana 46202-3275

DANIEL L. SEGAL, Department of Psychology, University of Colorado at Colorado Springs, Colorado Springs, Colorado 80933-7150

DARLENE STAFFELBACH, St. Vincent's Hospital Eating Disorder Program, Providence St. Vincent Hospital, Portland, Oregon 97225

WARREN W. TRYON, Department of Psychology, Fordham University, Bronx, New York 10458-5198

MARTA VALDEZ-MENCHANCA, University of California at Santa Barbara, Santa Barbara, California 93106

PATRICIA VAN OPPEN, Department of Psychiatry, Valeriuskliniek 1075 BG, Amsterdam, The Netherlands

THOMAS L. WHITMAN, Department of Psychology, University of Notre Dame, Notre Dame, Indiana 46556

ARTHUR N. WIENS, Oregon Health Sciences University, Portland, Oregon 97201

WILLIAM H. WILSON, Department of Psychiatry, Oregon Health Sciences University, Portland, Oregon 97201

JAMIE M. WINTER, Department of Psychology, University of Notre Dame, Notre Dame, Indiana 46556

DAVID L. WOLITZKY, Department of Psychology, New York University, New York, New York 10003-6634

ILIZABETH WOLLHEIM, California School of Professional Psychology, Fresno, California 93727

MICHAEL J. ZVOLENSKY, Department of Psychology, West Virginia University, Morgantown, West Virginia 26506-6040

Preface to the First Edition

Although senior undergraduate psychology students and first year master's- and doctoral-level students frequently take courses in advanced abnormal psychology, it has been almost two decades since a book by this title has appeared. Professors teaching this course have had a wide variety of texts to select from that touch on various aspects of psychopathology, but none has been as comprehensive for the student as the present volume. Not only are basic concepts and models included, but there are specific sections dealing with childhood and adolescent disorders, adult and geriatric disorders, child treatment, and adult treatment. We believe the professor and advanced student alike will benefit from having all the requisite material under one cover.

Our book contains 26 chapters presented in five parts, each part preceded by an editors' introduction. The chapters reflect updates in the classification of disorders (i.e., DSM-IV). In Part I (Basic Concepts and Models), the chapters include diagnosis and classfication, assessment strategies, research methods, the psychoanalystic model, the behavioral model, and the biological model. Parts II (Childhood and Adolescent Disorders) and III (Adult and Older Adult Disorders), each containing seven chapters, represent the bulk of the book. To ensure cross-chapter consistency, each of these chapters on psychopathology follows an identical format, with the following basic sections: description of the disorder, epidemiology, clinical picture (with case description), course and prognosis, familial and genetic patterns, and diagnostic considerations. Parts IV and V—on Child Treatment and Adult Treatment, respectively— each contain three chapters that deal with the major modes of therapy: dynamic psychotherapy, behavior therapy, and pharmacological interventions. Thus, the student will gain an understanding not only of childhood and adult psychopathology, but of the existing strategies for remediation of such psychopathology as well.

Many individuals have contributed to the fruition of our efforts here. First, we thank our eminent contributors, who took time out from their busy schedules to partake in this project. We thank Burt G. Bolton, as well, for his technical expertise with respect to the manuscript. Finally, but hardly least, we again thank our friend and editor at Plenum, Eliot Werner, who appreciated the timeliness of our project.

VINCENT B. VAN HASSELT
MICHEL HERSEN

Fort Lauderdale, Florida

Preface to the Second Edition

Our book is directed to senior undergraduate psychology students and first year master's- and doctoral-level students who take courses in advanced abnormal psychology. Professors teaching this course have had a wide variety of texts to select from that touch on various aspects of psychopathology, but none has been as comprehensive for the student as the present volume. Not only are basic concepts and models included, but there are specific sections dealing with childhood and adolescent disorders, adult and geriatric disorders, child treatment, and adult treatment. We believe the professor and advanced student alike will benefit from having all the requisite material under one cover.

The Second Edition of our book contains 27 chapters presented in five parts, each part preceded by an editors' introduction. The chapters reflect updates in the classification of disorders (i.e., DSM-IV). In Part I (Basic Concepts and Models), the chapters include diagnosis and classification, assessment strategies, research methods, the psychoanalytic model, the behavioral model, and the biological model. Parts II (Childhood and Adolescent Disorders) and III (Adult and Older Adult Disorders), containing seven and eight chapters, respectively, represent the bulk of the book. To ensure cross-chapter consistency, each of these chapters on psychopathology follows an identical format, with the following basic sections: description of the disorder, epidemiology, clinical picture (with case description), course and prognosis, familial and genetic patterns, and diagnostic considerations. Parts IV and V—on Child Treatment and Adult Treatment, respectively—each contain three chapters that deal with the major modes of therapy: dynamic psychotherapy, behavior therapy, and pharmacological interventions. Thus, the student will gain an understanding not only of childhood and adult psychopathology, but of the existing strategies for remediation of such psychopathology as well.

Many individuals have contributed to the fruition of our efforts here. First, we thank our eminent contributors, who took time out from their busy schedules to partake in this project. We thank Carole Londerée, Alexander Duncan, and Erika Qualls. Finally, but hardly least of all, we again thank our friend and editor at Kluwer Academic/Plenum Publishers, Eliot Werner, who appreciated the timeliness of our project.

MICHEL HERSEN
VINCENT B. VAN HASSELT

Forest Grove, Oregon
Fort Lauderdale, Florida

Contents

Part I. Basic Concepts and Models

Part II. Childhood and Adolescent Disorders

Part III. Adult and Older Adult Disorders

Part IV. Child Treatment

Basic Concepts and Models: Introductory Comments

Over time the discipline of abnormal psychology has become more complex, particularly as it adduces data from its sister disciplines, such as epidemiology, genetics, sociology, anthropology, and biology. Adding to such complexity is the status of theory in this area. Absence of theoretical unity is especially striking, given the distinct and, at times, contradictory expositions from those of psychoanalytic, behavioral, and biological persuasions. But in spite of such complexity and contradiction, there are some very basic data that the student of abnormal psychology must learn, and these are concerned with diagnosis and classification, assessment strategies, and research methods. Moreover, the student should be familiar with the three basic models of abnormal behavior: psychoanalytic, behavioral, and biological. Part I of this book, therefore, is devoted to an outline of these basic issues and models.

In Chapter 1, Daniel L. Segal and Frederick L. Coolidge discuss the historical roots of the diagnosis and classification of abnormal behavior, describe the current DSM-IV system, and highlight current controversies in the field. The authors show how the boundaries of mental illness have been subject to marked historical changes, as new disorders, conditions, theoretical underpinnings, and classification systems evolve regularly. Despite its imperfections, the DSM-IV represents clearly an important advance on its historical predecessors. This system is, and will continue to be, used in the psychiatric care of those with psychiatric problems. The authors prognosticate that the multiaxial system will continue in the next edition of the DSM, although minor adjustments to existing axes are likely to occur and additional axes may be added. For example, a new axis of defensive functioning (defense mechanisms) may be formalized based on its appearance in the DSM-IV Appendix B: Criteria Sets and Axes Provided for Further Study. As presently conceptualized, the Defensive Functioning Scale allows for clinicians to list in order up to seven of the specific defenses used by the patient (e.g., humor, dissociation, idealization, projection, acting out) and then list the predominant defensive level shown by the patient (e.g., high adaptive level, disavowal level, level of defensive dysregulation).

In Chapter 2, which focuses on assessment principles, Arthur N. Wiens, Erin A. Mueller, and James E. Bryan show how assessment strategies discussed can be expected to lead to a diagnosis of a patient's condition. They note that a great deal of thought has gone into identifying criteria for diagnoses and sources of unreliability in diagnostic formulations. Five sources of unreliability in making diagnoses are considered: subject variance, occasion variance, information variance, observation variance, and criterion variance. Wiens and his colleagues predict that unstructured assessment clinical interviews of the past will be replaced in the future by structured interview schedules for routine clinical assessment. This shift is supported by trends toward use of operational criteria for diagnosis, well-defined taxonomies, almost exclusive use of structured examinations in research settings, and the growing influence of clinician-researchers. Further, the demand for accountability has also forced a problem-oriented type of record keeping system in most institutions, with emphasis on branch-logic systems of clinical decision making and progress notes that reflect resolution of symptom-syndromes and changes in problem status rather than changes in psychodynamics.

In Chapter 3, F. Dudley McGlynn outlines the research methods carried out to study the numerous aspects of psychopathology. In addition to considering science and explanation in psychopathology and validity in research on psychopathology, McGlynn describes in detail research on etiology and on intervention. He notes that psychological research on intervention takes the form of case studies, intrasubject replication experiments, cognitive behavior therapy outcome research, behavior therapy analog research, comparative psychotherapy outcome research, meta-analyses, and psychotherapy process research. Behavior therapy analog research can accomplish strong internal validity; cognitive behavior therapy outcome research can approach acceptable external validity. He argues that yields from process research and comparative psychotherapy outcome research have been unimpressive.

In Chapter 4, Howard D. Lerner and Joshua Ehrlich introduce the reader to psycho-analytic theory and trace historically its developments since Freud into the various "overlapping models of the mind." Three primary models are presented: modern structural theory, self-psychology, and object relations theory. The authors document how each of the models has its unique focus on personality, development, psychopathology, and therapy.

In Chapter 5, the behavioral model of abnormal psychology is articulated by Warren W. Tryon. He underscores the imperative of learning which, of course, presupposes memory, and argues that all psychological development entails learning and memory and that divergent models differ only in the way they understand learning and memory. He shows how recent developments in learning and memory, referred to as Neural Network Learning Theory, promise to unify the behavioral and cognitive models of learning and memory and provide a unified theoretical understanding of abnormal psychology.

Operant conditioning is a form of R-S rather than S-R learning theory where consequences select (edit) response distributions. The resulting skewed distributions have either a higher or lower mean depending upon whether low or high values have been deleted. This developmental process enables behavior to "evolve" over time: ontogenetic evolution. Relationships that define various forms of operant conditioning are summarized. Tryon identifies pairs of operant conditions that are inherently problematic. He categorizes four possibilities for maintaining problematic behavior that might be diagnosed from samples of current behavior. The main treatment implication is to modify the offending contingency.

In addition to operant theory, the importance of the therapeutic relationship as fundamental to all clinical intervention is emphasized. The responsibility of the therapist to engage clients is accentuated, and recommendations for increasing one's Engagement Quotient are provided.

Finally, in Chapter 6, exciting new discoveries in the field are presented by Doil D. Montgomery and Pamela M. Planthara in support of the biological model. The authors note that certain specific pathologies do have underlying biological mechanisms associated with them. What seems to be the most parsimonious explanation is that genetics provides a general template for neural development, which is modified by the experiences of the individual. We inherit propensities that place limits on behavior. Yet the constraints may be altered by impoverished or enriched environments or by intense or sustained interventions. Recent information about neural development indicates that during embryonic development only approximately one-half of the neurons produced will survive development of the nervous system. These findings, combined with evidence from animal studies, indicate that the major determinant as to which nerve cells die and which survive depends upon which neurons are activated by experiences. The cells that are activated by experience survive and form connections with other neurons, whereas those that are not activated die. This provides powerful support for the role early experiences have upon neural development and subsequent behavior. The authors underscore that additional data are being rapidly addressed through new assay techniques of chemistry of tissue and new imaging techniques of neural and chromosomal tissue. There is great promise for a better understanding of the biology of behavior, which is likely to help direct early optimum experiences and specific interventions at multiple levels to facilitate an individual's development.

Diagnosis and Classification

DANIEL L. SEGAL AND FREDERICK L. COOLIDGE

INTRODUCTION

Coupled with exploratory behavior, the desire to understand and to classify the things in one's environment appears to be an inherent human trait. The word *diagnosis* itself comes from the Greek words *dia*, meaning apart, and *gnosis*, meaning to know, thus promoting the idea that to know or understand a condition one must be able to discriminate it from other conditions. The twentieth century psychologist Jean Piaget (1896–1980) postulated that the essence of the beginnings of knowledge in humans begins with the dual abilities of assimilating observations into existing categories and accommodating information that does not fit into existing categories by creating new ones (Piaget, 1932). The earliest roots of the diagnosis and classification of abnormal behavior, no doubt, stretch back into the very dawn of human consciousness and the rise of societal behavior. Acculturation processes and their evolutionary advantages over solitary existence probably served as a major impetus for the necessity of humans to decide who was capable of following the rules of society, who might be excused from them (perhaps the very young or very old), and who would not. For example, the contemporary Inuit North Americans describe, in their own language, a kind of antisocial personality disordered individual as "his mind knows what to do but he does not do it" (Murphy, 1976). In this introductory chapter, the major issues regarding the diagnosis and classification of abnormal behavior are analyzed. We first discuss the purposes of diagnosis and then provide a historical overview of diagnosis and classification. Next, we describe the current classification system and conclude with a discussion of criticisms and limitations of diagnosis and classification.

Definitions

The concepts of diagnosis and classification, as well as assessment and testing, are all intertwined. The word diagnosis can be used to mean the identification and labeling, analyzing the causes of, or classifying and grouping abnormal behaviors. Classification most often refers

DANIEL L. SEGAL AND FREDERICK L. COOLIDGE • Department of Psychology, University of Colorado at Colorado Springs, Colorado Springs, Colorado 80933-7150.

Advanced Abnormal Psychology, Second Edition, edited by Hersen and Van Hasselt. Kluwer Academic/Plenum Publishers, New York, 2001.

to the creation and maintenance of a formal system of distinct groupings, whereas assessment may refer to the observation, examination, and gathering of relevant data.

The assessment, diagnosis, and classification of abnormal behaviors provide the foundation of a scientific approach for their greater understanding. When reliable and valid categories are established, discussions may begin as to the causes, nature, and treatment of those disordered behaviors. The classification system may be further expanded when the diagnostic process addresses behaviors that do not fit neatly into existing categories. Part of this process is the important ability to generalize from what has been observed.

Purposes and Features of Diagnosis

A number of benefits result from application of formal diagnostic labels to clinical phenomena. Diagnostic labels help professionals communicate with one another about cases. For instance, much can be communicated from one professional to another by stating that an individual has symptoms of borderline personality disorder. Knowledge of disorders and symptoms also helps clinicians organize information elicited from patients. For example, if an individual presents with frequent crying spells, anhedonia, and overeating, a clinician may probe about the presence or absence of other symptoms of major depression (e.g., sleep disturbance, concentration problems, suicidal impulses) to confirm or rule out the diagnosis. Diagnosis is sometimes used to determine the legal status of an individual. For example, neuropsychological evaluations are often conducted to determine one's competency or ability to make medical and financial decisions. Other evaluations focus on the psychological competence of an individual; for example, when a psychotic individual commits a crime. Diagnosis can help the seriously mentally ill person be placed in a mental health facility rather than a jail.

Another important aspect of diagnosis is that (in a good science) it should determine treatment. Similar to the medical model in which a diagnosis of strep throat implies the successful treatment by a course of antibiotic medications, diagnosis in mental health often influences the type of therapy provided. In fact, in recent years the field has provided many empirically validated psychological treatments of specific mental disorders (see excellent review by DeRubeis & Crits-Cristoph, 1998). For example, efficacious treatments for major depression include cognitive therapy, behavior therapy, and interpersonal therapy. Unfortunately, empirically validated psychological treatments are not currently available for many disorders (e.g., bipolar disorder, anorexia nervosa, dissociative identity disorder). Diagnosis is also important because it affects one's ability to receive reimbursement for mental health services from insurance companies. It is a sad reality that some insurance companies pay for services for some disorders and refuse to pay for others. A final purpose of diagnosis is that it can be used to enhance research about causes and treatments of mental disorders. Indeed, if investigators can accurately group similar people together, research can be conducted to examine common environmental or biological causes and the most effective intervention strategies.

Several other points about diagnosis should also be highlighted here. First, persons with a particular diagnosis (e.g., depression) need not exhibit identical features, although they should present with certain cardinal symptoms (e.g., either depressed mood or anhedonia). Indeed, criteria for many disorders (according to the current diagnostic guide, the *Diagnostic and Statistical Manual for Mental Disorders*, DSM-IV, APA, 1994) are polythetic, which means that an individual must meet a minimum number of symptoms to be diagnosable, but not all symptoms need be present (e.g., five of nine symptoms must be present to diagnose major depression). This allows some variation among people with the same disorder. Second, individuals with the same disorder should have a similar history in some areas; for example, a typical age of onset, prognosis, and common comorbid conditions. Other important information about a diagnosis includes prevalence and course data; the extent of its genetic loading (i.e. whether it consistently runs in families, concordance rates among twins); the extent to which it is affected by psychosocial forces; the extent to which it varies according to gender, age, and culture; the types of subtypes and/or specifiers; associated laboratory findings, physical examination findings, and general medical conditions; and information about differential diagnosis. Fortunately, information about many of these areas is provided in the text of DSM-IV for each disorder.

Historical Overview of Diagnosis and Classification

Ancient Roots

It may be surmised that the tripartite system (assessment, diagnosis, and classification) began its evolution with the ancient Egyptians. The Edwin Smith Surgical Papyrus (Breasted, 1991) dates to about 1650 B.C.E. and was based on an even earlier work. This hieroglyphic medical manuscript served as a diagnosis and treatment manual for head injuries. It presents case reports of 48 head-injured patients who were first examined (assessment), then diagnosed and classified (head injury, treatable or not), and then, in treatable cases, a treatment was suggested. Because clinical psychology has generally followed a medical model, it comes as no surprise that today abnormal behavior is still assessed (usually by clinical interviews and psychological tests), a diagnosis is proposed, and treatment plans are suggested.

Perhaps, one of the earliest aspects of evaluating abnormal behavior began with its causes. One early suspicion for the cause of abnormal behavior was a supernatural or divine influence. The practice of trephination, drilling a hole in a person's skull, dates back at least 10,000 years and may have been an attempt to change a person's abnormal behavior by releasing them from supernaturally evil spirits, although this may be pure conjecture. What is known is that trephination was practiced in many places in the world, including Europe, the Middle East, and South America, and that many patients lived long after their operations (Finger, 1994). Even today, the concept of a divine etiology for mental illness is not uncommon. The idea that sinful behaviors are punishable by God through mental illnesses remains popular.

Early Mesopotamian writings and later Chinese and Greek treatises began to recognize two sources for abnormal behavior: supernatural/divine causes and environmental influences on various organs of the body, like the heart. Interestingly, not until much later (about 500 B.C.E.) was the brain considered an undeniable cause of human behavior. This tradition also may have derived from Egyptian practices. In mummification, Egyptians removed what they considered to be important organs: the liver, lungs, stomach, and intestines. They were placed in separate vessels called canopic jars. The heart was considered too important to remove, and the brain was considered irrelevant and was usually drained from the skull (Finger, 1994).

Greek Traditions

The ancient Greeks, such as Hippocrates (460–377 B.C.E.), began important new and long-influential traditions in diagnosing and classifying abnormal behavior. The writings attributed to Hippocrates (Hippocrates, 1952) strongly countered supernatural influences as a cause of abnormal behavior. Hippocrates clearly established that abnormal behavior was caused primarily by the interaction of environmental factors (like climatic variables such as heat, cold, humidity, and dryness) upon the human brain. This latter important contribution was not universally accepted. Even two thousand years later, people still looked to supernatural or divine causes for abnormal behavior. Still, Hippocrates was eminently clear:

> Men ought to know that from nothing else but the brain come joys, delights, laughter and sports, and sorrows, griefs, despondency, and lamentations. And by this, in an especial manner, we acquire wisdom and knowledge, and see and hear, and know what are foul and what are fair, what are bad and what are good.... And by the same organ we become mad and delirious, and fears and terrors assail us, some by night, and some by day, and dreams and untimely wanderings. And cares that are not suitable.... All of these things we endure from the brain, when it is not healthy, but is more hot, more cold, more moist or more dry than natural.... And we become mad from its humidity. (1952 translation, p. 336)

As noted earlier, Hippocrates' belief in the brain's susceptibility to external factors reflected a modification of ancient earlier ideas that air, water, earth, and fire caused abnormal behavior. Hippocrates associated the four elements with four conditions (dryness, moisture, cold, and warmth) that, in turn, influenced four bodily fluids of yellow and black bile, blood, and phlegm. These four fluids formed Hippocrates' humoral theory; that is, differences in individual behavior could be attributed to excesses or deficiencies of the four body fluids or humors. Hippocrates' descriptions of their actions are also vivid:

> As long as the brain is at rest, the man enjoys his reason, but the depravement of the brain arises from phlegm and bile, either of which you may recognize in this manner: Those who are mad from phlegm are quiet, and do not cry out nor make a noise; but those from bile are vociferous, malignant, and will not be quiet, but are always doing something improper. (1952 translation, p. 337)

Of course, treatment for these ailments centered about the reduction of these excess fluids or cooling them, like the induction of vomiting, the use of laxatives for purging, and the use of drugs like opium.

Hippocrates and his followers had a profound effect upon later diagnosis and classification by fighting the long popular notions of supernatural and divine control upon human behavior. They also emphasized the brain, and not the heart, as the premier instigator of all behavior, and, finally, they recognized that external forces (like climate) and internal forces (like digestion and diet) on the brain played a prominent role in abnormal behavior. Hippocrates' beliefs, as noted earlier, were not universally accepted even by the Greek philosopher Plato (427–347 B.C.E.) or his disciple Aristotle (384–322 B.C.E.) nearly 100 years later (Aristotle, 1952; Plato, 1952). The notion that the heart was the seat of emotion and memory was difficult to dislodge after a 2,000-year prehistory and so was the notion of divine influences. For example, Plato ascribed specific mental diseases (such as mania, hysteria, and hallucinatory delirium) to specific evil gods. He also proposed that beneficial gods could intervene against the influence of evil gods and even instill positive mental changes. Through Plato's influence, the soul became the nucleus of a person's personality, although he still believed that bodily humors could cause abnormal behavior through poor diet, drugs, and climate. It is also interesting to note that a differentiation was made at this time between acute and chronic mental illnesses. For example, debates arose as to whether cauliflower and basil either caused acute madness or whether they alleviated it (Roccatagliata, 1986).

In 342 B.C.E., Aristotle was appointed to head a faculty of learned people to educate Alexander the Great, and when the latter became king, he financed Aristotle's research. Aristotle, as an empiricist and excellent observer, broke with the thinking of Plato that parts of the body justified the existence of the whole. Aristotle thought that the total organism justified the existence of the parts and that they were all reciprocally connected. In a manner, Aristotle heralded a psychosomatic theory of abnormal behavior. Unfortunately, Aristotle also promoted natural heat as a major producer of pathological mental and physical states and, unlike Plato, reverted to the heart as the seat of thinking and emotion. The brain, Aristotle wrote, was "a residue lacking any sensitive faculty" (Roccatagliata, 1986, p. 106).

Through Aristotle's works and influence, classification of abnormal behavior began to expand, although not in any clear formal manner. Descriptions were made of many prototypes of modern psychopathological states like mania, melancholy, confusion, delirium, mental torpor, obsessions, anxiety, pathological fears, and cyclothymic psychosis. Generally, all of these disorders were thought to be caused by psychosomatic humoral processes, that is, heat and cold (chief among the causative agents) affected the bodily fluids which subsequently affected behavior.

Roman Traditions

After the death of Aristotle in 322 B.C.E., Theophrastus (372–287 B.C.E.) assumed direction of Aristotle's school. While Aristotle was alive, he and Theophrastus collaborated frequently, and Theophrastus wrote on a variety of topics such as the effects of various drugs on mental states, marriage, child-raising, alcoholism, melancholy, epilepsy, and, interestingly, on people's character or temperaments. In the latter work, he described 30 different characters or personalities that were differentiated on the basis of more fundamental personality traits like superstitious beliefs or vanity. Theophrastus also reestablished the idea that the brain is the seat of the intellect, and he advanced the diagnosis and classification of abnormal behavior in some sophisticated ways, even by current standards (Edmonds, 1929).

In his writing, *On Character*, Theophrastus established the beginnings of the concepts for personality disorders. The Greek writer Homer, centuries earlier, had adopted a similar stance by ascribing to some of his characters a single dominant personality trait, such as the "brave Hector" or the "crafty Ulysses." Theophrastus went beyond Homer's single master trait by describing how an individual's character might express itself in a variety of situations. Each of his 30 characters was dominated by a single but primary trait such as lying, flattering, talkativeness, cheapness, tactlessness, surliness, discontentedness, and rudeness. His description of the cheap person (penurious) overlaps many of the general and associated features of the modern obsessive–compulsive personality disorder, such as stinginess with money, compliments, and affection; excessive devotion to work; rigidity; and inflexibility. His character dominated by superstitious beliefs may be a forerunner of the schizotypal personality disorder, his lying character may herald the antisocial personality disorder, his flatterer may be the narcissistic personality disorder, and his discontented character may have features of both the passive-aggressive and the depressive personality disorders.

With the death of Alexander the Great in 323 B.C.E., there began a steady decline of interest in medicine and other sciences in Greece. Many of the Greek-trained physicians then turned to Rome and the Roman Empire for further study and support. Galen (130–200 A.D.; 1952 translation), a Greek-born and trained physician, became one of the most famous of the later Roman physicians and remained one of Hippocrates' chief supporters. He defended Hippocrates' theory of body humors against critics who advanced their own theories of humors and vapors in the human body. To Galen's credit, he emphasized that the origin of the intellect was the brain, including imagination, intelligence, and memory, and there were hints in his writings that the brain might have areas that were localized by their function. Galen's chief legacy may be his classification of people into at least two psychological types:

the melancholic and the sanguine. The melancholic type has many modern counterparts, including the introvert, the dysthymic person, and the depressive personality disorder. The sanguine type serves as a model for the modern concept of extroversion. Galen recognized, like Hippocrates before him, that human behavior can be affected by diet and climate, and Galen is often credited with the biological influences on human behavior now known as temperaments; that is, biological predispositions to act in consistent ways.

Dark Ages and the Renaissance

Galen began, however, an unfortunate legacy that spaces in the brain, the ventricles, contained "spirits" that were the essence of brain function, and he thought that no brain injury would have consequences unless the ventricles were also penetrated. By about the third or fourth century, the "Dark Ages" began in Western Europe and persisted for about 1,000 years. There was a further decline in the sciences as the Catholic church hierarchy played a greater role in many aspects of common life. The belief in supernatural effects on behavior flourished. Sinful behavior became an accepted causative agent of abnormal behavior, and ironically, it still is today. Insanity was also believed to have been caused by demons and witches. One popular "diagnostic manual" of the time was the *Malleus Malificarum* (*The Hammer of Witches*), which presented methods for identifying and assessing witches, such as tying the accused woman's hands and feet together and throwing her into a river. If she floated, she was a witch. There were, however, pockets of cultures in the rest of the world that still venerated the works of Hippocrates, Aristotle, and Galen (Cohen, Swerdlik, & Phillips, 1996).

With the onset of the Renaissance, a renewed interest in the brain began, and foremost among these brain scholars was Leonardo da Vinci (1472–1519). Although the pope had forbidden human autopsies, da Vinci conducted more than 300 of them and made more than 1,500 drawings of the human body and brain. He conducted experiments with cattle brains to make anatomically correct drawings of the ventricles, but consistent with the thinking of the time, he also classified various brain functions to the ventricles (Finger, 1994). da Vinci, whether intentionally or not, began a rich tradition of anatomical descriptions of the brain that may have reached an ironic zenith about 300 years later in the work of Austrian anatomist and physician Franz Gall (1758–1828).

The zeitgeist of psychological classification at the beginning of Gall's life was to classify human behavior based on facial characteristics or physiognomy. Gall, in his own writings, claims that at the age of nine, he discovered his theory of brain localization. A friend of his at school was very good at memorization, and he had *les yeux a fleur de tete* or bulging eyes. Gall decided that his friend's bulging eyes were due to overdeveloped frontal lobes, and thus, was born Gall's theory of phrenology. In Vienna in 1781, Gall began giving popular public lectures. Church authorities worked to pass legislation prohibiting Gall's public lectures, and he then moved to Paris to continue his work. Although the French Academy of Sciences soundly rejected Gall's notion that skull indentations and bumps reflected human temperaments, he was well received within certain circles and was lavishly supported (Finger, 1994).

Age of Enlightenment

As noted earlier, the desire to classify people according to categories and to ascribe consistent behaviors associated with these categories appears to be a deep and meaningful human trait. Consistent with this human need, the pseudoscience, phrenology, was and is not alone in the world of beliefs. Astrology, the belief that stars and planets influence people's lives, is probably the most ancient of human trait classification systems. Palmistry is perhaps equally ancient and also draws upon the influence of celestial objects, reflecting human characters and directing one's ultimate fate. Other pseudosciences also gained prominence during the late 1700s, including graphology, the purported ability to predict human character from one's handwriting.

It is no small irony that these pseudosciences flourished along with a virtual wealth of new and valuable medical and scientific findings from such eminent scientists as the Italian physiologist Galvani, the Italian physicist Volta, the English chemists Dalton and Priestley, the English philosopher and mathematician Sir Isaac Newton, the French writer Voltaire, and the Swedish physician and botanist Linnaeus. In 1735, Linnaeus classified all then known botanical and animal specimens into genus and species. He also gave people the name *Homo sapiens* and placed them in the order of primates.

This entire period from the 1600s through the early 1800s was to be known as the epoch of enlightenment, and yet it was not a period without contradictions and paradoxes. For instance, the treatment of mentally ill people was horrendous. Few mentally ill people were cared for in any systematic fashion anywhere in the world. Most became vagrants, often begging for their food. Dangerous or troublesome patients were often jailed, locked, and chained in wards of poorhouses or orphanages. One eminent German physician warned his students that they risked losing their own sanity if they spent too much time in treating mental patients. However, the enlightenment also led to a wave of moral uplift and revolt (Alexander & Selesnick, 1966).

The French physician Philippe Pinel (1745–1826) served as the director of psychiatric hospitals at Bicêtre and Salpetriere in France. Observations of his patients led him to classify psychotic illnesses into the melancholias (depressions), manias without delirium, manias with delirium, and dementia. He was also able to recognize and describe differences in disturbances of attention, memory, judgment, and emotion. He followed the general sentiment of the late 1700s and early 1800s that abnormal behavior was caused by metabolic disturbances or lesions in the central nervous system. A distinction began of viewing mental illnesses as *organic*, with a strongly suspected physiological cause, or as *functional*, such as bad habits acquired through a poor psychological environment. Pinel, himself, believed that mental illness was the result of hereditary influences, coupled with poor life experiences. He emphasized to his students that mental illness was a natural phenomenon and could be studied just like the natural sciences. He urged his students and physicians to live among the insane to make careful observations and, only after that, to begin a systematic presentation of their data. Pinel instituted humanistic reforms that he called "moral treatment." Such reforms would spread over Europe and even to America. Pinel was later often referred to as the man who took the chains off the limbs of the insane. Whether he literally removed these chains remains debatable; however, there is little question as to the influence of his moral reforms (Alexander & Selesnick, 1966).

Despite better descriptions of mental illness and a greater appreciation for the need for systematic categorization, treatments remained bizarre and cruel. Because vague Hippocratic humoral notions about the etiologies of mental illness still flourished, mentally ill patients were often blood-let, given emetics to make them vomit, given laxatives to purge them, drenched continually in cold water, and confined for minutes in a spinning chair. Most of these treatments were designed to restore some vaguely understood chemical or magnetic balance. Thus, despite general advances in the other sciences and despite a moral revolution in the conditions for housing the mentally ill, the frontline treatments often remained barbaric.

The English psychiatrist James Prichard (1786–1848) created the distinction between antisocial behavior, such as lying, gambling, and drug use and other forms of insanity more typically found in mental hospitals. Prichard (1835) called this behavior "moral insanity," and this general category of disorders would later be called character disorders or personality disorders. The word *character* is derived from the Greek word *to engrave*, implying that the behaviors in question are deeply and permanently engraved so that change is unlikely or extremely difficult. Even until the early twentieth century, most character disorders remained largely unstudied entities. Until the mid-twentieth century, the bulk of personality disorder research was upon the psychopath or sociopath, now known as the antisocial personality disorder.

Modern Era

In 1850, Austrian physician Morel (1809–1873) stated that there was too much of an emphasis on the organic causes of mental illness and not enough study of the emotional aspects of the patients. He also (rightly) believed that the abuse of drugs like alcohol could interact with one's heredity to create mental illnesses. While reviewing some case histories of mental patients whose insanity began in adolescence, Morel concluded that they had a hereditary disease that led unremittingly to complete deterioration. He named the illness "demence precoce" (early dementia; Alexander & Selesnick, 1966).

In 1883, highly influential German psychologist Wilhelm Wundt encouraged one of his students, Emil Kraepelin (1856–1926), to publish a book *Compendium Der Psychiatrie* (*Compendium of Psychiatry*). This work, well written and organized, later blossomed into four volumes of over 2,400 pages. In the textbook's 4th edition in 1893, Kraepelin included the concept of dementia praecox, which at that time remained a specifically adolescent disease that progressed into a dementia. Later, Kraepelin would present variations, such as catatonia (for patients who alternated between muteness and violence) and dementia paranoides (for patients who had delusions of persecution and paranoia). Kraepelin also thought that most of these conditions were rarely curable and usually led to complete deterioration and feeble-mindedness. Kraepelin did differentiate dementia praecox from manic-depressive psychoses on the basis of the prognosis: He thought patients with dementia praecox rarely recovered, whereas patients with manic-depressive psychoses often recovered (Kraepelin, 1919/1971).

As for functional psychological disturbances that Kraepelin called "psychic causes," he thought that they were more often products of an underlying organic disease rather than a cause. He did admit that there might be a small group of illnesses that have a psychic origin. He gave examples of personality change after an accident (which he called accident neuroses) and combat neuroses. Nevertheless, he felt that a decisive factor in the development of insanity was a person's heredity. Kraepelin was impressed with the geneticist Mendel's work and urged those in the mental health field to research the influence and transmission of heritable psychological states (Kraepelin, 1917/1962).

With Sigmund Freud's (1856–1939) publication of *Studies in Hysteria* (with Josef Breuer) in 1895/1957 and *The Interpretation of Dreams* in 1900/1965, the psychiatric community began to focus on the treatment of mental illness, as well as upon less severe psychopathologies, such as the neuroses and psychophysiological disorders. Freud and Breuer offered the revolutionary idea that hysterical patients were suffering from an unconscious traumatic memory. The secret to curing these symptoms would be to allow the patients to talk about, rediscover, and reexamine the traumatic event. Hysteria would later, in Freud's time, become known as a hysterical neurosis or conversion neurosis. It is now classified in the category of somatoform disorders and is called a conversion disorder.

It has been suggested that the world's attention to Freud and his "talking cure" (psychoanalysis) in the early 1900s pushed Kraepelin and his contributions into the background (Harms, 1971). The truth of this assertion is difficult to measure, but it is likely that diagnostic systems such as those of Kraepelin and other Europeans had been focused upon the more severe psychopathologies like those afflicting the patients in mental institutions. Freud's development of a "talking cure" may have developed because he focused on the less severe psychopathologies such as neuroses that, of course, were more amenable to his new methods of uncovering repressed material by free association and dream analysis. Freud's imprint upon the modern diagnostic system persisted strongly, even until 1980 when the American Psychiatric Association modified its psychoanalytic focus to a more behavioral one. Until 1980, the diagnostic classification of neuroses was based firmly upon Freud's work and his classification of neurotic types, including anxious, hysterical, phobic, depressive, and neurasthenic.

Freud, however, was not the first to use the term *neurosis*. William Cullen (1712–1790), a physiologist at the University of Edinburgh, published a four-volume textbook classifying all then known mental diseases in 1777. He used the general term neurosis to imply a mental disease not caused by a lesion or localized pathology. He also described various categories of neuroses, including an amazingly accurate description of an anxiety attack. Cullen did, however, ultimately view the cause of neuroses as a function of a physiological breakdown (Alexander & Selesnick, 1966). Clearly, it was Freud, more than a hundred years later, who changed the paradigm from the idea that the etiology of neuroses had physiological bases to psychological and, sometimes, traumatic ones.

Foundations of the Current Diagnostic System

In 1911, Swiss psychiatrist Eugen Bleuler (1857–1939) coined the word *schizophrenia* (split mind), and that term eventually replaced Kraepelin's use of dementia praecox. Bleuler used the term *split mind* to indicate a fragmenting of the thought processes, a lack of coherence between thought and emotion, and a split from reality (not multiple personalities as is sometimes erroneously believed). Bleuler was impressed with Freud's emphasis on the psychological aspects of mental illness. Although Bleuler believed that mental illness had an organic etiology, nevertheless, he thought that psychotic symptoms could be better understood by comparing them to mental processes of normal people. He also felt that the ultimate outcome of Kraepelin's dementia praecox was not always a full-blown dementia (or feeble-mindedness in their terminology). The latter belief was, in part, the genesis for Bleuler's change of terminology to schizophrenia.

As further evidence of Freud's influence, Bleuler also thought that psychotic symptoms reflected archaic, unconscious, wishful symbolic thinking processes, and he called this specific aspect *autistic thinking*. He also described the disturbances in the expression of emotion in schizophrenia, including bizarre and inappropriate affect, and he made observations of ambivalent thinking. Thus, for Bleuler, the essential symptoms of schizophrenia became loose, fragmented associations in thinking, autistic thought processes, disturbed affect, and ambivalence (Alexander & Selesnick, 1966).

In spite of Bleuler's important addition to classification, Kraepelin's compendium became the single most influential diagnostic classification system in history. It was unrivaled in European countries, and it would even impact the development of a diagnostic classification system in America. In May, 1917, the American Medico-Psychological Association (now the American Psychiatric Association) drew up and adopted the first American diagnostic classification system and took responsibility for its maintenance and publication. Based upon much of Kraepelin's system, its original purpose was to gather descriptive statistical data from mental hospitals.

As noted previously, personality disorders had been largely unstudied diagnoses (other than psychopathy) until the early twentieth century. In 1923, German psychiatrist Kurt Schneider (1950) published a text on psychopathologic personalities, and this work came to serve as a major basis for the current conception of personality disorders. He made a number of substantial contributions to this area. First, he did not view "psychopathologic personalities" (his term for personality disorders) as necessary precursors to other or more severe mental disturbances but saw them as coexistent entities. This contribution heralded the multiaxial diagnostic classification system that was introduced by the American Psychiatric Association in 1980. Second, he saw personality disorders as developing in childhood and continuing into adulthood. Third, he described 10 different psychopathologic personalities commonly seen in psychiatric settings, some of which have greatly influenced current personality disorder diagnoses such as his depressive personality (depressive personality disorder), anankastic personality (obsessive–compulsive personality disorder), attention-seeking personality (histrionic personality disorder), labile personality (borderline personality disorder), and the affectionless personality (antisocial personality disorder).

The Current Classification System (DSM-IV)

Development of the Diagnostic and Statistical Manual of Mental Disorders

There were only minor revisions of the 1917 version of the American Psychiatric Association's diagnostic classification system in 1933 and 1942. However, with the advent of another world war, the United States military was faced with a need for a more sophisticated diagnostic classification system. It was estimated that 90% of those unfit for military service did not fit within the diagnostic nomenclature. In the 1940s, the Army, Navy, and Veterans Administration all created independent systems of classification. From about 1948 to 1951, the American Psychiatric Association worked feverishly to create a single revised system, and the result of this monumental work was the publication in 1952 of the *Diagnostic and Statistical Manual of Mental Disorders* (*DSM-I*; APA, 1952). The DSM-I then consisted of seven major diagnostic categories including acute and chronic brain disorders, mental deficiency, psychotic disorders, psychophysiological disorders, psychoneuroses, personality disorders, and transient situational disorders. It should be noted that the DSM-I reflected only an American tradition. The international variant at that time was the ICD-6, published by the World Health Organization.

The DSM-I was revised in 1968 (*DSM-II*) which was similar to DSM-I with slight improvements in terminology. Major improvements in diagnosis and classification occurred in 1980 with the publication of DSM-III, including the use of explicit diagnostic criteria and a descriptive approach that attempted to be neutral (as opposed to being psychoanalytic) with respect to etiological theories. Perhaps the most important innovation was the application of a *multiaxial system*, which requires judgments on each of five axes and consequently prompts clinicians to evaluate a wide range of information. DSM-III-R (1987) corrected inconsistencies in DSM-III but did not create an additional quantum leap like the DSM-III. In 1994, the current version, DSM-IV, was published backed by an extensive revision process that included comprehensive and systematic reviews of the scientific literature, reanalyses of already collected data sets, and extensive issue-focused field trials designed to assess the reliability and performance of each criteria set.

The DSM-IV Multiaxial System

The major innovation in DSM-III, the development of a multiaxial system, was kept and improved upon in DSM-III-R and DSM-IV. In the multiaxial system, each person is rated on five distinct dimensions or axes, each of which refers to a different domain of the person's functioning. Although only Axis I and Axis II cover the classification of abnormal behavior, the inclusion of Axes III–V indicates awareness that factors other than a person's symptoms should be considered in a thorough assessment. Indeed, each domain is important because it can help the clinician understand the experience of the person more fully, plan treatment, and predict the outcome. According to DSM-IV (APA, 1994), the multiaxial system also provides a convenient and standard format for organizing and communicating clinical information, for capturing the complexity of clinical phenomena, and for describing potentially important differences in functioning among persons with the same diagnosis. Each axis is briefly described next.

AXIS I: CLINICAL DISORDERS AND OTHER CONDITIONS THAT MAY BE A FOCUS OF CLINICAL ATTENTION

All disorders and conditions experienced by the patient are reported on Axis I, except personality disorders and mental retardation, which are coded on Axis II. Axis I is comprised of 16 broad categories under which specific disorders are subsumed. Table 1 presents the 16

TABLE 1. DSM-IV Axis I Categories[a]

Category	Example(s) of disorder	# of disorders
Disorders Usually First Diagnosed in Infancy, Childhood, or Adolescence	Autistic Disorder; Pica	40
Delirium, Dementia, and Amnestic and Other Cognitive Disorders	Dementia of the Alzheimer's Type, With Early Onset	16
Mental Disorders Due to a General Medical Condition Not Elsewhere Classified	Personality Change Due to ... [Indicate the General Medical Condition]	3
Substance-Related Disorders	Alcohol Abuse; Polysubstance Dependence	114
Schizophrenia and Other Psychotic Disorders	Schizoaffective Disorder; Delusional Disorder	8
Mood Disorders	Major Depressive Disorder; Bipolar I Disorder	9
Anxiety Disorders	Obsessive–Compulsive Disorder; Generalized Anxiety Disorder	11
Somatoform Disorders	Conversion Disorder; Hypochondriasis	7
Factitious Disorders	Factitious Disorder with Predominantly Psychological Signs and Symptoms	2
Dissociative Disorders	Dissociative Amnesia; Dissociative Identity Disorder	5
Sexual and Gender Identity Disorders	Hypoactive Sexual Desire Disorder; Pedophilia	29
Eating Disorders	Anorexia Nervosa; Bulimia Nervosa	3
Sleep Disorders	Narcolepsy; Sleep Terror Disorder	13
Impulse-Control Disorders Not Elsewhere Classified	Kelptomania; Trichotillomania	6
Adjustment Disorders	Adjustment Disorder With Depressed Mood	6 types
Other Conditions That May Be a Focus of Clinical Attention	Sibling Relational Problem; Academic Problem	32

[a]Adapted from *Diagnostic and Statistical Manual of Mental Disorders*, 4th ed. Washington, DC: American Psychiatric Association, 1994.

categories along with examples of specific disorders in each category. As can be seen in Table 1, 15 of the 16 categories describe diagnosable mental *disorders*. However, the final category, Other Conditions That May Be a Focus of Clinical Attention, describe not mental disorders but rather conditions that may prompt the need for psychological intervention. Examples include parent–child relational problems, malingering, bereavement, and phase of life problems.

AXIS II: PERSONALITY DISORDERS AND MENTAL RETARDATION

Personality disorders are inflexible and maladaptive patterns of behavior reflecting extreme variants of normal personality traits that have become rigid and dysfunctional. Eleven personality disorders are standard in DSM-IV: paranoid, schizoid, schizotypal, antisocial, borderline, histrionic, narcissistic, avoidant, dependent, and obsessive–compulsive personality disorder, as well as personality disorder not otherwise specified. Two other personality disorders, depressive and passive-aggressive personality disorder, are included in Appendix B for Further Study. The evolution of the personality disorder diagnosis across versions of the DSM reveals a rich and sometime ironic history (see Coolidge & Segal, 1998, for a complete analysis). Interestingly, prominent dysfunctional personality traits can also be listed in Axis II when symptoms are noteworthy but below diagnostic threshold. Significant uses of various defense mechanisms can also be listed on Axis II, although this technique appears uncommon in clinical practice.

AXIS III: GENERAL MEDICAL CONDITIONS

On this axis, the diagnostician notes any current physical disorders (e.g., cirrhosis of liver, diabetes, brain tumors, cancer) that could be relevant to understanding or managing the patient's psychological difficulties. It is advisable to list all important medical conditions experienced by the patient and be inclusive rather than exclusive.

AXIS IV: PSYCHOSOCIAL AND ENVIRONMENTAL PROBLEMS

All social and environmental problems (stressors) experienced by the patient are reported on Axis IV. One should note as many as are judged relevant. Examples of stressors include recently divorced, inadequate finances, illiteracy, recent death of mother, threat of job loss, and living in a high crime neighborhood. The possibilities for stressors are endless, and all that affect the client should be reported. According to DSM-IV convention, it is typical to note only those problems that have been present during the *year preceding* the current evaluation. However, the clinician can note stressors occurring *prior* to the previous year if they contribute significantly to the mental disorder or have become a focus of treatment. For example, childhood sexual abuse may be an important factor in the development of Posttraumatic Stress Disorder, and it should be noted as a current stressor.

AXIS V: GLOBAL ASSESSMENT OF FUNCTIONING (GAF)

GAF Scale ratings are recorded on Axis V. Here, the clinician's judgment of the client's overall level of functioning is described on a 0–100 scale, on which higher numbers indicate better functioning. Explicit descriptions of functioning in ten point increments are provided in the DSM-IV (the GAF Scale appears on page 32). For example, a GAF range of 31–40 indicates "some impairment in reality testing or communication"; scores ranging from 51–60 suggest "moderate symptoms or moderate difficulty in social, occupational, or school functioning"; and scores between 71 and 80 denote mild symptoms that are "transient and expectable reactions to psychosocial stressors" with slight functional impairment (APA, 1994, p. 32). Typically, current GAF ratings are provided on a multiaxial diagnosis, and the common variants also include the highest GAF in the past year or at some other relevant time, such as at discharge from an inpatient unit. GAF scale ratings (albeit subjective) are useful in describing the overall level of impairment of a patient, tracking clinical progress of a patient over time, and predicting prognosis.

CRITICISMS AND LIMITATIONS OF DIAGNOSIS AND CLASSIFICATION

It is safe to say that the current psychiatric classification system (the DSM-IV) is the most sophisticated and comprehensive diagnostic manual ever created. However, classification and the DSM remain far from perfect. Criticisms of modern classification center around several areas, namely, concerns about reliability, validity, cultural relevance of the DSM, and categorical classification of the DSM. First, however, we discuss briefly the issue of whether or not mental illness actually exists.

Is Mental Illness a Myth?

In a bold and controversial article, influential theorist Thomas Szasz (1960) posed a fundamental challenge to professionals who were engaged in the study of abnormal behavior. Essentially, Szasz argued that mental illness is a myth, that is, there is no such thing as mental illness. He posited that the term has outlived its utility and should be discarded similar to the fate of the concept of demonic possession that dominated during the Middle Ages. Szasz suggested that professionals use the term "mental illness" as a descriptive *label* for behaviors that members of a society find unusual, deviant, unpleasant, or annoying. He also suggested that the term is used to supply a *cause* for these irritating behaviors, suggesting the presence of circular reasoning. Rather than calling such problems mental illness, he suggested a more gentle term, namely "problems in living" which most (ordinary) people likely would experience due to the complexities of life. Although Szasz generated a healthy debate about this topic, mainstream psychology and psychiatry essentially rejected his thesis; diagnosis remains as a necessary component of psychological science and practice. However, Szasz's cautions about the limitations of diagnosis are still important. For example, he warned that all diagnostic labels are inherently value-laden, made by people who looked at the behavior or symptom, and decided that it is not within their society's limits. With such value judgments come the possibility of discrimination and bias. Szasz also expressed reservations about the value of diagnosis because it could encourage diagnosed individuals to shirk responsibility for their behavior and blame it on their illness.

Reliability of Psychiatric Diagnosis

Reliability refers to consistency, stability, and dependability of measurement. Indeed, the reliability of psychiatric diagnosis is a fundamental prerequisite for a valid psychiatric classification scheme. The most relevant type of reliability for psychiatric diagnosis is inter-rater reliability, which refers to the extent of agreement between two or more clinicians who examine the same patient. Independent ratings can be done at the same time in a joint interview, or videotaped interviews can be rated post hoc. Imagine the not so uncommon dilemma in clinical practice when different clinicians arrive at a different diagnosis for the same patient. That unfortunate individual likely would not feel confident in any given treatment plan (or clinician for that matter).

Another relevant form of reliability is test–retest reliability, which refers to the extent to which a diagnosis remains consistent over a discrete time interval. In this type of design, the same patient is rated at two distinct times. Test–retest data are often subject to debates about interpretations because some psychological disorders change naturally over time, which would result in lower test–retest values. Moreover, much anecdotal evidence supports the notion that many patients report inconsistent information from day to day and interview to interview. An advantage of the test–retest method is that it approximates "true clinical practice" because patients in some settings are examined at multiple times. Reliability data is typically reported by statistics of percentage agreement and/or the kappa index. Kappa is a better choice, however, because, unlike percentage agreement, kappa corrects for chance levels of agreement (Fleiss, 1981). Kappa coefficients range from −1.00 (perfect disagreement) to +1.00 (perfect agreement), and 0 indicates agreement no better or worse than chance. Kappas above .70 are generally considered strong agreement.

Historically, psychiatric practice and research have been hampered by poor reliability of psychiatric diagnosis. Studies in the 1950s and 1960s documented consistently poor and unacceptable reliability (e.g., Spitzer, Endicott, & Robins, 1975). Credible findings from most early investigations were lacking even for the best-known disorders, such as major depression and schizophrenia (Grove, 1987). Such disheartening unreliability of the DSM-I (APA, 1952) and DSM-II (APA, 1968) systems was a significant cause of professional concern among clinicians and researchers alike.

Two primary reasons have been identified to account for this historically lamentable state of affairs. The first targets the diagnostic criteria themselves, suggesting that poorly defined criteria were major culprits in poor reliability (Ward, Beck, Mendelson, Mock, & Erbaugh, 1962). In their classic report, Ward et al. reported that 80% of all diagnostic disagreements were attributed to inadequate diagnostic criteria. Unfortunately, early classification systems (such as the DSM and DSM-II) lacked explicit diagnostic criteria for most disorders. Clinicians faced the formidable task of rating general or vague symptoms that often represented a theoretical construct (often psychoanalytic in nature) that was difficult to operationalize. The second factor accounting for historically poor reliability involves the lack of standardization of questions that are posed to patients to evaluate psychiatric symptoms and ultimately to arrive at a diagnosis. Before standardized structured interviews, the unstructured clinical interview prevailed. With unstructured interviews, clinicians were entirely responsible for asking whatever questions they decided were necessary for them to reach a diagnostic conclusion. The amount and kind of information gathered, as well as the way clinicians probed and assessed symptoms during an interview, was largely determined by their theoretical model, view of psychopathology, training, and interpersonal style, all of which can vary widely from clinician to clinician.

These barriers to reliability were subsequently addressed and ameliorated by clinicians and researchers during the last 20 years. The problem of nebulous criteria was partially addressed with the publication of DSM-III (APA, 1980), which, as discussed earlier, greatly operationalized criteria in clear behavioral terms, took a more descriptive and atheoretical approach to symptoms, and introduced the multiaxial format. These innovations have continued to be refined in subsequent versions of DSM. The problem of unstandardized questioning was addressed by the development of structured interviews, which provided standardized questions, as well as guidelines for categorizing or coding responses (Segal, 1997). According to Segal, adoption of such procedures served to (1) increase the coverage of many disorders that previously might have been ignored, (2) enhance the diagnostician's ability to determine accurately if a particular symptom is present or absent, and (3) reduce the variability among interviewers. In summary, the introduction of operationalized, specified, empirically derived, and standardized criteria for mental disorders in conjunction with the construction of standardized structured diagnostic interviews has revolutionized the diagnostic process and improved reliability (and validity). Currently, reliability for most major diagnoses is good, indicating that the field has satisfactorily addressed this issue, at least for most disorders. Despite adequate levels of reliability, it is almost never 100% reliable, suggesting that there still are inconsistencies in the way diagnoses are decided.

Validity of Psychiatric Diagnosis

Whereas reliability refers to reproducibility and stability, validity refers to the extent to which a diagnosis is meaningful (e.g., the extent to which it tells us something important about the typical symptom presentation, etiology, pathogenesis, course, and response to treatment for a particular diagnosis). Validity is strongly related to reliability (conceptually, as well as statistically). Acceptable levels of reliability must be confirmed *before* conclusions about validity can be drawn. In other words, reliability is a necessary but not sufficient condition for validity. Without adequate reliability, the issue of validity becomes moot; by definition, the diagnosis is worthless if it cannot be measured accurately. It should be noted, however, that strong reliability does not guarantee validity because it is possible for clinicians to agree perfectly but be incorrect about all cases. As a case in point, clinicians could all agree that a particular client is "neurotic," but this vague and outdated term would tell them little about the specific nature of the problem, the probable cause of it, and efficacious treatment strategies.

Compared with reliability, validity is much harder to gauge and document accurately, and thus represents a formidable challenge for our field. According to Leckliter and Matarazzo (1994), the validity of a diagnosis is established by three lines of evidence: evidence related to statistically established clusters of behavior that form a diagnostic condition; evidence related to the etiology of a disorder (i.e., individuals with the same disorder have a similar environmental background); and evidence related to the treatment of specific disorders with specific interventions. Although investigative attention in these areas is strong, the lack of diagnostic validity is presently considered among the most serious issues facing the mental health community. Validity is especially problematic for personality disorders, which continue to be plagued with poorer reliability and validity coefficients than most Axis I disorders. Also, there is an absence of a cogent atheoretical rationale for the individual personality disorders (Livesley, 1998). There is also a debate among clinical researchers as to the validity of the three clusters of personality disorders (odd-eccentric, dramatic-erratic, anxious-fearful) proposed by the DSM system. Clearly, research on the validity of diagnosis is a top priority for our field.

Cultural Relevance of the DSM-IV

A lofty goal of the DSM-IV was that it would be relevant in a wide variety of contexts and to individuals with diverse cultural and ethnic backgrounds in the United States and internationally. Many efforts were made in this regard during preparation of the DSM-IV. Clearly, DSM-IV is an improvement over earlier editions. For example, international experts were involved to ensure a wide pool of information on cultural factors in psychopathology and diagnosis (APA, 1994). Greater compatibility was achieved between the DSM-IV and another major classification system, the World Health Organization's International Classification of Diseases 10th edition (ICD-10). Information about specific cultural features (e.g., how different cultural backgrounds affect the content, form, and expression of symptoms; cross-cultural prevalence information) has been included in the description of some mental disorders.

Perhaps most importantly, a glossary of many culture-bound disorders is included in Appendix I of the DSM-IV: Outline for Cultural Formulation and Glossary of Culture-Bound Syndromes. In this section, information is provided about the names of culture-bound syndromes, the cultures in which it occurs, and a description of the main psychopathologic features. As an example, the disorder "koro" is described as having a probable Malaysian origin and is defined as "an episode of sudden and intense anxiety that the penis (or, in females, the vulva and nipples) will recede into the body and possibly cause death" (APA, 1994, p. 846). In all, 25 conditions are discussed, which is an important beginning to increasing the cross-cultural validity of the DSM.

Despite these improvements, criticisms of the DSM-IV in this area have been expressed. Thakker and Ward (1998) cogently argue that DSM-IV still has an (incorrect) implicit assumption that its primary syndromes represent universal disorders. They suggest that this underlying thesis of the universality of disorders is based on Western conceptions of disease, which are inherently problematic and have limited cross-cultural relevance. As a case in point, Thakker and Ward point out that some mental disorders are rarely found outside the West (e.g., anorexia nervosa, dissociative identity disorder). They also review literature suggesting that some disorders, particularly schizophrenia and depression, do have significant cross-cultural variations, contrary to earlier views. As the DSM system gains increased acceptance worldwide, clearly, further research on the impact of culture on abnormal behavior is warranted as are refinements in future editions of the manual.

Categorical Classification of the DSM-IV

DSM-IV acknowledges that diagnosis is based on a categorical model (APA, 1994). A categorical model assumes a "Yes/No" or "Sick/Well" approach in which individuals either have the disorder (i.e. they meet criteria, they are diagnosable) or they do not (despite possibly having several symptoms but not enough to meet formal criteria). In contrast, the dimensional approach classifies clinical presentations based on quantitative descriptions of various domains of functioning, such as the degree of mania or body image distortion. In this approach, disordered behaviors fall on the same continuum with normal behaviors and are not something entirely different, as the categorical approach suggests. The dimensional approach also allows for a description of clinical presentations that do not have clear boundaries.

In a recent critique of the categorical model, Widiger (1997) notes that justification for this model comes from several sources: medicine uses a categorical model, categorical diagnosis is simple to understand, and clinical decisions are often categorical (e.g., the need to hospitalize a suicidal person). However, Widiger highlights many problems of the categorical model and concludes his analysis with a recommendation for a gradual conversion to a more dimensional approach to classification. According to Widiger, one problem of the categorical model is the substantial comorbidity of mental disorders, which raises the question of whether a single disorder is actually present instead of the co-occurrence of several distinct disorders. For example, among those with a personality disorder, comorbidity with additional personality disorders and clinical disorders (such as depression) is the rule rather than the exception.

Another inadequacy is the clinical reality that some patients who receive mental health treatment do not fit into any of the neat categories, suggesting poor clinical utility of some diagnoses. In the future, it is possible that a combination of categorical and dimensional models may coexist, which would draw on the benefits of both approaches. (For a complete discussion of this issue, see Widiger, 1997.) One empirical question to be addressed is whether some disorders truly are exclusively categorical, that is, do some types of psychiatric illnesses represent something completely, qualitatively different from normal functioning? The opposite question is whether all forms of mental illness are extreme variants of normal behaviors. In any case, serious attention is likely to be paid to this issue when the next revision of DSM takes place.

Summary

In this chapter, we discussed the historical roots of the diagnosis and classification of abnormal behavior, described the current DSM-IV system, and highlighted current controversies in the field. We emphasized how our views on the boundaries of mental illness have been subject to marked historical changes, as new disorders, conditions, theoretical underpinnings, and classification systems evolve regularly. Despite its imperfections, the DSM-IV represents clearly an important advance on its historical predecessors. This system is, and will continue to be, used in the psychiatric care of those with psychiatric problems. But what will the future bring? It is unlikely that wholesale changes in the system will be made in the near future, although the limited addition of new empirically supported disorders and the elimination of empirically weak disorders (e.g., possibly passive–aggressive personality disorder, premenstrual dysphoric disorder) will continue. If recent history is any guide, a new version of DSM (likely DSM-V) will appear in the coming decade (there was a seven-year interval between the publication of DSM-III in 1980 and DSM-III-R in 1987, and seven more years between DSM-III-R and DSM-IV in 1994).

The multiaxial system will surely continue in the next edition, although minor adjustments to existing axes could occur and additional axes may be added. For example, a new axis of defensive functioning (defense mechanisms) could be formalized based on its appearance in the DSM-IV Appendix B: Criteria Sets and Axes Provided for Further Study. As presently conceptualized, the Defensive Functioning Scale allows clinicians to list in order up to seven of the specific defenses used by the patient (e.g., humor, dissociation, idealization, projection, acting out) and then list the predominant defensive level shown by the patient (e.g., high adaptive level, disavowal level, level of defensive dysregulation). Research will bear out whether this axis (and other proposed disorders in Appendix B) will be included as official components of the DSM. We conclude our chapter with a caution: time and time again, academics evaluate the current scientific knowledge base and believe that their science represents "the truth." With the passage of time, however, crude notions and incorrect ideas become painfully obvious. We should view our current conceptualizations of diagnosis and classification in mental health with a grain of salt, firm in our knowledge that the future will bring about advances that cannot even be imagined now.

References

Alexander, F. G., & Selesnick, S. T. (1966). *The history of psychiatry: An evaluation of psychiatric thought and practice from prehistoric times to the present.* New York: Harper & Row.

American Psychiatric Association. (1952). *Diagnostic and statistical manual of mental disorders.* Washington, DC: Author.

American Psychiatric Association. (1968). *Diagnostic and statistical manual of mental disorders* (2nd ed.). Washington, D.C.: Author.

American Psychiatric Association. (1980). *Diagnostic and statistical manual of mental disorders* (3rd ed.). Washington, D.C.: Author.

American Psychiatric Association. (1987). *Diagnostic and statistical manual of mental disorders* (3rd ed. Rev.). Washington, D.C.: Author.

American Psychiatric Association. (1994). *Diagnostic and statistical manual of mental disorders* (4th ed.). Washington, D.C.: Author.

Aristotle (1952). The writings of Aristotle. In M. J. Adler (Ed.), *Great books of the western world*. Chicago: Britannica.

Breasted, J. H. (Ed. and Trans.). (1991). *The Edwin Smith surgical papyrus*. Chicago: University of Chicago Press.

Breuer, J., & Freud, S. (1957). *Studies on hysteria* (J. Strachey, Ed. and Trans.). New York: Basic Books (original work published 1895).

Cohen, R. J., Swerdlik, M. E., & Phillips, S. M. (1996). *Psychological testing and assessment: An introduction to tests and measurements*. Mountain View, CA: Mayfield.

Coolidge, F. L. & Segal, D. L. (1998). Evolution of the personality disorder diagnosis in the Diagnostic and Statistical Manual of Mental Disorders. *Clinical Psychology Review, 18*, 585–599.

DeRubeis, R. J., & Crits-Cristoph, P. (1998). Empirically supported individual and group psychological treatments for adult mental disorders. *Journal of Consulting and Clinical Psychology, 66*, 37–52.

Edmonds, J. M. (Ed. and Trans.). (1929). *The characters of Theophrastus*. Cambridge, MA: Harvard University Press.

Finger, S. (1994). *Origins of neuroscience: A history of explorations into brain function*. New York: Oxford University Press.

Fleiss, J. L. (1981). *Statistical methods for rates and proportions*, 2nd ed. New York: Wiley.

Freud, S. (1965). *The interpretation of dreams*. New York: Avon (original work published 1900).

Galen (1952). On the natural faculties. In M. J. Adler (Ed.), *Great books of the western world*. Chicago: Britannica.

Grove, W. M. (1987). The reliability of psychiatric diagnosis. In C. G. Last & M. Hersen (Eds.), *Issues in diagnostic research* (pp. 99–119). New York: Plenum.

Harms, E. (1971). Emil Kraepelin's dementia praecox concept: An introduction. As cited in Kraepelin, E. (1919). Dementia praecox and paraphrenia (R. M. Barclay, Trans.). In G. M. Robertson (Ed.), *Dementia praecox and paraphrenia* (pp. viii–xviii). Huntington, NY: Robert E. Krieger (original work published 1919).

Hippocrates (1952). Hippocratic writings. In M. J. Adler (Ed.), *Great books of the western world*. Chicago: Britannica.

Kraepelin, E. (1962). *One hundred years of psychiatry*. New York: Philosophical Library (original work published 1917).

Kraepelin, E. (1971). Dementia praecox and paraphrenia (R. M. Barclay, Trans.). In G. M. Robertson (Ed.), *Dementia praecox and paraphrenia*. Huntington, NY: Robert E. Krieger (original work published 1919).

Leckliter, I. N., & Matarazzo, J. D. (1994). Diagnosis and classification. In V. B. Van Hasselt & M. Hersen (Eds.), *Advanced abnormal psychology* (pp. 3–18). New York: Plenum.

Livesley, W. J. (1998). Suggestions for a framework for an empirically based classification system of personality disorder. *Canadian Journal of Psychiatry, 43*, 137–147.

Murphy, J. M. (1976). Psychiatric labeling in cross-cultural perspective: Similar kinds of disturbed behavior appear to be labeled abnormal in diverse cultures. *Science, 191*, 1019–1028.

Piaget, J. (1932). *The moral judgment of the child*. New York: Harcourt, Brace & World.

Plato (1952). The writings of Plato. In M. J. Adler (Ed.), *Great books of the western world*. Chicago: Britannica.

Prichard, J. C. (1835). *A treatise on insanity*. London: Sherwood, Gilbert & Piper.

Roccatagliata, G. (1986). *A history of ancient psychiatry*. Westport, CT: Greenwood Press.

Schneider, K. (1950). *Psychopathic personalities* (9th ed., English translation). London: Cassell (original work published 1923).

Segal, D. L. (1997). Structured interviewing and DSM classification. In S. M. Turner & M. Hersen (Eds.), *Adult psychopathology and diagnosis* (3rd ed., pp. 25–57). New York: Wiley.

Spitzer, R. L., Endicott, J., & Robins, E. (1975). Clinical criteria for psychiatric diagnosis and DSM-III. *American Journal of Psychiatry, 132*, 1187–1192.

Szasz, T. S. (1960). The myth of mental illness. *American Psychologist, 15*, 113–118.

Thakker, J., & Ward, T. (1998). Culture and classification: The cross-cultural application of the DSM-IV. *Clinical Psychology Review, 18*, 501–529.

Ward, C.H., Beck, A.T., Mendelson, M., Mock, J.E., & Erbaugh, J.K. (1962). The psychiatric nomenclature: Reasons for diagnostic disagreement. *Archives of General Psychiatry, 7*, 198–205.

Widiger, T. A. (1997). Mental disorders as discrete clinical conditions: Dimensional versus categorical classification. In S. Turner & M. Hersen (Eds.), *Adult psychopathology and diagnosis*, 3rd ed. (pp. 3–23). New York: Wiley.

2

Assessment Strategies

Arthur N. Wiens, Erin A. Mueller, and James E. Bryan

Introduction

We begin this chapter with a quote from a report issued by the Psychological Assessment Work Group (Meyer, Finn, Eyde, Kay, Kubiszyn, Moreland, Eisman, & Dies, 1998). The report had two parts: Part I was on "Benefits and costs of psychological assessment in healthcare delivery"; Part II was on "Problems and limitations in the use of psychological assessment in contemporary healthcare delivery." The Work Group was created by the Board of Professional Affairs, American Psychological Association. Meyer et al. (1998) wrote,

> Many psychologists consider thorough, formal assessment to be one of their most valuable tools for evaluating a new client. The assessment process—integrating the results of several carefully selected tests with relevant history information and observation—enables the sophisticated clinician to form an accurate, in-depth understanding of the patient; formulate the most appropriate and cost-effective treatment plan; and later, monitor the course of intervention. Unfortunately, the value of psychological assessment is not always recognized outside the profession of psychology. As a cost-containment strategy, many managed healthcare organizations have recently become reluctant to permit physicians to refer clients who need assessments or have refused to pay for this time-consuming but uniquely valuable process. This seems to be a penny-wise but pound-foolish policy because improperly diagnosed patients get inappropriate or inadequate treatment, causing more problems and expense down the road. (p. 4)

Clinical psychologists have long favored objective psychological assessment with a variety of psychological instruments to help decide which forms of treatment will be most helpful to a patient. Comprehensive patient assessment can help in formulating a diagnosis that is currently required for patient care reimbursement; identifying urgent care issues (e.g., suicidal ideation and intent, psychosis); assessing character traits (i.e., Axis II diagnoses) that affect prognosis and preferred treatment modalities; and providing a problem list of behaviors/symptoms and their severity to guide decisions about the necessary level of care. Psychologists have assumed that psychological assessment (with psychometric testing) can achieve

Arthur N. Wiens, Erin A. Mueller, and James E. Bryan • Oregon Health Sciences University, Portland, Oregon 97201.

Advanced Abnormal Psychology, Second Edition, edited by Hersen and Van Hasselt. Kluwer Academic / Plenum Publishers, New York, 2001.

assessment goals more objectively and quickly than just a clinical interview or any other form of clinical assessment.

The earliest psychological tests tended to be measures of cognitive ability (e.g., the Binet tests) and were met with early success. They increased decision-making accuracy. They reduced bias because of "objectivity" and "data orientation." This was especially true in industrial and military settings where individual interviewing and case histories were too expensive and time-consuming. The early successes created the expectation that personality and diagnostic classifications could also be assessed by using the same psychometric model.

Over time, two paradigms developed, namely, "psychometric testing" and "psychological assessment." Psychometric testing assumes that psychological tests provide data that are useful without regard for context. For example, based on normative findings, the descriptive meaning associated with a scaled score of 10 on the Arithmetic subtest from the Wechsler Adult Intelligence Scale-Third Edition (WAIS-III: Wechsler, 1997) is that a person possesses "average skills in mental calculations." The goal of psychometric testing is to attain more data, and the end product is a series of trait or ability descriptions. The two strengths of this approach are that it is relatively quick and it can improve decision-making accuracy. Three weaknesses of this approach are that it is inappropriate for diagnosis, the score descriptions do not account for context, and it is a poor method for assessing personality.

Psychological assessment assumes the use of psychological test data, but the data are placed within a context. Matarazzo (1990) made a strong case for placing data within a context in his presidential address to the APA which he entitled "Psychological assessment versus psychological testing." The goals of psychological assessment include creation of a comprehensive picture of the individual, increased decision-making accuracy, and generation of solutions to problems facing clinicians. The end product is a comprehensive review of the individual in context. Three strengths are that the review is comprehensive, it accounts for unique context and history, and it provides a basis for diagnosis and treatment recommendations. Three weaknesses are that it is time-consuming, it requires a highly educated and trained clinician experienced in integrating many sources of knowledge (e.g., test construction, personality, other measures, history), and it is still not 100% reliable. As noted by Meyer et al. (1998),

> The clinician's focus is not on obtaining a single test score or even a series of scores. Rather, the focus is on taking a variety of test-derived pieces of information, obtained from multiple methods of assessment, and placing the data in the context of historical information, referral information, and behavioral observations made during the testing and interview process, in order to generate a cohesive and comprehensive understanding of the person being evaluated. The clinician must then communicate this understanding to the patient, his or her significant others, and referral sources in a frank but interpersonally sensitive and therapeutic manner. (p. 8)

Meyer et al. (1998) illustrate their point with an example. The meaning of a WAIS-III Arithmetic subtest scaled score of 10 varies when it is put within the context of the individual. Although a scaled score of 10 on the WAIS-III subtests is accepted as an "average" performance, the meaning of this individual score varies when all information is considered as a whole. Meyer et al. (1998) note that an experienced psychologist takes into account all data points, not just the scaled score of 10, when formulating hypotheses with regard to the individual's potential diagnoses and appropriate treatment recommendations.

They continue their example further with two specific case scenarios (Meyer et al., 1998). In the first case, achieving a WAIS-III Arithmetic scaled score of 10 for the individual who recently suffered a head injury may suggest that he, or she, incurred a "precipitous decline in auditory attention span and the capacity to manually manipulate information" (p. 8). However, in the second case of a head-injured individual who has completed cognitive remediation, the scaled score of 10 may indicate a significant improvement in cognitive functioning since his, or her, post-injury status. The authors emphasize the advanced level of skill required to make such differentiations. Meyer et al. (1998) offer further clarification:

> By analogy, the medical counterpart to psychological testing occurs when technicians or medical personnel obtain scores on a blood pressure gauge, thermometer, or blood test. The medical counterpart to psychological assessment occurs when a physician takes the information from various tests and places them in the context of the symptomatic presentation and history of the patient to understand the full scope of his or her condition accurately. In medicine as in psychology, many different conditions can lead to an identical score on a particular test (e.g., many illnesses can produce a fever of 101°F) and the task is to use a range of test-derived sources of information in combination with the patient's history and presenting complaints to disentangle the competing possibilities. (p. 8)

Given the variety of questions addressed in comprehensive psychological assessment, it seems clear that many different assessment strategies have to be employed.

Assessment Strategies

Interviewing

The Clinical Interview

The topics to be covered in an initial clinical interview are relatively consistent from one clinician to the next. The general objective is to obtain a careful history that can be the foundation for diagnosing and treating the patient's disorder. More specific objectives of the clinical interview are to understand the individual patient's personality characteristics, including both strengths and weaknesses; to obtain insight into the nature of the patient's relationships with those closest, both past and present; and to obtain a reasonably comprehensive picture of the patient's development from the formative years to the present.

In preparing a written record of a clinical interview, most clinicians begin by presenting *identifying information*, such as the patient's name, age, marital status, sex, occupation, race, place of residence and circumstances of living, history of prior clinical contacts, and referral and information sources. The *chief complaint*, or the problem for which the patient seeks professional help, is usually reviewed next and is stated in the patient's own words or in the words of the person supplying this information (e.g., a parent in the case of a child patient). The intensity and duration of the presenting problem is noted, specifically the length of time each symptom has existed and whether there have been changes in quality and quantity from a previous state. It is also useful to include a description of the patient's appearance and behavior.

In reviewing *present illness* or presenting problem, the clinician looks for the earliest and most disabling behavior or symptoms and whether there were any precipitating factors leading to the chief complaint. Often, the precipitating or stress factors associated with the onset of symptoms may be subtle and require the clinician to draw on knowledge of behavior and psychopathology, as well as a typical life history, to help with inquiry regarding relevant life changes. The clinician should also report how the problems have affected the patient's life activities. It is important to review *past health history* for both physical and psychological problems; for example, physical illnesses that might be affecting the patient's emotional state.

Prior episodes of emotional and mental disturbances should be described. The clinician also needs to inquire about and report prescribed and nonprescribed medication and alcohol and drug use. Possible organic mental syndromes must be noted.

Personal and social history usually includes information about the patient's parents and other family members and any history of psychological or physical problems. The account of the patient's own childhood and developmental experiences may be detailed. Educational and occupational histories are noted, as well as social, marital, military, legal, and other experiences. The personal history should provide a comprehensive portrait independent of the patient's illness (Siassi, 1984). The mental status examination is also included in the initial clinical interview but will be reviewed separately later. The section of the interview on initial impressions or *findings* should include deductions made by the clinician from all sources available to this point regarding the patient's past history, description of the present problems, and the results of the clinician's examination as determined from the mental status examination, the results of psychological testing, contributions of family members and significant others, educational and employment history, and so on. Finally, *recommendations* are presented about what kind of treatment the patient should receive for what problems and target symptoms.

MENTAL STATUS EXAMINATION

The mental status examination is reviewed under the following headings: general appearance and behavior; mood, feelings, and affect; perception; speech and thought; sensorium and cognition; judgment; insight; and reliability.

An example of a mental status examination report that was printed from responses recorded in a structured interview (Harrell, 1984) is presented here:

> Ms. Doe was generally cooperative with the interviewer although her specific interactions were defensive. Level of consciousness during the interview was unimpaired. She was not under the influence of alcohol or drugs. Ms. Doe was oriented to time, place, person, and situation. No apparent deficits were evidenced in attention and concentration. Comprehension of simple commands was unimpaired. There was evidence of impairment in short term memory. No indications of amnesia were present. Current intellectual level appeared to be average and fund of information was below average. Current intellectual functioning appears to be consistent with that evidenced prior to the onset of the present condition. Abstract thinking appeared intact. No impairment was evidenced in simple computational skills. There was no evidence of specific neurological impairment. Examination of perceptual processes did not reveal any illusions, hallucinations, or other perceptual dysfunctions. No unusual aspects of thought content were noted. There was no evidence of phobias. The predominant mood during the evaluation was moderate anger which was consistent with thought content. Secondary moods included mild depression. Generally, affective reactions were appropriate to status or complaints. Appropriate variability in affective reactions was observed. There was no evidence of significant cyclic mood changes. There was no indication that Ms. Doe is currently at risk for suicide. Current risk of danger to others appears to be low. No current self-destructive behavior patterns were identified. Level of impulse control was estimated to be limited and judgment generally appeared to be below average. Level of insight was characterized by some awareness of problems with some denial.

COMMUNICATION BETWEEN DOCTOR AND PATIENT

Although a treatise on the importance of the doctor–patient relationship is beyond the scope of this chapter, it is necessary to point out that a clinical interview, or mental status examination, cannot be validly conducted unless reasonable rapport is established and the doctor and patient are listening to each other.

In a study of more than 1000 encounters between internists and patients, Beckman and Frankel (1984) reported that most people are interrupted by their physicians within the first 18 seconds of beginning to explain what is wrong with them. This practice often prevents people from completing the purpose of their visit.

Typically, people go to their physicians with about three concerns, and the most troubling complaint is not always presented first. No relationship was found between the order of presentation and the importance of the complaint. This finding challenges the prevailing hypothesis that the first complaint is the most important. Once interrupted early in the encounter, patients rarely return to any additional concerns. The researchers found no differences between male and female doctors in the tendency to interrupt and control the interview. They also found that an encounter averages about 15 minutes in the United States and about half that in Great Britain.

The doctor–patient encounter can be made more useful if patients think beforehand about what they want to say and get out of the visit and take more control of the interview. It appears that older people are less willing to assert themselves in this manner than younger people and thus they may be at particular risk for not having their concerns heard. Basically, patients want clinicians who will work with them and who will understand them, and a very important strategy in assessment in abnormal psychology is establishing rapport or a working relationship between doctor and patient.

Structured Interviews

A major source of unreliability in the diagnosis of psychological disorders is the variability of information about a patient that is available to a given clinician. For example, some clinicians may talk with patients' families, and others may not. Similarly, some clinicians may ask questions concerning areas of functioning and symptoms, and other clinicians may not.

To deal with such information variance, psychologists and psychiatrists have developed structured clinical interviews that reduce that portion of the unreliability variance based on different interviewing styles and coverage. The structured clinical interview is used routinely in clinical research and increasingly in daily clinical patient examinations. A structured clinical interview essentially outlines a list of target behaviors, symptoms, and events to be covered and some guidelines or rules for conducting the interview and recording the data. Interview schedules vary. Some offer only general and flexible guidelines, and others have strict and detailed rules (i.e., some are semistructured and others are highly structured). With the latter, wording and sequence of questions, recording responses, and rating responses are all specified and defined. The interviewer may be regarded as an interchangeable piece of the assessment machinery. Clinical judgment in eliciting and recording information is minimized and, given the same patient, different interviewers should obtain the same information. The impact of computers in standardized interviewing also appears decisive because they allow efficient retrieval of information. Computers can also be used to apply an algorithm to yield reliable diagnoses from raw data.

Diagnostic Interview Schedule (DIS)

The DIS (Robins, Helzer, Croughan, & Ratcliff, 1981) is a fully structured interview schedule designed to enable clinicians to make consistent and accurate DSM-III psychiatric diagnoses. It was designed to be administered by persons not professionally trained in clinical psychiatry or psychology, and all of the questions and the probes to be used are fully explained. It reminds interviewers not to omit critical questions and presents well-tested phrasing for symptoms that are difficult to explain or potentially embarrassing to patients. Questions about symptoms cover both their presence or absence and severity (e.g., taking medication for the symptoms, seeing a professional about the symptom, and having the symptom significantly interfere with one's life). In addition, the interview ascertains whether the symptom was explained entirely by physical illness or injury or is a complication of the use of medication, illicit drugs, or alcohol. The age at which a given diagnostic symptom first appeared is also determined, along with the most recent experience of the symptom. These questions are designed to help determine whether a disorder is current (i.e., the last two weeks, the last month, the last six months, or the last year). Demographic information including age, sex, occupation, race, education, marital status, and history of treatment is also determined. Current functioning is evaluated by the ability to work or attend school, maintain an active social life, act as head or cohead of a household, and get along without professional care for physical or emotional problems within the last 12 months.

Aside from a few open-ended questions at the start of the interview to allow the interviewee the opportunity to voice the chief complaint and to give the interviewer some background for understanding answers to close-ended questions, the interview is completely precoded. Symptoms assessed by the computer are precoded at five levels: (a) negative, the problem has never occurred; (b) present, but so minimal as to be of no diagnostic significance; (c) present and meets criteria for severity, but not relevant to the psychiatric diagnosis in question because every occurrence resulted from the direct or side effects of prescribed, over-the-counter, or illicit drugs or alcohol; (d) present and meets criteria for severity but not relevant to the psychiatric diagnosis in question because every occurrence resulted from medical illness or injury; and (e) present, meets criteria for severity, and is relevant to the psychiatric diagnosis under consideration.

The DIS has been translated into different languages, and its use is now underway, or planned, in about 20 different countries. Cross-national comparisons in psychiatric and psychological epidemiology are possible due to the growing number of population surveys in various countries that have used the DIS. Similarly, cross-cultural surveys of anxiety disorders and prevalence and symptomatic expression and risk factors in alcoholism have been planned.

Computerization of the DIS makes direct patient administration possible either in its entirety (18 sections) or one section at a time. The computer printout lists all DSM-III diagnoses for which the patient meets the criteria. It also presents additional information about each diagnosis, including the recency of symptoms, duration, and age of onset. In addition, the printout lists for the clinician what other diagnoses must be ruled out before this diagnosis can be assigned according to the DSM-III hierarchy. Eighteen diagnostic categories are surveyed, including both Axis I and Axis II disorders.

We have been using the Computerized-DIS (Blouin, 1985) in our clinic for some time. As part of our assessment strategy, we wanted to include a replicable procedure that clinicians/researchers in other settings could duplicate exactly if they wished to replicate our clinical data. As one example, we have been using the DIS routinely in examining fibromyalgia patients. This is an illustration of a particular patient population in which we assumed that psychological factors had an important role either as an etiological factor in the development of the illness or as a consequence of suffering from it.

To date, after more than 100 physician-referred examinations and consultations, all patients have been able to complete the DIS. Our patients appear to be willing and perhaps welcome the opportunity to respond to the various questions about their health status and history. Time at the computer screen to complete the DIS has varied from about 45 minutes to more than two hours, depending on how many different question branches the patient's responses lead to.

PSYCHOLOGICAL/SOCIAL HISTORY REPORT

Another standardized data collection questionnaire that we use routinely is the Psychological/Social History Report (Rainwater & Coe, 1988). Questions are in a multiple-choice response format which permits computer scoring of the responses with a narrative printout of the results. Question categories include family/developmental experiences, educational experiences, employment experiences, military history, alcohol and drug use history, medical history, marriage history, diet, psychological history, and presenting problems. As with many questionnaires, the patient is asked to respond to many more questions than a face-to-face interviewer might have patience to pursue. Responding to such an array and variety of questions prevents overlooking a critical problem area in the patient's life that might later turn out to be a critical assessment omission.

Young, O'Brien, Gutterman, and Cohen (1987) found that structured interviews increase the number of clinical observations (e.g., number of problem areas) and the amount of relevant patient information that is recorded by a factor of 2. Clinicians using structured interviews are not limited to the presenting symptoms in their diagnostic formulations; thus, their results have higher reliability. Interviewers using structured interviews consider themselves equally as empathic as when using free-flowing interviews. With practice, they can use structured interviews with increasing efficiency, so that this method requires about the same amount of time as traditional clinical interviews.

AutoSCID II

The AutoSCID II (First, Gibbon, Williams, & Spitzer, 1991) is a computer-administered version of the "Structured Clinical Interview for DSM-III-R Personality Questionnaire." It has been designed to assist in assessing personality disorders and can be used to collect diagnostically relevant historical data directly from the patient using SCID II PQ questions. The clinician can be prompted by the responses the patient has made to the screening questions to inquire further about evidence for the different personality disorders. It can be used to screen for the presence of adult Axis II disorders, as identified in the DSM-III-R.

This diagnostic approach to personality disorder views personality traits as enduring patterns of perceiving, relating to, and thinking about the environment and oneself, which are exhibited in a wide range of important social and personal contexts. Only when personality traits are inflexible and maladaptive and cause either significant functional impairment or subjective distress do they constitute personality disorders (DSM-III-R, American Psychiatric Association, 1987). To be rated as present, there must be evidence that the described characteristic is pathological, persistent, and pervasive. Pathological characteristics must be beyond those experiences that one would expect to see in nearly everyone; for example, social anxiety would have to be clearly extreme. To be diagnosed, a characteristic should have been present during a period of at least five years. The characteristic should also be apparent in a variety of contexts, such as at work and at home or in different relationships.

COMPUTER-ADMINISTERED INTERVIEWS

Computers have long played a significant role in assessment. Much modern test construction has depended on the availability of computing resources. As test administration itself became more feasible with the advent of microcomputers, one of the questions raised concerned the comparability of data obtained with traditional paper-and-pencil administration and computerized administration. Lukin, Dowd, Plake, and Kraft (1985) obtained no significant differences between scores on measures of anxiety, depression, and psychological reactance across these two administration formats. Most important, while producing results comparable to the paper-and-pencil assessment, computerized administration was preferred over the paper-and-pencil administration by 85% of the subjects.

More recently, Choca and Morris (1992) compared a computerized version of the Halstead Category Test to the standard projector version of the test using neurologically impaired adult patients. Every subject was tested with both versions and the order of administration was alternated. Results indicated that the difference in the mean number of errors between the two versions of the test was not significant. Scores obtained with the two versions were similar to what would be expected from a test–retest administration of the same instrument. The authors note that one advantage of the computerized version is that it assures an error-free administration of the test. Second, the computer version allows collecting additional data as the test is administered, such as the reaction time and the number of perseverations when a previous rule is inappropriately used. Finally, it may eventually be possible to show that prompts from the examiner do not make a significant difference in the eventual outcome. If this were the case, the computer version would have the added advantage of requiring a considerably shorter time commitment from the examiner (Choca & Morris, 1992).

There is evidence (e.g., Giannetti, 1987) that automated self-reports have advantages for both clinical practice and research. Patients accept and enjoy responding to on-line computerized questionnaires and frequently prefer them to clinical interviews or paper-and-pencil questionnaires. Even chronic and disturbed inpatients can answer computer-presented questions without assistance. There are indications that respondents are more likely to report socially undesirable behavior to a computer (e.g., reporting greater alcohol consumption to computers than to interviewers). Self-report and interviewer-collected history data show high agreement. Finally, completing interviews by computer rather than by traditional means may save cost.

Adams and Heaton (1987) called attention to a further administrative/research role of computers in clinical practice: creating and maintaining an informational database. This database might include information about patient demographics, referral sources, historical data, criterion test results (e.g., imaging data), psychological test findings, and clinical outcome. Such information is valuable in documenting the sources of patients, their demographic and base-rate profiles, the relationship of neuropsychological tests to other results, and the impact of testing or other services on patient outcome. These data are of importance in quality assurance and in evaluative research. External reviewers and third-party agencies increasingly request data showing the accuracy of diagnosis and relationship to hospital/clinic utilization, more appropriate care, and improved outcome. Practice data are important to have in view of the current climate in health services delivery. Once this view is accepted, it follows that the optimal way to gain control of the quality and accuracy of such data is to implement one's own system to generate the data.

Information from Family Members and Other Collaterals

The clinical usefulness of psychological test results is determined by its relationship to the person's functioning in everyday life. Literature regarding the "ecological validity" of psychological assessment consistently compares psychometric test data to other measures of real-world functioning (e.g., Baird, Brown, Adams, & Schatz, 1987). Information obtained from others who live with and know the person is essential to understanding the nature of the condition and predicting its long-term effects. Such information from family members and others closely involved with the person ("collaterals") can serve many purposes.

In diagnosis, other persons can help describe changes in the person's functioning, in terms of deterioration of general social roles (e.g., employment status and quality, domestic responsibilities, recreation and activity level), or global change in personality and emotional style. Such significant others can also help specify clinically significant symptoms that may not emerge through psychometric methods or that individuals may not recognize or acknowledge themselves (e.g., the "positive spouse sign" is familiar to interviewers of early-stage dementia patients, when the spouse points out significant deficits that the patient minimizes or fails to mention).

In terms of ongoing behavior management, family members may be able to alert the clinician to specific problematic or at-risk behaviors requiring rapid attention. The degree of discrepancy between family members' and patients' ratings of functioning on the same measure can be informative. Discrepancies may point to the patients' lack of awareness of symptoms, as well as to possible hypervigilance and overinvolvement of the relatives. As a source of outcome data, the same measures can be administered to relatives over time, before and after treatment, and at successive intervals afterward. Family members may be able to describe the effectiveness of interventions and provide suggestions to apply methods better to their own situation.

Family rating methods typically address global estimation of adjustment and role function, as well as more specific important behaviors and cognitive/emotional symptoms. They represent a systematic means of gaining highly relevant dispositional information about the person and complementing clinical psychometric information, or supplementing it when complete testing may not be possible. Issues of psychometric reliability and validity are central to their meaningfulness and usefulness. These are commonly in the form of self-administered paper-and-pencil measures, as well as structured face-to-face or telephone interviews. Some of the more commonly employed measures are described here.

SELF-ADMINISTERED MEASURES

These are completed by the collateral member alone and typically involve scoring the level of functioning on a variety of general and specific items. The *Katz Adjustment Scale-Relatives Form* (Hogarty & Katz, 1971) is a measure of quality of life for both patient and relative. It has been used in a wide variety of studies involving health care conditions that compromise everyday functioning. The relative rates two areas: (1) the person's current level of performance across a wide variety of daily social role functions, and (2) their estimation of how well they feel the person is meeting what they *expect* of them in that capacity. This provides both a measure of level of function, as well as of discrepancy, from the relative's expectations.

COGNITIVE BEHAVIOR RATING SCALES

The Cognitive Behavior Rating Scales (Williams, 1987) address common sequelae of neurological conditions. The rater indicates the presence and degree of severity of a range of emotional and behavioral symptoms, neurological signs, and cognitive deficits. These are organized under nine scales entitled Language Deficit, Apraxia, Disorientation, Agitation, Need for Routine, Depression, Higher Cognitive Deficits, Memory Disorder, and Diffuse Dementia.

Briefer and more behaviorally specific rating forms have been developed with particular purposes in mind. An example is the *Patient Competency Rating Form* developed by Prigatano (1986) as part of a comprehensive neuropsychological rehabilitation program. This measure rates observations of the patient's ability to perform a variety of daily living skills, from hygiene to cooking, and the degree of difficulty that is presented by emotional and cognitive symptoms. The *Disability Rating Scale* (Rappaport, Hall, Hopkins, Belleza, & Cope, 1982) is a similar brief measure of self-care, cognitive level, and occupational functioning designed for head-injured patients in clinic and at home.

FAMILY INTERVIEW MEASURES

Other family rating systems are placed in the context of a structured interview. This permits rating the same sorts of areas noted before but in a more qualitative and content-oriented format of contact with the family member. The *Vineland Adaptive Rating Scales* (Sparrow, Balla, & Cicchetti, 1984) are among the most widely used in this regard. They allow obtaining highly useful information about the adaptive functioning of impaired and mentally retarded persons which cannot be as clearly described by test data, particularly for severely impaired persons. They are scaled by norm group and age equivalence in four broad domains: communication, socialization, motor skills, and maladaptive behavior. This format allows estimating the general level of function in each area, as well as drawing a profile of adaptive strengths and weaknesses in the person's daily living.

Other behaviorally oriented interviews include the *Social Behavior Assessment Schedule* (Platt, Weyman, Hirsch, & Hewett, 1980), designed to assess the extent of dysfunction of schizophrenic patients and its impact on persons who live with them. In this format, the family member is asked to rate the degree of severity of a variety of behavioral and psychiatric-symptom-related areas, along with the extent to which they find those symptoms distressing to them. This has been applied to other populations, such as the head-injured, and used as a measure of subjective burden involved in caregiving for such persons at home (Bryan & Strachan, 1992). *The Burden Interview* (Zarit, Orr, & Zarit, 1985) is a brief, symptom-focused rating system also designed to assess the degree of distress associated with caring for dementia patients.

Observed Interactions

PARENT–CHILD INTERACTION

The opportunity to observe individuals interacting with each other often provides a great deal of information about each of the individuals, as well as their relationship. Observed interaction is often of critical importance in evaluating children, whose behavior may in large part reflect the stimulus values and reinforcement behaviors of the parents. Robinson and Eyberg (1981) asserted that direct observation is a critical component of clinical child assessment and described an observational system to do such assessment.

They described a study in which they standardized and validated the Dyadic Parent–Child Interaction Coding System (DPICS), a comprehensive observational system for conduct problem children. Both parent and child behaviors are observed and coded. Each parent (i.e., mother and father if available) was observed in two five-minute interactions with each child in a playroom. There were two types of interaction. In the child-directed interaction, the parent was instructed to allow the child to choose any activity and to play along with the child. In the parent-directed interaction, the parent was instructed to select an activity and keep the child playing according to the parent's rules.

Interrater reliability was assessed; the mean reliability coefficient for parent behaviors was .91 and for child behaviors, .92. Validity was investigated by examining differences between normal and conduct problem families. Parents of conduct problem children made more critical statements and direct commands and gave fewer descriptive questions than parents of normal children. In addition, the conduct problem parents gave a higher percentage of direct commands to their children than did normals. The conduct problem children demonstrated more whining, yelling, and noncompliance than normal children. For example, the average normal child noncomplied 6.1 times, whereas the average conduct problem child noncomplied 14.2 times during 10 minutes of observation. The DPICS correctly classified 94% of families and predicted 61% of the variance in the parents' report of home behavior problems.

Robinson and Eyberg (1981) suggest that continuous recording contributes to validity and utility by providing a complete account of all behavior and allows collecting data in less time than typically required by interval sampling methods. They also note that the structure of the situations permits both the parent and the child to proceed naturally under varying degrees of parental control, thus maximizing the possibility of observing interactional dysfunction in conduct problem families. The authors explicitly acknowledge that characteristics of the parent, as well as those of the child, contribute to the diagnosis of a conduct problem. Finally, they point out that their observational procedure can be used serially to guide the course of treatment and to document treatment change.

The DPICS has been used clinically in different assessment situations. As already noted, it can be used to assess conduct problems between parent and child and to monitor change with treatment intervention. It has also been used in clinical assessment when there are clinical/forensic questions such as determining child custody and terminating parental rights. The generation and availability of empirical observation data can be useful in such decision making.

INPATIENT WARD OBSERVATION METHODS

Among the most important sources of information regarding patients is observation of how they function while in the hospital. Structured inpatient rating scales have been developed for interpreting and organizing the inpatient observation information sensibly. These typically place high value upon being brief and convenient, while also seeking to adapt acceptable levels of reliability and validity. The best known of these methods have evolved from the experiences with inpatient psychiatry. They tend to be structured around diagnostically significant behaviors and related observable symptoms. Clinically, they are used to help diagnose and track changes in patients' mental state and functional status over time. They are also used to help establish the validity of diagnostic systems through research on large groups of patients by using the wealth of available information from patients within a controlled setting.

The most common inpatient psychiatric rating methods have been in use for decades. They include the *Brief Psychiatric Rating Scale* (BPRS; Overall & Gorham, 1962), the *Present State Examination* (Wing, Cooper, & Sartorius, 1974), and the *Nurses' Observation Scale for Inpatient Evaluation* (NOSIE; Honigfeld, Gillis, & Klett, 1966). They enjoy widespread use and their psychometric and diagnostic discriminatory properties are continuously refined. These typically rate both the global level of functioning and specific descriptive subscales.

Recent modifications of the BPRS include the development of an 18-item format in which the clinicians rate items described by one or two sentences on a scale of "very mild" to "severe." The BPRS-18 includes the following six scales: Anxiety-Depression; Lack of Energy; Thought Disturbance; Hostility-Suspiciousness; and Schizophrenia (including unusual thought content, hallucinations, blunted affect, and emotional withdrawal). Hafkenscheid (1991) found that the thought disturbance, schizophrenia, and global scales had adequate reliability and discriminatory power. The NOSIE has also been found convenient and sensitive to clinical change. Recent studies have reported good reliability and identified six main factors: Social Competence, Social Interest, Personal Neatness, Irritability, Psychoticism, Retardation, and Depression (Dingemans, Bleeker, & Frohn-DeWinter, 1984).

These scales have been adopted in current research on "positive" and "negative" symptoms in diagnostic subtypes of schizophrenia. Positive symptoms involve abnormal and maladaptive functions such as hallucinations, bizarre behavior, and disturbed thought. Negative symptoms relate to the absence or lack of aspects of normal functioning and include lack of initiative, social withdrawal, the flat affect, and impoverishment of thought and speech. Dingemans (1990) found that both the BPRS and NOSIE contributed to reliable identification of positive symptoms, although negative symptoms were less consistently measured. Greater use of these scales to track patient progress and operationalize diagnostic constructs is expected.

Special Assessment Situations

QUALITY OF LIFE ASSESSMENT

Advances in the effectiveness and expense of clinical health procedures have raised pressing questions about how and when they should be applied. The benefits versus costs of medical procedures are the focus of crucial economic and biomedical ethical decision making. The concept of *quality of life* has evolved as the measure of worth to be balanced against the efforts, costs, and risks of intervention methods. The impact on the quality of life of recipients is addressed at many levels. These range from political/social resource distribution to measures of the effectiveness of drug, surgical, or psychological treatment to clinical contact with individual patients involving the ongoing assessment of their progress and response. Quality of life is further used as an outcome measure in individual and epidemiological studies and as the basis for establishing standards of care in many areas.

Although a crucial construct, quality of life is also broad and vague. It is generally agreed that it can best be conceived as a multidimensional construct, an aggregate of distinguishable and closely related factors that affect response to the disease and/or treatment. Definitions of the construct typically include

1. physical aspects, including mobility, pain, and appearance;
2. psychological and emotional aspects, including cognitive/intellectual function, self-esteem, and sense of subjective well-being; and
3. social aspects, including role functioning, contact versus isolation, and reciprocation in relationships (Siegrist & Junge, 1989).

Shumaker, Anderson, and Czajkowski (1990) have further added productivity and intimate involvement with others as relevant dimensions. Spilker (1990) has proposed a system-based definition that couches the safety, efficiency, and cost of treatment in terms of outcomes of physical status, psychological well-being, social interactions, and economic status. The patient's values, beliefs, and judgments represent moderating factors that also affect outcome.

Given the broad definition and wide range of applications of this construct, its meaning is being established through specific uses and measurement strategies. Shumaker et al. (1990) recommend a hypothesis-testing approach, with emphasis upon the specific areas considered relevant to a particular treatment. "Quality of life" seems all-encompassing, whereas prediction about the types of expected effects forces the examiner to consider which dimensions are most relevant to the clinical trial.

Considerable attention has been given to the psychometric foundations of measures of the quality of life. Objective, reliable, and standardized measurement is especially important in such a value-laden area. As a result, most measures emphasize the types of specific dimensions mentioned before. Some approaches include all of them within a single instrument, whereas other authors advocate a battery of individual tests. To be useful and meaningful, such measures must meet standards of reliability and validity (in all forms). Further, they must be sensitive indicators of change that provide information about which dimensions are affected by treatment, in which directions, and at which times.

A variety of approaches have been employed in quality of life assessment. They include scaled observer ratings and triangulation of information from different sources, such as family members, co-workers, and physicians (Siegrist & Junge, 1989). The self-report questionnaire format is by far the most common due to many advantages of data collection, cost-efficiency, and applicability to a range of patients. It is most effective compared to other indices of physical, psychological, and social functioning, including ratings by physicians and others who know the person well.

Many self-report measures have been developed, the most common of which will be summarized as examples of the types of dimensions addressed and questions utilized. The *General Health Questionnaire* (Goldberg, 1979) is a 60-item scale developed as a screening measure of somatic symptoms, mood and affective states, subjective feelings of distress, and social interactions. The *Symptom Checklist-90-Revised* (Derogatis, 1983), is a similar 90-item rating scale of symptoms primarily in nine psychiatric categories and yields both separate scale scores and a Global Symptom Index. The *Chronic Illness Problem Inventory* (Kames, Naliboff, Heinrich, & Schag, 1984), permits rating perceived severity of limitation in a wide range of areas of daily functioning among persons affected by debilitating illnesses. The *Quality of Life Scale* (Burkhardt, Woods, Schultz, & Tiebarth, 1989) is a brief, 16-item scale that yields a summary satisfaction score regarding broad areas of life. Specific scales such as the *Quality of Life Rating Scale* (Walker, Blankenship, Ditty, & Lynch, 1987), a nine-item Likert-scaled measure designed for clients within a head-injury rehabilitation program, have been developed for more circumscribed populations.

QUALITY OF WELL-BEING SCALE

The Quality of Well-Being Scale, developed by Kaplan and Anderson (1990), is a functional health scale completed by the clinician. It consists of three scales that focus on elementary aspects of daily functioning: Social role activity, Physical activity, and Mobility. These provide a description of the level of general function, and an extensive list of 25 specific symptoms that can impede function is also included. Each of the functional levels and symptom is assigned a "preference weight," which then comprise a global quality of well-being score. Preference weighting of this sort has been used as the basis for health-care cost-utility analysis, placing relative weighted value upon types of symptom combinations. They are the basis of actuarial systems that employ indexes, such as "quality-adjust life-years," or QALY's.

The Outcome Questionnaire (OQ; Lambert, Lunnen, Umphress, Hansen, & Burlingame, 1994) is a 45-item self-report questionnaire designed to measure progress in psychotherapy. Patient progress is measured along three dimensions of mental health functioning that are consistent with the *Diagnostic and Statistical Manual of Mental Disorders*, Fourth Edition (DSM-IV; American Psychiatric Association, 1994) diagnostic guidelines. They are as follows: Subjective Discomfort, Interpersonal Relationships, and Social Role Performance. This brief questionnaire can be completed by the patient in less than 10 minutes. The OQ is used by several national insurance carriers that are responsible for more than 30 million lives.

Psychological Testing

We have saved our discussion of psychological testing as the last topic in our brief and selective overview of psychological assessment activities. This is not because we consider it the least important. Indeed, to the contrary, it is the most important of a psychologist's assessment activities, and we do not consider that any psychological assessment consultation is complete unless, or until, some form of psychological testing has been done and some testing data have been recorded.

STANDARD OF CARE

In our discussion of psychological testing, we want to introduce several assessment concepts and strategies that have become the norm in clinical practice. The first issue we want to highlight can be labeled "standard of care." Psychologists are no longer "islands of practice" unto themselves. Under our almost universal third-party coverage, insurance companies want to know the quality of care for which they are paying. Similarly, because of the expansion of malpractice complaints, both patients and their attorneys want to know what are accepted standards of care and whether the patient's care was at such a level.

Quality of care and patient satisfaction are defined by patient perceptions and expectations perhaps even more than by standards established by the profession. We have already discussed the importance of doctor–patient communication. Two additional very important components of patient satisfaction are accessibility and availability of services. Our clinic has tried to attend to timely availability to patients and has established and monitored efforts toward this goal.

TIMELINESS

An important assessment strategy is to respond promptly to a request for a psychological consultation. Many inpatients are hospitalized for relatively short periods of time and, if psychological consultation findings and/or recommendations are to be included in decision making about the patient, the consultation assessment needs to take place within 24 hours. For outpatient consultations, the patient should also be contacted within 24 hours to arrange a mutually convenient appointment time, ideally within two weeks.

QUALITY ASSURANCE

In our health-care setting, as in most others where hospital or other health facility accreditation is involved, we must show what efforts we make to monitor, evaluate, and improve clinical services. One aspect of this monitoring and evaluative function is to have established standards of care and then to assess whether we are delivering services according to that standard. Standards of care are clearly involved when we consider what constitutes acceptable psychological testing in response to various consultation referrals.

For example, our clinical faculty has established a standard of care in assessing questions of intellectual ability level in patients. When seeing a patient for such a referral question, the core procedures include the use of an intelligence test, an academic achievement test, and a review of the patient's educational history with a review of school transcripts when these can be obtained. In our Quality Assurance monitoring, we review records to confirm that these core procedures have indeed been completed.

TESTING PROTOCOLS FOR DIFFERENT PATIENT GROUPS

We have no doubt that, in time and in the interests of establishing and assuring appropriate standards of care, testing protocols appropriate to various patient groups and to various referral questions will be established. Although practicing psychologists have long discussed the uniqueness of each patient, the advantages of flexible testing, and the desirability of tailoring assessment to each individual, such approaches to assessment raise some important questions in our minds. For example, one cannot know what relationship scores from one test have to scores from another test unless the tests have been used consistently and systematically with each other so that, through research or extensive experience, such relationships can be identified. When different tests are used with each patient, it is not possible to observe or establish patterns of test response within a given patient group.

It is also important to observe standard testing procedures. As pointed out by Faust, Ziskin, and Hiers (1991), when a clinician alters standard instructions or test procedures, then short of research on these changes, one does not know how this impacts test scores or what scores would have been achieved had the standard instructions been used.

When consistent test protocols are not used with particular patient groups or referral questions, it becomes more difficult to determine effectiveness or accuracy across different assessment cases. One has essentially performed a unique set of procedures with every individual and must conduct a separate "experiment" for each case seen (Faust et al., 1991). Overall, an approach that allows different assessment procedures among a given diagnostic category of patients is likely to result in significant variability across different clinicians, is quite difficult to evaluate scientifically, and seems open to examiner bias.

As an assessment strategy in our clinic, we have developed testing protocols for different patient groups. One of these consists of patients referred from a Rheumatology Clinic with a presumed diagnosis of fibromyalgia. The treatment of most fibromyalgia patients requires some form of psychological intervention. Thus, many of these patients are seen for psychological evaluation when they are accepted into our university hospital treatment program (Bennett, Campbell, Burckhardt, Clark, O'Reilly, & Wiens, 1991). We wanted a psychological test battery that would reproduce assessment procedures used by other clinicians/investigators and that could be replicated by other clinicians in turn. We chose the following procedures to constitute our protocol: Clinical Interview, C-DIS, Psychological/Social History Questionnaire, MMPI, Cornell Medical Index Health Questionnaire, the Shipley Institute of Living

Scale, and a Quality of Life Inventory. We have been able to describe the psychological characteristics of this patient population to a number of different professional audiences.

As a second example and in concert with clinicians in our Occupational Health Clinic and Department of Neurology, we believe that behavioral and neurophysiological changes may be the earliest and sometimes the only indicators of acute or chronic neurotoxicity, that is, we view behavior as a sensitive indicator of central nervous system impairment. The literature has suggested that neurotoxins interfere with at least four distinct aspects of central nervous system functions: memory, visuomotor performance, affect, and verbal concept formation. We have proposed measuring behavior by neuropsychological tests for objectively assessing early neurological deficit and for detecting preclinical nervous system changes resulting from environmental or occupational exposure to neurotoxic agents. The core psychological test protocol that we selected for our neurobehavioral examination is as follows: WAIS-III, MMPI, Halstead–Reitan Neuropsychology Test Battery (15 subtests), Rey Auditory Verbal Learning Test, Rey–Osterreith Complex Figure Test, Cornell Medical Index Health Questionnaire, and a Structured Interview. The interview has a number of foci: previous health history, medications, use of alcohol/drugs, present symptoms and history, general orientation, physical appearance and gait, speech, affect, personality characteristics, and general competence to handle daily activities. We have been able to describe the modal cognitive, personality, and physical complaints of these patients and to differentiate among them: (a) those who show no identifiable emotional or cognitive dysfunction, (b) those who show primarily emotional-characterological concerns and no significant evidence of cognitive impairment, (c) those who have a history of episodes of emotional dysfunction and show evidence of cognitive impairment, and (d) those who have evidence of cognitive impairment as the primary finding. We do not believe that we could have made the observations that we have of this patient group without a standardized testing protocol.

NEUROPSYCHOLOGICAL ASSESSMENT

A final consideration is related to the neuropsychological evaluation, that is, examiner qualifications. Currently, there is debate within the field of psychology with regard to who is qualified to conduct a neuropsychological evaluation. Bigler and Clement (1997) note,

> Practicing neuropsychologists are well aware that familiarity with test instruments is only one of many skills needed to perform an evaluation. A knowledge of the commonly seen clinical syndromes, such as vascular disorder, traumatic injury, tumor, infectious processes, and many others, is a critical component of the knowledge base necessary to perform a competent neuropsychological assessment. (p. 49)

Historically, neuropsychologists were trained to use test batteries to determine if the patient was "organic" and to identify the location of the brain lesion (Bigler & Clement, 1997). Today neuropsychologists are expected to provide a comprehensive evaluation of the patient's cognitive and emotional functioning. This requires clinicians to be well trained in psychological testing, and they must also be well schooled in functional neuroanatomy and brain imaging data (e.g., MRI, CT, PET, SPECT).

SUMMARY

The assessment strategies that we have been discussing can be expected to lead to a diagnosis of a patient's condition. A great deal of thought has gone into identifying criteria for diagnoses and sources of unreliability in diagnostic formulations. Spitzer, Endicott, and Robins (1975) noted five sources of unreliability and then determined that two of them contributed most heavily to diagnostic unreliability. The first source of unreliability they noted was *subject variance*, which occurs when patients actually have different conditions at different times. They gave the example of the patient who may show alcohol intoxication on admission to a hospital but develop "delirium tremens" several days later. A second source of unreliability is *occasion variance*, which occurs when patients are in different stages of the same condition at different times. An example of this would be a patient with a bipolar disorder who is depressed during one period of illness and manic during another. A third source of unreliability is *information variance*, which occurs when clinicians have different sources of information about their patients. Examples here include information from clinicians who talk with patients' families and those who do not, or information from interviewers who question patients concerning areas of functioning and symptoms about which other interviewers do not ask. A fourth area of unreliability is *observation variance*, which occurs when clinicians notice different things, although presumably observing the same patient behavior. Clinicians may disagree on whether a patient was tearful, hard to follow, or hallucinating. A fifth source of unreliability is *criterion variance*, which occurs when clinicians use varying diagnostic criteria (e.g., whether a formal thought disorder is necessary for the diagnosis of schizophrenia or precludes a diagnosis of affective disorder).

Spitzer et al. (1975) concluded that the largest source of diagnostic variability by far was criterion variance. Their efforts in the development of DSM-III diagnostic criteria obviously reflected their confidence in this conclusion. Their research efforts to reduce information variance (the second most important source of unreliability) led to the development of structured clinical interviews that reduce that portion of the unreliability variance based on different interviewing styles and coverage.

We can predict that the unstructured assessment clinical interviews of the past will be replaced in the future by structured interview schedules for routine clinical assessment. This shift is supported by trends toward the use of operational criteria for diagnosis, well-defined taxonomies, almost exclusive use of structured examinations in research settings, and the growing influence of clinician-researchers. Further, the demand for accountability has also forced a problem-oriented type of record keeping system in most institutions, with emphasis on branch-logic systems of clinical decision making, and progress notes that reflect resolution of symptom-syndromes and changes in problem status, rather than changes in psychodynamics. Finally, the impact of computers appears decisive in that they allow more efficient retrieval of information than possible with records of noncomputerized narrative clinical interviews. Computers can also be used to apply an algorithm to yield highly reliable diagnoses from raw data (Siassi, 1984).

The comprehensiveness of the information that can be collected with structured interviews has led to their use in routine clinical practice. The availability of personal computers is contributing to their increased use in patient self-administration of various structured interviews, including psychosocial history interviews and diagnostic interviews. Using assessment strategies that allow patients to contribute data about themselves ever more directly, it should be possible to reduce information variance even more in the future. We have attempted to illustrate both the principles and techniques of assessment strategies in the practice of abnormal psychology. What we still have to research is how such expanded information bases can be used most validly in assessment/diagnosis and in assisting the persons who come to us for help.

Of course, while we are researching extant assessment procedures and strategies, new ones are developing. A prominent example is in the area of *telehealth* which is making the physical isolation of rural communities less of an obstacle to quality health care. Physicians can examine a patient while linked by video to an expert consultant at a distant medical center.

Urban radiologists and dermatologists can review medical images transmitted over telephone lines. An anecdotal example concerns an urban dermatologist who calls up a color image of a sore thumb on his computer screen and magnifies it a hundred times. He recognizes the growth as a tumor that later turns out to be a melanoma. Unfortunately, the patients' primary care physician, based in a small rural town, had for months misdiagnosed the growth as a wart.

An active telehealth network in Oregon is used for three things: administrative conferences, educational offerings, and clinical consultations. These uses apply to mental health. Eastern Oregon has only a handful of "circuit-riding" mental health professionals, who may drive hundreds of miles between clinics. Educational programs are offered to mental health providers, thus reducing their isolation. Clinical consultation is provided for predischarge planning and legal process hearings. Telehealth programs are proliferating in medicine, and we expect that clinical psychologists will become much more involved in them as time passes.

REFERENCES

Adams, K. M., & Heaton, R. K. (1987). Computerized neuropsychological assessment: Issues and applications. In J. N. Butcher (Ed.), *Computerized psychological assessment* (pp. 355–365). New York: Basic Books.

American Psychiatric Association. (1987). *Diagnostic and statistical manual of mental disorders* (3rd ed., revised). Washington, DC: Author.

American Psychiatric Association. (1994). *Diagnostic and statistical manual of mental disorders* (4th ed). Washington, DC: Author.

Baird, A. D., Brown, G. G., Adams, K., & Schatz, M. W. (1987). Neuropsychological deficits and real-world dysfunction in cerebral revascularization candidates. *Journal of Clinical and Experimental Neuropsychology, 9,* 407–422.

Beckman, H. B., & Frankel, R. M. (1984). The effect of physician behavior on the collection of data. *Annals of Internal Medicine, 101,* 692–696.

Bennett, R. M., Campbell, S., Burckhardt, C., Clark, S., O'Reilly, C., & Wiens, A. N. (1991). A multidisciplinary approach to fibromyalgia management. *The Journal of Musculoskeletal Medicine, 8,* 21–31.

Bigler, E. D., & Clement, P. F. (1997). *Diagnostic clinical neuropsychology,* 3rd ed. Austin: University of Texas Press.

Blouin, A. (1985). *Computerized psychiatric diagnosis: Manual.* Ottawa, Canada: Ottawa Civic Hospital.

Bryan, J. E., & Strachan, A. M. (1992). Expressed emotion, coping, and subjective burden in family caregivers of the closed head injured. *Journal of Clinical and Experimental Neuropsychology, 14,* 29.

Burkhardt, C. S., Woods, S. L., Schultz, A. A., & Tiebarth, P. M. (1989). Quality of life in adults with a chronic illness: A psychometric study. *Research in Nursing and Health, 12,* 347–354.

Choca, J., & Morris, J. (1992). Administering the Category Test by computer: Equivalence of results. *The Clinical Neuropsychologist, 6,* 9–15.

Derogatis, L. R. (1983). *SCL-90-R: Administration, scoring, and procedures manual.* Towson, MD: Clinical Psychometric Research.

Dingemans, P. M. (1990). The Brief Psychiatric Rating Scale (BPRS) and the Nurses' Observation Scale for Inpatient Evaluation (NOSIE) in the evaluation of positive and negative symptoms. *Journal of Clinical Psychology, 46,* 168–174.

Dingemans, P. M., Bleeker, J. A. C., & Frohn-DeWinter, M. L. (1984). A cross-cultural study of the reliability and factorial dimensions of the Nurses' Observation Scale for Inpatient Evaluations (NOSIE). *Journal of Clinical Psychology, 40,* 169–172.

Faust, D., Ziskin, J., & Hiers, J. B. (1991). *Brain damage claims: Coping with neuropsychological evidence,* Vol. I. Los Angeles: Law and Psychology Press.

First, M. B., Gibbon, M., Williams, J. B. W., & Spitzer, R. L. (1991). *AutoSCID II for Personality Disorders.* Toronto: Multi-Health Systems, Inc. & American Psychiatric Association.

Giannetti, R. A. (1987). The GOLPH psychosocial history: Response-contingent data acquisition and reporting. In J. N. Butcher (Ed.), *Computerized psychological assessment* (pp. 124–144). New York: Basic Books.

Goldberg, D. (1979). *Manual of the general health questionnaire.* Windsor, England: NFER Publishing.

Hafkenscheid, A. (1991). Psychometric evaluation of a standardized and expanded Brief Psychiatric Rating Scale. *Acta Psychiatrica Scandinavica, 84,* 294–300.

Harrell, T. H. (1984). *Intake Evaluation Checklist: Clinician Version*. Indialantic, FL: Psychologistics, Inc.

Hogarty, G. E., & Katz, M. M. (1971). Norms of adjustment and social behavior. *Archives of General Psychiatry, 25,* 470–480.

Honigfeld, G., Gillis, R., & Klett, J. (1966). NOSIE-30: A treatment-sensitive ward behavior scale. *Psychological Reports, 19,* 180–182.

Kames, L. D., Naliboff, B. D., Heinrich, R. L., & Schag, C. C. (1984). The chronic illness problem inventory: Problem-oriented psychosocial assessment of patients with chronic illness. *International Journal of Psychology Medicine, 14,* 65–75.

Kaplan, R. M., & Anderson, J. P. (1990). The general health policy model: An integrated approach. In B. Spilker (Ed.), *Quality of life assessments in clinical trials* (pp. 131–149). New York: Raven Press.

Lambert, M. J., Lunnen, K., Umphress, V., Hansen, N. B., & Burlingame, G. (1994). *Administration and scoring manual for the outcome questionnaire* (OQ-45.1). Salt Lake City, UT: IHC Center for Behavioral Healthcare Efficacy.

Lukin, M. E., Dowd, E. T., Plake, B. S., & Kraft, R. G. (1985). Comparing computerized versus traditional psychological assessment. *Computers in Human Behavior, 1,* 49–58.

Matarazzo, J. D. (1990). Psychological assessment versus psychological testing. *American Psychologist, 45,* 999–1017.

Meyer, G. J., Finn, S. E., Eyde, L. D., Kay, G. G., Kubiszyn, T. W., Moreland, K. L., Eisman, E. J., & Dies, R. R. (1998). *Benefits and costs of psychological assessment in healthcare delivery: Report of the Board of Professional Affairs Psychological Assessment Work Group, Part I*. Washington, DC: American Psychological Association.

Overall, J. E., & Gorham, D. (1962). Brief psychiatric rating scale. *Psychological Reports, 10,* 799–812.

Platt, S., Weyman, A., Hirsch, S., & Hewett, S. (1980). The Social Behavior Assessment Schedule (SBAS): Rationale, contents, scoring, and reliability of a new interview schedule. *Social Psychiatry, 15,* 43–55.

Prigatano, G. (1986). *Neuropsychological rehabilitation*. Baltimore: Johns Hopkins University Press.

Rainwater, G. D., & Coe, D. S. (1988). *Psychological/social history report: Manual*. Melbourne, FL: Psychometric Software, Inc.

Rappaport, M., Hall, K. M., Hopkins, K., Belleza, T., & Cope, D. N. (1982). Disability Rating Scale for severe head trauma: Coma to community. *Archives of Physical Medicine and Rehabilitation, 63,* 118–123.

Robins, L. N., Helzer, J. E., Croughan, J., & Ratcliff, K. (1981). National Institute of Mental Health Diagnostic Interview Schedule. *Archives of General Psychiatry, 38,* 381–389.

Robinson, E. A., & Eyberg, S. M. (1981). The Dyadic Parent–Child Interaction Coding System: Standardization and validation. *Journal of Consulting and Clinical Psychology, 49,* 245–250.

Shumaker, S., Anderson, R. T., & Czajkowski, S. M. (1990). Psychological tests and scales. In B. Spilker (Ed.), *Quality of life assessments in clinical trials* (pp. 95–113). New York: Raven Press.

Siassi, I. (1984). Psychiatric interview and mental status examination. In G. Goldstein & M. Hersen (Eds.), *Handbook of psychological assessment* (pp. 259–275). Elmsford, NY: Pergamon.

Siegrist, J., & Junge, A. (1989). Conceptual and methodological problems in research on the quality of life in clinical medicine. *Social Sciences Medicine, 29,* 463–468.

Sparrow, S. S., Balla, D. A., & Cicchetti, D. (1984). *Vineland Adaptive Behavior Scales*. Circle Pines, MN: American Guidance Service, Inc.

Spilker, B. (1990). Introduction. In B. Spilker (Ed.), *Quality of life assessments in clinical trials* (pp. 3–9). New York: Raven Press.

Spitzer, R. G., Endicott, J., & Robins, E. (1975). Clinical criteria for diagnosis and DSM-III. *American Journal of Psychiatry, 132,* 1187–1192.

Walker, D. E., Blankenship, V., Ditty, J. A., & Lynch, K. P. (1987). Prediction of recovery for closed-head-injured adults: An evaluation of the MMPI, the Adaptive Behavior Scale, and a "Quality of Life" Rating Scale. *Journal of Clinical Psychology, 43,* 699–707.

Wechsler, D. (1997). *WAIS-III: Wechsler Adult Intelligence Scale-Third Edition*. San Antonio, TX: Psychological Corporation.

Williams, J. M. (1987). *Cognitive Behavior Rating Scales: Manual*. Odessa, FL: Psychological Assessment Resources, Inc.

Wing, J., Cooper, J., & Sartorius, N. (1974). *The measurement and classification of psychiatric symptoms*. Cambridge, England: Cambridge University Press.

Young, G., O'Brien, J. D., Gutterman, E. M., & Cohen, P. (1987). Structured diagnostic interviews for children and adolescents. *Journal of the American Academy of Child and Adolescent Psychiatry, 26,* 611–620.

Zarit, S. H., Orr, N. K., & Zarit, J. M. (1985). *The hidden victims of Alzheimer's disease: Families under stress*. New York: New York University Press.

3

Research Methods

F. Dudley McGlynn

Introduction

Psychology began as an attempt to understand consciousness scientifically, as an attempt to discover the basic elements of consciousness, and then to describe how those elements combine to form consciousness as given. The first psychology failed and was replaced by alternative psychologies, that is, the classical "schools" of functionalism, behaviorism, and Gestalt psychology. None of the alternative psychologies won the day. Psychology became fragmented into "miniature systems" or clusters of narrow research problems and specialized methods (e.g., general and special theories of learning, perception, and emotion). As a result, modern psychology encompasses an astonishingly diverse array of problems and methods (Staats, 1991).

The history of psychopathology is much the same as that of general psychology. Biological, psychodynamic, behavioral, cognitive, and developmental approaches have struggled for ascendancy but none has won the day. As a legacy, modern psychopathology embodies a confusing mixture of theories that are manifestly incompatible and research methods that mirror disparate scientific assumptions. Commonalities across the various approaches to research in psychopathology can be found only by focusing on the most basic levels of scientific activity.

Science as a Rationo-Empirical Method

Fundamentally "the scientific method" is an amalgam of two ancient approaches in epistemology or the philosophy of knowledge. An epistemic position, known as rationalism, is defined by the proposition that knowledge is arrived at by thought; perfect knowledge exists only at the level of ideas. An epistemic position, known as empiricism, is defined by the proposition that knowledge is arrived at by observation; practical knowledge exists at the level of perception. Science is an amalgam because thought and observation are linked in various ways so as to provide statements about natural phenomena. The statements are best described

F. Dudley McGlynn • Department of Psychology, Auburn University, Auburn, Alabama 36849-5214.

Advanced Abnormal Psychology, Second Edition, edited by Hersen and Van Hasselt. Kluwer Academic/Plenum Publishers, New York, 2001.

as rationo-empirical statements because they usually have both rational (conceptual) and empirical (observable) implications.

Description and Explanation

The business of the scientific psychologist is to make statements about behavior. The business of the psychopathologist is to make statements about those subsets of behavior that are said to manifest or to reflect psychopathology. In general, the rationo-empirical statements made by psychopathologists have to do with description and explanation of those behaviors.

Differences between description and explanation have occupied the attention of many writers (e.g., Kearney, 1971; Westfall, 1977) as have differences between approaches to explanation (e.g., Hempel & Oppenheim, 1948; Marx, 1963; Popper, 1959; Turner, 1967). Description and explanation both consist of rationo-empirical statements, but descriptive and explanatory statements have different emphases. Scientific descriptions are statements that portray events along with other events or conditions that precede, accompany, or follow them. As such, scientific descriptions are predominantly empirical in emphasis; they are "if-then" statements about observed states of affairs. Scientific explanations are empirical "if-then" statements also, but they convey something more; they convey the rational implication that the presence of the "if" term is meaningfully related to the presence of the "then" term.

The nature of the meaningful relationship between the "if" and "then" terms in explanatory statements is at issue in philosophical analyses of the concept of causality. In necessity theories of causation (e.g., Aristotle), the "if-then" relationship is one of necessity; causation exists when the presence of the "if" term is deemed necessary to the presence of the "then" term. In regularity theories of causation (e.g., Hume, 1739/1978), the "if-then" relationship is one of constant conjunction; causality exists when the "if" and "then" terms always occur together. In manipulability theories of causation (e.g., Collingwood, 1940), the relationship is one of production; causality exists when the "then" term can be produced by manipulating the "if" term. Modern theories of causation usually involve elaborations or constraints on classical views such as those mentioned before (see White, 1990). As one example, Bunge (1963) developed the view that Collingwood's production and causation are not equivalent; causation instantiates the more general principle of production.

Explanation in Psychopathology

Several approaches to causal explanation are encountered frequently in psychopathology. For psychopathology researchers working within the biological perspective, an explanation is an "if-then" statement in which the "if" term is stated with a vocabulary that is more molecular or more "basic" than the vocabulary of the "then" term. For example, when an "if" term from anatomy (such as microorganismic infection of the brain) precedes a "then" term about behavior (such as disorganized speech), an explanation of the behavior has been achieved. Biological explanations of behavior are *reductive* (Marx, 1963). Taken along with their scientific contexts, they tend to imply regularity theories of causation.

For psychopathology researchers working with the family-systems perspective, an explanation is an "if-then" statement in which the "if" term is stated with a vocabulary that is more molar or less "basic" than is the vocabulary of the "then" term. For example, when an "if" term from family-systems theory (such as expressed emotion) precedes a "then" term about behavior (such as hospital recidivism), an explanation of the behavior has been achieved.

Family-systems explanations of behavior are *constructive* (Marx, 1963). Taken along with their scientific contexts, they also imply regularity theories of causation.

For researchers working within the behavioral perspective, an explanation is an "if-then" statement in which the "if" term describes the procedures or conditions that are necessary and sufficient to produce or control the behavior in the "then" term. For example, explanatory terms such as positive reinforcement, negative reinforcement, and punishment refer to means of controlling rates of behaviors by arranging for the behaviors to produce specified outcomes. Behavioral explanations are constructive explanations that clearly imply productive/generative theories of causation.

Some approaches to explanation in psychopathology are conspicuous by their absence. From the perspective of information theory, as one example, an explanation of a phenomenon is a statement that reduces uncertainty, a statement that provides information about the phenomenon above and beyond the information contained in its description (Attneave, 1959). The concept of explanation as uncertainty reduction is of considerable potential value in psychopathology because it focuses attention on the emptiness of some explanations. When a given array of behaviors is explained with a term such as "personality disorder" or even "schizophrenia," does that explanation tell us anything about the behaviors we did not already know? If not, then should we learn to avoid certain superficially explanatory uses of our terms?

Arguments over the propriety of alternative approaches to explanation in psychopathology are clearly possible. The biological scientist can argue that the behavioral scientist's explanations are merely descriptive. The behavioral scientist can argue that the biologist's explanations are naively reductionistic. The information theorists can challenge other theorists to show that they are doing something more than restating the same information in a different vocabulary.

VALIDITY IN RESEARCH ON PSYCHOPATHOLOGY

Concern over scientific validity cuts across all varieties of the rationo-empirical method. Four types of validity are customarily distinguished: internal validity, external validity, theoretical validity, and statistical validity (Cook & Campbell, 1979).

Internal Validity

The dimension of internal validity refers to the degree to which changes in the phenomena under study are known to be related to the research variable(s) of interest, not to other factors. Internal validity is conceptualized as a dimension because different research strategies yield different degrees of internal validity. Retrospective case studies (later), for example, are low on the dimension of internal validity because the case study writers do nothing to rule out unknown influences on the phenomena of interest in the case. Well-executed experiments (later), on the other hand, are high on the dimension of internal validity because experimenters bring to bear procedural and/or statistical controls over unknown influences on the experimental phenomena of interest. Other research strategies usually fall in between retrospective case studies and experiments along the dimension of internal validity. For example, in quasi experiments (later), some controls over unwanted influence on experimental phenomena are absent, but efforts are made to identify such deficiencies and to chronicle their implications for interpreting quasi-experimental data.

External Validity

External validity refers to the degree to which the rationo-empirical statements produced by research are accurate when they are applied in contexts other than the research contexts used to produce them. Again, external validity is a dimension because different research strategies afford different levels of external validity. Retrospective case studies are low on the dimension of external validity because they provide no information at all about other contexts in which the statements yielded by the case might be applicable. Experiments also tend to be low on the dimension of external validity; the procedures used to maximize internal validity tend to produce artificiality with respect to the naturalistic phenomena that experimental events represent. Quasi experiments can be relatively high on the dimension of external validity compared to experiments because there is less emphasis on maximizing internal validity in quasi experiments.

Theoretical Validity

Theoretical validity refers to the degree to which the procedures used in research satisfactorily represent the constructs of one or more theories and/or the events that the theories purport to explain. In much scientific research, a theory is used to arrive at a hypothesis or a prediction about what will happen in an experiment or other empirical undertaking. The empirical work is then conducted, and the theory is retained, modified, or discarded in the light of the results. This rationo-empirical approach can succeed only insofar as the rational implications of the theory are captured faithfully by the empirical features and products of the research. For example, a general theory maintains that the behaviors of sociopathic humans reflect subtle neurological peculiarities. Gorenstein and Newman (1980) tested hypotheses based on that theory by experimenting with specified behaviors among rats whose brains they had damaged surgically. The issue of theoretical validity revolves around the degree to which the empirical connections between experimental lesions and behaviors among rats faithfully represent the rational (theoretical) connections between neurological peculiarities and sociopathic conduct among humans.

Statistical Validity

According to the discipline of mathematical statistics, valid inference from observations made on research samples (e.g., 30 schizophrenic subjects vs. 30 normal subjects) to observations that might be made on sampled populations (e.g., schizophrenics vs. normals at large) requires that the numbers used in statistical calculations be obtained in certain ways and have certain properties. For example, the numbers should be obtained from random independent samples of the target population, they should be normally distributed, and they should be based on measurement (number-assignment) operations such that the sizes of differences between the phenomena designated by all pairs of adjacent numbers are the same. According to the traditional account, a given inference is statistically valid to the extent that the above desiderata have been met. Empirical work has shown, however, that some statistical inferences are valid even when these desiderata are not met. A statistic is said to be "robust" when the conclusions it produces are not influenced unduly by numbers that violate the theoretical assumptions of mathematical statistics. In practice, statistical errors are rife within the research literature in psychology and psychopathology. In principle, a given research product is statistically valid either when the numbers used in statistical analyses meet the requirements of mathematical statistics or when the statistics used are robust.

Relationships among Types of Validity

Internal validity is important fundamentally; internal validity permits statements about what leads to what. Statistical validity is also important fundamentally (in research paradigms that make use of inferential statistics); statistical validity is the basis of valid inference from observed samples to the populations those samples represent. External validity is not important fundamentally; it becomes important when the purpose of the research is to afford statements that are applicable directly to one or more real-world contexts (e.g., clinics, hospitals). Theoretical validity is not important fundamentally either; it becomes important when the purpose of the research is to afford statements that pertain to the empirical value of one or more theories. Different research methods and goals place different emphases on the four dimensions of validity; the various types of validity cannot be achieved simultaneously. In turn, overall validity in a scientific arena derives from the cumulation of findings that are produced by heterogeneous research methods that complement one another along the various dimensions of validity.

RESEARCH ON ETIOLOGY

Psychopathology research takes place in many different arenas, for example, the arenas of etiology (the study of causes), epidemiology (the study of population prevalence), taxonomy (the study of classification), intervention, and prevention. In each arena, research methods that are basically the same are adapted to serve special purposes. The arenas of etiology and intervention are used here to organize the narrative. Within the section on etiological research, activities are subdivided into four general methods: case studies, correlational methods, quasi experiments, and experiments. Each method occupies a legitimate place in the psychopathologist's armamentarium and, as noted above, the various methods play complementary roles in producing valid knowledge.

The Retrospective Case Study

The case study method has played an influential role in the history of psychopathology. Case studies reported during the middle of the nineteenth century initiated interest in an apparent constellation of behavioral phenomena that would later be called schizophrenia (Bleuler, 1911). A case study of the Genain quadruplets (Rosenthal, 1963) stirred interest subsequently in a genetic contribution to the phenomena of schizophrenia. The cases of Little Hans (Freud, 1909), and of Anna O. (Breuer & Freud, 1895) influenced the formulation of psychoanalytic theory and the "talking cure" for psychoneuroses.

An etiologic case study is a narrative that describes a patient's symptoms and the circumstances that presumably brought the symptoms about, usually interpreted from some systematic theoretical perspective (e.g., psychoanalysis, conditioning theory, genetics). Scientific work can be divided into the contexts of discovery and confirmation (Marx, 1963). Within the scientific context of discovery, the case study has considerable merit. Indeed, the case study is the only method that holds the promise of portraying the ontogeny of psychopathology in all its subtlety and complexity. Within the scientific context of confirmation, however, the retrospective case study is sorely lacking. Among other shortcomings, case study data are acquired without the observational conditions that are necessary to afford trustworthy statements about what leads to what. Case studies also are open to major biases introduced by reporters' theoretical orientations. Notable of the latter problem is the ease with which behavioral theorists (Wolpe & Rachman, 1960) challenged the putative evidence for psychodynamic etiology in the case of Little Hans.

Correlational Research

Most research on the etiology of psychopathology is nonexperimental, often called "correlational" research. In nonexperimental research, measures are taken of historical and/or biological and/or psychological variables, and then mathematical relationships among the measures are described. In univariate correlational research, one etiologic variable and one measure of psychopathology are of interest. In multivariate correlational research, many etiologic and psychopathologic variables are related simultaneously. There are numerous statistical variations in "correlational" research, and some of the variations are quite sophisticated arithmetically. In general, however, correlational research belongs in the scientific context of discovery. Correlational research affords statements about relationships between etiologic and psychopathological variables, but the statements need to be confirmed by other methods. Only some subsets of correlational methodology are overviewed here, and only a few examples are provided. Examples appear throughout the text; the narrative here should assist in understanding methodological terminology in those examples.

Ex Post Facto Comparisons

In experimental research (later), the phenomena of interest are created by what the experimenter does. In nonexperimental research, the phenomena of interest are brought to the investigator by the research subject; they have already been created. Most ex post facto (after the fact) comparison research seeks to discover how the phenomena of interest were created by discovering one or more potentially causal differences between persons who manifest the phenomena and persons who do not. Even though psychopathologists from all theoretical perspectives use ex post facto comparisons, they are particularly common in the biological literature.

The study of genetic influences on psychopathology provides many examples of ex post facto comparisons in the biological literature. In *family pedigree studies* of genetic influence, the incidences of psychopathologies among the blood relatives of affected persons (probands) are compared with the incidences of the same psychopathologies or of related conditions among the blood relatives of unaffected persons. Higher incidences among the relatives of affected persons suggest genetic influence. For example, schizophrenia is more common among the relatives of probands diagnosed with schizophrenia than among the population at large (Parnas et al., 1993) and the prevalence of schizophrenia increases as the genetic relationship to the proband becomes closer (Gottesman, 1991). In *twin studies* of genetic influence, the incidences of psychopathologies among genetically identical twins are compared with the incidences of psychopathologies among fraternal twins whose genes are no more alike than those of other siblings. Higher concordance among identical-twin pairs than among fraternal-twin pairs suggests genetic influence. For example, the concordance rate in one report for schizophrenia was 48% among identical-twin pairs but only 17% among fraternal-twin pairs (Gottesman, 1991). In *adoption studies* of genetic influence, the life histories of adoptees who were later diagnosed with schizophrenia are studied so that the incidences of schizophrenia among biological versus adoptive relatives can be compared. In the best known example, Kety and his colleagues (e.g., Kety et al., 1978; Kety, 1988) identified 33 adoptees diagnosed with schizophrenia and 33 similar adoptees not diagnosed with schizophrenia among 5,500 adults. Then, they located and interviewed 365 biological and adoptive relatives of the 66 adoptees. Among the biological relatives of the schizophrenic adoptees, 14% were schizophrenic; among the adoptive relatives, only 2.7% were schizophrenic.

Study of the neuropathology in schizophrenia also provides many examples of ex post facto comparisons in the biological literature. The first modern work was reported by Johnstone et al. (1976). In that work, 13 people diagnosed with schizophrenia and observed via computerized axial tomography (CAT) had relatively large brain ventricles by contrast with eight normal subjects. Since that time, CAT scans, magnetic resonance imaging (MRI), positron emission tomography (PET), and postmortem examinations have yielded a great many post hoc comparisons of potentially causal differences between the brains of schizophrenics and the brains of others. There have been comparisons of ventricular size (Andreason et al., 1990), of overall brain size (Marsh et al., 1994), of the sizes of various lobes (Suddath et al., 1990), of the sizes of the basal ganglia and limbic structures (Bogerts et al., 1990), and so forth (see Chua & McKenna, 1995). For the most part, these comparisons failed to produce reliable differences between the brains of people diagnosed with schizophrenia and the brains of people with whom they have been compared.

Ex post facto comparisons sometimes involve more than one comparison variable. When a researcher is interested in several factors that might act in concert to produce differences between clinical groups or subgroups and others, a multivariate (later) technique, known as discriminant analysis, can be used. In discriminant analysis, values for groups of variables are used to form a composite score, called the discriminant function, that discriminates between the comparison groups as much as possible and quantifies the importance of each variable to the optimal discrimination. Discriminant analysis is similar to a multiple regression procedure (later) in which the criterion variable is categorical (i.e., each research subject is assigned to one category or another). For example, Foy and his colleagues (Foy et al., 1984; Foy & Card, 1987) used a discriminant function approach to understanding combat-related posttraumatic stress disorder (PTSD). In the 1987 study, combat veterans who did and did not merit a research diagnosis of PTSD were identified with 88% accuracy via a discriminant function that included eight variables, for example, tension, alcohol abuse, suicidal thoughts, and marital problems. The nature of the discriminant function suggested that the current diagnostic criteria for PTSD are incomplete.

Ex post facto comparisons rarely produce clear-cut differences. Furthermore, even if clear-cut differences were produced, causal interpretations of those differences would be problematic. Ex post facto comparisons are low on the dimension of internal validity because numerous unknown but potentially important factors can be confounded with the variables that are the focus of research. Ex post facto comparisons also fail to reveal the direction or temporal flow of causal relationships among the phenomena of interest. For example, an observed difference between the brains of persons diagnosed with schizophrenia and the brains of others might reflect a history of taking neuroleptic medication that is unique to those with the schizophrenia diagnosis (i.e., the brain difference might be a *result* of the diagnosis).

Beyond the inherent shortcomings of ex post facto comparisons, many are weakened unnecessarily by using diagnostic categories to form comparison groups. For example, a group of people diagnosed with schizophrenia will include individuals whose symptomatic behaviors do not overlap. A comparison group of nonschizophrenics probably will include individuals whose behaviors overlap some of the behaviors seen among the diagnosed schizophrenics. Hence it is unclear what behaviors are explained by results from ex post facto comparisons across diagnostic groups.

In principle, the substantive yield from ex post facto comparisons can be improved by using relatively homogenous comparison groups. Jones et al. (1994), for example, used the relatively narrow Research Diagnostic Criteria (Spitzer, Endicott, & Robins, 1978) to identify a group of 121 schizophrenics whose brains were compared with those of 67 normal volunteers. Lewis (1990), as another example, studied separate subgroups among diagnosed schizophrenics by using the presence/absence of positive symptoms (Crowe, 1985), by using indexes of illness chronicity, and by using classification based on response to treatment. Persons (1986) argued that, in general, ex post facto comparisons should be made across relatively discrete behavioral categories such as the presence or absence of thought disorder. This is a cogent argument because the recommended comparisons focus relatively more attention on the behaviors of subjects and less attention on the behaviors of diagnosticians.

SIMPLE CORRELATION AND SIMPLE REGRESSION

Simple correlation research uses only two variables. For example, mothers and their children might be asked to rate, on a scale of 1 to 7, the degree to which they are frightened by each item on a list of objects or events such as dogs, spiders, dental visits, thunder. Then, a coefficient of correlation can be calculated to quantify the extent to which the mothers and their children provided similar fear-intensity ratings for the various items. A coefficient of +1.00 indicates that the fear ratings of the mothers and their children were exactly the same. A coefficient of −1.00 indicates that the fear ratings of mothers and their children were exactly opposite. A coefficient of 0.00 indicates that no relationship at all exists between the fear ratings of mothers and those of their children. The mathematical model of simple correlation assumes only that the two variables are somehow mutually interdependent; none of the philosophical bases of causality is addressed. A large positive correlation between the fear ratings of mothers and those of their children might prompt research on the extent to which maternal fears influence children's fears, on the extent to which children's fears influence maternal fears, or on the extent to which fears among mothers and their children are shaped by other factors that mothers and their children have in common.

Simple regression research likewise uses only two variables; values for a predictor variable are given and are used to predict values for a criterion variable. Unlike the mathematical model of correlation, the mathematical model of regression assumes that values for the criterion variable in some way depend on values for the predictor variable. Hence, research narratives say that one variable "predicts" or "explains" the other. At the level of calculation, however, simple regression is the same as simple correlation. Hence, words such as prediction and explanation have no important causal implication.

MULTIPLE CORRELATION AND MULTIPLE REGRESSION

Customary descriptions of the experimental method state that the effects of one (independent) variable on another (dependent) variable are studied, and effects on the dependent variable from other factors are ruled out. In brief, the classical method isolates and studies the influence of one variable at a time. Because of advances in mathematical statistics during the past several decades, multivariate techniques now exist that permit the study of effects from many variables simultaneously. Multivariate techniques are often associated with nonexperimental research. However, mathematically equivalent multivariate techniques are available for analyzing complex data sets from experimental work.

The multivariate techniques of multiple correlation and multiple regression are used to describe the strongest linear covariations that exist between two or more variables on one side of an "if-then" relationship and one variable on the other side of the relationship. The mathematical models are simple extensions of the two-variable model just described. In general, multiple correlation and multiple regression are used to form the "best" (i.e., the most highly correlated or most predictive) composites from among the groups of two or more variables and to describe linear relationships between those composites and the single variable on the other side of the "if-then" relationship. For example, McNeal and Berryman (1989) studied the components of dental phobia by describing the "best" predictors of scores for dental fear among self-reports about other fears. Self-reported dental fear scores were used as the criterion variable for a multiple regression procedure in which the composite predictor variable was made up potentially of scores for fear of pain, of being closed in, of mutilation, and of social scrutiny. Among males, the best composite prediction of dental fear scores was afforded by scores for fear of pain and fear of being closed in. Among females, the best composite prediction of dental fear scores was afforded when scores for fear of mutilation were added in. Scores for fear of scrutiny were not useful for predicting dental fear scores among respondents of either sex.

OTHER CORRELATIONAL METHODS

There are several special-purpose mathematical approaches to understanding linear relationships among multiple nonexperimental measures. One of these, discriminant analysis, was discussed earlier. Another is termed canonical correlation. As noted, multiple correlation and multiple regression extend their simple models by identifying groups of two or more variables on one side of an "if-then" relationship that yield the strongest correlation or regression with respect to a single variable on the other side of the "if-then" relationship. The method of canonical correlation extends the simple models still further by finding the strongest linear associations or best possible predictions that exist among composites or groups of variables on both sides of the "if-then" statement.

Another special-purpose approach is called loglinear analysis. Multiple regression is not robust when the measures used violate the assumptions of mathematical statistics (earlier). At the same time, much multivariate research in psychopathology uses categorical assignments that constitute measurement violations (e.g., diagnosis, gender, assignment to one research condition versus another). Loglinear analysis is a method for describing multivariate relationships among large numbers of categorical variables (Marascuilo & Busk, 1987).

Another set of correlational techniques is called factor analysis. Researchers in psychopathology often deal with numerous variables (e.g., scores on tests or test items about personality or psychopathology; measures of symptoms of anxiety, depression, or schizophrenia). Factor analysis is a group of procedures by which a set of variables can be reduced in number to form a smaller set of intercorrelated variables called latent variables or factors. In general, factor analysis simplifies research by reducing the numbers of variables, but often there is the implication that the latent variables (factors) exist apart from the larger set of variables from which they were derived. For example, factor analyses have identified three clusters of schizophrenic symptoms that are relatively independent of one another: (1) hallucinations and delusions; (2) emotional unresponsiveness, reduced capacity for pleasure, poverty of speech, apathy, and social withdrawal; and (3) disorganized and bizarre behavior, thought disorder, and inappropriate emotion (Buchanan & Carpenter, 1994). In turn, these factors have been used frequently to form relatively homogenous groups for ex post facto comparisons of the brains of schizophrenics versus the brains of others (earlier). The results of the comparisons point to different neural substrates for hallucinations and delusions (e.g., Silbersweig et al., 1995) than for negative symptoms such as poverty of speech and social withdrawal (e.g., Tamminga et al., 1992).

Another multivariate technique that has recently become popular is called structural equation modeling, causal modeling, or covariance structure analysis. Structural modeling is a rationo-empirical method that is used to test and compare theories about "causal mechanisms" that might account for patterns of linear covariation in nonexperimental data. In structural modeling, the data are factor analytically derived latent variables or factors. The hypotheses are theoretically derived statements about the ways the latent variables should be related to one another and to the measured variables. The mathematical treatment boils down to regression analysis (earlier) using factor scores (e.g., Bentler, 1985).

Comment

There are methods for multivariate analysis of nonexperimental data sets other than those described earlier (e.g., cluster analysis, multidimensional scaling). There also are many nuances involved in applying the approaches just reviewed. Advances in statistics, the availability of computer software packages, and the availability of personal computers have made correlational research attractive. Perhaps correlational research is too attractive. Very frequently the numbers used in nonexperimental research have dubious or demonstrably weak empirical meaning. Certainly the scientific product of nonexperimental research, even research using the most sophisticated mathematics, can be no better than the empirical quality of the numbers that are analyzed. Therefore, considerable attention should be paid to the research conditions under which the numbers for nonexperimental analyses are acquired. In addition, considerable caution should be used when encountering words such as explanation, prediction, and cause as they are used in the context of multivariate, nonexperimental research. The meanings of such words are quite narrow, and the use of such words can be misleading.

Quasi-Experimental Research

The generic feature of "correlational research" is that the investigator has no influence on the phenomena studied or on any of the factors that might affect the phenomena studied. The identifying feature of experimental research (later) is that, in principle at least, the investigator produces the phenomenon studied and has control over all of the factors that might influence that phenomenon. The term quasi-experimental research denotes a general experimental strategy that falls in between correlational and experimental research; the investigator influences some phenomenon of interest but has incomplete control over the various factors that might influence that phenomenon (Cook & Campbell, 1979).

There are several experimental strategies that deal in various ways with influential factors that cannot be controlled. In general, a causal relationship between two variables is argued when one variable precedes the other in time, when a credible scientific theory of the relationship between the two variables exists, and when alternative explanations of the relationship have been ruled out. As such, the causal appeal rests on weak versions of both conjunction and necessity as characteristics of the "if-then" relationship.

Some interesting quasi-experimental work has been done in connection with information-processing theories that seek to elucidate panic disorder (see McNally, 1990, 1994). The work begins with some theory of the way information processing among panic sufferers differs from information processing among others. The theory is then used to design an experimental task on which panic sufferers and others should perform differently if the theory is correct. Finally the relevant task performances are compared, and the theory is retained, discarded, or modified in the light of results from the comparison.

According to one general theory, panic attacks arise initially from catastrophic misinterpretation of normally benign bodily events (Clark, 1988). Mathews and his colleagues proposed, in addition, that the catastrophic response to benign bodily signals is part of a more general tendency among panic sufferers to allocate attentional resources disproportionately to potential threats. The postulated attentional bias for threat has been studied quasiexperimentally in two ways. Burgess et al. (1981) compared the performances of agoraphobic patients versus normal controls in a dichotic listening task. Subjects were presented with different prose passages to each ear after being instructed to attend to and repeat aloud only one of the passages. Subjects were asked also to detect out-of-context threat words and out-of-context neutral words that were being presented to either ear. By contrast with the normal subjects, agoraphobic subjects detected more threat words than neutral words in the passage they were not repeating. This result can be taken to mean that the agoraphobics displayed an attentional bias for threat information. Several investigators have compared the performances of panic patients versus comparison subjects in quasiexperiments using the Stroop color-naming paradigm. In the Stroop paradigm, words are printed in various colors. Subjects are asked to ignore the word and to name the print color as quickly as possible. The datum of interest is the latency to color naming; relatively long latencies to color naming presumably reflect interference with color-information processing brought about by unwanted processing of word meaning. As an example, Ehlers, Margraf, Davies, and Roth (1988) found that, by contrast with normal subjects, panic patients and nonclinical panickers showed relatively long color-naming latencies for words related to physical threat. Again, the result can be taken to mean that the panic sufferers displayed an attentional bias for threat information.

The term quasi-experimental research is somewhat unfortunate because it implies that the research is not quite experimental or not quite good enough. In fact behavioral investigators who work with actual experiments (later) often fail to control all of the variables that might influence the phenomena studied. Hence, the differences that exist between quasi-experiments and experiments are not so clear-cut as the customary distinction implies. The strength of quasi-experimental design strategy is that it prompts investigators to identify systematically any uncontrolled influences and to take them into account in interpreting data. For example, Campbell and Stanley (1966) listed eight sources of unwanted influence that can compromise internal validity and four sources of unwanted influence that can threaten external validity.

Experimental Research

The paradigm of the experiment begins with producing some phenomenon of interest under carefully controlled conditions of observation. Then, the effects of one or more manipulated ("independent") variables on the phenomenon are studied, and other potential sources of influence on the phenomenon are taken into account in one way or another. Two examples of this sort of work are the production of fear of snakes among monkeys by vicarious fear experiences (Mineka et al., 1984), and attempts to produce delusions, compulsions, and dissociation via hypnotic induction (Hilgard, 1977; Kihlstrom, 1979).

The important aspect of true experiments in psychopathology is that the phenomena of interest are produced by something the experimenter does to subjects; they are not brought to the laboratory by subjects then studied by the experimenter after the fact. In principle, an ability to produce and control psychopathological phenomena demonstrates that the phenomena are understood. Indeed, control over a phenomenon amounts to explanation of that phenomenon from the philosophical vantage point of radical behaviorism (e.g., Skinner, 1953), and control over a phenomenon instantiates the argument (Collingwood, 1940) that production is a viable basis for causal interpretations of "if-then" relationships.

Ethical considerations preclude attempts to produce bona fide psychopathology in humans. Therefore, the experimental psychopathologist must be content with animal models or with subclinical human analogs. In the case of animal models, the fact of phyletic discontinuity imposes inherent limits on the accuracy of rationo-empirical statements made about humans. Similar problems arise with subclinical human models. The human experimental psychopathologist is ethically prohibited from producing the exact phenomena of interest. Therefore, room always exists for questioning the accuracy of experimental approximations.

A related problem is that the production of any phenomenon in an experiment requires considerable knowledge, or at least agreement, about the nature of the phenomenon that is produced. The state of our knowledge about the events of psychopathology augurs against routine agreement about when those events have been reproduced satisfactorily. Finally, experiments often have an artificial character. As noted earlier, the procedures that are necessary to create controlled conditions for observation (internal validity) often have the collateral effect of weakening the real-world accuracy (external validity) of the statements produced by the experiment.

Notwithstanding criticisms such as those, the experimental production of phenomena that are germane to understanding psychopathology is worthwhile. This would be especially true if experimental psychopathologists would fundamentally shift the focus of their efforts. Many criticisms of experimental psychopathology boil down to allegations of suspect external validity with respect to events in naturalistic and clinical settings. The traditional response to concern over external invalidity has been to match experimental events to clinical events as carefully as feasible (Abramson & Seligman, 1977). Problematically, the matching strategy runs aground on several of the issues described earlier (e.g., clinic matching requires knowledgeable agreement about the events being matched). An alternative to the clinic matching approach is to articulate experimental purposes that circumvent concern over external validity. One way to circumvent the issue of external validity is to place experimental psychopathology in the scientific context of discovery, not of scientific confirmation (Marx, 1963). When experimental work is placed explicitly in the scientific context of discovery, the rationo-empirical statements produced by the work are not judged in terms of external validity. Rather, the statements are judged in terms of whether they prompt confirmatory research that is relatively high on the dimension of external validity, for example, quasi-experimental research using clinical patients and settings. Another way to circumvent the problematic external validity of experimentally produced statements is to orient experimentation explicitly toward theoretical hypothesis testing. When experimental work is used to test theory, the statements produced are judged in terms of theoretical validity, not external validity. A given theory can be tested with experiments that are high on the dimension of internal validity and with quasi-experiments that are high on the dimension of external validity. In this way, theories, experiments, quasi-experiments, and other methods can be interlaced to produce rationo-empirical statements that are based on controlled and externally valid research without attempting to meet the ill-conceived requirement of achieving internal validity and external validity simultaneously.

RESEARCH ON INTERVENTION

The remainder of this narrative is about research on psychological intervention. Various approaches to research are discussed: simple case studies, intrasubject replication experiments, cognitive behavior therapy outcome experiments, behavior therapy analogue experiments, comparative psychotherapy outcome experiments, psychotherapy process research, and meta-analytic methods.

The Case Study Method

The case study has always been a basic and important aspect of research on intervention. During the past century, intervention case studies have evolved from little more than short stories to legitimate pieces of research. In the contemporary case report, considerable detail is provided about how the presenting problem was measured, about how the treatment was conducted, and about how any beneficial changes were documented. Of course, there are differences of opinion about the desiderata of measurement and reporting. An illustrative case of a young man was reported by Zeitlin and Polivy (1995). One class of presenting symptoms was obsessional thinking about being bad, about contributing to the deaths of his parents, and about disappointing his foster parents. Another class of presenting symptoms was coprophagia, ingestion of (his own) feces that, in this case, was experienced as anxiety reducing. Treatment for the obsessional thinking entailed an approach known as "imaginal flooding." In brief, imaginal flooding took the form of prolonged imagining and orally depicting five anxiety-provoking scenes or vignettes in which he had disappointed his foster parents, had caused the suicide of his natural father, etc. The scenes were imagined in order of increasing aversiveness, and each was repeated and prolonged until the act of imagining it was not associated with anxious discomfort. Treatment for coprophagia entailed an approach known as "flooding plus response prevention" (see Steketee & Foa, 1985). In brief, various cues for coprophagic urges were placed prominently in the patient's day-to-day environment, and he was instructed to confront the cues and then resist their associated urges. The effects of treatment were assessed solely via the patient's self-reports; through a one-year telephone follow-up, obsessional thinking about natural and foster parents had subsided along with coprophagic urges and actions.

Clearly, case studies such as the one described fall very low on the dimension of internal validity. Many unknown factors can coincide with intervention and influence measures of the presumed effects of intervention. Examples of such factors are cycles in the targeted problem and the effects of repeated evaluation on measures of the targeted problem. Case studies are also low on the dimension of external validity because they provide no data about interventions applied by other therapists, interventions applied to other patients, etc. As with the etiologic case study, therefore, intervention case studies belong in the scientific context of discovery. Case studies suggest therapeutic possibilities that must be confirmed by more rigorous research before their implications are accepted.

Intrasubject Replication Methodology

Intrasubject replication methodology (sometimes called single-subject methodology) is a general approach to psychological science (Johnston & Pennypacker, 1993). It is based on the cogent argument that most behavioral research methods are designed to afford rationo-empirical statements about populations or population samples, not statements about the individuals who comprise those populations and samples. It is intended to be a corrective methodology that permits statements about individuals.

Intrasubject replication methodology is well-suited to the intervention case study (Hersen & Barlow, 1976) and has been used routinely for a quarter century by workers in the tradition known as behavior therapy. In general, intrasubject replication research seeks to demonstrate repeated changes in behavior that are meaningfully related to changes in the subject's environment (or to changes in some other variable such as the initiation of treatment). Repeated changes in behavior that track repeated changes in the environment are used to argue that the environmental changes produced the behavioral changes, that is, the behavioral change was not produced by some unknown and temporally coincident factor. The reversal experiment exemplifies one common intrasubject replication research strategy. In a reversal experiment, some behavioral influence condition is introduced after a period of recording the behavior of interest. Then, the influence condition is withdrawn and later reintroduced while the behavior of interest is still monitored. The argument that the influence condition is responsible for the behavioral change is supported when behavioral change tracks the introduction, withdrawal, and reintroduction of the condition. O'Brien, Bugle, and Azrin (1972), for example, taught and motivated a severely retarded six-year old to eat with appropriate utensils. Correct and incorrect eating behaviors were recorded reliably from samples taken during a 66-meal sequence of eight phases in which one or both of two interventions were alternated with four phases of no intervention. Graphic display of percent-correct eating behaviors across the sequence of phases showed clearly that one of the two interventions produced correct eating, whereas the other intervention had no effect.

The multiple baselines across behaviors experiment exemplifies another common intrasubject replication research strategy. A multiple baselines across behaviors experiment begins with simultaneous recording of three or more behaviors through time. As the experiment unfolds, each behavior is subject to a behavioral influence condition sequentially while simultaneous recording of all behaviors continues. The argument that the influence condition is responsible for the behavioral change is supported when behavioral change tracks the sequential introduction of the condition. Mizes (1985), for example, used multiple baselines across behaviors (abdominal tensing, leg raising, and discharge-criterion behaviors such as walking down a hallway) to study behavioral influence over a bedridden patient diagnosed with conversion disorder. Behavioral influence was demonstrated when the frequency of each class of behaviors was increased in turn by reward in the form of contingent parental visits.

Each intrasubject replication strategy has strengths and weaknesses. The intrasubject reversal strategy, for example, can be used only when the effects of treatment are transient. Permanent or long-lasting treatment effects preclude a return of behavior to untreated levels when treatment is withdrawn and forestall the opportunity to demonstrate the controlling effects of reinstituted treatment. Intrasubject multiple baselines experiments can be used to evaluate permanent or long-lasting interventions, but they require that the three or more target behaviors be relatively independent. If the target behaviors covary too closely, then successful intervention with one will also influence the others and will preclude opportunities to demonstrate the orderly sequence of intervention/behavioral change correspondences that is required by the logic of the experimental strategy.

Cognitive Behavior Therapy Outcome Research

Cognitive behavior therapy often involves using fairly well-defined intervention procedures or sets of procedural "packages" to influence fairly well-defined problem behaviors. For example, procedures such as guided exposure (Marks, 1981) and interoceptive exposure

(Barlow, Craske, Cerny, & Klosko, 1989) are used to influence measures of agoraphobia and panic. In the most simple cognitive behavior therapy outcome experiment, one group of patients is assessed and treated and another group of patients is assessed simultaneously but not treated. Differences in the simultaneously assessed target behaviors of treated versus untreated participants are construed as reflecting influence from some aspect(s) of the experimental treatment and/or treatment context. A simple treatment versus no-treatment experiment can demonstrate the effectiveness of an intervention-in-context provided that the experimental treatment and context are faithful representations of clinical treatments and contexts and that the experimental measures are externally valid indexes of adaptively significant naturalistic performances. This is so because data from patients who are assessed but untreated afford means of taking into account potential confounds such as cycles in the target behaviors and effects of assessment procedures on assessment results. However, treatment versus no-treatment comparisons do not permit conclusions about the specific effects of the treatments used because of the potential for effects from contexts per se. Therefore, research strategies have evolved to separate the effects of treatments from the effects of the clinical contexts in which treatments are imbedded.

One historically prominent strategy for distinguishing between treatment effects and context effects is the use of the "psychological placebo" (Thorne, 1950). In experiments that use a psychological placebo, one (control) group of patients is treated with a set of procedures that theoretically should not influence measures of the target behavior of interest, and another (experimental) group of patients receives the experimental treatment. In principle, data from patients exposed to the placebo quantify the effects of context; values that represent context effects are subtracted from values that represent overall treatment effects to yield net scores that quantify the effects of treatment procedures per se. In the first prominent use of the psychological placebo, Paul (1966) used subjects who suffered from fear of public speaking to compare the effects of a treatment known as systematic desensitization (Wolpe, 1958) to the effects of psychotherapy and the effects of a placebo regimen called pseudodesensitization.

In practice, the psychological placebo strategy was problematic (see Kazdin & Wilcoxon, 1976). Therefore, it was replaced with other approaches to distinguishing between treatment effects and context effects. The main contemporary strategy is, simply, to compare the effects of two or more treatments that are provided in the same context. In this way the effects of context presumably are equated and any differences between treatment effects are, inferentially, due to the differing procedures. Contemporary research also provides comparative data acquired from patients who are simultaneously assessed but temporarily untreated (e.g., those on a waiting list for treatment).

Behavior therapy outcome experiments have been used to evaluate the effects of competing treatments and also to evaluate the effects of combined treatments. For example, the effects of behavioral and cognitive treatments alone and in combination on panic disorder (Kleiner, Marshall, & Spivack, 1987) and social phobia (Mattick, Peters, & Clarke, 1989) have been described experimentally as have the separate and combined effects of behavioral and pharmacological approaches to treating specific phobia (Marshall & Segal, 1986). When researchers wish to compare several treatments across multiple measures of outcome, multivariate statistics of the type described earlier are used, for example, multivariate analysis of variance.

Behavior Therapy Analog Research

Because of ethical constraints on dealing with patients and practical limitations associated with research in clinical settings, cognitive behavior therapy outcome research is often low on the dimension of internal validity. Therefore, a need exists for research that uses subjects other than patients and takes place in contexts other than clinics. The term "analog research" is used to refer to such efforts. Some analog research uses animal subjects. For example, Delprato (1973) used aversively conditioned rats to evaluate the effects of an experimental "treatment" that was analogous to a clinical treatment known as systematic desensitization (Wolpe, 1958). Similarly, Baum and his colleagues used aversively conditioned rats to study the effects of experimental treatments that mirror a clinical approach known as in vivo flooding (see Thyer, Baum, & Reid, 1988).

Most behavior therapy analog research has used nonclinical human subjects, persons who are not patients but who are recruited for research by media solicitations or in some other way. For example, Lang and Lazovik (1963) used snake-fearful college students to evaluate the effects of an experimental version of Wolpe's (1958) systematic desensitization. A major potential benefit of behavior therapy analog research is enhanced internal validity relative to clinic-based investigations. This is so because analog researchers have relatively more freedom to control the experimental events to which subjects are exposed, that is, subjects in analog experiments can be more readily left untreated or exposed to psychological placebos (earlier), and they can be treated with standardized materials, etc. The inherent weakness in behavior therapy analog research is in external validity. This is so by definition; interventions, subjects, and intervention targets are purposeful approximations of treatments, patients, and behavioral phenomena in the clinic.

Much controversy has surrounded the value of behavior therapy analog research. Mainly, the controversy has been about external validity. Bernstein and Paul (1971) argued incorrectly that analog investigations must be high on the dimension of external validity to be worthwhile. At the same time, many of the early analog researchers made inaccurate statements about the clinical implications of empirical generalizations based on their findings. Most of the controversy was unnecessary. The proper role of analog behavior therapy research is that of producing empirical generalizations that are high on the dimension of internal validity and, often, on the dimension of theoretical validity. These validity goals can be accomplished by analog methods. In turn, internally valid analog research and externally valid clinical outcome research should play complementary roles in building the body of knowledge about how and when behavior therapy works.

Comparative Psychotherapy Outcome Research

Comparative psychotherapy outcome research pits psychotherapies against one another to decide which therapies are best. The work proceeds by assessing patients' problems, randomly assigning patients to treatment conditions, conducting somewhat standardized versions of the different treatments, and reassessing patients' problems to afford comparisons of therapeutic change. In principle, comparative psychotherapy outcome research is straightforward and has much to recommend it as a means of choosing psychotherapeutic approaches. This is particularly true given contemporary advances in methodology (e.g., the availability of treatment manuals that regularize research psychotherapies). Comparative psychotherapy outcome research also provides opportunities to study the psychotherapy process (later) and to develop theory in the psychotherapy arena.

In practice, however, there are significant reasons to question the ultimate value of comparative psychotherapy outcome research. There are several hundred versions of "psychotherapy" that stand as candidates for comparative-outcome evaluation. Each evaluative research program would be expensive and time-consuming. The effects of various therapies on measures of outcome often are too small to permit actuarial tests based on feasible numbers of patients to reveal actual differences between them (Kazdin & Bass, 1989). The number of potential confounds across compared treatments is very large, sufficiently large to raise questions about the degree to which random assignment of feasible numbers of patients' controls for all of them (Hsu, 1989). Furthermore, comparative psychotherapy outcome research does not use straightforward treatment procedures and does not target clear-cut outcome measures (such as the discrete target behaviors used in cognitive behavior therapy research). Rather, manualized treatments are subject to idiosyncratic distortions, and dependent variables take the forms of patient and therapist ratings of improvement, of changes in psychometric measures of complex constructs such as self-esteem, etc. In general, therefore, comparative psychotherapy outcome research is more problematic than research on the effects of cognitive behavior therapy (see Kazdin, 1986). Not surprisingly, the empirical yield from psychotherapy investigations has not been comparable to that produced by research (earlier) in the behavior therapy tradition.

Meta-Analysis

For reasons such as those just mentioned, individual psychotherapy outcome experiments do not suffice to determine how well a particular intervention works or how it compares with competing interventions. Rather, knowledge about the comparative efficacy of an intervention emerges slowly through the accumulation of information from multiple comparative-outcome experiments involving different therapists, different patients, different settings, and different outcome measures, etc. The term meta-analysis refers to a set of statistical methods through which heterogeneous information from diverse procedural sources can be standardized and pooled for comparison purposes. In the psychotherapy outcome arena, meta-analysis has been used typically to compare the magnitudes of therapeutic benefits, termed effect sizes, that are associated with different therapy approaches (e.g., Smith, Glass, & Miller, 1980). Meta-analysis has also been used to compare psychological and medical interventions. For example, Gould et al. (1997) undertook a meta-analysis of results from cognitive-behavioral versus pharmacological treatments for social phobia. The results from 24 studies involving 1079 patients showed an average treatment-effect size of .74 for cognitive behavioral treatment and an average treatment-effect size of .62 for pharmacotherapy. These values were significantly different from zero and not significantly different from each other. The authors recommended group-administered cognitive-behavioral treatment based on cost-effectiveness projections.

Psychotherapy Process Research

Psychotherapy process research seeks to explain how psychotherapy works by identifying the events or other aspects of psychotherapy sessions that are important and by describing how the identified events affect patients beneficially (Mahrer & Nadler, 1986). Some researchers have defined as important those psychotherapeutic events that presumably are related to improvement on treatment-outcome criteria (Orlinsky & Howard, 1978). Other researchers have identified as important those psychotherapeutic events that are demonstrably related to positive evaluations of therapy sessions by patients and/or therapists (e.g., Stiles, 1980). Still others have deemed important those psychotherapeutic events that comport well with some theory of therapeutic practice (e.g., Greenberg, 1986) or with some theory about the psychological determinants of the patient's problems. In the latter case, for example, if excessive self-criticism is construed theoretically as a determinant of the patient's problem, then events that signal reduced self-criticism are defined as important (Rice & Greenberg, 1984).

Most research on the important events in psychotherapy has used a "frequency approach" (Russell & Trull, 1986) to describe patient and therapist vocalizations during therapy sessions. The work begins by developing language-category systems and coding strategies (Russell & Stiles, 1979). Content-category systems, for example, classify vocalizations by their denotative, connotative, referential, or metaphorical meanings (e.g., death, mother, sexual anxiety, dependence). Given a language-category system and a coding strategy, work with the frequency approach continues by recording the frequencies with which therapists and/ or patients exhibit the coded language variables during and across psychotherapy sessions.

At best, the frequency approach provides tallies of the frequencies with which various classes of vocalizations occur during psychotherapy sessions. The frequency approach tells investigators nothing about the way the patient's vocalizations influence the therapist's vocalizations or vice versa. That is a lethal shortcoming because moment-to-moment reciprocal influences between patients and therapists presumably are at the core of psychotherapy.

Some psychotherapy process researchers have attempted to redress weaknesses in the frequency approach by using sequential analysis methods (Sackett, 1979) to describe serial dependencies between the vocalizations of therapists and patients. Sequential analysis in psychotherapy process research begins with the derivation of language categories such as those used in the frequency approach (before). Then, simultaneous times series descriptions (language category sequences) of the vocalizations of the patient and therapist, as their interactions unfold through time, are examined for serial dependencies between the two sets of time series variables. For example, a serial dependency between the language of a patient and the language of a therapist exists if changes in the patient's voice-quality categorization occurs a disproportionately high number of times immediately after a specific category of a therapist's vocalization, for example, interpretation.

Time series descriptions of the psychotherapy process are limited in several ways. As one example, the coding systems for patient and therapist behaviors necessarily have a preliminary character; time series work seeks to elucidate the psychotherapy process, but something must be known already about the psychotherapy process to develop the codes for time-series description. As a second example, time-series description is ordinarily restricted to dependencies between events in one time-series variable and the immediately preceding events in the other. Hence temporally delayed influence is missed, and the flow through time of psychotherapeutic transactions is chopped into bits and pieces. In principle, a method known as lagged sequential analysis can be used to identify dependencies between events in one time series variable and events in another that are further back in time than the immediately preceding one, for example, a patient's response to something the therapist said five minutes earlier. However, lagged sequential analysis does not solve the problem of describing multielement sequences as psychotherapy proceeds through time (Russell & Trull, 1986).

Summary

Scientific research produces rationo-empirical statements about phenomena of interest. The rationo-empirical statements of interest to psychopathologists are descriptions and explanations of behaviors that manifest or reflect psychopathology. The statements are judged in terms of four types of validity: internal, external, theoretical, and statistical validity. The various types of validity are rarely if ever achieved simultaneously; rather, overall validity in a scientific arena evolves out of the methodological complementarity that inheres in diverse research methods.

The arenas of etiology and intervention were chosen to characterize research in psychopathology. Research on etiology takes the forms of case studies, nonexperimental research, quasi-experimental research, and actual experiments. A type of nonexperimental research known as the ex post facto comparison is prevalent. It is an inherently weak method that often is compromised further by the use of diagnostic categories to form groups for ex post facto comparisons.

Psychological research on intervention takes the forms of case studies, intrasubject replication experiments, cognitive behavior therapy outcome research, behavior therapy analog research, comparative psychotherapy outcome research, meta-analyses, and psychotherapy process research. Behavior therapy analog research can achieve strong internal validity; cognitive behavior therapy outcome research can approach acceptable external validity. The yields from psychotherapy process research and comparative psychotherapy outcome research have been unimpressive.

REFERENCES

Abramson, L. Y., & Seligman, M. E. P. (1977). Modeling psychopathology in the laboratory: History and rationale. In J. P. Maser & M. E. P. Seligman (Eds.), *Psychopathology: Experimental models* (pp. 1–26). San Francisco: Freeman.

Andreason, N. C., Swayze, V. W., Flaum, M., et al. (1990). Ventricular enlargement in schizophrenia evaluated with computed tomographic scanning. *Archives of General Psychiatry, 47,* 1008–1115.

Attneave, F. (1959). *Applications of information theory to psychology: A summary of basic concepts, methods, and results.* New York: Holt, Rinehart & Winston.

Barlow, D. H., Craske, M. G., Cerny, J. A., & Klosko, J. S. (1989). Behavioral treatment of panic disorder. *Behavior Therapy, 20,* 261–282.

Bentler, P. (1985). *Theory and implementation of EQS: A structural equation program.* Los Angeles: BMDP Statistical Software.

Bernstein, D. A., & Paul, G. L. (1971). Some comments on therapy analogue research with small animal "phobias." *Journal of Behavior Therapy and Experimental Psychiatry, 2,* 225–237.

Bleuler, E. (1911). *Dementia praecox: oder gruppe der schizophrenien.* In Aschaffenburg Handbuch der Psychiatrie, Spezieller Teil 4., Abt: I, Vienna: F. Deuticke.

Bogerts, B., Falkai, P., Haupts, M., Greve, B., Ernst, S., Tapernon-Franz, U., & Heinmann, U. (1990). Post-mortem volume measurements of limbic system and basal ganglia structures in chronic schizophrenics. *Schizophrenia Research, 3,* 295–301.

Breuer, J., & Freud, S. (1895). *Studien uber hysterie.* Vienna: Franz Deuticke.

Buchanan, R. W., & Carpenter, W. T., Jr., (1994). Domains of psychopathology: An approach to the reduction of heterogeneity in schizophrenia. *Journal of Nervous and Mental Disease, 182,* 193–204.

Bunge, M. (1963). *Causality: The place of the causal principle in modern science.* Cleveland, OH: World.

Burgess, I. S., Jones, L. M., Robertson, S. A., Radcliffe, W. N., & Emerson, E. (1981). The degree of control exerted by phobic and non-phobic verbal stimuli over the recognition behaviour of phobia and non-phobic subjects. *Behaviour Research and Therapy, 19,* 233–243.

Campbell, D. T., & Stanley, J. C. (1966). *Experimental and quasi-experimental designs for research.* Chicago: Rand McNally.

Chua, S. E., & McKenna P. J. (1995). Schizophrenia—a brain disease? A critical review of structural and functional cerebral abnormality in the disorder. *British Journal of Psychiatry, 166,* 563–582.

Clark, D. M. (1988). A cognitive model of panic attacks. In S. Rachman & J. D. Maser (Eds.), *Panic: Psychological perspectives* (pp. 71–89). Hillsdale, NJ: Erlbaum.

Collingwood, R. G. (1940). *An essay on metaphysics.* Oxford, England: Clarendon Press.

Cook, T. D., & Campell, D. T. (1979). *Quasi experimentation: Design and analysis issues for field settings.* Chicago: Rand McNally.

Crow, T. J. (1985). The two syndrome concept: Origins and current status. *Schizophrenia Bulletin, 11,* 471–486.

Delprato, D. J. (1973). An animal analogue to systematic desensitization and elimination of avoidance. *Behaviour Research and Therapy, 11*, 49–55.

Ehlers, A., Margraf, J., Davies, S. & Roth, W. T. (1988). Selective processing of threat cues in subjects with panic attacks. *Cognition and Emotion, 2*, 201–219.

Foy, D. W., & Card, J. J. (1987). Combat-related posttraumatic stress disorder etiology: Replicated findings in a national sample of Vietnam-era men. *Journal of Clinical Psychology, 43*, 28–31.

Foy, D. W., Sipprelle, R. C., Rueger, D. B., & Carroll, E. M. (1984). Etiology of post-traumatic stress disorder in Vietnam veterans: Analysis of premilitary, military, and combat exposure influences. *Journal of Consulting and Clinical Psychology, 52*, 79–87.

Freud, S. (1909). Analysis of a phobia in a five-year-old boy. In *Collected works of Sigmund Freud*, Vol. 10. London: Hogarth, 1956.

Gorenstein, E. E., & Newman, J. P. (1980). Disinhibitory psychopathology: A new perspective and a model for research. *Psychological Review, 87*, 305–315.

Gottesman, I. I. (1991). *Schizophrenia genesis: The origins of madness*. New York: Freeman.

Gould, R. A., Buckminster, S., Pollack, H. H., Otto, M. W., & Yap, L. (1997). Cognitive-behavioral and pharmacological treatment for social phobia: A meta-analysis. *Clinical Psychology: Science and Practice, 4*, 291–306.

Greenberg, L. (1986). Change process research. *Journal of Consulting and Clinical Psychology, 54*, 4–9.

Hempel, C. G., & Oppenheim, P. (1948). Studies in the logic of explanation. *Philosophy of Science, 15*, 135–175.

Hersen, M., & Barlow, D. H. (1976). *Single-case experimental designs: Strategies for studying behavior change*. New York: Pergamon.

Hilgard, E. H. (1977). *Divided consciousness: Multiple controls in human thought and action*. New York: Wiley-Interscience.

Hsu, L. M. (1989). Random sampling, randomization, and equivalence of contrasted groups in psychotherapy outcome research. *Journal of Consulting and Clinical Psychology, 57*, 131–137.

Hume, D. (1978). *A treatise of human nature*. Oxford, England: Oxford University Press (original work published in 1739).

Johnston, J. M., & Pennypacker, H. (1993). *Strategies and tactics of behavioral research*, 2nd ed. Hillsdale, NJ: Erlbaum.

Johnstone, E. C., Crow, T. J., Frith, C. D., Husband, J., & Kreel, L. (1976). Cerebral ventricular size and cognitive impairment in chronic schizophrenia. *Lancet, ii*, 924–926.

Jones, P. B., Harvey, I., Lewis, S. W., Toone, B. K., Van Os, J., Williams, M., & Murray, R. M. (1994). Cerebral ventricle dimensions as risk factors for schizophrenia and affective psychosis. *Psychological Medicine, 24*, 995–1011.

Kazdin, A. E. (1986). Comparative outcome studies of psychotherapy: Methodological issues and strategies. *Journal of Consulting and Clinical Psychology, 54*, 95–105.

Kazdin, A. E., & Bass, D. (1989). Power to detect differences between alternative treatments in comparative psychotherapy outcome research. *Journal of Consulting and Clinical Psychology, 57*, 138–147.

Kazdin, A. E., & Wilcoxon, L. A. (1976). Systematic desensitization and nonspecific treatment effects: A methodological evaluation. *Psychological Bulletin, 83*, 729–758.

Kearney, H. (1971). *Science and change*. New York: McGraw-Hill.

Kety, S. (1988). Schizophrenic illness in the families of schizophrenic adoptees: Findings from the Danish national sample. *Schizophrenia Bulletin, 14*, 217–222.

Kety, S., Rosenthal, D., Wender, P. H., Schulsinger, F., & Jacobsen, B. (1978). The biologic and adoptive families of adopted individuals who become schizophrenic: Prevalence of mental illness and other characteristics. In L. C. Wynn, R. L. Cromwell, & S. Matysse (Eds.), *The nature of schizophrenia: New approaches to research and treatment*. New York: Wiley.

Kihlstrom, J. F. (1979). Hypnosis and psychopathology: Retrospect and prospect. *Journal of Abnormal Psychology, 88*, 459–473.

Kleiner, L., Marshall, W. L., & Spevack, M. (1987). Training in problem solving and exposure treatment for agoraphobics with panic attacks. *Journal of Anxiety Disorders, 1*, 219–238.

Lang, P. J., & Lazovik, A. D. (1963). Experimental desensitization of a phobia. *Journal of Abnormal and Social Psychology, 66*, 519–525.

Lewis, S. W. (1990). Computerized tomography in schizophrenia 15 years on. *British Journal of Psychiatry, 157*, 16–24.

Mahrer, A. R., & Nadler, W. P. (1986). Good moments in psychotherapy: A preliminary review, a list, and some promising research avenues. *Journal of Consulting and Clinical Psychology, 54*, 10–15.

Marascuilo, L. A., & Busk, P. L. (1987). Loglinear analysis: A way to study main effects and interactions for multidimensional contingency tables with categorical data. *Journal of Counseling Psychology, 34*, 433–455.

Marks, I. M. (1981). *Cure and care of neurosis: Theory and practice of behavioral psychotherapy*. New York: Wiley.

Marsh, I., Suddath, R. I., Higgins, N., & Weinberger, D. R. (1994). Medial temporal lobe structures in schizophrenia: Relationship of size to duration of illness. *Schizophrenia Research, 11*, 225–238.

Marshall, W. L., & Segal, Z. (1986). Phobias and anxiety. In M. Hersen (Ed.), *Pharmacological and behavioral treatment: An integrative approach* (pp. 260–288). New York: Wiley.

Marx, M. H. (1963). *Theories in contemporary psychology*. New York: Macmillan.

Mattick, R. P., Peters, L., & Clarke, J. C. (1989). Exposure and cognitive restructuring for social phobia: A controlled study. *Behavior Therapy, 20*, 3–23.

McNally, R. J. (1990). Psychological approaches to panic disorder: A review. *Psychological Bulletin, 108*, 403–419.

McNally, R. J. (1994). *Panic disorder: A critical analysis*. New York: Guilford.

McNeal, D. W., & Berryman, M. L. (1989). Components of dental fear in adults? *Behaviour Research and Therapy, 27*, 233–236.

Mineka, S., Davidson, M., Cook, M., & Keir, R. (1984). Observational conditioning of snake fear in rhesus monkeys. *Journal of Abnormal Psychology, 93*, 355–372.

Mizes, J. S. (1985). The use of contingent reinforcement in the treatment of a conversion disorder. *Journal of Behavior Therapy and Experimental Psychiatry, 16*, 341–346.

O' Brien, F., Bugle, C., & Azrin, N. H. (1972). Training and maintaining a retarded child's proper eating. *Journal of Applied Behavior Analysis, 5*, 67–72.

Orlinsky, D. E., & Howard, K. I. (1978). The relation of process to outcome in psychotherapy. In S. L. Garfield & A. E. Bergin (Eds.), *Handbook of psychotherapy and behavior change* (pp. 283–329). New York: Wiley.

Parnas, J., Cannon, T. D., Jacobsen, B., Schulsinger, H., Schulsinger, F., & Mednick, S. S. (1993). Lifetime DSM-III-R diagnostic outcomes in the offspring of schizophrenic mothers. *Archives of General Psychiatry, 50*, 707–714.

Paul, G. L. (1966). *Insight vs. desensitization in psychotherapy*. Stanford, CA: Stanford University Press.

Persons, J. (1986). The advantages of studying psychological phenomena rather than psychiatric diagnosis. *American Psychologist, 41*, 1252–1260.

Popper, K. R. (1959). *The logic of scientific discovery*. London: Hutchinson.

Rice, L. N., & Greenberg, L. S. (1984). The new research paradigm. In L. N. Rice & L. S. Greenberg (Eds.), *Patterns of change: Intensive analysis of psychotherapy process* (pp. 7–25). New York: Guilford.

Rosenthal, D. (Ed.) (1963). *The Genain quadruplets*. New York: Basic Books.

Russell, R. L., & Stiles, W. B. (1979). Categories for classifying language in psychotherapy. *Psychological Bulletin, 86*, 404–419.

Russell, R. L., & Trull, T. J. (1986). Sequential analysis of language variables in psychotherapy process. *Journal of Consulting and Clinical Psychology, 54*, 16–21.

Sackett, G. P. (1979). The lag sequential analysis of contingency and cyclicity in behavioral interaction. In J. D. Osofsky (Ed.), *Handbook of infant development* (pp. 623–649). New York: Wiley.

Silbersweig, D. A., Stern, E., Frith, C. D., Cahill, C., Holmes, A., Grootoonk, S., Seaward, J., McKenna, P., Chua, S. E., Schnorr, L., Jones, T., & Frackowiak, R. S. J. (1995). A functional neuroanatomy of hallucinations in schizophrenia. *Nature, 378*, 176–179.

Skinner, B. F. (1953). *Science and human behavior*. New York: Macmillan.

Smith, M. L., Glass, G. V., & Miller, T. I. (1980). *The benefits of psychotherapy*. Baltimore: Johns Hopkins University Press.

Spitzer, R. L., Endicott, J., & Robins, E. (1978). *Research diagnostic criteria for a selected group of functional disorders*. New York: Biometric Research, New York State Psychiatric Institute.

Staats, A. W. (1991). Unified positivism and unification psychology: Fad or new field? *American Psychologist, 46*, 899–912.

Steketee, G., & Foa, E. B. (1985). Obsessive–compulsive disorder. In D. H. Barlow (Ed.), *Clinical handbook of psychological disorders* (pp. 69–144). New York: Guilford.

Stiles, W. B. (1980). Measurement of the impact of psychotherapy sessions. *Journal of Consulting and Clinical Psychology, 48*, 176–185.

Suddath, R. L., Christison, G. W., Torrey, E. F., et al. (1990). Anatomical abnormalities in the brains of monozygotic twins discordant for schizophrenia. *New England Journal of Medicine, 322*, 789–794.

Tamminga, C. A., Thaker, G. K., Buchanan, R. W., Kirckpatrick, B., Carpenter, W. T., Jr., & Chase, T. (1992). Limbic system abnormalities identified in schizophrenia using positron emission tomography with fluorodeoxyglucose and neocortical alterations with the deficit syndrome. *Archives of General Psychiatry, 49*, 522–530.

Thorne, F. C. (1950). Rules of evidence in the evaluation of the effect of psychotherapy. *Journal of Clinical Psychology, 8*, 38–41.

Thyer, B. A., Baum, M., & Reid, L. D. (1988). Exposure techniques in the reduction of fear: A comparative review of the procedure in animals and humans. *Advances in Behaviour Research and Therapy, 10*, 105–127.

Turner, M. B. (1967). *Philosophy and the science of behavior*. New York: Appleton-Century-Crofts.

Westfall, R. S. (1977). *The construction of modern science*. Cambridge, England: Cambridge University Press.

White, P. A. (1990). Ideas about causation in philosophy and psychology. *Psychological Bulletin, 108*, 3–18.

Wolpe, J. (1958). *Psychotherapy by reciprocal inhibition*. Stanford, CA: Stanford University Press.

Wolpe, J., & Rachman, S. (1960). Psychoanalytic "evidence," a critique based on Freud's case of Little Hans. *Journal of Nervous and Mental Disease, 131*, 135–147.

Zeitlin, S. B., & Polivy, J. (1995). Coprophagia as a manifestation of obsessive–compulsive disorder: A case report. *Journal of Behavior Therapy and Experimental Psychiatry, 26*, 57–64.

4

Psychoanalytic Model

Howard D. Lerner and Joshua Ehrlich

Introduction

Psychoanalysis is a comprehensive theory of personality. It provides rich conceptual frameworks for understanding personality development through the life cycle, the complex workings of the human mind, and psychopathology. Psychoanalysis is also a procedure: a method of studying the mind and a form of psychotherapy. In this chapter we explore psychoanalysis both as a theory of personality and as a psychological treatment.

Writing and practicing between 1890 and 1939, Sigmund Freud, the founder of psychoanalysis, offered people a revolutionary way to view themselves. He suggested that mental life is vastly more complex than psychologists previously had assumed. His illumination of unconscious thought processes dramatically expanded the depth and range of psychology and altered our understanding of human nature. Of all disciplines within psychology, only psychoanalysis deals with the full range of human experience: loss, lust, guilt, sadism, bodily sensation, self-destructiveness, unconscious and conscious fantasy, dreams, mortality, the influence of childhood experience, and humor.

The impact of psychoanalysis on popular thought in the past century has been immense. It has influenced theories and values in childrearing, education, sexuality, human relationships, the arts, and other domains of human experience. Terms such as *libido*, *identification*, and *defense*, which originated with Freud, are now part of everyday language.

Psychoanalysis continues to be associated with Freud in many people's minds, but it has, in fact, evolved enormously in the sixty years since Freud's death. For instance, research in infant and child development has influenced psychoanalytic thinking profoundly. New insights into the early role of the mother and father have altered theory and practice. Pointed critiques of Freud's understanding of female development have led to revisions in theory and treatment. Brilliant clinicians and theorists such as Melanie Klein, Anna Freud, and, more recently, Heinz Kohut and Otto Kernberg have revised and expanded psychoanalytic theory and influenced clinical practice.

Howard D. Lerner and Joshua Ehrlich • Department of Psychiatry, University of Michigan, Ann Arbor, Michigan 48104. *Current address for Howard D. Lerner*: Ann Arbor, Michigan 48104

Advanced Abnormal Psychology, Second Edition, edited by Hersen and Van Hasselt. Kluwer Academic/Plenum Publishers, New York, 2001.

In recent decades, psychoanalysts, confronted by criticism both from inside and outside psychoanalysis, have subjected themselves to increasing self-scrutiny in an effort to find a more meaningful role in the communities in which they live and practice. As one important example, confronted with critiques of its tendency to pathologize homosexuality, psycho-analysts have begun to revise traditional theories of psychosexual development to be more flexible and inclusive. Psychoanalysts also have focused increasing attention on the psycho-logical impact of immigration (Akthar, 1995) and on the role of race in psychotherapy (Holmes, 1992). Parallel with these developments, psychoanalytic institutes, the training ground for psychoanalysts, have become more broad-based. In America, where psycho-analysis was once almost exclusively the domain of physicians, psychoanalytic institutes now offer training opportunities for psychologists, social workers, academicians, and others.

In a parallel development, psychoanalysts have increasingly sought bridges to other disciplines within psychology and psychiatry. For instance, Stern (1985) offered a rich integra-tion of infant research and psychoanalysis. Shevrin and his colleagues (1996) offered a compelling bridge between psychoanalysis, neurophysiology, and cognitive psychology, uti-lizing laboratory-based experimental methods. Reiser (1984) explored the relationship be-tween developments in neurobiology and psychoanalysis. As new theoretical developments take hold in psychiatry and psychology—attachment theory is one example—they influence psychoanalysts' understanding of personality and inform their approaches to treatment.

THE FOUR PSYCHOLOGIES OF PSYCHOANALYSIS

In approaching psychopathology from the perspective of psychoanalytic theory, it is crucial to understand that psychoanalysis does not offer a single, coherent theoretical system. Psychoanalysis is not the monolithic, uniform, "grand" theory it is often purported to be. To begin, Freud, through the course of his writings, advanced evolving, often divergent, concep-tualizations of the human mind to account for new observed clinical phenomena. Of even greater importance, psychoanalysis, as noted, has undergone enormous revisions and transfor-mations that have drastically altered Freud's original ideas.

As psychoanalytic theory has evolved, divergences in the understanding of early devel-opment, psychopathology, treatment, and more fundamentally, the nature of the human mind, have led to the development of different theoretical approaches or models within psycho-analysis. In fact, psychoanalysis today can be thought of as a loose-fitting mosaic of several complementary submodels, each of which furnishes concepts and formulations for observing and understanding important dimensions of personality development and functioning, Within contemporary psychoanalytic thought, four conceptual approaches—modern structural the-ory, self-psychology, object relations theory, and intersubjective theory—are most influential. Each theory or model offers a coherent account of early development and psychopathology, and emanating from these, of the way treatment should proceed.

BASIC ASSUMPTIONS OF THE FOUR PSYCHOANALYTIC MODELS

The four models, which we explore at length, are neither mutually exclusive nor exhaus-tive. Each offers a coherent model that can stand alone but can most fruitfully be thought of as overlapping each of the others. Several areas of convergence are most important. First, a continuum concept of psychopathology underlies all psychoanalytic approaches. It is widely thought that all mental disorders lie on a continuum, in which psychosis and neurosis (or relative mental health) are at opposite ends. The continuum concept stresses the similarities and differences among all disorders. The model further implies that any individual can move along the continuum, depending on life circumstances and crises.

A second area of substantial agreement between theories is that early childhood development is crucial to later functioning. Adults reenact early childhood experiences and fantasy in their adult life. All psychoanalytic models view the parent–child relationship as critical.

Third, all psychoanalytic models appreciate the profound significance of unconscious mental processes—unconscious thinking, memories, feelings, and fantasies—in determining behavior and personal meanings. Emphasizing unconscious mental processes, psychoanalytic theorists place relatively less emphasis on overt behavior and focus a sharper lens on underlying structures and meanings.

A fourth area of convergence involves the approach to treatment. All psychoanalytic theorists advocate an intensive, long-term form of psychotherapy that involves using free association, a relatively neutral or objective stance on the part of the therapist, and the reenactment of childhood experiences, fantasy, and conflict in relationship to the analyst. The notion of the repetition of the past in the present in the relationship to the analyst is termed "transference." Transference is central to all psychoanalytic treatments. The working-through and understanding of the transference is viewed by theorists as the crucial therapeutic task within all four psychoanalytic psychologies.

A fifth area of significant convergence among theorists involves the significance of theory and clinical data. Since the formative days of psychoanalysis, its theory has been intimately connected with clinical observation and with the techniques of the psychoanalytic method. This is not to say, however, that psychoanalysis has not been influenced by other disciplines. In fact, contributions from other disciplines, such as cognitive psychology, the neurosciences, and infant research, have informed contemporary psychoanalytic theorizing.

MODERN STRUCTURAL THEORY

History

Freud offered models of the mind that gradually evolved—from the topographical (unconscious and conscious) to the structural (ego, superego, and id). Modern structural theory, an enormously complex, rich theoretical system, represents a refinement and elaboration of Freud's original structural theory. Structural theory, above all, is a conflict theory. From the perspective of structural theory, all psychic phenomena, including psychopathology, are manifestations of conflict. Recognizing and effecting shifts in conflicts are the main tasks of treatment. Some psychoanalysts believe that psychoanalytic theory is, above all, a conflict theory, and some question whether nonconflict models (such as self-psychology) are psychoanalytic at all. Many structural theorists integrate self psychology and other conceptual frameworks into their theoretical understanding and clinical work.

In broadest strokes, Freud first proposed a model that involved conflict between the conscious and unconscious (the topographical model). The structural model, which posited conflict between the three agencies of the mind—ego, superego, and id—represented a more complex, refined approach to psychic functioning. Arlow (1991) summarized this model succinctly:

> The ego is the final arbiter over the conflicting claims or derivative expressions of the instinctual drives, collectively designated as the id, and moral imperatives and ideal aspirations collectively designated as the superego. In its role as mediator, the ego integrates the realistic concerns of the individual for survival, adaptation, and inner harmony. (p. 4)

Boesky (1990) details how, in the last 50 years, psychoanalysis has gradually elaborated Freud's structural model, although the tripartite structure of superego, ego, and id remains its cornerstone.

The Compromise Formation and the Components of Psychic Conflict

As structural theory has evolved, the concept of *compromise formation* moved to the fore and became the central theoretical construct in the explication of psychic functioning, including psychopathology. The most prominent proponent of modern structural theory, Charles Brenner, a New York-based psychoanalyst, offered the most influential contributions to the understanding of compromise formation. Brenner's *The Mind in Conflict* (1982) became the most important single contribution to modern structural theory.

According to structural theory, the mind is constantly in a state of dynamic tension. The term "drive derivative" is used because drives are thought to be biological; the term "derivative" indicates the psychological representation of the biological drives. The ego functions oppose these drive derivatives sufficiently to ward off experiences of unpleasure (anxiety and/or depressive affect). The consequence of this dynamic tension is always a compromise between the competing components of the mind, termed a *compromise formation*.

All compromise formations have four components: (1) a drive derivative, (2) anxiety and/or depressive affect, (3) defense, and (4) an aspect of superego functioning. According to Brenner (1982), *all* psychic phenomena—moods, wishes, dreams, fantasies, plans, etc.—represent compromise formations, that is, all psychic phenomena represent compromises between the derivative of an instinctual drive, the accompanying depressive and/or anxious affect, defense, and an aspect of superego functioning. All manifestations of psychopathology represent compromise formations, too, according to modern structural theory. Following we illuminate each component of the compromise formation, explore how the compromise formation works, and then explore pathological compromise formations.

Drive Derivative

Within structural theory, instinctual drives are viewed as the force that propels fundamental drives, sexual and aggressive. As our discussion of self-psychology will suggest, the notion of primary instinctual drives is controversial. The controversy over drives extends beyond the scope of this discussion. In exploring structural theory, it is essential to understand that instinctual drives are viewed as primary motivators of human behavior, that they are seen as existing from early on in psychic development, and that manifestations, or representations of these drives (drive derivatives), are believed to play an integral role in all psychic conflict.

Anxiety and/or Depressive Effect

The second component of the compromise function is anxiety and/or depressive effect. According to Brenner (1982), affects (what we commonly call emotions) are complex psychic phenomena that contain sensations of pleasure or unpleasure (or a combination of the two), plus ideas. Structural theory posits an intrinsic tension in all people's lives between the wish for gratification of instinctual drives and feelings of unpleasure that such drives often arouse. Unpleasure can take the form of a fear of a future occurrence (anxiety) or a repetition of a previously experienced catastrophe (depression). The fundamental tension between drive and unpleasure stood as the centerpiece of Freud's conflict theory.

"CALAMITIES OF CHILDHOOD"

Why do instinctual drives often arouse unpleasure and thus produce intrapsychic conflict? The answer, according to structural theory, is rooted in what are termed the "calamities of childhood"—imagined dangers with which all children attempt to cope in play and fantasy. The ideas bound up with all sensations of unpleasure can be traced to the "calamities of childhood": object loss (the loss of a parent), loss of love, castration, and superego condemnation. The "calamities of childhood" represent normative developmental experiences for the child that involve intense feelings of unpleasure (anxiety and/or depressive affect). When psychoanalysts describe "calamities of childhood," they are describing fantasied experiences, purely intrapsychic events, although these may become entangled with events in reality (e.g., castration fears may be heightened by having surgery as a child; fear of loss of a parent's love may be exacerbated by a parent's withdrawal from a child). It is essential to have some understanding of the "calamities of childhood" because they provide the crucial links between childhood experiences and fantasies and adult psychic functioning, including psychopathology.

Development

Structural theorists have focused most attention on what they term *oedipal development* during childhood and its impact on all ensuing development. Neurotic (as opposed to more severe) difficulties are usually associated with oedipal-level conflicts. According to Brenner (1982), oedipal development occurs approximately between the years 2½ and 5. Psychological development is enormously complex during this time, but a brief summary will suffice here. In normal development, the oedipal triangle takes place when the daughter is attached to the father (an attachment that includes aggressive, competitive wishes directed toward the mother and sexual wishes directed toward the father) and fears that the mother will punish her for this attachment. The opposite situation occurs for the boy through his attachment to the mother and his fears of his father's retaliation. A principal "calamity" during oedipal development involves the fear of or fantasied experience of castration (or bodily harm). This is often evident in the child's play, dreams, and fantasies. Other calamitous worries—fears of losing the parents' love or of losing the parents altogether—also abound in the fantasy-filled minds of young children grappling with the intensity of their own aggressive and sexual wishes and the complex world that surrounds them. Fantasies, wishes—and also fears—from the oedipal period of development *persist* in psychic life from childhood onward. Often these contribute significantly to adolescent and adult psychological difficulties, as we will describe.

Now, we are ready to look at the emergence of the compromise formation. According to structural theory, drive derivatives that press for gratification often arouse anxiety or depressive affect (which is intrinsically bound up with one or more of the calamities of childhood). When this occurs, the ego, which seeks to facilitate gratification of drives and also to reduce anxiety or depressive affect, opposes the expression of the drive by implementing a defense. The dynamic tension between the drive derivative and the defense forms the centerpiece of the compromise formation. The compromise formation, according to Brenner (1982), functions to allow the greatest degree of satisfaction of drive derivatives without arousing too much anxiety and/or depressive affect. Brenner suggests that the ego functions as a mediator of satisfaction unless the drive derivatives arouse unpleasure; then the ego functions appear as defenses.

Defenses

According to Brenner (1982), defenses, the third component of the compromise formation, are aspects of mental functioning that can be defined only in terms of their function or consequence: the reduction of anxiety or depressive affect aroused by a drive derivative. Certain defenses—repression, denial, sublimation—have become well known within the popular culture. The final component of the compromise formation, an aspect of superego functioning, involves the moral component of each compromise formation. The superego contribution to compromise formation often involves the experience of guilt.

An example of a compromise formation from everyday life might be helpful here. A college student, a young man, has a crush on his teacher, a female professor in her forties. His frankly sexual wishes toward her (a sexual drive derivative) arouse anxiety because they are associated with forbidden incestuous wishes from his childhood (thus, the childhood calamity associated with his anxiety is the fear of castration; the superego component involves his feeling of guilt). Therefore, he implements a defense, denial, against these sexual wishes. If one were to ask him about sexual wishes toward his professor, he would answer in all honesty that he does not harbor such wishes because, in fact, they never enter consciousness. He is, however, able to entertain with pleasure the fantasy of kissing the teacher just once at the end of the school year. He also has a sexual dream about her two times, in which she appears in disguised form. His sexual wishes, in other words, achieve *a degree* of satisfaction. To return to the compromise formation, this young man achieves a compromise between the gratification of the drive derivative (the sexual wish toward the professor) and the unpleasure associated with the drive derivative (anxiety, which is tied to fears of castration). This whole process is unconscious, though the young man may, at moments, be aware of feeling slightly anxious in this teacher's classroom without knowing why.

Pathological Compromise Formations and the Structural Approach to Neurosis

Not all compromise formations work, that is, they might not achieve a reasonable balance between the expression of the drive and the need to maintain unpleasure within tolerable limits. Brenner (1982) suggests that a compromise formation is pathological when a combination of any of the following conditions exists: too much restriction of gratification of drive derivatives; too much anxiety or depressive affect; too much inhibition of one's capacity to exert mastery in the world; too great a tendency to injure or destroy oneself or too great a conflict with those around one. In the instance of the young man, for example, the student's anxiety about his sexual wishes might become so intense that he withdraws from the class the woman professor teaches. Or, because of his guilt about his sexual wishes, he might begin failing the class in an unconscious effort to atone. In such instances, we would suggest that the compromise formations—catalyzed by his sexual wishes toward his professor—are pathological.

As suggested, structural theorists since Freud have focused most attention on neurotic difficulties, which they believe are rooted predominantly in oedipal development. The possible roots of neurotic conflict within childhood are complex and multi-determined by and as varied as the individuals who have them. We have talked briefly about oedipal-level conflict. In discussing the emergence of conflict in childhood, the structural theorists tend to place less emphasis on external circumstances—for instance, unempathic parenting—than on the powerful impact of instinctual drives and unconscious fantasy. They differ profoundly in this from the self-psychologists. Structural theorists stress that normative developmental experiences are often internalized in profoundly distorted ways because of the intensity of the child's wishes, the impact of defensive efforts, and the level of the child's cognitive functioning (Tyson, 1991).

As a common example, a 5-year-old boy, who is angrily competing with his father, often projects his hostile, destructive wishes onto his father in an effort to disown them. In his own mind, then, his *father* is the angry one even when, in reality, the father may be a benign, nonhostile presence in the boy's life. The boy might internalize an image of himself in violent conflict with a destructive man, who is bent on harming him. This, in fact, is often the critical feature in the development of castration anxiety. The child projects his or her own aggressive wishes onto the parent and then fears retaliation. The intensity of the child's own instinctual drives, the primitive nature of his or her defenses (projecting wishes), and his or her limited cognitive capacities combine to create a monster in the child's mind. Selma Fraiberg (1959), in her book *The Magic Years*, poignantly describes how preschoolers, through magical thinking, develop fears and phobias in response to everyday occurrences. What is crucial is that these childhood experiences often reverberate throughout life. A girl's unconscious fear about a woman's retaliation may reemerge when she competes with other girls on the ballfield (which she unconsciously associates with competing against her mother) or, later, attempts to consummate a sexual relationship with a man (which she unconsciously associates with the forbidden sexual wish for the father).

Structural theorists emphasize the power of wishes, primitive thinking, and unconscious fantasy, but they do not deny that childhood events in reality can profoundly affect children. They stress, however, that the children do not internalize events, as *they are*, but filter them through the lens of their own wishes and fears. As a fairly common example, a single mother might sleep in a bed with her son following a divorce and, because she is lonely, might place him in the role of the man of the household, despite his age. Such an experience often makes boys acutely anxious because they fantasize that they have, in fact, won the oedipal competition. Then, they live in dread of the father's retaliation. Such boys, anxious in childhood, may develop significant inhibitions in the sexual realm and in self-assertion. What is crucial here is that the meaning of the life event, according to the structural theorist, can only be understood in the context of the child's fantasy life.

Clinical Example of Neurosis

As a more in-depth example of the structural view of neurotic-level functioning, let us look at M.T., a 32-year-old graduate student at a major university.

M.T. struggled intensely with worries about his competence in many domains in his life: in work, in athletics, and, most painfully, in terms of his sexual functioning and attractiveness to women. Although he was successful as a student (he was close to completing his doctorate), managed his day-to-day life with relative ease, and had engaged in two, generally positive, long-term relationships with women, he still worried about his adequacy and competence and suffered from chronic, mild depressive symptoms and, at times, from painful feelings of anxiety.

In reflecting on his intimate relationships with women, M.T. related that he had longstanding fears that "something bad" might happen. Further exploration suggested that these fears were associated with fiercely critical and aggressive thoughts that welled up inside him when he engaged in close heterosexual relationships. He worked hard to suppress these thoughts but was unable to do so. A gentle man, who, in fact, had never been violent in reality, M.T. took a harsh view of himself as a "jerk" and "insensitive" because he harbored such thoughts.

Constantly worried that he might hurt others' feelings, M.T. tended to assume a passive stance in his relationships. He let women take the lead, both in the bedroom and other domains, and worked, sometimes desperately, to inhibit any overt expression of anger. In school and on the ballfield (he played intramural soccer), he functioned adequately, but he tended to inhibit himself because he worried about asserting himself, which felt like an aggressive act. Thus, he failed to come close to achieving his potential.

Historically, M.T.'s neurotic difficulties appeared bound up to a great extent in his trouble negotiating the triadic relationship with his mother and father. As a boy, M.T. had aligned himself closely with his mother, who, he described, served as his "confidante." His father tended to be angry and, at times, explosive; he frightened M.T. and angered M.T.'s mother. While M.T. had admired certain qualities of his father—his outgoing style and competitive drive—he had feared aligning himself with him for fear of losing his alliance with his mother. M.T. described how furious he had been at his father for demanding so much attention from family members and also for denigrating him. Afraid of how angry he felt, however, he tended to retreat from confrontation with his father and to seek a safe haven in his mother's arms. Unconsciously, it appeared, he felt profoundly guilty for what he experienced as having a closer relationship with his mother than his father did.

As an adult, in an unconscious defensive maneuver, M.T. shifted back and forth between these two primary identifications. At moments, he identified with his father and his father's competitive, self-assertive strivings. Then, anxious about his emerging aggressive wishes and fears of alienating the woman, he shifted to an identification of what he experienced as the woman's "softer features." From this position, he suffered less anxiety about his aggressive wishes, but also found himself unable to assert himself fully—sexual or otherwise. He felt inhibited, according to his own description, and out of touch with his masculinity.

In returning to the notion of compromise formation, we see how in typical neurotic ways, M.T.'s compromise formations were what Brenner would term pathological. He suffered from feelings of anxiety and depression, which appeared tied to his inability to adequately modulate his aggressive wishes. His guilt (emanating from the superego component of his compromise formations) led him to inhibit himself, so that he failed to perform with the mastery and pleasure expected were he less conflicted.

The Structural Approach to Severe Psychopathology

Where the self-psychologists placed most emphasis on an explication of narcissistic disorders, and object relations theorists, at least recently, emphasized borderline disorders, structural theorists, as the previous discussion should suggest, focused most attention on neurotic disorders. The structural theory of intrapsychic conflict that involves drive and defense offers a powerful model for illuminating such common neurotic difficulties as inhibitions of sexual and aggressive wishes and excessive guilt. Critics, such as Kohut, argue, however, that structural theory is less adequate in explaining more severe psychopathology.

In contrast to the self-psychologists and object relations theorists who tend to stress that *deficits* in psychic structure underlie severe psychopathology (e.g., the self-psychologists speak of an "impoverished" or inadequate self-structure), structural theorists tend to stress *conflict* in the etiology of severe psychopathology. And, as one would expect, all symptoms represent pathological compromise formations.

As an example of this approach, we turn briefly to a segment of a psychoanalysis of a woman who had borderline tendencies, that was conducted by a psychoanalyst whose predominant approach is structural (Willock, 1991). The patient, a woman in her late twenties, was often depressed, chronically anxious, had no friends, showed significant impairments in her parenting, and was locked into a miserable marriage in which she functioned as an "obedient slave." In the analysis, typical of borderline patients, she quickly developed an intense transference to the analyst which involved painful fears of separation and the troubling experience of not being able to remember the analyst during her separation from him during the weekends. In contrast to the object relations theorist, who might view her inability to recall the analyst as originating in a developmental deficit involving a lack of object constancy or evocative memory, Willock felt that her difficulty emanated from a *conflict*. As he interpreted to the patient, she failed to remember him because, were she to allow herself to picture him, she would feel a more terrible longing that she could not be with him. In other words, according to the analysts, the "not remembering" was a symptom of conflict. It represented a defensive effort by the patient to fend off intensely painful feelings about her separation from the analyst. In a similar fashion, structural theorists tend to view the borderline's subjective experience of "emptiness" or inner "deadness" as manifestations of psychic conflict, as opposed to a symptom of deficient psychic structure.

As biological psychiatry has come to dominate the contemporary understanding of severe psychopathology, especially psychotic disorders and major depressive disorders, structural theorists have sought to integrate biological approaches with their understanding of conflict and its ubiquitous role in psychic life. Structural theorists recognize that constitutional impairments often contribute to such severe disorders as schizophrenia, but they continue to focus on the manifestations of conflict in understanding the patient's psychic life. Willock (1990) summarized his approach succinctly: "No matter what organic impairments are present in the psychoses, they still manifest themselves through the patient's mind ..." (p. 1078).

The Structural Approach to Treatment

The structural approach to psychoanalytic treatment follows directly from the conceptual model of the compromise formation. In the most basic terms, the analyst, by interpreting the patient's defenses, seeks to facilitate the emergence of different transferences in relation to the analyst. These transferences are understood in terms of compromise formations. They contain derivatives of instinctual drives (now directed toward the analyst), defenses, affects, and a superego component.

The analyst's central task is to help patients gradually understand how they construct the world according to childhood experience and fantasy: how, for example, people inhibit themselves because of unconscious fears of retaliation for sexual thoughts or how people behave in self-destructive ways because of guilt due to aggressive wishes. Where Freud in his early writing and Freudian theorists focused on making the unconscious conscious (the "cathartic method"), modern structural theorists have a more complex, ambitious task. They seek to help patients understand *all* aspects of their mental functioning, beginning with an understanding, through gradual, painstaking analysis, of how they seek to fend off feelings of unpleasure by a variety of defensive maneuvers.

This should not be viewed as a dry, intellectual approach that involves one person who offers didactic seminars to a compliant patient. The analyst's persistent interpretation of defenses facilitates the emergence of intense affects and painful confrontations for patients with their own primitive wishes and fantasies. Interpretation is generally seen useful only when conflicts have emerged, usually with emotional intensity, in the transference. At the same time, the structural theorist does emphasize *insight*. Where the self-psychologist and object relations theorist tend to stress the role of the therapeutic relationship itself in therapeutic change, the structural theorist traditionally focuses on the mutative role of *interpretation*. Properly timed interpretations in the context of the transference can produce shifts in the dynamic tension of the compromise formation, according to structural theory. Patients, for instance, might come to allow themselves more gratification of drive derivatives with less guilt and inhibition, or might come to assert themselves more actively without precipitating conflict with others.

As an example, let us return briefly to our young college student, sitting, mildly anxious, in the class of the woman professor. Let us imagine one aspect of a psychoanalytic treatment with him. Gradually, through the analyst's consistent interpretation of his denial about his sexual wishes toward the professor (and, perhaps, other older women), he comes to understand that he, indeed, harbors such wishes and that they make him intensely uncomfortable. Over time, he comes to understand, perhaps through a persistent anxiety-provoking fantasy that his male analyst will attack him for having sexual thoughts, that his anxiety resides in castration fears. As he comes to understand his fear of his analyst, he might come to see that this unfounded fear is rooted in childhood fantasy, tied to his parents, that his sexual wishes for his mother would elicit his father's wrath. As he gains this insight, he becomes more comfortable with his sexual fantasies. He finds that he is freer to enjoy sex and that he worries less that something is somehow wrong with him for his sexual desires.

Emblematic of the ongoing evolution of psychoanalysis, the modern structural approach to treatment has gradually shifted in recent years. In part, this is due to the influence of the more relational approaches within psychoanalysis, for example, self-psychology, and object relations theories. Where structural theorists traditionally have viewed the analyst as more contained and distant, modern-day structural theorists see the analyst as more engaged, as part of a powerful interpersonal field. This shift is perhaps most apparent in the approach to countertransference. Countertransference—which, in general terms, refers to the analyst's emotional reactions to the patient—was once viewed as an interference, something that analysts were encouraged to analyze within themselves and get under control. Today, even the more traditional structural theorist views countertransference as meaningful, as offering important information about the patient and also about the analyst.

A related, clinically rich concept that has emerged in recent years is *enactment*. Enactment refers to "symbolic interactions between analyst and patient which have unconscious meanings to both" (Chused, 1991). Analysts, engaged in listening to patients and also attending to their own thoughts and feelings, often become aware that they have been pulled out of an ordinary analytic stance. Understanding what has happened can become an extremely useful source of information about the patient (and the analyst). As an example, analysts might find that they are offering interpretations in a subtly critical manner, not typical of the way they usually work. They might recognize that patients, prone to feelings of guilt and evoking attacks by others, have unconsciously elicited punishing stances in analysts. To refer back to the example of the college student, a young man such as this, anxious about his own self-assertion, might elicit in the analyst a tendency to take control of the sessions and spare the young man the anxiety of having more control over his own analysis. When analysts recognize that they are assuming such roles, they can use them to help patients better understand how they deal with analysts and with others in their lives.

The increasing focus on countertransference and enactment has led to a type of clinical presentation that has new focus. Instead of discussing the patient from the position of an objective observer, the analyst presents the complex, subtle enactments that occur between patient and analyst. This entails a level of self-disclosure on the part of the analyst that was rare previously. Ted Jacobs (1991) described in detail how his self-analysis helped him understand himself and his patients better. Judith Chused (1991) offers a rich clinical presentation of her analysis with a school-age girl and her exploration of the way her own intense emotional reactions allowed her to develop a meaningful therapeutic relationship with this troubled youngster. James McLaughlin (1991) offers a poignant, in-depth study of how his own conflicts, rooted in his own painful childhood experiences, led him into a therapeutic bind with an analytic patient. While focusing on interpretation and the central role of conflict and unconscious fantasy, these prominent analysts also incorporate the notion of enactment as central to the psychoanalytic process.

SELF-PSYCHOLOGY

History

Self-psychology, one of the newest of the four conceptual frameworks that we are exploring, offers an approach to human development—and to psychopathology and its treatment—that diverges sharply from the theory of drives and conflicts rooted in Freud's structural model. The emergence of self-psychology as an important contemporary psychoanalytic approach can be attributed to the contributions of Heinz Kohut, a Chicago-based psychoanalyst, who died in 1981. Kohut's central contributions—*The Analysis of the Self* (1971) and *The Restoration of the Self* (1977)—stand as the cornerstone of self-psychology. Kohut's work has been elaborated on and expanded by his followers, and, in turn, it has had an enormous influence on the field in general and on relational models in particular. It still stands as the definitive conceptualization of the self-psychological approach.

Kohut's most important theoretical contribution was to bring to the fore the central role of narcissism in psychological functioning (Wallerstein, 1983). The myth of *Narcissus* encompasses many of the themes elaborated by Kohut. Narcissus, a handsome young man, was much loved by the nymphs, including Echo, who was painfully rejected by him. The gods vowed to punish him for his callousness by causing him to fall in love with his own image reflected in a pool. However, the mirror-like image fragmented each time that Narcissus reached out to embrace it, causing him to pine away in melancholia and ultimately to die.

The concept of narcissism has a long, varied history within psychoanalysis. It also has come to assume important meanings within the popular culture. In fact, many social critics believe we live in a "culture of narcissism." Here, we use the functional definition offered by Stolorow (1975): the "structural cohesiveness, temporal stability, and positive affective coloring of the self-representation." In simpler terms, it means a consistent, relatively realistic sense of one's self through time and across different situations. Adler (1989) suggested that Kohut's contributions to narcissistic disorders shifted the term "narcissistic" from being pejorative, meaning "entitled," to a concept that spoke to an individual's sense of incompleteness and low self-esteem.

Kohut believed that classical psychoanalytic formulations, which focused on biological drives and conflict, offered little toward understanding the role that narcissism plays in healthy and pathological development. He offered a comprehensive, psychologically based developmental theory that explored the vicissitudes of narcissistic development in early childhood and the maintenance of narcissism throughout the life cycle. Kohut and his followers have emphasized the role that the caregiver's empathy toward the young child plays in the development of the child's—and subsequent adult's—healthy sense of self. Kohut's emphasis and careful explication of narcissism catalyzed significant interest in it within psychoanalysis, both as it pertained to early development (the caregiver's empathy toward the child) and also to the treatment situation (the analyst's empathy toward the patient).

Kohut's conceptual framework is termed self-psychology because he places the development of the self at the center of his theory. The "core of the personality," according to Kohut and Wolf (1978), the self is "an independent centre of initiative and independent recipient of impressions." In contrast to the structural theory, which views instinctual drives (e.g., aggressive, sexual) as the primary motivator behind all human behavior, self-psychology is based on the motivational primacy of self-experience. The individual is concerned with maintaining a vital, complete, nonfragmented sense of self (Stolorow, 1983). From the perspective of self-psychology, manifestations of infantile instinctual drives (e.g., destructive rage, sexual "fixations") are not primary, but emerge when the self has been threatened in some way. As an important example, the structural model tends to view aggression as an instinctual given. In contrast, self-psychology tends to view the emergence of aggression as secondary to narcissistic trauma or injury. Structural theorists have criticized self-psychologists for failing to fully appreciate what they believe is the formative role of inborn sexual and aggressive drives in early development and in the development of psychopathology.

Development

In the self-psychologist's theory of development, the caregiver's capacity to respond empathically to the child's psychological needs is central. Empathy, the tool by which we know others, according to Kohut (1977), is the origin of psychological life. Without an empathic caregiver responding to the infant as though it already had a self, it is unlikely that the infant would develop a sense of self. According to this view, the child is born with innate potentials, and the environment responds selectively to them, channeling innate givens into what is referred to as a "nuclear self." In brief, the birth of the self, according to self psychologists, is a function of caregiving empathy that mobilizes the child's constitutional endowments. Kohut terms the caregiver of the infant and child a "self-object," because the developing child, who has not yet established a firm sense of self, experiences the parenting figure as part of the self (in an effort to facilitate understanding of this central and complex notion, Kohut and Wolf (1978) suggest that infants and developing children expect to control the self-object in a manner similar to adults' expectations of controlling their own mind and body).

According to Kohut and Wolf (1978), the child has two overriding emotional needs in relation to the caregiver. First, the child requires the self-object to "confirm the child's innate sense of vigor, greatness, and perfection" (p. 414). This is termed a "mirroring" self-object. It refers to the child's need for caregivers who can appreciate and affirm its special qualities and respond with pleasure to its initiatives. Second, "the child needs a self-object to whom the child can look up and with whom he can merge as an image of calmness, infallibility, and omnipotence" (p. 414). This is termed the "idealizing" self-object. In day-to-day terms, this refers to children's need for calm, capable parents whose sense of themselves in the world is secure and who can provide the children with a sense of stability and self-confidence with which the children can safely identify.

In ordinary, "good-enough" circumstances, the parents can provide the child sufficiently with the self-object functions described so that the child develops a positive, healthy self. The caregivers' calm and self-confidence and also their pleasure and affirmation of the child is gradually internalized by children as they develop, so that they can maintain, relatively consistently, a sense of self-confidence, enthusiasm, and positive feeling, despite life's inevitable frustrations and disappointments. If individuals have developed firmly established selves, according to Kohut and Wolf (1978), they can tolerate wide swings of self-esteem and cope with the dejection of failure and the exhilaration of success, experiences that often lead to acute psychological distress in those who have more precariously established selves.

The gradual processes through which the child internalizes the parental functions of helping the child maintain narcissistic equilibrium are termed "transmuting internalization." These occur when the child's sense of calm and omnipotence is disturbed by the inevitable minor failures in the caregivers' response. For example, a parent does not understand why an infant is crying and thus is unable to temporarily soothe it, or, at a particular moment, a parent fails to pay attention to a child who is urgently seeking affirmation. In response to these ordinary "empathic failures," the child attempts to maintain a sense of narcissistic perfection by establishing grandiose or exhibitionistic images of the self or by attributing narcissistic perfection to the parenting figure. Gradually, however, the child relinquishes these ideal images of its own, as well as the caregiver's narcissistic perfection. In so doing, it slowly acquires increments of inner psychological structure. To put it in other terms, repeated, tolerable disappointments in the caregiver lead the child over time to develop the capacity for self-soothing and the modulation of tension and to an increasing capacity to regulate its own self-esteem. These ideas carry over to treatment. In psychoanalysis from a self-psychological perspective, the analyst is seen as invariably repeating prior insults to the patient's self-esteem. How such experiences are dealt with in the treatment is vital to the process. Analysts must be keenly aware of the way their own narcissistic, self-aggrandizing tendencies lead to subtle, yet powerful, exploitations of patients that are similar to the patients' past traumatic experiences.

Disorders of the Self

Kohut's view of psychopathology grew directly out of his developmental theory. In contrast to ordinary, nontraumatic lapses in empathy that contribute to internalizing parental functions and, gradually, the development of a healthy self, serious, persistent failures in parental empathy lead to narcissistic traumas, that is, they create injuries to the self. Single traumatic incidents are rarely critical in the development of disorders of the self. Instead, ongoing failures of the caregivers to provide the child with adequate mirroring and idealizing self-objects are critical. These failures potentially lead to a weakened or defective self, the core of psychopathology in narcissistic individuals. If the self-object responses are not optimally frustrating—that is, if they are excessively frustrating, stimulating, or depriving—the vulnerable self of the child is threatened and is forced to erect defenses to protect itself. Kohut referred to this threat as "disintegration anxiety," the fear of loss of self. The fear of the loss of sense of who one is, according to self psychologists, is the deepest form of human anxiety that underlies all psychopathology. All psychopathology, according to this view, ultimately results from arrested self-development, implying the failure of necessary self-objects.

As examples of ongoing failures in empathy that self psychologists describe, one might consider a chronically angry father who is struggling with feelings of inadequacy and constantly derides his son, a toddler, for not being more competent every time the boy tries something new (e.g., putting on a shirt, drawing). One might envision the experience of a one-year-old daughter of a chronically anxious, overburdened mother, who cannot sit still for more than a few minutes at a time. When the child wishes to be held at vulnerable moments, it is put down after a few seconds because the mother is too preoccupied to respond appropriately. In essence, the parents' own self pathology prohibits them from attending to the child's developmental needs for mirroring and idealizing self-objects. When "good enough" self-objects are lacking, the child develops an inadequate sense of self. It fails to develop those internal structures that allow it to regulate its own narcissistic equilibrium. Instead, the child (and, later, the adult) retains an archaic grandiosity in the wish to continue the fusion with an omnipotent self-object to maintain an archaic sense of self as a defense against painful states of anxiety and depression (Blatt & Lerner, 1991). Often, the self-perceptions of these individuals are fragmented and discontinuous, and they seek in others the replacement for the psychological structures that they lack (an urgent search for affirmation, for instance, and mirroring). Drug addiction is viewed as a self-disorder in which the drug is used to fill the missing gap in psychological structure. According to this view, parents of the addict failed to perform, as a self-object, their tension-regulating and other functions, resulting in a traumatic disappointment in the idealizing self-object. Eating disorders, particularly bulimia and overeating, are seen in a similar fashion.

In the gravest instances of what self-psychologists term "disturbances of the self," the individual develops a chronic psychosis. This occurs, according to Kohut and Wolf (1978), when the self is noncohesive, lacking in even the most basic capacities for self-esteem regulation. Psychotic disorders are viewed as the outcome of inherent biological tendencies, of a childhood lacking in even minimally effective mirroring, or the combination of both biological and environmental factors. On the continuum of primary disorders of the self, borderline states represent the second most severe disturbance. According to Kohut and Wolf (1978), borderline states emanate from the permanent breakup or enfeeblement of the self. In contrast to the more blatant manifestations of psychotic disorders, borderline disorders are more muted, more subject to an overlay of complex defense mechanisms. From the self-psychological perspective, borderline states are rooted in part in the caregiver's chronic inability to understand the developing child's need to establish autonomy. This psychological view of borderline disorders has been criticized by many in the field for failing to take heed of the central role of overwhelming aggressive impulses in the formation of the disorder (e.g., Adler, 1989).

Many disorders of the self, resulting from unempathic caregiving during infancy and childhood, are less severe than the psychotic and borderline disorders noted previously. Although psychoanalysts tend to avoid diagnostic labelling, Kohut and Wolf (1978) offer a subtyping of self disorders, although they caution that these groupings do not do justice to the complexity of any one individual's clinical presentation. These classifications are considered useful because they tie particular problems in child development to their later behavioral and experiential manifestations. The "understimulated self" arises in the face of insufficient stimulation from caregivers in childhood. Individuals who have understimulated selves experience themselves as boring, apathetic, and lacking in vitality. They seek excitement in an effort to ward off feelings of deadness and depression. An understimulated toddler might engage in head banging or hair pulling, a school-aged child in compulsive masturbation, an adolescent in dangerous, daredevil activities, and an adult in a range of perverse sexual and addictive behaviors. The "overstimulated self" results from unempathic overstimulation during childhood, especially excessive responses to the child's grandiose-exhibitionistic strivings. Overwhelmed by unrealistic fantasies of greatness, which produce acute anxiety, individuals with overstimulated selves urgently seek to avoid situations in which they might be the center of attention and often suffer from severe inhibitions. A "fragmented self" develops in individuals to whom caregivers were unable to offer integrating responses. States of fragmentation, which often arise in response to an experience of lack of empathy in others, vary in degree. More severe manifestations include profound anxiety and hypochondriacal worry.

THE UNDERSTIMULATED SELF: A CLINICAL EXAMPLE

> R.D., a 14-year-old high school student, was referred for treatment by his school guidance counselor and local police. Recently, both the parents and police began to accumulate evidence that R.D. was responsible for stealing more than $23,000 from relatives and neighbors through a series of break-ins. He was also suspected of dealing and using drugs. Interestingly, these allegations were always difficult to prove and, despite an early history of head-banging, erratic school performance, and large deposits into his bank account, R.D.'s behavior only recently had come to the attention of his parents. R.D.'s history reveals that he was adopted at six weeks of age. His mother recalls that he had severe diaper rash and never smiled. Indeed, upon meeting R.D., the therapist was struck by how sad, depressed, empty and apathetic he appeared. The little that he did have to say was that he felt that he had no problems, was doing fine in school, and really had no interest in anything. It became increasingly apparent that R.D.'s late night break-ins, operation of a gambling ring, and use of drugs were desperate attempts to create excitement to ward off the subjective experience of deadness. Despite good social skills, he preferred to be alone, and every step along the way he would recklessly sabotage his own achievements and skills. For example, he used his lucrative baseball card collection as a front for stolen money. Once this was uncovered, he seemed to lose any interest that he had in collecting baseball cards.

Self-psychologists, beginning with Kohut, have focused most attention on individuals who have disorders of narcissism. Such individuals have severe difficulties in maintaining self-esteem. Interpersonally, these narcissistic individuals are extremely sensitive to what they experience as disappointments, failures, and slights. Kohut and Wolf (1978), again with cautions about oversimplification, offer a typology of narcissistic personality types. The "mirror-hungry personality" urgently seeks affirmation and approval from others. Chronically seeking to counteract painful feelings of worthlessness, these individuals persistently exhibit themselves in an effort to induce self-objects to admire them and thus bolster their self-esteem. "Ideal-hungry personalities" constantly search for relationships with others whom they can admire for their intelligence, wealth, beauty, or other attributes. Usually, however, this new self-object relationship cannot fill the individuals' powerful sense of deficiency and, disappointed, they set out once again to find a "special someone" in whose glory they can bask. "Alter ego personalities" seek relationships with self-objects who, by conforming to the self's values, appearance and options affirm the existence of the self. "Merger-hungry personalities" control others in relationships in an attempt to find in others the structure they lack for their own fragmented self. "Contact-shunning personalities" avoid others because their need for others is so great. They fear rejection and, on a deeper level, fear that their selves will be lost in the yearned-for fusion with the self-object.

Throughout life, individuals who have narcissistic disorders unconsciously and generally without success, seek to repair long-standing deficits in their selves through current relationships. Extraordinarily vulnerable to rejection and disappointment and, in essence, seeking the impossible in their relationships (that current relationships can somehow repair the damage done by nonempathic self-objects during childhood), these individuals often have short-lived or shallow and extremely frustrating relationships. Absorption in their own desperate psychological needs contributes to their interpersonal difficulties because much of the time they are unable to focus empathically on the needs of others. The outward qualities that characterize many individuals who have narcissistic disorders—self-absorption, aloofness, arrogance, grandiosity, ragefulness—often make it difficult for others, including clinicians, to maintain empathy with them and to recall that these personality characteristics, in fact, represent an effort to contend with intense feelings of worthlessness, depression, and incompleteness.

Mirror-Hungry Personality: A Clinical Example

A.E., a 23-year-old graduate student, was initially referred for treatment because of anorexia nervosa. She was painfully thin, like a waif. She reported secluding herself in her dorm room, only to emerge at dinner time to parade herself through the dining hall "to be seen by everyone" as she took a small salad and once again retreated to her room. She became even more secluded as her friends pleaded with her to eat. Her history revealed that her father died suddenly when she was ten years old, and that she had an overly close, enmeshed relationship with her mother, in which A.E. actually mothered the mother. She reported that as a little girl she would frequently come home from school, eager to tell her mother about her excellent grades or success in basketball. But the mother, rather than listening with pride, habitually steered the conversation from A.E. to herself, and frequently began to talk about either her own needs at the moment or her own previous successes, which overshadowed those of her daughter. What emerged in her treatment was A.E.'s self-righteous demands for exclusive attention, praise, and reassurance. This was surprising in the sense that she presented herself as being painfully shy and inhibited and, in her own words, "always putting other people's needs ahead of my own." Because of A.E.'s experience that her own needs would not be echoed with understanding and empathy, she felt deep shame, which, in turn, led her to suppress all of her needs—including the need to eat—which she manifested in her eating disorder, depression, and hopeless withdrawal. Her "parading" through the dining hall in the dorm was an angrily expressed exhibitionistic demand that the "wrongs" that had been done to her be set right.

The Self-Psychology Approach to Treatment

In keeping with his reformulation of psychopathology as "developmental arrest" due to self-object failure, Kohut viewed the treatment process as a means by which the arrested self can complete its developmental task with a new self-object experience. This process revolves around the therapeutic mobilization of the developmentally arrested self, the use of the therapist as a "good enough" self-object that was missing in development, and the "transmuting internalization" of the self-object therapist into psychological structure.

Within treatment, the self-psychologist focuses on the emergence of a "self-object transference" within the therapeutic relationship. This occurs when the patient revives, in relation to the analyst, a childhood need for either mirroring or idealizing, a need that had been insufficiently responded to empathically by the original caregivers. In the mirroring transference, patients seek the acceptance and confirmation from the analyst that they failed to receive earlier in life. In the idealizing transference, the patient seeks merger with the analyst as an idealized source of strength and calmness. Kohut and Wolf (1978) stress the need for the analyst to maintain a calm, empathic stance in the face of the narcissistic patient's often rageful and incessant demands. The analyst must be alert not to exhort, attempt to educate, or blame the patient for what appears to be unreasonable behavior:

But if he can show to the patient who demands praise that, despite the availability of average external responses he must continue to "fish for compliments" because the hopeless need of the unmirrored child in him remains unassuaged, and if he can show to the raging patient the helplessness and hopelessness that lies behind his rages, can show him that indeed his rage is the direct consequence of the fact that he can not assert his demands effectively, then the old needs will slowly begin to make their appearance more openly as the patient becomes more empathic with himself. (p. 423)

As the patients' old needs gradually reemerge in the treatment situation, analysts can assist patients to understand how unfulfilled needs from childhood continue to dominate their current lives. Most importantly, the analyst assumes a new self-object function for the patient. By offering patients a mirroring and idealizing self-object—and analyzing their empathic failures and their effect on patients—analysts facilitate the process of internalization of parental functions that have been incomplete in the patients' childhoods.

OBJECT RELATIONS THEORY

History

The history of psychoanalysis has been punctuated by theoretical debates, but no debate has been as wide ranging and has had such profound implications as that involving what is called object relations theory. Object relations theorists address how significant early formative relationships become internalized and affect our subsequent experience of ourselves and other people. What aspects of our relationships determine whom we choose as lovers, spouses, or friends? What is the dynamic nature of our internal object world? How does it evolve and what are the implications for treatment? What is biologically innate in the psychology of the person, and what is modulated by direct environmental experience, especially experience within interpersonal relationships? What is the nature of motivation? Is it the pressure of instinctual wishes and drives or seeking relationships with other people?

Interest in the study of object relations evolved as Freud's interest extended beyond basic biological predispositions to include the cultural and family context and their influence on psychological development. His interest in the superego, defined as the internalization of cultural prohibitions and values, led him to a fuller appreciation of the family as a mediating force in the transmission of cultural values. Freud focused increasing attention on the role of parents in shaping psychological development. Development came to be viewed as a consequence of the caregiving patterns of significant people in the child's early environment. Later, knowledge gained from psychoanalytic work with children and the observation of normal and disrupted development of infants and children contributed further to the psychoanalytic appreciation and understanding of early developmental phases, their role in normal personality development, and the occurrence of psychopathology throughout the life cycle.

Object relations theories work to account for personality development, psychopathology, and treatment on the basis of internalization of relationships with others. Many consider Melanie Klein to be, historically, the central figure in the development of object relations theory. As an aside, it should be noted that many of the most influential theorists in psychoanalysis have been women, such as Klein, Anna Freud, Helena Deutsch, Karen Horney, Clara Thompson, Annie Reich, Edith Jacobson, and Margaret Mahler. Melanie Klein was particularly attentive to the influence of drives, especially aggression and anxiety in children. Inborn aggression and what she referred to as the "paranoid-schizoid" and "depressive" developmental positions (not stages) led to the development of what she referred to as "fragmented internal objects." The internal world, according to Klein, provides the basis for the child's subsequent perceptions and interpersonal relationships. Internal objects develop, according to Klein, from extreme experiences of good and bad that were originally attributed to fragmented, part properties of the mother, such as the mother's breast. These representations become increasingly differentiated, integrated, and realistic with development. Internal objects are not exact replicas of external objects and experiences but are always embellished by the infant's drives and fantasies which are externalized (projected) and then reinternalized (introjected). This process of successive projections and introjections enable internal objects to become increasingly integrated and realistic. The term "object" in object relations theory refers to the distinction between internal and external people and also to the fact that we never perceive and experience others precisely for who they are.

Klein's interest in the child's development of internal objects stressed the symbolizing activity of the child. Within her theories, there is an inextricable link between the experiences of love and hate in early relationships and the development of cognitive processes. Perhaps more than anything else, Melanie Klein reminds us that we live in two worlds, including an internal world that is as real and as central as the external world. This internal world is a "place," a life space, in which meaning is generated. The reality of this internal world is the origin of personal meaning, which is then expressed in the quality of interpersonal relationships established in the external world through the life cycle.

Object Representation

As noted earlier, our sense of who we are in relation to others begins in infancy and evolves throughout life. A key concept in object relations theory is that of "object representation." Broadly defined, according to Blatt and Lerner (1991), object representation refers to conscious and unconscious mental schemata—including cognitive, affective, and experiential components—of significant interpersonal encounters. Beginning as vague, diffuse, variable experiences of pleasure and unpleasure, schemas gradually develop into differentiated, consistent, relatively realistic representations of the self and the world of other people. The earliest forms of representation are based on those action sequences and behaviors associated with the gratification of basic needs; later forms are based on specific perceptual and functional features of the self in relationship to caregiving agents; higher forms are more symbolic and conceptual. There is constant and reciprocal interaction between past and present interpersonal relationships and the development of representations. Schemas evolve both developmentally and in psychoanalytic treatment from the internalization of interpersonal relationships. New levels of object representation and self-representation provide a revised internal landscape and organization for subsequent interpersonal relationships. The psychoanalytic concept of object representation overlaps, in important and exciting ways, cognitive psychologists' research on mental schemata.

Object relations theory is not a unitary theory. It is, rather, a way of thinking, a movement within psychoanalysis that represents the convergence of two sources of information—the clinical observation of patients in psychoanalysis and psychotherapy and systematic observation of infants in relation to their mothers. The most influential developmental studies in the United States on object relations have been those of Margaret Mahler and her colleagues, summarized in the book *The Psychological Birth of the Human Infant* (1975). Other investigators, such as Bowlby (1969, 1973), convincingly illustrated the importance of early mother–infant bonding and attachment in establishing a sense of self and others. The cognitive studies of Jean Piaget have had a profound impact on object relations theory in general and on theories of the development of object representations in particular. These seminal psychoanalytic observations were integrated by Kernberg (1975, 1976) in his theoretical approach to psychopathology. The mental processes he observed in patients who had borderline personality organizations (patients located in the middle of the psychopathology continuum between neurosis and psychosis) have striking parallels to the behavior of children in certain phases of development.

Development

Object-relational thinking views attachment as a central phenomenon, and increasingly, in line with infant research, assumes that infants are preprogrammed from birth for human contact and to form relationships with caretakers. There is considerable evidence from converging lines of investigation across disciplines that newborns come into the world with more sophisticated equipment hardwired than previously thought. But, as Winnicott (1949) stated in his deceptively simple, yet evocative way, "There is no such thing as a baby." This is to say, we cannot conceptualize the infant apart from its caregivers. Many findings from parent observational and experimental infant research and neurobiological studies confirm the existence of motivational systems of competence and mastery in the child. Tronick and Gianino (1986), on the basis of careful observations of infant–mother interactions, found that the successful joint repair of interactive or communicative mismatches by mother and child is experienced by the child as "affectance." Novick and Novick (1996), in a major contribution, extended these findings to the area of competence, mastery, and self-esteem. According to the Novicks, the child's real capacity to elicit appropriate responses from the caregiver is the root of feelings of competence, affectance, and reality-based self-esteem. The capacity of the mother–infant dyad to repair inevitable breaches in the empathic tie is also an important source of feelings of competence and positive self-esteem. The capacity for pleasure depends on and is regulated by the ability of each partner in the couple in interaction with the other, which leads in turn to the experience of having an actual effect on the other.

Many object-relations theories of development stem from the observational studies of Mahler and her colleagues, who formulated their findings in terms of what is called "separation-individuation theory." Based on the study of severely disturbed infants, Mahler, Klein, and Bergman (1975) conducted a 10-year observational study of normal children and their mothers. These children entered the study in their first few months of life. Psychoanalytically trained researchers observed them, both alone and in interaction with their mothers, through their third year. The remarkable series of detailed and empathic observations were then used to delineate what Mahler called "the psychological birth of the human infant."

According to these investigators, the infant, after the first few months of life, develops a dawning awareness of self and others. The child and mother then begin to form two poles of a dyadic unity of symbiosis (2–6 months). Slowly differentiating from the mother, the infant enters the separation-individuation phase and its specific subphases: differentiation, practicing, and rapprochement. The child becomes increasingly aware of the mother as a separate agent during the differentiation or "hatching" subphase (6–10 months). With increased motor and cognitive skills, the child, during the practicing subphase (10–16 months), appears to be intoxicated, in a "love affair with the world." Taken with its own sense of power, the child easily "darts away" from the mother, as if she were not needed. Yet, with increased growth, there is an awareness of separateness and helplessness which ushers in the all-important subphase of rapprochement (16–24 months). The child is then observed moving back and forth, separating and returning, willful yet dependent. As what is termed the "rapprochement crisis" resolves, the child begins to display confidence in the mother's continued loving presence, despite her occasional absences. The ability to retain an image or representation of the mother as a caring, gratifying presence, but also frustrating, is called emotional object constancy (24–36 months). With this, the child develops an increasingly stable, more complex sense of individuality, along with an increasingly stable and realistic sense of significant others.

Borderline Personality

Extensive clinical and research studies of the borderline personality during the past 30 years have played a significant role in the development of object relations theory. Developmentally, borderline disorders display conflicts and issues that appear consistent with the rapprochement subphase. Kernberg, in two major books, *Borderline Conditions and Pathological Narcissism* (1975) and *Object Relations Theory and Clinical Psycho-analysis* (1976), as well as in numerous publications, advanced the most thorough psychoanalytic understanding of people who had what he termed "borderline personality organization." He described these individuals as having certain symptoms, personality characteristics, and developmental features in common. For more than 50 years, the term "borderline" referred to people who were thought to have features of both neurosis and psychosis, and who seemed to shift back and forth erratically between the two. Kernberg argued instead that these individuals have a remarkably specific and stable form of psychopathology. They were thought to be "stable in their instability." In terms of symptoms, they are impulsive, intensely angry, and prone to addictions, promiscuity, and reckless, self-defeating behaviors; prone to intense, often short-lived but intense chaotic relationships; and chronically plagued with diffuse anxiety.

Glenn Close's portrayal of Alex in the movie *Fatal Attraction* offers an excellent example and caricature of the borderline individual. Unlike more neurotic individuals, Alex could not maintain relationships with others by expressing warmth, concern, and dedication. It is extremely difficult for such individuals to maintain empathy and understanding in a relationship, once conflicts arise. Yet, paradoxically, they are unable to separate or take perspective. As a result, the relationships of borderline individuals are often chaotic and embellished with either idealization or depreciation. As with Alex, manipulation often replaces empathy as a way of relating to others. These individuals tend to overreact to internal stimuli, often aggressively and self-destructively. Underneath the often contradictory, misleading, and vexing clinical picture of the borderline patient, according to Kernberg, lie remarkably specific and relatively stable forms of coping, specific defensive operations, and highly pathological and "split" internalized self- and object representations. The poor coping skills of borderline individuals are termed "ego weakness," which consists of difficulty in modulating anxiety, regulating the intensity of emotions, a lack of impulse control, and poor social judgment.

According to Kernberg, a characteristic feature of the borderline individual is intense aggression. Because of either constitutional predisposition to aggression, excessive frustration during development, and/or trauma, such as sexual, physical and emotional abuse, these individuals tend to split off internalized good self- and object representations from bad self- and object representations. Further, they tend to project excessively bad (aggressive) self- and object representations onto other people. The combination of splitting and projection leads to an incapacity to integrate good and bad self- and object representations during the rapprochement subphase of development.

From a psychoanalytic perspective, the category of borderline personality organization is broad and includes individuals thought to be schizoid (excessively withdrawn), paranoid (extremely suspicious and distrustful), antisocial or psychopathic personalities, and who are thought to have multiple personality disorders. These disorders, it is thought, exhibit similar underlying internal object relations, ego weakness, and what is termed "primitive defensive operations," such as splitting, excessive projection, idealization, and devaluation. It should also be stated that these symptoms often exist alongside some very admirable skills and talents. Again, Glenn Close's portrayal of Alex in *Fatal Attraction* illustrates the paradox of the way outstanding intellectual and work functions can coexist with other more primitive features of the personality.

CLINICAL EXAMPLES OF BORDERLINE PERSONALITY

The impulsivity of many borderline individuals resembles that of toddlers. Without fully considering consequences, they may swiftly move toward what seems gratifying at the moment in an effort to forget what is frustrating.

> R.G., a 19-year-old female college student, was told to learn a more efficient laboratory procedure by her physics instructor. The professor valued her and was trying to help. However, RG could not experience the help while simultaneously tolerating the frustration of feeling criticized and needing to learn something new. She forgot that she was an honor student who had a history of success in laboratory sciences. She impulsively dropped the class, drank excessively, and sought out friends for comfort and to complain to. A week later, feeling lonely, bored, and anxious about what she did, she returned to the professor in an attempt to get back into the class. Her life away from the lab now became frustrating, and the class once again "looked good."

Individuals such as RG often turn to drugs, alcohol, or brief sexual encounters in frantic attempts to soothe pain and gratify needs. When the drugs or sexual relationships cause frustration and lower self-esteem, they impulsively leave them, only to return. This is similar to what observers of infants have noted about the "rapprochement" child's movement away from and back to the mother. This movement also extends to treatment. Often these individuals seek treatment to escape feelings of loneliness and emptiness. While initially feeling safe and less alone, once they find therapy frustrating, they seemingly forget its good aspects and leave treatment just as quickly as they entered it.

This sudden shifting of self- and object representations also causes difficulty in relationships. Borderline individuals often experience new relationships as "all good" and gratifying and are prone to form intense infatuations that can be extremely exciting. However, these quickly fall apart because the individual who has a borderline personality lacks object consistency—the ability to recall good memories when frustrated. In *Fatal Attraction*, Alex's explosive shifts in mood around any separation from her lover illustrate the consequence of a lack of object constancy in the object relations of a borderline patient.

When individuals who have a borderline personality feel unloved in a relationship, they desperately attempt to change their feelings, often by manipulating others. They believe they could feel good, if only the other could "make it happen." When ungratified or frustrated, they throw tantrums, threaten, and even make suicide attempts. As can be seen in the case of Alex, the suicide attempt is often prompted by a separation and is less an attempt to kill oneself than to manipulatively force the return of the all-good object and to punish the all-bad object. These individuals are unable to recognize that the person whom they experience as ignoring them or not loving them at one moment, is the same person they felt loved by at previous moments. The intense anger of borderline individuals also derives from splits in the internal experience of self in relationship to others. The intense sadism seen in Alex—exemplified by her blowing up her lover's car, kidnapping his daughter, and boiling the daughter's pet rabbit—all demonstrate what is termed in the literature "borderline rage."

Identity disturbance, characteristic of borderline personality organization, stems from an absence of object constancy and internal splitting along all-good and all-bad dimensions. Many individuals actually describe themselves as having a "good self" and a "bad self.

> R.B., a 20-year-old student, had a history of academic success and did well in school as long as he was in a structured situation in which his assignments were clear and his professors supportive. On weekends, however, he experienced feelings of loss of identity and desperately sought contact and soothing through alcohol abuse, dangerous relationships, and compulsive exercising.

In the absence of object constancy, such individuals cannot maintain a sense of well-being if relationships are even temporarily frustrating. When they are feeling deprived or alone, they cannot recall that life is generally satisfying and that people care about them. They may feel exhilarated with a supportive person. The extremes of all-good and all-bad self–other experiences make the borderline individual prone to constantly shifting moods.

The all-bad self–other state can often precipitate extremes of stimulating, self-damaging acts.

> One 19-year-old student felt so enraged at her boyfriend, whom she experienced as ignoring her, that she repeatedly leaped off the top of her bunk bed, hurling herself against the wall and onto the floor. She binged and drank wildly and then attempted to force herself to throw up. In an attempt to focus herself and gain control, she painstakingly removed all of the "fuzz" from a peach pit.

Adler (1985), among others, has suggested that the early history of borderline patients includes parents who are unable to empathize, soothe, and confirm confidently, so that the child does not have the opportunity to learn or internalize this function. As a result, individuals who have a borderline disorder cannot empathize with others, self-soothe, or regulate the intensity of their own feelings. Masterson and Rinsley (1975) described a classic pattern that it is thought takes place during the rapprochement subphase in borderline families. During this subphase, it is critically important for the child to separate from and return to the mother and for the mother to be steady and empathic. The mothers of borderline patients need to cling to their children to meet their own frustrated dependency needs and offer excessive approval, support, and love for clinging behavior. They are threatened by separation and become "attacking, critical, hostile, angry, withdrawing supplies and approval in the face of assertiveness or other efforts toward separation-individuation" (p. 169). This behavior reinforces the child's all-good and all-bad split object representations and also leads the child to feel abandoned for behaving maturely and to constantly seek overly enmeshed, clinging, dependent relationships.

Psychotic Personality Organization

Individuals who have psychotic personality organizations are even more unable to maintain a stable integration of self- and object representations. This seriously undermines their capacity to appraise themselves and other people realistically over time and in different situations. Similar to the borderline individuals, those who have psychotic-level personality organizations employ a range of "primitive" defenses which further undermine their coping skills. The reasons for using these defensive operations, however, are different in borderline and psychotic individuals. According to Kernberg (1975), splitting and other defenses protect the borderline individual from intolerable feelings of ambivalence and the overwhelming rage that interferes with all significant relationships. In contrast, the psychotic individual uses these defenses in an effort to avoid the experience of disintegration, merger, and loss of boundaries. Merger refers to the internal fusion or blurring of self- and object representations. The regressive experience of merger manifests itself in a total and frightening loss of reality testing, in delusions, hallucinations, and confusion between self and others.

Object relations theory has illuminated how and when people develop a sense of reality, as well as how they lose and regain it. The ability to adapt to the world and experience daily events requires a capacity to distinguish between self and other and yet to remain in relationship to the other. Without contrast, that is, separateness, there is fusion and symbiotic oneness—an inability to develop a self in relationship to another. Without the sense of differentiation and contrast, these individuals develop self–other boundary confusion or psychosis.

As the self-image dissolves and becomes swallowed up by the image of the other, the psychotic persons can literally feel themselves disappearing into the other. This loss of self is catastrophic and is experienced in terms of ceasing to exist, a disintegration. Consequently, although psychotic patients seek fusion, they also fear and avoid it. Burnham and her colleagues (1969) characterized this tendency among psychotic patients as the "need–fear dilemma."

> One 18-year-old psychotic young man in the throes of the "need–fear dilemma," was brought to the emergency room by his mother. With one hand he grasped the mother's hand like an infant, while with the other he attempted to hit her.
>
> The dorm-room of an 18-year-old freshman was described as a "virtual altar" to his mother, with her pictures and letters arranged in an almost religious fashion. He complained of feeling "lost, isolated, listless, distant from others, and unable to concentrate." As his disjointed speech, hallucinations and withdrawal gradually increased in school, he began to behave in increasingly bizarre ways, which culminated with him attacking his mother with a knife. His delusional beliefs, visual hallucinations and concrete thinking represented desperate attempts to maintain a boundary or distinction between self and other, between himself and his mother.

The Object Relations Approach to Treatment

Clinical psychoanalytic work within the object relations approach is based on a number of theories that converge in their view of development and psychopathology as products of the internalization of formative interpersonal relationships. As a result, treatment focuses on the manifestations of these internalizations in relationships in general and the relationship to the therapist in particular (transference). Object relations theory has not drastically changed psychoanalysis as much as it has subtly influenced its focus. This influence comes from insights into interpersonal and internal development, which has helped provide better therapeutic maps for exploration of borderline and psychotic conditions. Object relations theory has also focused on new aspects of the therapist–patient interaction. Over time, as we will see in our section on relational models, this approach has become increasingly popular and influential.

Formulations about therapeutic action—that is, what is therapeutic in psychoanalysis—increasingly consider therapy a significant interpersonal relationship in which the treatment relationship itself becomes the mediator for the patient's development. If the internalization of object relations results in the formation of psychological structures during normal development, then the internalization of significant interactions between the patient and the therapist plays an important role in the therapeutic process. The therapist becomes available as a "new object" by eliminating, step by step, the interpersonal distortions (transference) that interfere with the establishment of new, healthier object relationships. It is the internalization of new and relatively undistorted relations with the therapist that leads to therapeutic change.

The formulations in clinical examples presented in this chapter suggest that there are different types of distortions in the representational world in various forms or levels of psychopathology. These differences are expressed in the therapeutic process in terms of the nature of the therapeutic relationship, that is, the transference. Given a good-enough psychotherapeutic environment—the "holding environment"—reminiscent of the early mother–infant relationship, treatment interventions are aimed at promoting differentiation and integration. They facilitate the patient's evolving awareness of self as having a coherent identity, and they assist in the development of a fuller and deeper appreciation of others.

THE INTERSUBJECTIVE AND RELATIONAL PERSPECTIVES

Stolorow, Atwood, and Brandschaft (1994), among others, refer to a "new paradigm" developing in psychoanalysis. Mitchell (1988) refers to it as "relational-model theorizing"; infancy researchers (Beebe, Jaffe, & Lachmann, 1992) call it a "dyadic systems perspective"; Hoffman (1991) terms it "social constructivism"; and Stolorow and his colleagues (1992) call it "intersubjectivity theory." According to this "new paradigm," observers and their language are thought of as inextricably linked to the observed, and the impact of therapists and their organizing activity on the unfolding of the therapeutic relationship itself become a focus of analytic inquiry and reflection. The psychoanalyst views the individual's associations less as products of isolated, internal intrapsychic mechanisms and more as forming at the interface of interacting worlds of experience.

Greenberg and Mitchell (1983), in a landmark book, originally identified a "relational model" in psychoanalysis as an alternative to what they referred to as "classical drive theory." These authors suggested that: "… the most significant tension in the history of psychoanalytic ideas has been the dialectic between the original Freudian model … and an alternative comprehensive model … which evolves structure solely from the individual's relations with other people" (p. 20). Although even the most traditional psychoanalytic thinkers today have all but abandoned "drive theory," it appears that the essential tension within psychoanalysis between the "new paradigm" and other models revolves around the relative focus on the internal or intrapsychic models versus interactional, relational, or intersubjective models. The so-called "new paradigm" has a powerful influence on psychoanalytic theory and clinical practice. The relational or intersubjective perspective does not represent one coherent theory, but relational thinkers believe in a common outlook in which human relationships play a superordinate role in development, in the evolution of personality and of psychopathology, as well as in the practice of psychoanalytic therapy.

What is the relational perspective? According to Ghent (1992),

> Relational theorists have in common an interest in the intrapsychic as well as the interpersonal, but the intrapsychic is seen as constituted largely by the internalization of interpersonal experience mediated by the constraints imposed by biologically organized templates and delimiters. Relational theorists

tend also to share a view in which both reality and fantasy, both outer world and inner world, both the interpersonal and the intrapsychic, play immensely important and interactive roles in human life. Relational theorists do not substitute a naive environmentalism for drive theory. Due weight is given to what the individual brings to the interaction: temperament, bodily events, physiological responsivity, distinctive patterns of regulation and sensitivity.

The Relational Approach to Psychopathology

Relational thinkers tend to agree that clinical phenomena cannot be understood psychoanalytically apart from the intersubjective context or relational matrix in which they arise. Although this perspective can be applied to all forms and levels of psychopathology, we will focus on formulating the borderline personality disorder in relational terms. Relational and intersubjective theorists criticize the view that the term "borderline" designates a distinct personality structure rooted in intense conflicts and primitive defenses. Rather, relational theorists propose an alternative formulation of borderline phenomena largely from a developmental and self-psychological perspective, focusing on the particular stresses in relationships that elicit borderline defenses. In essence, what is referred to as "borderline" does not reside in a pathological condition located solely in the patient. Rather, what is thought to be borderline lies in phenomena arising in an intersubjective field or relational matrix consisting of a vulnerable self and a failing "archaic self-object" (the experience of a nonempathic caregiver rated in the past).

Brandschaft and Stolorow (1987) offer an intersubjective view of the borderline personality disorder. They suggest that the intense, often contradictory emotions that these patients express within the transference in psychotherapy and in particular, their virulent negative reactions indicate specific structural weaknesses and vulnerabilities rooted in early developmental interferences. Early needs for mirroring and idealizing become revived in the therapeutic transference, carrying with them hopes for a resuming development. When these needs are responded to and understood empathically, intense positive reactions follow. Likewise, when these needs are not recognized, understood, or responded to empathically, intense negative reactions ensue. The intense hostility and angry reactions of the borderline individual, it is thought, encapsulate memories of specific traumatic childhood experiences. In this sense, the term "borderline" is not seen as a pathological condition located exclusively within the patient. Rather, according to Brandchaft and Stolorow (1987) "... it refers to a phenomenon arising in an intersubjective field—a field consisting of a precarious, vulnerable self and a failing, archaic self-object. Viewing treatment as an intersubjective field, the patient's psychopathology is thought of as being codetermined by the patient's disorder of self and the therapist's capacity to understand and empathize with it."

Ingmar Bergmann's classic movie *Persona* will serve as a clinical illustration of the relational or intersubjective perspective. The movie illustrates the mental breakdown of a somewhat childish but decent young woman, a nurse responsible for the care of a psychologically severely ill woman presenting what could best be described as a narcissistic personality. The young nurse, subjected to intense criticism, virulent depreciation, and exploitation by the other woman, gradually broke down. She could not face the fact that the ill woman only responded to the nurse's love with hatred and was unable to acknowledge any loving or other human feeling toward her. It appeared that the sick woman could live only if and when she could destroy what was valuable in the nurse, although in the process she destroyed herself as a human being. In a dramatic segment, the nurse generated an intense hatred for the sick woman and mistreated her cruelly. If we consider the nurse as a therapist and the ill woman the patient, we can consider the movie from a relational point of view. Rather than seeing the sick woman as cruel and sadistic, an intersubjective or relational therapist might attempt to empathize with the woman's traumatic loss (the illness) and disintegration and regression as a way of protecting herself against any involvement with others for fear of getting hurt. Thinking of the nurse as the therapist, there was every indication that the nurse required the patient's responsiveness to maintain her own self-esteem and to regulate her own feelings. When frustrated, the nurse demonstrated her own narcissistic vulnerability and tendency toward borderline rage. In a similar fashion, the movie *Fatal Attraction* can be viewed from a relational perspective. Such a perspective would emphasize the ways Alex, "the other woman," was genuinely deceived, used and exploited by a highly self-centered, narcissistic husband who "cheated" on his devoted wife.

Relational and intersubjective theories have extended far beyond the clinical situation to include a distinct blend of American psychoanalytic feminism that has dealt with issues of sex and gender, as well as political theory and social criticism. Relational writers have shown a particular interest in studying and treating adults who suffered childhood sexual abuse. Davis and Frawley (1994) attempted to reconcile psychoanalysis with recent research on trauma. These investigations led the authors to propose that psychoanalysis reintroduce the notion of "dissociation." The phenomenon of dissociation, the splitting off of certain, often traumatic, experiences so as to preserve and protect the internal object world, is an important defense for those who have been traumatized in general and abused in particular. This treatment recognizes that therapy cannot take place in the verbal domain of interpretation alone but requires the active participation of the therapist, as patients replay the pivotal self- and object relational schemata of their traumatic childhoods.

The range and depth of issues addressed by relational clinicians and theorists are presenting a serious challenge to more traditional psychoanalytic theories. Although such challenges are far from new, they have invigorated and enlivened psychoanalytic debate and have contributed to an important shift toward a recognition of the centrality of relationships in human development and personality structure.

SUMMARY

This chapter was designed to provide an overview of modern psychoanalytic theory and practice. It emphasizes that psychoanalysis does not represent a single, monolithic theory but instead is comprised of several different theories of the mind that stand on their own in providing a coherent approach to human development and therapeutic practice and also influence one another. It explores in some detail four of the most prominent psychoanalytic theories: modern structural theory, self-psychology, the object relations theories, and the intersubjective theories. This chapter should make clear that psychoanalysis is an evolving enterprise. The theory is evolving as it is fertilized and cross-fertilized from within and also from without—from neurosciences, feminist theory, cognitive science, infant research, and other disciplines. Practice, too, is evolving as psychoanalytic institutes become more broad-based and attentive to a wider range of issues that need to be addressed within the larger community. Although it interacts with other disciplines, psychoanalysis remains unique in its focus on intensive, in-depth therapy, the central role of the unconscious, the formative impact of childhood experience and fantasy on the adult, and the centrality of human relationships. It is also unique in its attention to the full range of human experience.

REFERENCES

Adler, G. (1985). *Borderline psychopathology and its treatment*. New York: Jason Aronson.

Adler, G. (1989). Uses and limitations of Kohut's self psychology in the treatment of borderline patients. *Journal of the American Psychoanalytic Association, 37*, 761–785.

Akthar, S. (1995). A third individuation: Immigration, identity, and psychiatric process. *Journal of the American Psychoanalytic Association, 43*, 1051–1084.

Arlow, J. A. (1991). Conflict, trauma, and deficit. In S. Dowling (Ed.), *Conflict and compromise: Therapeutic implications* (pp. 3–14). Madison, CT: International Universities Press.

Beebe, B., Jaffe, J., & Lachmann, F. M. (1992). A didactic systems view of communication. In N. S. Skolnick & S. C. Warshaw (Eds.), *Relational perspectives in psychoanalysis* (pp. 61–28). Hillsdale, NJ: The Analytic Press.

Blatt, S. J., & Lerner, H. (1991). Psychodynamic perspectives on personality theory. In M. Hersen, A. E. Kazdin, & A. S. Bellack (Eds.), *The clinical psychology handbook*, 2nd ed. (pp. 147–169). New York: Pergamon.

Boesky, D. (1990). The psychoanalytic process and its components. *Psychoanalytic Quarterly, 59*, 550–584.

Bowlby, J. (1969). *Attachment and loss*, Vol. I: *Attachment*. New York: Basic Books.

Bowlby, J. (1973). *Attachment and loss*, Vol. II: *Separation: Anxiety and anger*. New York: Basic Books.

Brandschaft, B., & Stolorow, R. (1987). The borderline concept: An intersubjective viewpoint. In J. Grotstein, M. Solomon, & J. Lang (Eds.), *The borderline patient*, Vol. 2 (pp. 103–126). Hillsdale, NJ: The Analytic Press.

Brenner, C. (1982). *The mind in conflict*. New York: International Universities Press.

Burnham, D., Gladstone, A., & Gibson, R. (1969). *Schizophrenia and the need–fear dilemma*. New York: International Universities Press.

Chused, J. (1991). The evocative power of enactments. *Journal of the American Psychoanalytic Association, 39*, 615–640.

Davis, J. M., & Frawley, M. G. (1994). *Treating the adult survivor of childhood sexual abuse: A psychoanalytic perspective*. New York: Basic Books.

Fraiberg, S. (1959). *The magic years*. New York: Norton.

Ghent, E. (1992). Foreword. In N. J. Skolnick & S. C. Warshaw (Eds.), *Relational perspectives in psychoanalysis* (pp. xiii–xvii). Hillsdale, NJ: The Analytic Press.

Greenberg, J., & Mitchell, D. (1983). *Object relations and psychoanalytic theory*. Cambridge, MA: Harvard University Press.

Hoffman, I. Z. (1991). Discussion: Toward a social constructivist view of the psychoanalytic situation. *Psychoanalytic Dialogue, 1*, 74–105.

Holmes, D. (1992). Race and transference in psychoanalysis and psychotherapy. *International Journal of Psycho-Analysis, 73*, 1–12.

Jacobs, T. (1991). *The lure of the self*. Madison, CT: International Universities Press.

Kernberg, O. (1995). *Borderline conditions and pathological narcissism*. New York: Jason Aronson.

Kernberg, O. (1996). *Object relations theory and clinical psycho-analysis*. New York: Jason Aronson.

Kohut, H. (1971). *The analysis of the self*. New York: International Universities Press.

Kohut, H. (1977). *The restoration of the self*. New York: International Universities Press.

Kohut, H., & Wolf, E. S. (1978). The disorders of the self and their treatment: An outline. *International Journal of Psycho-Analysis, 59*, 413–425.

Mahler, M., Klein, F., & Bergman, A. (1975). *The psychoanalytic birth of the human infant*. New York: Basic Books.

Masterson, J., & Rinsley, D. (1975). The borderline syndrome, the role of the mother in the genesis and psychic structure of the borderline personality. *International Journal of Psycho-Analysis, 56*, 163–177.

McLaughlin, J. (1991). Clinical and theoretical aspects of enactment. *Journal of the American Psychoanalytic Association, 39*, 595–614.

Mitchell, S. A. (1988). *Relational concepts in psychoanalysis*. Cambridge, MA: Harvard University Press.

Mitchell, S. A., & Aron, L. (1999). Preface. In S. P. Mitchell & L. Aron (Eds.), *Relational psychoanalysis: The emergence of a tradition* (pp. ix–xx). Hillsdale, NJ: The Analytic Press.

Novick, J., & Novick, K. K. (1996). *Fearful symmetry: The development and treatment of sadomasochism*. New York: Jason Aronson.

Reiser, M. (1984). *Mind, brain, body: Toward a convergence of psychoanalysis and neurobiology*. New York: Basic Books.

Shevrin, H., Bond, J. A., Brakel, A. W., Hertel, R. K., & Williams, J. W. (1996). *Conscious and unconscious processes: Psychodynamic, cognitive, and neurophysiological convergences*. New York: Guilford.

Stern, D. N. (1985). *The interpersonal world of the infant*. New York: Basic Books.

Stolorow, R. (1975). Toward a functional definition of narcissism. *International Journal of Psycho-Analysis, 56*, 179–185.

Stolorow, R. (1983). Self-psychology—a structural psychology. In J. D. Lichtenberg and S. Kaplan (Eds.), *Reflections on self psychology* (pp. 287–296). Hillsdale, NJ: Erlbaum.

Stolorow, R., Atwood, G., & Brandschaft, B. (1988). *Psychoanalytic treatment: An intersubjective approach.* Hillsdale, NJ: The Analytic Press.

Stolorow, R., Brandschaft, B., & Atwood, G. (1992). *Contexts of being. The intersubjectivist foundation of psychological life.* Hillsdale, NJ: The Analytic Press.

Stolorow, R., Atwood, G., & Brandschaft, B. (1994). *The intersubjective perspective.* New York: Jason Aronson.

Tronick, E. Z., & Gianino, A. (1986). *Interactive mismatch and repair: Zero to three* (pp. 1–6).

Tyson, R. L. (1991). Psychological conflict in childhood. In S. Dowling (Ed.), *Conflict and compromise: Therapeutic implications* (pp. 31–48). Madison, CT: International Universities Press.

Wallerstein, R. S. (1983). Self psychology and "classical" psychoanalytic psychology—nature of their relationship. A review and overview. In J. D. Lichtenberg & S. Kaplan (Eds.), *Reflections on self psychology* (pp. 313–337). Hillsdale, NJ: Erlbaum.

Willock, M. D. (1990). Psychoanalytic concepts of the etiology of severe mental illness. *Journal of the American Psychoanalytic Association, 38,* 1049–1081.

Willock, M. D. (1991). Working with conflict and deficit in borderline and narcissistic patients. In S. Dowling (Ed.), *Conflict and compromise: Therapeutic implications* (pp. 77–94). Madison, CT: International Universities Press.

Winnicott, D. (1949/1981). The ordinary devoted mother. In M. Davis and D. Wallbridge (Eds.), *Boundary and space* (pp. 125–130). New York: Brunner/Mazel.

5

Behavioral Model

Warren W. Tryon

Introduction

Abnormal psychology is concerned with psychological and behavioral disorder. The medical model of abnormal psychology addresses etiology, diagnosis (including assessment), and treatment. The behavioral model of abnormal psychology described later also addresses these topics but in a substantively different manner. We consider each of these topics in the following sections. Briefly, etiology concerns the origins of disorder. Whereas the medical model looks for a pathogen of some kind, the behavioral model looks to principles of learning to find the causes of behavioral development, including both normal and abnormal outcomes. This means that abnormal behavior derives from a normal learning process but results in maladaptive outcomes. In other words, abnormal behavior is governed by the same laws of learning as normal behavior; abnormal behaviors are learned the same way as normal behaviors. Therefore, learning is the central causative process in the behavioral model. Learning implies memory, for without some way to retain what has been learned, development cannot be cumulative. Hence, learning and memory are the two primary psychological pillars upon which the behavioral model rests. It should be noted that all psychological explanations of normal and abnormal behavior, grounded in any and all psychological models, are based on learning and memory because there is no other way to implement psychological development. In other words, all psychological explanations (models) are based on an implied or explicit learning theory; they differ only in what is said to be learned and how learning is presumed to take place.[1] Operant and respondent conditioning are two traditional areas of learning research upon which the behavioral model rests, and therefore we cover these areas. Considerably more

---

[1] Formal recognition of learning and memory as the central psychological processes from which all psychological development flows is an important step toward theoretical unification. Behavioral models explicitly recognize these processes. Psychodynamic and cognitive models discuss the results of learning and thereby imply some form of learning theory. Explicit formulations about mechanisms of learning and memory are needed. Connectionist neural network models implement explicit theories of learning and memory to explain perception, cognition, and language acquisition in addition to operant and respondent conditioning. See Tryon (1993a, 1993b, 1994, 1995a, 1995b, 1995c, 1995d, 1996, 1998a, in press) for further comments by this author.

Warren W. Tryon • Department of Psychology, Fordham University, Bronx, New York 10458-5198.

Advanced Abnormal Psychology, Second Edition, edited by Hersen and Van Hasselt. Kluwer Academic/Plenum Publishers, New York, 2001.

attention is paid to operant conditioning because it plays a correspondingly larger role (cf. Ayllon, & McKittrick, 1982; Cohen, & Filipczak, 1971; Kazdin, 1977; Parker, 1996). We briefly consider recent developments in the field of learning called Neural Network Learning Theory (NNLT) that unifies animal and human learning from simple habit formation through complex cognitive processing, language development, and memory. Therefore, NNLT provides a comprehensive theoretical basis for learning that sets the occasion for unifying schools of behaviorism with mainstream psychology.

Most psychologists and psychiatrists rely on the *Diagnostic and Statistical Manual*, currently in its fourth edition (APA, 1994), for diagnosis. This atheoretical nonetiological medically based system is not very informative for those working from the behavioral model. Therefore, we consider an alternative diagnostic system based on a taxonomy of operant conditioning that identifies at least eight important diagnostic conditions, each of which has clear treatment implications to guide intervention. The happy result is that diagnosis leads to treatment recommendations.

The title of this chapter incorrectly suggests that a single, monolithic, unified and universally endorsed behavioral model based on a coherent universally endorsed behaviorism exists and that this chapter describes it. Unfortunately, behaviorism is a theoretical belief system much like Protestantism, or any other ism for that matter, in that it entails many different factions that continue to change over time. We begin this chapter with a brief review of what have been termed three generations of behaviorism (Staats, 1996) to illustrate the extent to which behaviorism has changed over time and is currently composed of divergent schools and camps. This chapter could have been written from any one of these perspectives. It is not possible to review them all adequately in a single chapter nor is that my intention. Critics of the behavioral model typically focus on first or second generation behaviorisms and ignore third generation behaviorism because it makes their task easier. I, on the other hand, attempt to draw on the strengths of each facet of the behavioral model plus neural network learning theory in an effort to present the "best" behavioral model.

A Short History of Behaviorism

Behaviorism is not a unified theoretical point of view. Bolles (1979) reviewed what he terms "The Classical Heritage" with separate chapters on Thorndike, Pavlov, Watson, Guthrie, Tolman, Hull, and Skinner. Malone (1990) more recently reviewed the same schools of behaviorism. Staats (1996, p. 1) identified three generations of behaviorism. We briefly review each of them.

First Generation

Staats (1996) attributes the first generation of behaviorism to John B. Watson (1913, 1930) and his earlier studies on conditioned emotional reactions with Raynor (Watson & Raynor, 1920). This initial statement of behaviorism is what most people think of. Watson contrasted his objective behavioral psychology to the then dominant introspective (subjective) American psychology of E. B. Titchener and William James. Psychology was to focus on behavior and behavior alone. Consciousness and other psychological states were considered neither definite nor scientifically usable. They reflected a mind–body dualism, and Watson was a materialistic monist. Explanations based on subjective states were to be replaced by objective scientific accounts of behavior. Stimuli and responses were operationally defined, and experimental designs were used to identify causal relationships among them. Pavlov's conditioned reflexes were highlighted, along with elementary principles of physiology. Watson acknowledged that some primitive behaviors evolved with our species, but he denied the existence of what were then and now called instincts, along with talent, handedness, temperament, mental abilities, and personality characteristics. Essentially all behaviors and emotional responses were learned, it was thought, through conditioning beginning with a *tabula rasa*. Watson assumed that every child is equally capable of learning every behavior and emotional response. Personality was considered the sum total of learned habits. Thought was viewed as self-talk. Watson was careful to deny that thought equaled laryngeal movement because he observed that people can think after their larynx has been removed. He maintained that muscular habits learned during speech acquisition were involved in thought.

Second Generation

Staats (1996, p. 2) associates Skinner (1938, 1945, 1953, 1957, 1966, 1969, 1971, 1974), Hull (1943), MacCorquodale and Meehl (1948), Spence (1944), and Tolman (1932) with behaviorism's second generation. The emphasis remains upon publicly observable behavior, that which can be videotaped. Much more will be said later about Skinner in the section on Operant Conditioning because he was such an influential proponent of behaviorism and because he was and is so frequently misunderstood.

Third Generation

Staats (1966, p. 3) identifies himself (Staats, 1964, 1968, 1971, 1975, 1981, 1986, 1993, 1996) with behaviorism's third generation. Although he initially termed this approach paradigmatic behaviorism, Tryon (1990) maintained that his efforts were more accurately termed psychological behaviorism and that became the title of a subsequent article (Staats, 1993) and the subtitle of his most recent book (Staats's, 1996). Staats uses the term unified positivism to describe this approach. He endorses the general values of science, including observation, measurement, and experimentation, and endorses general theory construction values of empirical definition, consistency, generalizability, and parsimony but is open to and actively encourages the use of psychological constructs. Basic Behavioral Repertoires (BBRs) constitute personality in his view. The following are some of the most prominent BBRs. The Verbal-Motor Repertoire involves the ability to understand language and use it to regulate behavior. The Verbal-Image Repertoire involves the ability of language to elicit a conditioned sensory response. The Verbal-Emotional Repertoire involves the ability of language to elicit emotions. The Verbal-Labeling Repertoire enables the person to respond verbally to external stimuli. The Verbal-Association Repertoire enables communication, problem solving, and mathematics. The Verbal-Imitation Repertoire enables language to govern behavior. The Verbal-Writing Repertoire connects language with written expression. The Sensory-Motor Repertoire connects stimuli with action. The Emotional-Motivational Repertoire entails affect and those factors that drive behavior. Standard psychological tests, such as IQ tests, are considered to entail standard behavioral samples. Performance on these tests quantifies specific BBRs. It should be easy to see why this approach is now termed psychological behaviorism.

Baldwin and Baldwin (1998) report that although early behaviorists focused their attention mainly on overt behavior, recent developments have stressed thinking, feeling, awareness, and self-efficacy (p. 332). They further assert that thinking is covert behavior (p. 333). They credit Homme (1965) with coining the term coverant to refer to thought as covert behavior.

Bandura (1977), Mahoney (1974), Michel (1981), Staats (1968, 1975), and Rosenthal and Zimmerman (1978) summarized research on covert operants. Martin and Pear (1999) describe "thinking" and "feeling" as "two fundamental behavioral categories" (p. 345). They criticize introductory psychology texts as incorrectly saying that practitioners of behavior modification ignore what goes on inside the person (p. 347). Martin and Pear (1999) write, "we assume that the principles and procedures of operant and respondent conditioning apply to private as well as to public behavior" (p. 348).

Cognition frequently entails the concept of equivalence, and behaviorists have recently developed methods for establishing equivalence. Sidman (1992), Sidman, Kirk, and Willson-Morris (1985), and Sidman and Tailby (1982) describe methods for producing equivalence classes. Plaud, Gaither, Weller, Bigwood, Barth, and von Duvillard (1998) describe the relevance of equivalence classes to behavior therapy. Behaviorists are now addressing clearly cognitive behaviors.

ETIOLOGY

Etiology involves the question of how behavioral disorder develops. The medical model describes normal functioning with one set of terms and explains abnormal functioning in terms of trauma or pathogens that interfere with normal functioning. The behavioral model differs primarily in that a single set of principles is used to describe both normal and abnormal behavior. One can argue that there is no such thing as *abnormal* behavior per se because all behavior is produced by the same "normal" learning principles, natural laws, that govern all behavior. Only the learned outcome is abnormal. By way of analogy, gravity causes all things to fall down. Sometimes gravity is "good" such as when fruit falls to the earth resulting in food for people and animals and causing seeds to be dispersed. At other times gravity is "bad" such as when objects fall from a construction site and injure or kill a passerby. Alternatively, we could describe gravity as "normal" when it leads to "good" outcomes and "abnormal" when it leads to "bad," but this is silly. Gravity per se is neither normal nor abnormal, nor is it good or bad. These evaluative terms describe gravity-related events. Learning principles are like gravity in that they sometimes lead to desirable outcomes and sometimes to undesirable outcomes. We begin our discussion of learning principles with operant conditioning because it formed an early basis of behavior therapy and continues as fundamental knowledge, although it is frequently misunderstood.

Operant Conditioning

GENERAL STATEMENT

Skinner is frequently thought of as a stimulus–response (S-R) psychologist. He is *not!* He is a response–stimulus (R-S) psychologist. Describing Skinner as a S-R theorist gets matters backwards. Skinner (1938) carefully distinguished his *operant* R-S psychology from Pavlov's *respondent* S-R psychology by emphasizing the organism's ability to *choose* whether or not to behave versus responding reflexively to stimuli. Operant conditioning is about choice; to respond or not respond, that is the question. We will see that choice is not really free even when it appears to be. In other words, operant conditioning involves environmental (social as well as physical) consequences that restrict choices and make them predictable. The greater the restriction, the more certain the outcome, the harder the determinism. Skinner (1971) addresses these matters at length in his book *Beyond Freedom and Dignity*.

What makes Skinner's approach to explaining behavior so radical and a major reason why he is so frequently misunderstood is that, like Darwin, he employed a novel and counter-intuitive form of explanation. We ordinarily think that causation occurs sequentially in time and that the cause *precedes* the effect. Therefore, one looks for causes *immediately before* the event. This is what S-R (respondent) psychology does. Conditioned stimuli occur immediately before conditional responses. Skinner's R-S (operant) approach entails looking for its cause *after* the behavioral event. There are two somewhat subtle issues here. First, although the consequence that follows an event (behavior) cannot be the cause of that behavioral instance, it does precede and therefore can influence future instances of the same behavior. Hence, this strategy can be used to explain all but the very first instance of a behavior and that encompasses the subject's entire life except for the moment during which the first instance occurred. The operant explanation for the first instance of a new behavior brings us to the second subtle issue which is that each behavior is actually a *class or distribution of behaviors*. Operants are technically classes of behaviors because it is not possible to exactly repeat the same behavior twice. Minor variations in response topography (form, intensity, duration) inevitably occur. For example, the force with which a rat or human presses a bar or button for a reinforcer will not be exactly the same every time. If a strain gauge is attached to the bar (button), repeated measurements will reveal that a *distribution* of forces was applied. All of these slightly different behaviors are included in the operant class of "bar press" or "button press." Consequences associated with previous instances of an operant causally influence (shape) the operant distribution and consequently the future probability of the operant under similar circumstances.[2] Consequences can gradually shape (edit) the response distribution until it is sufficiently different that a new name is needed. For example, rewarding more and more vigorous bar presses will result in a new behavior better called hitting or slamming than pressing. Hence, the first instance of hitting the bar can be said to have evolved from selective reinforcement of bar pressing. Darwin used the same principles of variation and selection to explain the origin of new species.

Sober (1984; pp. 99–100) illustrates the basic elements of selectionist causation by using a child's toy composed of a vertical cylinder that has three equally spaced inserts, like floors in an office building. Each floor has holes of different diameters cut into it. The top floor has large holes, the middle floor has medium holes, and the bottom floor has small holes. Four sets of colored balls are inserted from the top by the manufacturer, and the device is sealed. When the device is placed upright, the balls fall through the three sieves "selecting for" balls of various diameter. The largest balls exceed the diameter of even the largest holes in the top level and are "selected" to stay there. Those balls whose diameter is less than the width of the holes in the top layer but greater than the holes in the middle layer pass through the top sieve but not the middle one and are "selected" to stay there. Only the smallest balls make it to the bottom and are "selected" to be there.

A similar explanation pertains to the reason that the planets in our solar system orbit as they do and why the rings around Saturn are as we find them. In both cases, we observe what remains after a dynamic developmental period has ended. The systematic result appears to have been designed, to have purpose and intention, and we readily make such attributions because we focus on what remains rather than what initially was and what disappeared; both of which are currently unavailable for observation and therefore are not easily recognized as

---

[2]I refer to similar circumstances because it is theoretically impossible for exactly the same circumstances ever to occur twice except maybe under the most highly controlled laboratory conditions. Exact replications of circumstances probably never occur naturally.

causal variables. We more readily understand what we currently see as the product of direct creation, and this includes choices to behave one way versus another. Current attributions are readily understood as proximal causes, but the prior causal processes of variation and selection that gave rise to current attributions lie in the past and are frequently ignored because they are unavailable even through introspection. These distal causal factors that govern variation and selection frequently go unnoticed. Emphasis on salient proximal psychological mediators of behavior frequently has the unfortunate effect of terminating any further search for causal factors (selection and variation) because a strong impression has been created that all relevant causal factors have been identified. This is what Skinner meant when he said that intrapsychic explanations often get in the way of a more effective functional analytic explanation and why he did not accept "psychological" explanations (Skinner, 1977). The behavioral model focuses our attention on selection and the way it modifies behavioral variation over time. In other words, the behavioral model concerns itself with ontogenetic behavioral evolution.

Skinner's (1963, 1966, 1975, 1981, 1984a, 1984b) "evolutionary" explanation of onto-genetic behavioral development is the same functional argument that Darwin used to explain phylogenetic evolution. It is generally unknown that Darwin took a "black box" approach to biology just as Skinner did to psychology. Darwin had no choice in the matter because the science of genetics had yet to develop and consequently no proximal causal mechanism for the way variation came about and how natural selection could alter such variation was available. Consequently, acceptance of evolutionary theory by scientists was neither rapid nor without serious reservation. Bowler's (1983) book entitled *The Eclipse of Darwinism* details how Darwin's theory nearly became extinct (Catania, 1978, 1987). Although Darwin provided an ultimate causal explanation for the origin and extinction of species, he did not because he could not specify the proximal causal biological mechanisms by which variation and selection operated based on genetic mechanisms that were not yet understood. Mayr (1982) reported that scientific acceptance of Darwin's evolutionary theory waited more than *75 years* until the modern synthesis with population genetics occurred.

Failing to benefit from Darwin's experience, Skinner deliberately ignored questions about plausible proximal causal mechanisms by which selection (consequences) shapes behavioral variation. He attempted to limit psychology to a black box study of environment–behavior relationships and to leave to neuroscience all questions of proximal causal mechanisms by which behavior varies and environmental consequences exert their influence on behavior. He also correctly argued that formal theory was not necessary to experimentally identify lawful environment–behavior relationships (Skinner, 1950). Because this was all that psychology was supposed to do, no other role for theory was acknowledged. These actions confused and alienated many psychologists and made it difficult for them to appreciate that he used the same functional explanatory logic of variation and selection that Darwin had used and was now well accepted as scientifically valid. Skinner explained development in terms of ontogenetic (within the subject's life time) evolution. Tryon (1993b) discusses this issue at length. Herrnstein (1989), under the heading *Ontogenetic Parallel to Natural Selection*, wrote, "I refer to reinforcement theory. First, I describe the theory qualitatively, then I show that its mathematical structure is *identical* with that of evolution by natural selection, to the extent that those structures are known at the present time" (p. 41; emphasis added). He further stated that "Reinforcement, like evolution, is a matter of variation and selection" (p. 42). His discussion of conditioning followed under the heading "A Formal Theory of Selection" (pp. 44–54). Herrnstein maintained that "... the central theory of modern behaviourism displaces purpose in the analysis of individual behaviour by a formal structure that is the ontogenetic parallel to natural selection in evolution" (p. 41). Donahoe (1984) concurs that Skinner's ontogenetic evolution faces the same intellectual impediments as Darwin's phylogenetic evolution. The absence of proximal causal explanations for the way behavioral variation and selection work have, and continue to preclude broad acceptance of Skinner's functional explanations (Tryon, 1993b). Recent advances described later called Neural Network Learning Theory (NNLT) promise to provide the requisite proximal causal mechanisms and may consequently set the stage for much broader acceptance of Skinner's contributions.

A CLOSER LOOK AT SELECTION

Now, we consider variation and selection in greater detail. Repeated measurements of any behavior (or any variable for that matter) yield a distribution when measurement is sufficiently accurate and fine-grained (precise). A statistical distribution can be graphed by following the directions in any basic statistics book. Such a figure identifies the different possible measurement values along the horizontal x-axis (abscissa) and the frequency with which they occur along the vertical y-axis (ordinate). A bell-shaped normal curve frequently results where the average value lies near the middle of the measurement scale. The mean of this distribution can be increased or decreased (changed) by selection. If we delete the lowest 10% of the data points, the new mean will be larger than the original mean. If we delete the highest 10% of the data points, the new mean will be lower than the original mean. Behavioral genetic studies of selective breeding are informative. We talk about shaping a behavior, but we are actually shaping a distribution of instances of that behavior. For example, consider the distribution of the number of trials it takes for a group of rats to learn to run a maze correctly. Some take more trials than others. Tryon (1931) created a strain of "maze bright" rats by selectively breeding the males and females who took the fewest trials to learn to run a maze and a strain of "maze dull" rats by selectively breeding the males and females who took the most trials to learn to run a maze. As expected, the average number of trials to run the maze correctly decreased over generations for the "maze bright" strain and increased for the "maze dull" strain. Selection was the key causal factor here. DeFries, Gervais, and Thomas (1978) measured open field activity in mice. They mated the more active males with the more active females and the less active males with the less active females. Such selective breading produced a strain of high-activity and a strain of low-activity mice over 30 generations resulting in two nonoverlapping activity distributions. Again, selection was the causal variable. Other examples can be taken from nature. Consider a distribution of the running speed of cheetahs eons ago. The slower ones were less likely to survive and successfully raise young, thereby leaving the faster cats to breed. Over time, the average running speed of cheetahs increased.

Skinner argued that an analogous process occurs with behavior. For example, dogs greet their owners each time they come home and necessarily do so in various ways. Likewise, the owner's pet greeting behaviors also vary. Presume that owners respond to their pets on most days except for those times when the dogs greet in the least vigorous way. The dogs are therefore attended to on most days except when they greet in the least vigorous way. The result of this *selective* experience is to increase (reinforce) the more vigorous forms of greeting and decrease (extinguish) the less vigorous forms of greetings thereby changing (increasing) the average vigor of the dogs' greetings and thereby increasing the probability of being attended to by their owners.

The owners' behaviors, as we previously said, are not constant which means that on some days they are less attentive than on other days. These inattentive days mean that sometimes the dogs go unnoticed unless they use especially vigorous greetings. This experience removes an even larger segment of the dogs' less vigorous greeting behaviors thereby restricting the dogs' options to more aggressive forms of greeting behavior. The owners may take evasive actions to avoid the pets' new behavior that requires even more aggressive greeting behavior by the dogs to get responses. However, the pet owner's response may no longer be friendly. The dog may be punished for being too rough. Or, the owner may respond positively and therefore reinforce this new more aggressive greeting. This increases the average vigor of greeting and teaches that a range of even more aggressive greeting behavior may need to be displayed in future to get their owner's attention. We can clearly see a problem developing here but neither the pet nor its owner is likely to be aware of what is happening. Attributions will be made about the dog's character, about its instincts, and about almost everything but the ontogenetic evolutionary process that systematically shaped the undesirable behavior. The pet owner will blame the dog and their strong feelings may result in punishing the dog by the owner for *its* "bad" behavior. This is very confusing for the dog because it did only what was necessary to get attention. Punishment will reduce the intensity of the greeting behavior especially if it is administered swiftly, intensely, and consistently but such actions create undesirable long-term effects (from both the owner's and dog's perspectives). Unfortunately, punishment rapidly achieves short-term objectives of behavioral suppression that reinforces the user, thereby increasing the probability of using punishment in the future. An opposite example could be constructed where instances of behaviors at the low end of the greeting distribution are reinforced and those at the high end are extinguished, thereby resulting in a lower mean.

Reinforcement is Skinner's way of talking about selection. A reinforcer increases the future probability that the target behavior will occur under similar circumstances. Systematic selection over time, called shaping, causes behavioral development by shaping the distribution of one or more behaviors. This process is continually at work whether or not we are aware of it. Shaping can be positive, for example, when parents and teachers use it to augment academic, social, or athletic skills, or it can be negative as illustrated by the coercive family process whereby children are taught to use aversive methods to modify the behavior of family, friends, and teachers (Patterson, 1979, 1982, 1997). Martin and Pear (1999) contains sections beginning with the word "Pitfalls" where they explain how various forms of selection lead to behavioral problems with or without awareness by the participants. A comprehensive presentation of these selection methods (conditioning) is provided later under the heading "Taxonomy of Instrumental Conditioning."

MELIORATION

Herrnstein (1990) and Herrnstein and Vaughn (1980) use the term melioration to describe the importance of momentary consequences on behavior; organisms tend to maximize current outcomes. The authors maintain that reinforcement, natural selection, is a local rather than global phenomenon in that it pertains to the moment, rather than long-term outcome. Overeating, alcoholism, promiscuity, sedentariness, crime, and drug addiction are examples of short-term benefits that outweigh long-term costs for many people. Hence, melioration is a good model of human behavioral disorder, despite its development in the animal laboratory.

Respondent Conditioning

Pavlov was a physiologist, not a psychologist. The full title of his book is *Conditioned Reflexes: An Investigation of the Physiological Activity of the Cerebral Cortex*. We might say that Pavlov was the first neuropsychologist because he was interested in the way the cerebral cortex mediates learned behavior. He sought to study how the frontal lobes governed the acquisition and modification of simple behaviors. Frequently called classical conditioning, respondent conditioning is more descriptive because it is concerned with the way subjects respond to stimuli.

Anrep created a major misunderstanding when he mistranslated Pavlov's (1927/1960) Russian word condition*al* as the English word condition*ed*. Hence he wrote about condition*ed* reflexes rather than condition*al* reflexes. The minor change of two letters in one word renders a world of difference in meaning. Conditional reflexes, like conditional probability, depend on other factors. When these factors are no longer present (extinction), the conditional reflex decreases and may disappear.

Operant and respondent conditioning are often considered quite different. There are at least two reasons for questioning this view. First, Tryon (1976a) demonstrates that respondent conditioning is formally equivalent to two simultaneous operant reinforcement contingencies (see more about this later). Second, Donahoe (1991) and Donahoe and Palmer (1994, pp. 49–52) note that operant and respondent conditioning procedures appear similar to the subject even though they appear different to psychologists, because environmental stimuli are always present and the subject is always behaving thereby creating an ongoing S-R stream. Presenting a biologically active uncondition*al* stimulus (UCS) classically conditions the preceding stimulus and operantly conditions the preceding response, thereby making both procedures part of the same learning experience.

Modern day neuropsychologists such as LeDoux (1996) study how fear, escape, and avoidance are learned and how the brain forms corresponding memories based on respondent conditioning. Rescorla (1987, 1988) has written two very important articles summarizing the goal-oriented information processing nature of respondent conditioning. Respondent conditioning can be considered another mechanism by which behavioral selection occurs. For example, rats naturally prefer dark spaces. If shock is delivered while a rat is in a dark place, it can be made to fear the dark and "choose" to avoid dark places in future.

Neural Network Learning Theory

Advances in learning theory have recently been made that are important to the behavioral model, the cognitive model, and all of psychology. These developments have been referred to as Connectionist Neural Networks (CNNs), Artificial Neural Networks (ANNs), and Parallel Distributed Processing (PDP). I have written about these developments and their significance for behavior therapy and psychology under the heading Neural Network Learning Theory (NNLT) to emphasize the unification of neuroscience and psychology that this approach entails (Tryon, 1993a, 1993b, 1994, 1995a, 1995b, 1995c, 1995d, 1996, 1998a, 1999). Various books on this topic are also available (Churchland & Sejnowski, 1992; Commons, Grossberg, & Staddon, 1991; Dayhoff, 1990; Grossberg, 1988; Hertz, Krogh, & Palmer, 1991; Kahanna, 1990; Levine, 1991; Lisboa, 1992; Martindale, 1991; Nelson & Illingworth, 1991; Pao, 1989; Ritter, Martinetz, & Schulten, 1992; Selverston, 1985; Wasserman, 1989) in addition to Rumelhart and McClelland's (1986) seminal two-volume work. NeuralWare's NeuralWorks Professional II/Plus™ software comes with more than 900 pages of documentation that describe several different types of neural networks. Tryon (1995a) lists other software vendors. SPSS now has a neural network module. Feldman and Ballard (1982) describe the general properties of connectionist models. Therefore, only a brief account is given here.

Neural Architecture

ANNs are composed of at least two, frequently three, and sometimes more layers of nodes that are first approximations to real neurons in that they (1) have structures analogous to dendrites along which input is received, (2) have structures analogous to axons along which output flows, and (3) simulate synapses that connect one neuron to another. Like real neurons,

ANNs summate inputs and become active, "fire," or not depending on whether their activation level exceeds a nonlinear sigmoidal activation (threshold) function.

LEARNING FUNCTION

Neuroscience has established that all human and animal learning, entails synaptic modification (Donahoe & Palmer, 1994; Kandel, 1989, 1991; Rosenzweig, 1996). Short-term and long-term memory learning entail different neurobiological processes too complicated to summarize here, but the same processes are found across the phylogenetic continuum which means that humans and animals learn in the same way at the biological level. Various learning functions, expressed as mathematical equations, exist for modifying connection weights that are analogous to synapses. Positive weights are excitatory, negative weights are inhibitory. Experience alters these weights, thereby changing the pattern of excitatory and inhibitory synaptic states across the network. Hebb (1949) was probably the first psychologist to suggest that learning entailed systematically changing "synaptic" weights, and therefore one such learning function is called the Hebbian learning function in his honor. These "synaptic" changes are primarily responsible for the development of functional capacity that we take as evidence of learning, though neural architecture plays an important role as well.

EMERGENT PROPERTIES

ANNs typically begin "life" with small random values for synaptic weights.[3] The simulated organism cannot do much of psychological or behavioral interest in this state. Experience modifies synaptic weights in accordance with a learning function so that the new weights lead to more effective behavior. Learning functions produce convergence between present and desired behavior. In other words, the pattern of synaptic weights converges toward a "best fit" state during the learning process. The term "best fit" is used here in a way that is similar to regression where a "best fitting" regression line is drawn through a data set to minimize the sum of squared differences between observed and predicted values. The "best fit" for synaptic weights corresponds to maximum (correct) performance. The final functional properties of the network are said to emerge through training as the pattern of synaptic weights converges on a "best fit" configuration. A very partial list of NNLT simulation explanations of operant conditioning includes Commons, Grossberg, and Staddon (1991), Donegan, Gluck, and Thompson (1989), Gluck and Thompson (1987), Grossberg and Levine (1987), Grossberg and Schmajuk (1987, 1989), Hawkins (1989), Kehoe (1988), Klopf (1988), and Sutton and Barto (1981).

OTHER PROPERTIES

ANNs respond holistically. The entire network forms memories and makes decisions. It does *not* use if-then logical rules to perform cognition, learn language, or perform any other complex task. It does *not* have a central processor and a separate memory storage system like

---

[3]Biological preparedness (Seligman & Hager, 1972) can be accomplished by presetting synaptic weights so that full functionality occurs readily with little or no training. Lions are genetically prepared to hunt and quickly learn to kill by observing their mothers do so. Synaptic weights for effective hunting behavior have apparently been set to approximately correct values, and little change is needed through learning. Spiders, on the other hand, know how to weave a web immediately upon hatching. Their synaptic weights have obviously been set genetically to "final" or "adult" levels.

computers and therefore differs radically from traditional information processing models although ANNs are parallel information processing systems of a kind. An ANN processes "experiences" associated with operant and respondent conditioning the same way that it processes all information. NNLT accounts for a wide variety of human and animal behavior, including cognition, and therefore fosters theoretical unification. Tryon (1995b, 1996) demonstrated that NNLT is completely consistent with important behavioral values and important cognitive values and thereby provides a theoretical perspective that synthesizes both the cognitive and behavioral models. Moreover, NNLT is highly compatible with neuroscience, thereby integrating psychology with biology. These remarkable theoretical advances may provide the basis for a unified psychology and will hopefully get us past chapters like the present one on models that emphasize a single point of view.

Behavioral Diagnosis

Medical diagnosis of infectious disease entails detecting a pathogen responsible for observed symptoms of the disease. Illness is viewed as a corruption of normal physiological processes. Behaviorism is based on learning principles that pertain equally well to normal and abnormal behavior; there is no counterpart to the pathogen. Maladaptive behavior is learned by the same "normal" learning principles as adaptive behavior. Learning principles are scientific laws and therefore are neither normal nor abnormal.

Diagnosis can be understood more broadly in a technological way as a process of identifying reasons for a current problem. For example, a computer malfunction can be *diagnosed* as the result of a faulty circuit board or incorrect software code. Similarly, behaviorists can diagnose behavioral disorder in terms of the unfortunate, unintended, unanticipated, and unwanted application of learning principles. We will mainly consider operant conditions that are known as sufficient causes of behavioral disorder organized as a taxonomy of operant conditioning.

An important therapeutic objective is substantial beneficial change. Identification of *modifiable* causal variables is primarily important because it enables clinicians to focus intervention on factors that can be altered to bring about the desired change. Not all causal variables are modifiable. Some original causal events, like childhood sexual abuse and other trauma, are historical and cannot be changed which is primarily the reason that behaviorists are less concerned with the past than the present. Behavior therapists focus on what can be changed to improve adjustment and enhance functioning. Haynes (1992), Haynes and O'Brien (1990), Haynes, Spain, and Oliveria (1993), Haynes, et al. (1993), and O'Brien and Haynes (1995) discuss ways of identifying clinically relevant causal variables that are beyond the scope of this chapter. We focus on the subset of causal variables known as reinforcement contingencies because they are important causes of behavior and behavioral change.

A Taxonomy of Operant Conditioning

Contingent relationships between behaviors and consequences are causal factors in all normal and abnormal behavioral change in animals and humans. Some of these contingent relationships strengthen behavior, whereas others weaken behavior. We use the term "reinforcement contingency" to refer to all of these relationships between behaviors and consequences. A vast scientific animal and human literature has clearly demonstrated that reinforcement contingencies have causal properties. This point is especially relevant to the contemporary search for empirically supported treatments. The taxonomy presented below organizes these effective methods of behavioral change into a system that can be used to describe the problem and to recommend corrective actions. Behavioral diagnosis thereby frequently leads to behavior therapy, which is much more than can be said for a DSM diagnosis. Hayes and Follette (1992) have called for at least supplementing DSM categorization with a functional analysis which is what using the taxonomy entails.

Single Contingencies

Woods (1974) used line diagrams to operationally define 16 instrumental (operant) conditioning procedures along with clear verbal definitions. He organized these principles into a taxonomy that I expanded (Tryon, 1976a, 1976b, 1998b). The most current version is shown in Table 1 and includes extinction. The marginal entries on the left distinguish between response emission and omission. One typically focuses on the emission, presence, of behavior, but sometimes it is more clinically important to focus on what is *not* happening, the omission of the target behavior[4] because behavioral disorder can frequently be defined in terms of what is not happening, as well as what is going on. For example, a child who is out-of-seat during class is also not following rules, not doing assignments, not paying attention, etc. Alternative treatment formulations frequently follow from these different perspectives. For example, focusing on the emission of out-of-seat behavior suggests decreasing this behavior. The result is a child who remains seated. This may meet the behavioral objective of the referring teacher or parent, but it is not the most productive outcome. Interest in what the child is not doing while out-of-seat can lead to the differential reinforcement of alternative behaviors, such as assignment completion, that sets the occasion for sitting in-seat, paying attention, following directions, and improving academic skills.

The next left marginal entry in Table 1 is positive and negative reinforcers. One must first determine whether a specified consequence functions as a positive or negative reinforcer (see reinforcer identification section later). This can be done in a pilot study. If behavior increases contingent on the presentation of the stimulus, then it is a positive reinforcer because it strengthens behavior. Because the word reinforce always means to strengthen, negative reinforcement also entails an increase in the frequency, intensity, and/or duration of behavior but in reverse. Instead of leaving the stimulus off and contingently turning it on, the stimulus is continuously on and contingently turned off. Such stimuli are frequently aversive, and their termination brings relief. Consequently, terminating such stimuli contingent on the emission of a response is called relief conditioning in Table 1. Nagging is one such stimulus. Its termination contingent on a response increases the probability of that behavior; nagging offset reinforces (strengthens) that behavior. We represent positive reinforcers with a plus (+) sign and negative reinforcers with a minus (−) sign.

The next three columns indicate whether there has been an onset, offset, or no change in stimuli which have previously been identified as positive or negative reinforcers. Reward conditioning is defined as the onset or increase of a positive reinforcer contingent on the emission of the target behavior. Its effect is to increase the frequency, rate, or probability of the target behavior. The other way to increase the frequency, rate, or probability of the target

---

[4]Our emphasis on emission over omission parallels our tendency to explain what we see in terms of creative purposive forces rather than in terms of what was initially present (variation) and what was removed (extinction); see our discussion of ontogenetic evolution.

TABLE 1. Taxonomy of Operant Conditioning[a]

		Consequent event unsignaled			Consequent event signaled		
		Onset or increase	No change	Offset or decrease	Onset of increase	No change	Offset or decrease
Response emission	Positive reinforcer +	E^+ ↑ Reward[b]	$E+$ ↓ Extinction	E_+ ↓ Penalty	sE^+ ↑ Signaled reward	$sE+$ ↓ Signaled extinction	sE_+ ↓ Signaled penalty
	Negative reinforcer −	E^- ↓ Punish	$E-$ ↓ Extinction	E_- ↑ Relief	sE^- ↓ Signaled punish	$sE-$ ↓ Signaled extinction	sE_- ↑ Signaled relief
Response omission	Positive reinforcer +	O^+ ↓ Omission reward	$O+$ ↑ Omission extinction	O_+ ↑ Omission penalty	sO^+ ↓ Signaled omission reward	$sO+$ ↑ Signaled extinction	sO_+ ↑ Signaled omission penalty
	Negative reinforcer −	O^- ↑ Omission punish	$O-$ ↑ Omission extinction	O_- ↓ Omission relief	sO^- ↑ Signaled omission punish	$sO-$ ↑ Signaled extinction	sO_- ↓ Signaled omission relief

[a]Expanded version of a taxonomy first published by Woods (1974).
[b]The term conditioning is assumed to follow each table entry.

behavior is through relief conditioning which is defined as the offset or decrease of a negative reinforcer such as when nagging terminates on compliance with a request. Patterson (1979, 1982, 1997) uses the term "coercion" to describe the psychological experience of having one's behavior modified by using relief conditioning. Penalty conditioning is defined as the offset or decrease of a positive reinforcer contingent on the emission of the target behavior such as when tokens are taken back; a fine. Its effect is to decrease the frequency, rate, or probability of the target behavior. The other way to decrease the frequency, rate, or probability of the target behavior is through punishment conditioning that is defined as the onset or increase of a negative reinforcer contingent on the emission of a response. These four basic procedures are also defined in terms of the omission of the target behavior in the lower left quadrant of Table 1. Extinction is a noncontingent condition that means that all contingent relationship relationships between behavior and consequences must be removed. The taxonomy reveals that there can be no onset or offset of either a positive or negative reinforcer contingent on either the emission or omission of the target response. Hence, extinction requires that four conditions *not occur simultaneously*. No wonder it is so difficult to extinguish behavior outside the laboratory!

Consequences may be signaled or unsignaled. Stimuli are always present and therefore always associated with consequences (Donahoe & Palmer, 1994, pp. 49–52), but some stimuli are consistently correlated with a consequence so that they predictively signal the consequence (reinforcer). These stimuli are termed discriminative stimuli because they help the organism discriminate between the occasions when a response will be reinforced and when it will not be reinforced. The role discriminative stimuli play in behavioral disorders is sufficient to justify their presence as a separate entry in the taxonomy.

The following notation has been developed to represent the conditioning procedures described. Capital E represents target response *emission*, whereas O represents its *omission*. The plus sign symbolizes a *positive* reinforcer, whereas the minus sign represents a *negative* reinforcer. The superscript position indicates *onset*, the subscript position indicates *offset*, and the middle position indicates *no change*. The upward arrow ($\uparrow$) indicates that the effect of the conditioning procedure is to *increase* the frequency, rate, or probability of the target behavior. The downward arrow ($\downarrow$) indicates that the effect of the conditioning procedure is to *decrease* the frequency, rate, or probability of the target behavior.

Reinforcer Identification

A reinforcer can be identified by interviewing the subject about likes and dislikes; what the person is willing to work for and what the person is willing to prevent or turn off. Reinforcers can also be identified by observation. Premack (1959) discovered that a higher frequency (more probable) behavior can be used to reinforce a less frequently (lower probable) behavior by making the opportunity to engage in the higher frequency behavior contingent upon some of the lower frequency behavior. For example, suppose that a child is observed to come home after school and go out to play with high probability and do homework with low probability. One can increase (reinforce) homework behavior by making access to play contingent upon doing a specified amount of homework. Instead, one can require a specified number of minutes of study time before playing, but this is less desirable because the child could appear busy without working just to comply with the rule (reinforcement contingency). Having to do a certain number of math problems or learn to spell a certain number of words motivates the child to complete the task as soon as possible. This practice reduces arguments and facilitates compliance. It is not necessary to understand why the child engages in the more frequent behavior to know that access to it will reinforce less frequently occurring behaviors. The child may engage in the more frequent behavior out of social pressure rather than desirability. No matter, your insisting on some of the less frequent behavior before engaging in the more frequent behavior will increase the rate of the less frequent behavior, the target behavior. I recall a related example of an elderly patient who was found alone in her room with high frequency and socialized at bingo games with low frequency. Bingo attendance was reinforced by allowing time alone only after attending bingo. This meant limiting private time to something less than its baseline (operant) rate so that it could be dispensed as a reinforcer. The effectiveness of this method is easily understood once it is realized that privacy is in short supply in institutions and being alone is something that the patient therefore valued but was discouraged doing by staff who valued program participation. This example raises ethical questions as to whether the patient's personal values or the staff's treatment values should prevail.

Timberlake and Farmer-Dougan (1991) present a disequilibrium extension of Premack's principle based on earlier research by Timberlake and Allison (1974) in which any behavior that is occurring below its free operant level can be used as a reinforcer. The free operant level of a behavior is the frequency (probability) with which it "naturally" occurs in a particular setting. It is the rate with which the behavior occurs without any intervention, the rate maintained by "natural" reinforcement. Assume that an observer records the frequency with which math and writing assignments are engaged in during a school period and thereby determines the free operant level of each. We ignore for the moment that this behavior is influenced (reinforced) by teacher behavior and assume that the teacher behaves in a consistent manner which leads to stable rates of math and writing behavior. Assume further than at some point the student's math work falls below its free operant level. This means that it can be used to reinforce writing or some other behavior by allowing the child to do math work only after first doing a prescribed amount of writing or some other behavior. This can be understood as follows. The teacher continues to require math work to be done but the child is additionally told that it will first have to do some other behavior before it can start their math homework. Hence, the child satisfies the new contingency to be able to satisfy the old, preexisting contingency. Konarski, Crowell, and Duggan (1985) used this method to reinforce various academic behaviors in developmentally delayed children.

Binary Contingencies

Contingencies can, and frequently do, occur in pairs. Tryon (1976a) examined all possible binary pairs of conditioning procedures and noted that some of them are benign, whereas others lead to at least eight models of behavioral disorder. Table 2 sorts Table 1 entries into a 2×2 matrix based on whether they accelerate (increase) or decelerate (decrease) the emission or omission of a target response.

BENIGN COMBINATIONS

Selecting one entry from the upper left and one from the lower right quadrant doubly strengthens behavior without conflict. Likewise, selecting one entry from the lower left and one from the upper right quadrant doubly weakens behavior. These combinations are compatible and therefore create no conflict.

NONCONTINGENT COMBINATIONS

Combining one contingency from the lower left and one from the lower right quadrant decelerates both the emission and omission of behavior and produces depressive symptoms known as learned helplessness (LH). The usual procedure is to combine punishment (E^-) and omission punishment (O^-) so that the subject is noncontingently shocked. In other words, the subject is punished for emitting the target response and punished for not emitting the target response which means that it is always punished. The associated downward arrow correctly indicates that this combination decreases the frequency, rate, or probability of behavior. The signaled version (sE^- and sO^-) was used in much of the classic work on experimental neurosis (Wolpe, 1958).

TABLE 2. Taxonomy of Binary Contingencies

	Emission	Omission	Noncontingent
Accelerate	$E^+ \uparrow^a$ E_- $sE^+ \uparrow$ sE_-	$O^+ \downarrow$ O_- $sO^+ \downarrow$ sO_-	$A(E) \cdot A(O) = A(E \cdot O) = A = \uparrow^c$
Decelerate	$E_+ \downarrow$ E^- $E+ \downarrow sE^-$ $sE_+ \downarrow sE^-$ $sE+ \downarrow sE^-$	$O_+ \uparrow$ O^- $O+ \uparrow$ O_- $sO_+ \uparrow sO^-$ $sO+ \uparrow sO_-$	$D(E) \cdot D(O) = D(E \cdot O) = D = \downarrow$
Approach-avoidance conflict	$A(E) \cdot D(E) = (AD)E$ $= DE = \downarrow_b$	$A(O) \cdot D(O) = (AD)O$ $= DO = \uparrow$	

[a]All pointers indicate the effect of the conditioning paradigm on the emission (presence) of a response. The $\uparrow$ pointer indicates that conditioning increases the frequency, rate, or probability of a response. The $\downarrow$ pointer indicates that conditioning decreases the frequency, rate, or probability of a response.
[b]AD = D because algebraically $+(-) = -$ which in this case = D = $\downarrow$.
[c]EO = 1 because emission and omission are inversely related.

Another example of the way one condition from the lower left and one from the lower right lead to behavioral disorder is noncontingent penalty conditioning (E^+ and O^+) which results in the noncontingent offset of positive reinforcement. Severe problems occur if the reinforcer is important enough. It has long been known that noncontingent offset (separation) of maternal presence and attention is sufficient to produce depression and if protracted, results in major developmental disabilities (Spitz, 1946; Harlow & Suomi, 1974; Seligman, 1995).

Combining one procedure from the upper left and another from the upper right quadrant also produces a noncontingent condition, but one that is far less traumatic. For example, noncontingent reward conditioning results by combining E^+ and O^+. The subject is rewarded whether or not the target behavior is emitted. Skinner (1948) used this procedure to create "superstitious" behavior in the pigeon by noncontingently activating a feeder on a fixed interval 15-second schedule. Subjects rarely complain about receiving reward regardless of behavior. However, Eisenberger and Cameron (1996) identified noncontingent reward as detrimental because subjects lose interest in "work" that has no relationship to reward.

APPROACH-AVOIDANCE CONFLICTS

Two forms of approach-avoidance conflicts are described in Table 2. The most frequent version is produced by combining one procedure from the upper left with another from the lower left quadrant; using the first column. For example, rewarding (E^+) and punishing (E^-) the subject for the same act creates a conflict over whether to emit the behavior or not. The downward arrow correctly indicates that such conditions typically decrease the frequency, rate, or probability of the target behavior.

Combining one condition from the upper right quadrant and one from the lower right quadrant creates the second type of approach-avoidance conflict. This conflict is far less well investigated but is remarkable in that it is associated with an upward arrow indicating that it strengthens behavior. Conflict and repetition are the core elements of what Mowrer (1948) called the Neurotic Paradox, that self-defeating behavior is self-perpetuating. One expects punishment to reduce behavior in which case neurosis should be self-limiting. However, this type of conflict, what used to be called neurosis, is self-perpetuating, as indicated by the upward arrow. The reader is referred to Tryon (1978) for further consideration of the neurotic paradox, but one point deserves emphasis here: the neurotic paradox appears to involve an approach-avoidance conflict with regard to the *omission* of behavior.

Classical Conditioning

Classical (respondent) conditioning is frequently viewed as different from operant (instrumental) conditioning. Tryon (1976a) demonstrated that classical conditioning can be formally analyzed into two operant contingencies that are scheduled simultaneously. For example, appetitive classical conditioning occurs when one combines sE^+ from the upper left and sO^+ from the upper right quadrant. A stimulus is presented and a reinforcer is given regardless of whether the target behavior is emitted or omitted, thereby always pairing the stimulus with the reinforcer. This combination of contingencies creates a special noncontingent case where the subject learns stimulus–reinforcer relationships. The associated upward indicator correctly predicts that classical appetitive conditioning strengthens behavior because the response becomes increasingly more likely in the presence of the stimulus with which it has been repeatedly paired.

Donahoe (1991) and Donahoe and Palmer (1994, pp. 49–52) observed that operant and respondent conditioning procedures appear similar to the subject even though they appear different to psychologists. Environmental stimuli are always present, and the subject is always behaving, thereby creating an ongoing S-R stream. By inserting a biologically active stimulus, UCS, the experimenter classically conditions the preceding stimulus and operantly conditions the preceding response; the subject cannot tell the difference. The two conditioning procedures are complementary. Classical conditioning controls stimulus–UCS relationships, whereas instrumental conditioning controls response–UCS relationships.

It is not generally appreciated that classical (respondent) appetitive conditioning entails helplessness because the CS is followed by the US whether or not the subject emits an instrumental response. Many appetitive classical conditioning studies were published without signs of depression before the learned helpless literature began. Therefore, noncontingency per se probably does not cause depression. It must be about important consequence.

Diagnostic System

At least eight diagnostic conditions stem from what has been discussed. Table 3 identifies the first four and Table 2 identifies the second four. Table 3 presents four ways in which the single contingencies (conditional relationships) between behaviors and consequences systematized in Table 1 can produce behavioral disorder.

Condition I pertains to the presence of contingencies that increase (support) the negative behaviors that set the occasion for referral. Any condition in Table 1 that has an upward arrow in conjunction with negative behaviors is diagnostic of this condition. The treatment implications are (1) to remove these conditions or (2) to replace them with conditions that have a downward arrow, or (3) to replace them with conditions that support positive behavior.

Condition II pertains to the absence of contingencies that decrease (inhibit) the negative behaviors that set the occasion for referral. The absence of all conditions in Table 1 that have a downward arrow in conjunction with negative behaviors is diagnostic of this condition. The primary treatment implication is to initiate one or more conditions that have a downward arrow in conjunction with negative behaviors.

Condition III pertains to the absence of contingencies that increase (support) positive behaviors. The absence of all conditions in Table 1 that have an upward arrow in conjunction with positive behaviors is diagnostic of this condition. The primary treatment implication is to initiate one or more conditions that have an upward arrow in conjunction with positive behaviors.

Condition IV pertains to the presence of contingencies that decrease (inhibit) positive behaviors. Any condition in Table 1 that has a downward arrow in conjunction with positive behaviors is diagnostic of this condition. The treatment implications are (1) to remove these conditions or (2) to replace them with conditions that have an upward arrow.

The remaining four diagnostic conditions entail pairs of reinforcement contingencies (conditional relationships) identified in Table 2. There are multiple combinations of reinforce-

TABLE 3. Four Diagnostic Conditions Based on the Presence
or Absence of Contingencies that Increase or Decrease Positive or Negative Behaviors

	Contingencies that increase (upward arrow)	Contingencies that decrease (downward arrow)
Presence of	Negative behavior is condition I	Positive behavior is condition IV
Absence of	Positive behavior is condition III	Negative behavior is condition II

ment contingencies that produce the same effect. Treatment implications are the same in all cases.

Condition V pertains to any of the combination of procedures in Table 2 that simultaneously *decelerate* the emission and omission of a response that results in learned helplessness. The primary treatment implication is to remove one or the other contingency.

Condition VI pertains to any of the combination of procedures in Table 2 that simultaneously accelerate and decelerate the *emission* of behavior that results in an approach-avoidance conflict. The primary treatment implication is to remove one or the other contingency, thereby resolving the conflict.

Condition VII pertains to any of the combination of procedures in Table 2 that simultaneously accelerate and decelerate the *omission* of behavior that results in the neurotic paradox of self-defeating behavior that is self-perpetuating. The primary treatment implication is to remove one or the other contingency, thereby resolving the conflict.

Condition VIII pertains to any of the combination of procedures in Table 2 that simultaneously *accelerate* the emission and omission of a response that results in superstitious behavior. The primary treatment implication is to remove one or the other contingency.

Advantages

The diagnostic taxonomy described has at least three advantages over the DSM series:

1. It is individually tailored to clients and their relationships with significant others. It centers on who does what to whom rather than with what people have. It is dynamic rather than static.
2. A positive diagnosis carries *etiological* implications because it involves conditions sufficient to maintain behavioral disorder. It is frequently reasonable to assume that these conditions preexisted for some time, perhaps even before the behavioral disorder occurred and fostered its development.
3. *Treatment recommendations follow from diagnostic findings.* Positive diagnoses frequently entail specific treatment implications. The ways in which behavioral assessment results in treatment planning are considered in the Behavioral Psychotherapy section later.

BEHAVIORAL ASSESSMENT

Functional analysis is theoretically central to behavioral therapy because it seeks to empirically identify causal variables regarding the problems that brought the client to seek treatment, but it is seldom practiced largely because the methodology for obtaining the necessary information is so difficult, demanding, and expensive to implement. Behavioral clinicians want to know what their clients do the other 167 hours each week when they are not in session but generally do not have the resources to obtain this information independent of client report. Bijou, Peterson, and Ault (1968), Iwata, Pace, Kalsher, Cowdery and Cataldo (1990), Mace and Lalli (1991), Sasso et al. (1992), and Tryon (1998b) describe these standard behavioral assessment procedures. Traditional behavioral observation methodology is too labor-intensive and time-consuming to be practical in most clinical settings. Target behaviors must be carefully defined and well described in an observer training manual that may have to be revised or extended to include a new patient. Pilot studies are frequently required to verify the adequacy of each behavioral code. Observers must be trained to observe these behaviors reliably. Observer reliability must be checked periodically because behaviors tend to "drift" apart (Tryon, 1989). This requires retraining and continued monitoring. Arrangements must be made for home and or school visits. Observers must travel to these sites. Data must be entered into the computer, frequently by hand, though this situation is improving (see later), and then analyzed (Suen & Ary, 1987). Methods used include calculating conditional probabilities (Patterson, 1982; Patterson & Cobb, 1973), transition matrices (Whitehurst, Fischel, De-Baryshe, Caulfield, & Falco, 1986), and regression analyses (Martin, Maccoby, Baran, & Jacklin, 1981) or cross tabulation (Schlundt, 1985; Schlundt, Johnson, & Jarrell, 1985; Schlundt, Virts, Sbrocco, Pope-Cordle & Hill, 1993). This entire process is time-consuming, technically demanding, and therefore quite costly. For example, Jacob, Tennenbaum, Bargiel, and Seilhamer (1995) report that their Home Interaction Scoring System takes 24 to 30 minutes to prepare and transcribe each minute of audio tape and another 24 minutes to rate each minute of tape after first training raters for 60 hours. Hence, approximately one hour is required to score each minute of tape! The resulting high cost, none of which is billable to third party payers, prompts clinicians to choose very carefully when to record and to obtain as little data as possible and that limits the comprehensiveness of the assessment. These are some of the reasons that behavioral observation has not been widely incorporated into clinical practice and why it is unlikely to be used very often in the foreseeable future. Computer-based observing/ recording systems have reduced some of the work involved (Busch & Ciocco, 1992; Eiler, Nelson, Jensen & Johnson, 1989; Farrell, 1986; Hile, 1991; Horner & Storey, 1989; Repp, Harman, Felce, Van Acker, & Karsh, 1989; Torgerson, 1977) but require a substantial investment in computer hardware and software and training in their use. For example, Noldus Information Technology retails an integrated system for behavioral observation. Observational codes can be entered into a notebook, desktop PC, or a handheld computer (Psion Workabout) while either observing the actual behavior or reviewing a videotape of the behavior. However, observer codes still need to be established, observers still need to be trained to produce reliable data, and they still require periodic recalibration because of observer drift. Observers still need to go to where the behavior is occurring or they need to obtain videotapes of the behavior, which they will subsequently score. This means that someone must set up a video camera and return the tape to the laboratory associated with the clinical practice. The labor costs of this process are even more substantial than the hardware and software costs. More practical options are needed if behavioral diagnoses are to be routinely made using the previously mentioned taxonomy. Now, we consider how this can be done.

Behavioral Samples (Specimens)

Behavioral samples can always be obtained by clinicians during therapy sessions by formally or informally coding or noting the client's behavior during the therapy hour. This information continues to provide an important basis for diagnosis and assessment by all clinicians. However, the behaviorally oriented clinician is also interested in how the client behaves outside of therapy during the other 167 hours of the week. Marital, family, and child-related problems often have important home components. More importantly, members of the couple or family have their own perspectives that frequently differ in important ways from the other person or other family members. Clinicians frequently want to know how distorted these self-reports are. Objective information about actual behavior in natural settings is almost always very informative.

Placing trained observers in the home or other setting for behavioral observation is always expensive and third-party financial support for this practice is unlikely, except for the few investigators fortunate enough to receive large Federal and/or private grants. Therefore, some means of inexpensively obtaining behavioral samples (specimens) is necessary. The Noldus system mentioned earlier was designed to facilitate the process of coding videotapes. Camcorders continue to increase in quality and decrease in price and that makes them attractive. Supercircuits Inc. (One Supercircuits Plaza, Lender, TX 78641) makes a small (2.0 × 1.6 × 1.0 in) lightweight (1.7 oz) battery-powered video camera and transmitter called MicroBug that transmits audio and video at 434 MHz (just below channel 14) to any TV within 700 feet. Data can then be recorded on videotape. Timing mechanisms can control when data will be recorded. Some video systems orient to the speaker's voice and therefore do not need especially wide angle lenses and placement in the corner of a room near the ceiling to capture events occurring everywhere within the room.

Audiotape technology is attractive because it is less expensive (more cost-effective) than videotape technology. Audio is less conspicuous than video and is not special and costly to install. High-quality, omnidirectional, amplified microphones have an impressive range and can clearly record conversations. It is remarkable how informative sounds are. One can tell a great deal about what people are doing by listening to the sounds they make and what they say. In the days before TV, large audiences regularly tuned their radios to hear and derive considerable pleasure from dramatic stories supported by sound effects. Soskin and John (1963) pioneered using FM telemetry to record the spontaneous speech of two husband-wife pairs 14 to 16 hours a day. Purcell and Brady (1966) used cigarette case size waist-worn FM devices to telemeter the speech of 13 asthmatic adolescents (8 boys, 5 girls) aged 12 to 16 years living with house parents in two cottages at a residential treatment and research center. They reported complete adaptation to the device within two to four days. Bernal, Gibson, Williams, and Pesses (1971) also successfully audiotaped behavior.

Johnson and Bolstad (1975) audiotaped family members at home with and without an observer present to evaluate observer reactivity and the possibility that the observer's presence alters the behavior being observed. Their observer agreement was .96 for child deviant behavior, .89 for parent negative behavior, and .91 for parent commands. Correlations between observer present and observer absent were .68 ($p < .01$) for child deviant behavior, .51 ($p < .05$) for parent negative behavior, and .48 ($p < .06$) for parent commands. Only the first two are statistically significant and account for 46% and 26% of the variance, leaving 54% and 74% of the variance unaccounted for. The third correlation accounts for just 23% of the variance leaving 77% of the variance unaccounted for. Because high interobserver agreement was obtained, it appears that the subsequent disagreements were due to reactive effects of the observer being present.

Johnson, Christensen, and Bellamy (1976) sampled child–family interactions at random and at parent-selected intervals in five homes by using small belt-worn FM transmitters. Audible clicks were recorded on a second track to coordinate subsequent coding of 16 behaviors. Most recording was done at breakfast, early evening, and late evening. Jacob, Tenenbaum, Bargiel, and Seilhamer's (1995) Home Interaction Scoring System is based on more than 500 audiotape recordings of mealtime conversations. I first learned about home audiotaping as a graduate student at Kent State University around 1968 from Professor Edwin Bixenstein who had been using this procedure for some time in his clinical practice. The modern version of this procedure is to place a cassette tape recorder that has a good quality omnidirectional amplified microphone and is autoreverse loaded with a 120-minute cassette in a central location such as on the table during meal time or in the living room or another room where instances of the target behavior reportedly occur. The tape recorder is turned on at one or more times of the day that are typically associated with problematic relationships and let run until either an event is recorded or the tape has reached its end, if the recorder does not have autoreverse. If no event has been recorded, then the tape is turned over to avoid rewinding and recording is continued. If a problem interaction (behavioral specimen) is recorded, then the tape is mailed to the therapist. This process continues until several instances of the problem are recorded. Arguments between couples and disputes between siblings or between parents and children are examples. This approach entails *critical event sampling* if the tape recorder runs continuously until an example of the problematic behavior is recorded, or *critical period sampling* if the tape recorder is on only during specified times of the day.

Clinical Use

Assessment methods must be practical and pertinent to treatment or they will not be used. Knowing who did what to whom is both theoretically and clinically relevant. This information is theoretically relevant because behaviorism continues to stress behavior–environment relationships and the social environment is as important as the physical environment. This information is clinically relevant because couples and families invariably disagree about what happened. Objective information about the actual events is especially helpful. The therapist can use it to better determine how behavioral principles currently maintain the problem behavior and by implication, the etiology of the problem behavior. The therapist can also use this information therapeutically in at least three ways. The first option is to have client's continue to tape record their interactions at home until one or more incidents have been recorded and to mail these tapes to the therapist for review. Much can be learned from these tapes including material that client's either fail to mention during therapy, are unaware of, or have substantially distorted. Therapists can discern aspects of relationships of which the participants are unaware. It also allows the therapist to gauge the extent to which each participant's perception, memory, and reporting differs from each other and from the therapist's view of events. The bias towards reporting negative events by depressed patients (Beck, Rush, Shaw, and Emery, 1979) called state- dependent (mood-congruent) recall (Blaney, 1986; Matt, Vazquez, & Campbell, 1992; Williams, Watts, MacLeod, & Mathews, 1988) is a good example.

A second option is to review tapes during therapy with one member of the couple or family at a time to help them better understand their part in the problem, whether it be a relationship with spouse or a relationship with a child. Both husband and wife can listen along with the therapist, or all family members can listen as the tape is reviewed. The tape focuses all parties on the actual events rather than inaccurate perceptions. Two factors are especially helpful. People sound different to themselves on tape than they do when speaking. The difference is due to bone conduction which is present when speaking and absent on tape. This provides some objectivity in that the voice in question almost seems like it is someone else speaking. A second factor favoring objectivity is that the tapes are reviewed several days or a week after the incident when both parties have regained their composure and obtained some "distance" from the events in question. Corollary to this principle is the fact that people are more objective when observing than when behaving because disturbing emotions are associated with problematic behaviors. It is very difficult to get people to focus on their maladaptive behavior when they are emotionally upset. Emotional distress and self-critical introspection are inversely related. Angry people frequently criticize and find fault with others and rarely reflect on ways they might change their behavior. This is why it is important for people to see themselves "misbehaving."

A third option is to have couples or families review the tapes before therapy to see how

TABLE 4. Observational Form for Identifying Operant Contingencies

Antecedent	Behavior	Consequence	Symbol
1. Mother tells Bill it is time to get up	2. Bill does not answer	3. Mother yells at Bill	sO^-
4. Mother yells at Bill	5. Bill says he will get up	6. Mother stops yelling	$sE\_$
7. Mother is silent	8. Bill continues to sleep	9. Mother yells louder for Bill to get up	O^-
10. Mother yells louder for Bill to get up	11. Bill gets up and moves slowly	12. Mother stops yelling	$sE\_$

much progress they can make on their own. The value of this is that it sets the stage for them to learn to analyze and repair their own behavioral problems; first in consultation with the therapist and then on their own.

Table 4 provides an observation form that can be used to code behavioral interactions formally or informally while reviewing the tapes. It is based on the Antecedent, Behavior, Consequence (ABC) methodology introduced by Bijou, Peterson, and Ault (1968) and more recently used effectively by Iwata, Pace, Kalsher, Cowdery and Cataldo (1990), Mace and Lalli (1991), and Sasso et al. (1992) for identifying clinically important variables. The objective here is to diagnose instances of contingencies defined in Table 1. Table 4 illustrates how a brief portion of a morning interaction between a nine-year-old boy and his mother were coded. The father's voice is conspicuously absent. It was subsequently learned that he leaves for work sufficiently early to avoid the problems recorded on tape. It is clearly desirable to replace his absence with effective parenting.

The definition of specific target behaviors, antecedents, and consequents and the definition of "critical incident" have purposely been left undefined because it is useful for the client, couple, or family to discuss specific definitions of particular behaviors with each other and with the therapist.

Omission Sampling

The methods previously mentioned pertain to the emission (presence) of behavior. Omission conditioning pertains to the absence of behavior. It is important to stress that the absence of behavior can be modified in the same ways as the presence of behavior.[4] For example, it is possible to reinforce nonsmoking by identifying those times when a person does not smoke and providing a positive consequence. Almost any other behavior than smoking can be ongoing when reinforcement is administered. I say almost any behavior other because one would not want to positively reinforce aggressive or other aversive behavior.

BEHAVIORAL PSYCHOTHERAPY

The final section of this chapter concerns the way the behavioral model and diagnostic taxonomy direct treatment. Among the many distortions of the behavioral model is that

---

[4]Our emphasis on emission over omission parallels our tendency to explain what we see in terms of creative purposive forces rather than in terms of what was initially present (variation) and what was removed (extinction); see our discussion of ontogenetic evolution.

behaviorists are uncaring people who do not relate personally to their clients or consider their relationship with clients useful in any way. Therefore, we begin with a consideration of the therapeutic working alliance and then discuss additional benefits derived from the application of scientific principles of behavior modification.

Therapeutic Alliance

Psychologists provide treatment in a face-to-face setting with few exceptions.[5] Clients frequently come to therapy out of perceived need, but typically half of those who come for their first visit do not return for their second visit, and only half of those who come the second time return a third time. Hence, psychotherapists in general do not seem to provide very attractive services. One response to this situation has been to maintain that psychotherapy is not for everyone and that it should be prescribed only for suitable clients. Another response is that therapists are partly responsible for engaging clients in treatment and establishing a strong working alliance, despite the fact that many clients have long-standing difficulty relating effectively to others. G. S. Tryon (1985) defined an Engagement Quotient (EQ) as the percentage of clients that returns for a second visit. She found that practicum students who have higher EQs received better supervisory evaluations than those who have lower EQs. Some personal characteristics such as higher GRE Verbal and Miller's Analogy scores and being older have been associated with higher EQs (Tryon & Tryon, 1986), but more trainable variables have been identified. For example, longer sessions, asking more questions to begin with, and providing more information about their conditions and what can be done as the session progresses facilitate engagement (G. S. Tryon, 1989a, 1989b, in press). Making clients feel comfortable in an accepting and supportive atmosphere, displaying accurate empathy, and providing them with an opportunity to learn to deal more effectively with their situations are fundamental facets of therapeutic engagement. A large literature exists on this topic that is beyond the scope of this chapter. Suffice it to say here that behaviorists also understand the importance of a "good bedside manner." It is frequently difficult for clients to try new behaviors and implement homework recommended by the therapist. Sometimes clients initially comply simply because they trust and like the therapist. Hopefully, positive outcomes reinforce new behavior that leads to therapeutic gains. Nonspecific therapeutic factors (i.e., the placebo effect) should be maximized in all reasonable ways.

What differentiates behaviorists from other therapists is their belief that more than a relationship can be brought to therapy. This includes empirically supported treatment packages and individually designed treatment plans based on principles of operant and respondent conditioning that are among the most thoroughly studied and well replicated scientifically validated phenomena in psychology.

Diagnostic Treatment Prescriptions

The DSM approach to diagnosis is not etiologically based and therefore does not, in principle, lead to treatment recommendations. Some treatment decisions have become common for some diagnostic groups such as the practice of prescribing lithium for manic

---

[5]Sometimes psychologists are called upon to devise contingencies to better manage residential clients in cottage or closed wards. Administrative decisions about contingencies are best informed by contacts with those whose behavior will be impacted by them but can be decided without such consultation. Relationship issues do not arise in the latter case and are not nearly as great in the former situation as they are when treatment is provided in one-on-one settings.

depression and cognitive behavior therapy for major depression, but these decisions are pragmatic rather than theoretically derived from diagnostic assessment. The system of behavioral diagnosis presented before differs in that it is etiologically related in the sense that it embodies causal principles that describe sufficient conditions for developing and maintaining behavioral disorder. Table 3 shows that behavioral clinicians are primarily concerned with the emission of negative behaviors and the omission of positive behaviors. In other words, behavioral excesses are especially problematic when they entail negative behaviors, and behavioral deficits are especially problematic when they entail positive behaviors.

The first four diagnostic conditions summarized in Table 3 pertain to problematic effects created by single reinforcement contingencies. Martin and Pear's (1999) use of the term "pitfalls" is appropriate here because these are ways in which unintended problematic behaviors develop. Condition I involves direct support for the very behaviors that constitute the referral basis. People are frequently unaware of the ways in which they cause or exacerbate problem behaviors. Treatment should (1) reduce or eliminate these contingencies, (2) replace them with inhibitory conditions (those with a downward arrow), and/or (3) support alternative positive behaviors. The absence of all inhibitory conditions relative to negative behaviors is the essence of Condition II. Treatment should provide some opposition to negative behaviors. Condition III identifies the absence of support for positive behaviors. Parents and teachers frequently expect that good behavior will just happen on its own because people should be good and that no special attention needs to be paid to it. A related concern is that positive reinforcement will "go to their heads" and "spoil their character." Some psychologists are concerned that external reinforcement reduces creativity and undermines intrinsic motivation but Eisenberger and Cameron (1996) have shown that only when rewards are given noncontingently is there a problem. I expect that authors who question the value of reward cash their pay checks without concern that they are impairing their own creativity and intrinsic motivation, yet they expect children and adolescents to work without external incentives. Curiously, they do not question paying adults for their labors. Condition IV entails actively opposing positive behaviors. Parents sometimes attempt to expropriate their children's future behavior by insisting that they develop in ways that the parent values, rather than make alternative socially positive choices, and will actively oppose such pursuits. For example, a father wanted his son to become a pharmacist because that was his unfilled dream and opposed his son's choice to become a banker. Each of these first four behavioral diagnostic conditions give rise to at least two treatment implications. The first implication is to stop, withdraw, or preclude the offending contingency. The second treatment implication is to substitute a more desirable contingency, including differential reinforcement of other (DRO) behavior.

Conditions V through VIII describe particular pairs of contingencies that are inherently problematic. Removing one of the two contingencies can treat learned helplessness (Condition V). Even better is to substitute conditions that produce learned optimism (Seligman, 1996). Approach-avoidance conflicts over the emission of behavior (Condition VI) can be resolved by removing one of the two contingencies. Approach-avoidance conflicts over the omission of behavior (Condition VII) are the least well understood of the diagnostic conditions. See Tryon (1978) for further comments. Superstitious behavior and appetitive respondent conditioning (Condition VIII) may be the least problematic conditions. The primary treatment implication of diagnosing any one of the latter four conditions is to terminate one of the two contingencies. Their combination is harmful. Retaining either one or the other of the pair will almost certainly be an improvement. The major exception is if the retained contingency supports one or more undesirable target behaviors in which case this must be changed as well.

Cognitive Restructuring

Much of modern behavior therapy entails cognitive restructuring. These therapeutic strategies can be divided roughly into two categories. One category entails the use of reason to counter the assumptions, conclusions, and reasons patients give for continuing to act in self-defeating ways or why they cannot possibly change. This approach was begun by Abramson, Seligman, and Teasdale (1978), Beck (1963, 1967a, 1967b, 1976, 1991), Beck and Emery (1985), Beck, Rush, Shaw, and Emery (1979), Mahoney (1977), and others and has recently culminated with Albert Ellis's (1993) redefinition of Rational Emotive Therapy (RET) as Rational Emotive Behavior Therapy (REBT).

The other category uses principles of operant conditioning to modify covert operants (thoughts) using the same principles reviewed earlier that have been found effective in modifying overt behavior. This approach is especially well articulated by Martin and Pear (1999). Skinner never approved of the cognitive revolution in psychology and addressed both the origins of cognitive thought (Skinner, 1977) and the reasons that he chose not to be a cognitive psychologist (Skinner, 1989).

Thoughts, feelings, and behaviors are interrelated. Reinforcement contingencies (environment–behavior relationships) influence cognition and affect. Therapists should address all three elements for maximum effectiveness. Contemporary concern with cognition has overshadowed interest in reinforcement conditions that have cognitive and affective effects. For example, persons who live under helpless conditions (Condition V) will develop hopeless cognitions and depressive affect. Purely cognitive treatments that leave these etiological conditions intact must almost certainly be either less effective or even possibly ineffective. We know that not all persons treated with cognitive restructuring recover completely. Perhaps this is because reinforcement contingencies have not been examined. Allowing important etiological factors to go untreated reduces long-term follow-up success rates. Clinicians of all theoretical persuasions who ignore reinforcement contingencies leave potent etiological factors unchanged. To this extent their treatment is symptomatic rather than root cause oriented.

SUMMARY

The behavioral model of abnormal psychology is based on learning that presumes memory. It can be argued that all psychological development entails learning and memory and that divergent models differ only in the way they understand learning and memory. Recent developments in learning and memory, referred to as Neural Network Learning Theory, promise to unify the behavioral and cognitive models of learning and memory and provide a unified theoretical understanding of abnormal psychology.

Operant conditioning is a form of R-S rather than S-R learning theory where consequences select (edit) response distributions. The resulting skewed distributions have either a higher or lower mean, depending upon whether low or high values have been deleted. This developmental process enables behavior to "evolve" over time, which is ontogenetic evolution. Table 1 summarizes the environment–behavior relationships that define various forms of operant conditioning. Table 2 identifies pairs of operant conditions that are inherently problematic. Table 3 categorizes four possibilities for maintaining problematic behavior that might be diagnosed on the basis of samples of current behavior. The main treatment implication is to modify the offending contingency. Table 2 identifies pairs of operant conditions that are known to be problematic. The main treatment implication is to remove one or the other contingency and then to inspect for the presence of the four conditions identified in Table 3.

Information about who does what to whom can be obtained from the interview, but more objective data can be obtained by observers. Unfortunately, observers are expensive to train and maintain, and presently there is no way to bill for their services. Therefore, technological alternatives such as home audiotaping are recommended. The therapist can review these tapes before or during a session to identify problematic interpersonal behaviors and recommend changes.

The importance of the therapeutic relationship as fundamental to all clinical intervention was emphasized. The responsibility of the therapist to engage clients was accentuated and recommendations for increasing one's Engagement Quotient were provided. Reinforcement contingencies are etiological factors. Therapists ignore them at their clients' expense.

REFERENCES

Abramson, L. Y., Seligman, M. E. P., & Teasdale, J. D. (1978). Learned helplessness in humans: Critique and reformulation. *Journal of Abnormal Psychology, 87,* 49–74.

American Psychiatric Association. (1994). *Diagnostic and statistical manual of mental disorders,* 4th ed. Washington, DC: Author.

Ayllon, T., & McKittrick, S. M. (1982). *How to set up a token economy.* Austin, TX: Pro-Ed.

Bandura, A. (1977). *Social learning theory.* Englewood Cliffs, NJ: Prentice-Hall.

Baldwin, J. E., & Baldwin, J. I. (1998). *Behavior principles in everyday life,* 3rd. ed.. Upper Saddle River, NJ: Prentice-Hall.

Beck, A. T. (1963). Thinking and depression. 1. Idiosyncratic content and cognitive distortions. *Archives of General Psychiatry, 9,* 324–333.

Beck, A. T. (1967a). *Depression: Causes and treatment.* Philadelphia: The University of Pennsylvania Press.

Beck, A. T. (1967b). *Depression: Clinical experimental, and theoretic aspects.* New York: Harper.

Beck, A. T. (1976). *Cognitive therapy and the emotional disorders.* New York: International Universities Press.

Beck, A. T. (1991). Cognitive therapy: A 30-year retrospective. *American Psychologist, 46,* 368–375.

Beck, A. T., & Emery, G. (1985). *Anxiety disorders and phobias: A cognitive perspective.* New York: Basic Books.

Beck, A. T., Rush, A. J., Shaw, B. F., & Emery, G. (1979). *Cognitive therapy of depression.* New York: Guilford.

Bernal, M. E., Gibson, D. M., Williams, D. E., & Pesses, D. I. (1971). A device for recording automatic audio tape recording. *Journal of Applied Behavior Analysis, 4,* 151–156.

Bijou, S. W., Peterson, R. F., & Ault, M. H. (1968). A method to integrate descriptive and experimental field studies at the level of data and empirical concepts. *Journal of Applied Behavior Analysis, 1,* 175–191.

Blaney, P. H. (1986). Affect and memory: A review. *Psychology Bulletin, 99,* 229–246.

Bolles, R. C. (1979). *Learning theory,* 2nd ed. New York: Holt, Rinehart and Winston.

Bowler, P. J. (1983). *The eclipse of Darwinism: Anti-Darwinian evolution theories in the decades around 1900.* Baltimore: The Johns Hopkins University Press.

Bush, J. P., & Ciocco, J. E. (1992). Behavioral coding and sequential analysis: The portable computer systems for observational use. *Behavioral Assessment, 14,* 191–197.

Catania, A. C. (1978). The psychology of learning: Some lessons from the Darwinian revolution. *Annals of the New York Academy of Sciences, 309,* 18–28.

Catania, A. C. (1987). Some Darwinian lessons for behavior analysis: A review of Bowler's *The Eclipse of Darwinism. Journal of the Experimental Analysis of Behavior, 47,* 249–257.

Churchland, P. S., & Sejnowski, T. J. (1992). *The computational brain.* Cambridge, MA: MIT Press.

Cohen, H. L., & Filipczak, J. (1971). *A new learning environment: A case for learning.* Boston: Authors Cooperative.

Commons, M. L., Grossberg, S., & Staddon, J. E. R. (1991). *Neural network models of conditioning and action.* Hillsdale, NJ: Erlbaum.

Dayhoff, J. (1990). *Neural network architectures.* New York: Van Nostrand Reinhold.

DeFries, J. C., Gervais, M. C., & Thomas, E. A. (1978). Response to 30 generations of selection for open-field activity in laboratory mice. *Behavior Genetics, 8,* 3–13.

Donahoe, J. W. (1984). Skinner—The Darwin of ontogeny? (pp. 487–488). In B. F. Skinner (1984a). *Selection by consequences. The Behavioral and Brain Sciences*, *7*, 477–510.

Donahoe, J. W. (1991). The selectionist approach to verbal behavior: Potential contributions of neuropsychology and connectionism. In L. J. Hayes & P. N. Chase (Eds.), *Dialogues on verbal behavior: The first international institute on verbal relations* (pp. 119–150). Reno, NV: Context Press.

Donahoe, J. W., & Palmer, D. C. (1989). The interpretation of complex human behavior: Some reactions to parallel distributed processing, J. L. McClelland, D. E. Rumelhart, and the PDP research group (Eds.). *Journal of the Experimental Analysis of Behavior*, *51*, 399–416.

Donahoe, J. W., & Palmer, D. C. (1994). *Learning and complex behavior*. Boston: Allyn and Bacon.

Donegan, N. H., Gluck, M. A., & Thompson, R. F. (1989). Integrating behavioral and biological models of classical conditioning. *The Psychology of Learning and Motivation*, *23*, 109–156.

Eiler, J. M., Nelson, W. W., Jensen, C. C., & Johnson, S. P. (1989). Automated data collection using bar code. *Behavior Research Methods, Instruments & Computers*, *21*, 53–58.

Eisenberger, R., & Cameron, J. (1996). Detrimental effects of reward: Reality or myth? *American Psychologist*, *51*, 1153–1166.

Ellis, A. (1993). Changing rational-emotive therapy (RET) to rational-emotive behavior therapy (REBT). *The Behavior Therapist*, *16*, 257–258.

Farrell, A. D. (1986). The microcomputer as a tool for behavioral assessment. *The Behavior Therapist*, *1*, 16–17.

Feldman, J. A., & Ballard, D. H. (1982). Connectionist models and their properties. *Cognitive Science*, *6*, 205–254.

Gluck, M. A., & Thompson, R. F. (1987). Modeling the neural substrates of associative learning and memory: A computational approach. *Psychological Review*, *94*, 176–191.

Grossberg, S. (1988). *Neural networks and natural intelligence*. Cambridge, MA: MIT Press.

Grossberg, S., & Levine, D. S. (1987). Neural dynamics of attentionally modulated Pavlovian conditioning: Blocking, interstimulus interval, and secondary reinforcement. *Applied Optics*, *26*, 5015–5030.

Grossberg, S., & Schmajuk, N. A. (1987). Neural dynamics of attentionally modulated Pavlovian conditioning: Conditioned reinforcement, inhibition, and opponent processing. *Psychobiology*, *15*, 195–240.

Grossberg, S., & Schmajuk, N. A. (1989). Neural dynamics of adaptive timing and temporal discrimination during associative learning. *Neural Networks*, *2*, 79–102.

Hayes, S. C., & Follette, W. C. (1992). Can functional analysis provide a substitute for syndromal classification? *Behavioral Assessment*, *14*, 345–365.

Haynes, S. N. (1992). *Models of causality in psychopathology: Toward synthetic, dynamic, and nonlinear models of causality in psychopathology*. New York: Allyn & Bacon.

Haynes, S. N., & O'Brien, W. H. (1990). Functional analysis in behavior therapy. *Clinical Psychology Review*, *10*, 649–668.

Haynes, S. N., Uchigakiuchi, P., Meyer, K., Orimoto, L., Blaine, D., & O'Brien, W. H. (1993). Functional analytic causal models and the design of treatment programs: Concepts and clinical applications with childhood behavior problems. *European Journal of Psychological Assessment*, *9*, 189–205.

Haynes, S. N., Spain, E. H., & Oliveria, J. (1993). Identifying causal relationships in clinical assessment. *Psychological Assessment*, *5*, 281–291.

Hawkins, R. D. (1989). A biologically realistic neural network model for higher order features of classical conditioning. In R. G. M. Morris (Ed.), *Parallel distributed processing: Implications for psychology and neurobiology* (pp. 214–247). Oxford, England: Clarendon Press.

Hebb, D. O. (1949). *The organization of behavior*. New York: Wiley.

Harlow, H. F., & Suomi, S. J. (1974). Induced depression in monkeys. *Behavioral Biology*, *12*, 273–296.

Herrnstein, R. J. (1989). Darwinism and behaviourism: Parallels and intersections. In A. Grafen (Ed.), *Evolution and its influence* (pp. 35–61). Oxford, England: Clarendon Press.

Herrnstein, R. J. (1990). Rational choice theory: Necessary but not sufficient. *American Psychologist*, *45*, 356–367.

Herrnstein, R. J., & Vaughn, W., Jr. (1980). Melioration and behavioral allocation. In J. E. R. Staddon (Ed.), *Limits to action: The allocation of individual behavior* (pp. 143–176). New York: Academic Press.

Hertz, J., Krogh, A., & Palmer, R. G. (1991). *Introduction to the theory of neural computation*. Reading, MA: Addison-Wesley.

Hile (1991). Hand-held behavioral observations: The observer. *Behavioral Assessment*, *13*, 187–196.

Homme, L. E. (1965). Perspectives in psychology: XXIV. Control of coverants, the operants of the mind. *The Psychological Record*, *15*, 501–511.

Horner, R. H., & Storey, K. (1989). Putting behavioral units back into the stream of behavior: A consumer report. *The Behavior Therapist*, *12*, 249–251.

Hull, C. L. (1943). *Principles of behavior*. New York: Appleton-Century-Crofts.

Iwata, B., Pace, G., Kalsher, M., Cowdery, G., & Cataldo, M. (1990). Experimental analysis and extinction of self-injurious escape behavior. *Journal of Applied Behavior Analysis, 23,* 11–27.

Jacob, T., Tennenbaum, D., Bargiel, K., & Seilhamer, R. A. (1995). Family interaction in the home: Development of a new coding system. *Behavior Modification, 19,* 147–169.

Johnson, S. M., & Bolstad, O. D. (1975). Reactivity to home observation: A comparison of audio recorded behavior with observers present or absent. *Journal of Applied Behavior Analysis, 8,* 181–185.

Johnson, S. M., Christensen, A., & Bellamy, G. T. (1976). Evaluation of family intervention through unobtrusive audio recordings: Experiences in "bugging" children. *Journal of Applied Behavior Analysis, 9,* 213–219.

Kahanna, T. (1990). *Foundations of neural networks.* Reading, MA: Addison-Wesley.

Kandel, E. R. (1989). Genes, nerve cells, and the remembrance of things past. *Journal of Neuropsychiatry, 1,* 103–125.

Kandel, E. R. (1991). Cellular mechanisms of learning and the biological basis of individuality. In E. R. Kandel, J. H. Schwartz, & T. M. Jessell (Eds.), *Principles of neural science* (pp. 1009–1031). Norwalk, CT: Appleton & Lange.

Kazdin, A. E. (1977). *The token economy: A review and evaluation.* New York: Plenum Press.

Kehoe, E. J. (1988). A layered network model of associative learning: Learning to learn and configuration. *Psychological Review, 95,* 411–433.

Klopf, A. H. (1988). A neuronal model of classical conditioning. *Psychobiology, 16,* 85–125.

Konarski, E. A., Jr., Crowell, C. R., & Duggan, L. M. (1985). The use of response deprivation to increase the academic performance of EMR students. *Applied Research in Mental Retardation, 6,* 15–31.

LeDoux, J. (1996). *The emotional brain: The mysterious underpinnings of emotional life.* New York: Simon & Schuster.

Levine, D. S. (1991). *Introduction to neural and cognitive modeling.* Hillsdale, NJ: Erlbaum.

Lisboa, P. G. (Ed.). (1992). *Neural networks: Current applications.* New York: Van Nostrand Reinhold.

Mace, F. C., & Lalli, J. S. (1991). Linking descriptive and experimental analyses in the treatment of bizarre speech. *Journal of Applied Behavior Analysis, 24,* 553–562.

MacCorquodale, K., & Meehl, P. E. (1948). On the distinction between hypothetical constructs and intervening variables. *Psychological Review, 55,* 95–107.

Mahoney, M. J. (1974). *Cognition and behavior modification.* Cambridge, MA: Ballinger.

Mahoney, M. J. (1977). Reflections on the cognitive-learning trend in psychotherapy. *American Psychologist, 32,* 5–13.

Malone, J. C. (1990). *Theories of learning: A historical approach.* Belmont, CA: Wadsworth.

Martin, J. A., Maccoby, E. E., Baran, K. W., & Jacklin, C. N. (1981). Sequential analysis of mother–child interaction at 18 months: A comparison of microanalytic methods. *Developmental Psychology, 17,* 146–157.

Martin, G., & Pear, J. (1999). *Behavior modification: What it is and how to do it,* 6th ed. Englewood Cliffs, NJ: Prentice-Hall.

Martindale, C. (1991). *Cognitive psychology: A neural-network approach.* Belmont, CA: Brooks/Cole.

Matt, G. E., Vazquez, C., & Campbell, W. K. (1992). Mood-congruent recall of affectively toned stimuli: A meta-analytic review. *Clinical Psychology Review, 12,* 227–255.

Mayr, E. (1982). *The growth of biological thought: Diversity, evolution, and inheritance.* Cambridge, MA: Harvard University Press.

Michel, W. (1981). *Introduction to personality,* 3rd ed. New York: Holt.

Mowrer, O. H. (1948). Learning theory and the neurotic paradox. *American Journal of Orthopsychiatry, 18,* 571–610.

Nelson, M. M., & Illingworth, W. T. (1991). *A practical guide to neural nets.* Reading, MA: Addison-Wesley.

O'Brien, W. H., & Haynes, S. N. (1995). Behavioral assessment. In L. A. Heiden & M. Hersen (Eds.), *Introduction to clinical psychology* (pp. 103–139). New York: Plenum.

Pao, Y. H. (1989). *Adaptive pattern recognition and neural networks.* Reading, MA: Addison-Wesley.

Parker, H. C. (1996). *Behavior management at home: A token economy program for children and teens.* Plantation, FL: Specialty Press.

Patterson, G. R. (1979). A performance theory for coercive family interaction. In R. B. Cairns (Ed.), *The analysis of social interactions: Methods, issues, and illustrations* (pp. 119–162). Hillsdale, NJ: Erlbaum.

Patterson, G. R. (1982). *A social learning approach*: Vol. 3. *Coercive family process.* Eugene, OR: Castalia.

Patterson, G. R. (1997). Performance models for parenting: A social interactional perspective. In J. E. Grusec & L. Kuczynski (Eds.), *Parenting and children's internalization of values: A handbook of contemporary theory.* New York: Wiley.

Patterson, G. R., & Cobb, J. A. (1973). Stimulus control for classes of noxious behaviors. In J. F. Knutson (Ed.), *The control of aggression: Implications from basic research.* Chicago: Aldine.

Pavlov, I. P. (1960). *Conditioned reflexes: An investigation of the physiological activity of the cerebral cortex* (G. V. Anrep, Trans.). New York: Dover (original work published 1927).

Plaud, J. J., Gaither, G. A., Weller, L. A, Bigwood, S. J., Barth, J., & von Duvillard, S. P. (1998). Rational-emotive behavior therapy and the formation of stimulus equivalence classes. *Journal of Clinical Psychology, 54*, 597–610.

Premack, D. (1959). Toward empirical behavioral laws. I: Positive reinforcement. *Psychological Review, 66*, 219–233.

Purcell, K., & Brady, K. (1965). Adaptation to the invasion of privacy: Monitoring behavior with a miniature radio transmitter. *Merrill–Palmer Quarterly, 12*, 242–254.

Repp, A. C., Harman, M. L., Felce, D., Van Acker, R., & Karsh, K. G. (1989). Conducting behavioral assessments on computer-collected data. *Behavioral Assessment, 11*, 249–268.

Rescorla, R. R. (1987). A Pavlovian analysis of goal-directed behavior. *American Psychologist, 42*, 119–129.

Rescorla, R. R. (1988). Pavlovian conditioning: Its not what you think it is. *American Psychologist, 43*, 151–160.

Ritter, H., Martinetz, T., & Schulten, K. (1992). *Neural computation and self-organizing maps: An introduction.* Reading, MA: Addison-Wesley.

Rosenthal, T. L., & Zimmerman, B. J. (1978). *Social learning and cognition.* New York: Academic.

Rosenzweig, M. R. (1996). Aspects of the search for neural mechanisms of memory. *Annual Review of Psychology, 47*, 1–32.

Rumelhart, D. E., & McClelland, J. L. (Eds.). (1986). *Parallel distributed processing: Explorations in the microstructure of cognition.* Cambridge, MA: MIT Press.

Sasso, G. M., Reimers, T. M., Cooper, L. J., Wacker, D., Berg, W., Steege, M., Kelly, L., & Allaire, A. (1992). Use of descriptive and experimental analyses to identify the functional properties of aberrant behavior in school settings. *Journal of Applied Behavior Analysis, 25*, 809–821.

Schlundt, D. G. (1985). An observational methodology for functional analysis. *Bulletin of the Society of Psychologists in Addictive Behaviors, 4*, 234–249.

Schlundt, D. G., Johnson, W. G., & Jarrell, M. P. (1985). A naturalistic functional analysis of eating behavior in bulimia and obesity. *Advances in Behavior Research and Therapy, 7*, 149–162.

Schlundt, D. G., Virts, K. L., Sbrocco, T., Pope-Cordle, J., & Hill. J. O. (1993). A sequential behavioral analysis of craving sweets in obese women. *Addictive Behaviors, 18*, 67–80.

Seligman, M. E. P. (1995). *Helplessness: On depression, development, and death*, 2nd ed. San Francisco: Freeman.

Seligman, M. E. P. (1996). *The optimistic child: A proven program to safeguard children against depression and build lifelong resilience.* New York: HarperCollins.

Seligman, M. E. P., & Hager, J. L. (Eds.). (1972). *The biological boundaries of learning.* New York: Appleton.

Selverston, A. I. (Ed.). (1985). *Model neural networks and behavior.* New York: Plenum.

Sidman, M. (1992). Adventitious control by the location of comparison stimuli in conditional discriminations. *Journal of the Experimental Analysis of Behavior, 58*, 173–182.

Sidman M., Kirk B., & Willson-Morris M. (1985). Six-member stimulus classes generated by conditional-discrimination procedures. *Journal of the Experimental Analysis of Behavior, 43*, 21–42.

Sidman, M., & Tailby, W. (1982). Conditional discrimination vs. matching to sample: An expansion of the testing paradigm. *Journal of the Experimental Analysis of Behavior, 37*, 5–22.

Skinner, B. F. (1938). *The behavior of organisms.* New York: Appleton.

Skinner, B. F. (1945). The operational analysis of psychological terms. *Psychological Review, 52*, 270–277.

Skinner, B. F. (1948). "Superstition" in the pigeon. *Journal of Experimental Psychology, 38*, 168–172.

Skinner, B. F. (1950). Are theories of learning necessary? *Psychological Review, 57*, 193–196.

Skinner, B. F. (1953). *Science and human behavior.* New York: Appleton-Century-Crofts.

Skinner, B. F. (1957). *Verbal behavior.* New York: Appleton-Century-Crofts.

Skinner, B. F. (1963). Operant behavior. *American Psychologist, 18*, 503–515.

Skinner, B. F. (1966). Phylogeny and ontogeny of behavior. *Science, 153*, 1205–1213.

Skinner, B. F. (1969). *Contingencies of reinforcement.* New York: Appleton-Century-Crofts.

Skinner, B. F. (1971). *Beyond freedom and dignity.* New York: Alfred A. Knopf.

Skinner, B. F. (1974). *About behaviorism.* New York: Alfred A. Knopf.

Skinner, B. F. (1975). The shaping of phylogenetic behavior. *The Journal of the Experimental Analysis of Behavior, 24*, 117–120.

Skinner, B. F. (1977). Why I am not a cognitive psychologist. *Behaviorism, 5*, 5–10.

Skinner, B. F. (1981). Selection by consequences. *Science, 213*, 501–504.

Skinner, B. F. (1984a). Selection by consequences. *The Behavioral and Brain Sciences, 7*, 477–510.

Skinner, B. F. (1984b). The evolution of behavior. *Journal of the Experimental Analysis of Behavior, 41*, 217–221.

Skinner, B. F. (1989). The origins of cognitive thought. *American Psychologist, 44*, 13–18.

Sober, E. (1984). *The nature of selection: Evolutionary theory in philosophical focus.* Cambridge, MA: MIT Press.

Soskin, W. F., & John, V. P. (1963). The study of spontaneous talk. In R. G. Barker (Ed.), *The stream of behavior* (pp. 228–281). New York: Appleton-Century-Crofts.

Spitz, R. A. (1946). Anaclitic depression: An inquiry into the genesis of psychotic conditions in early childhood. *The Psychoanalytic Study of the Child*, *2*, 142, 313.

Spence, K. W. (1944). The nature of theory construction in contemporary psychology. *Psychological Review*, *51*, 47–68.

Staats, A. W. (1964). *Human learning*. New York: Holt, Rinehart & Winston.

Staats, A. W. (1968). *Learning, language, and cognition*. New York: Holt, Rinehart & Winston.

Staats, A. W. (1971). *Child learning, intelligence, and personality*. New York: Harper & Row.

Staats, A. W. (1975). *Social behaviorism*. Homewood, IL: Dorsey.

Staats, A. W. (1981). Social behaviorism, unified theory, unified theory construction methods, and the zeitgeist of separatism. *American Psychologist*, *36*, 239– 256.

Staats, A. W. (1986). Behaviorism with a personality: The paradigmatic behavioral assessment approach. In R. O. Nelson & S. C. Hayes (Eds.), *Conceptual foundations of behavioral assessment*. New York: Guilford.

Staats, A. W. (1993). Psychological behaviorism: An overarching theory and a theory-construction methodology. *The General Psychologist*, *48*, 58–59.

Staats, A. W. (1996). *Behavior and personality: Psychological behaviorism*. New York: Springer.

Suen, H. K., & Ary, D. (1989). *Analyzing quantitative behavioral observation data*. Hillsdale, NJ: Erlbaum.

Sutton, R. S., & Barto, A. G. (1981). Toward a modern theory of adaptive networks: Expectation and prediction. *Psychological Review*, *88*, 135–170.

Timberlake, W., & Allison, J. (1974). Response deprivation: An empirical approach to instrumental performance. *Psychological Review*, *81*, 146–164.

Timberlake, W., & Farmer-Dougan, V. A. (1991). Reinforcement in applied settings: Figuring out ahead of time what will work. *Psychological Bulletin*, *110*, 379–391.

Tolman, E. C. (1932). *Purposive behavior in animals and man*. New York: Century.

Torgerson, L. (1977). Datamyte 900. *Behavior Research Methods and Instrumentation*, *9*, 405–406.

Tryon, G. S. (1985). The engagement quotient: One index of a basic counseling task. *Journal of College Student Personnel*, *26*, 351–354.

Tryon, G. S. (1989a). Study of variables related to client engagement using practicum trainees and experienced clinicians. *Psychotherapy*, *26*, 54–61.

Tryon, G. S. (1989b). A study of engagement and premature termination in a university counseling center. *Counseling Psychology Quarterly*, *2*, 437–447.

Tryon, G. S. (in press). Initial engagement of clients in counseling. In G. S. Tryon (Ed.), *Counseling based on process research*. Needham Heights, MA: Allyn & Bacon.

Tryon, G. S., & Tryon, W. W. (1986). Factors associated with clinical practicum trainees' engagement of clients in counseling. *Professional Psychology: Research and Practice*, *17*, 586–589.

Tryon, R. C. (1931). Studies in individual difference in maze ability. *Journal of Comparative Psychology*, *12*, 1–22, 95–115, 303–345, 401–420.

Tryon, W. W. (1976a). Models of behavior disorder: A formal analysis based on Woods's taxonomy of instrumental conditioning. *American Psychologist*, *31*, 509–518.

Tryon, W. W. (1976b). A system of behavioral diagnosis. *Professional Psychology*, *7*, 495–506.

Tryon, W. W. (1978). An operant explanation of Mowrer's neurotic paradox. *Behaviorism*, *6*, 203–211.

Tryon, W. W. (1989). Behavioral assessment and psychiatric diagnosis. In M. Hersen (Ed.). *Innovations in child behavior therapy* (pp. 35–56). New York: Springer.

Tryon, W. W. (1990). Why paradigmatic behaviorism should be retitled psychological behaviorism. *The Behavior Therapist*, *13*, 127–128.

Tryon, W. W. (1993a). Neural networks: I. Theoretical unification through connectionism. *Clinical Psychology Review*, *13*, 341–352.

Tryon, W. W. (1993b). Neural networks: II. Unified learning theory and behavioral psychotherapy. *Clinical Psychology Review*, *13*, 353–371.

Tryon, W. W. (1994). Synthesis not complementarity. *American Psychologist*, *49*, 892–893.

Tryon, W. W. (1995a). Neural networks for behavior therapists: What they are and why they are important. *Behavior Therapy*, *26*, 295–318.

Tryon, W. W. (1995b). Resolving the cognitive behavioral controversy. *The Behavior Therapist*, *18*, 83–86.

Tryon, W. W. (1995c). Synthesizing animal and human research via neural network learning theory. *Journal of Behavior Therapy and Experimental Psychiatry*, *26*, 303–312.

Tryon, W. W. (1995d). Synthesizing psychological schisms through connectionism. In A. Gilgen & F. Abraham (Eds.), *Chaos theory in psychology* (pp. 247–263). Westport, CT: Praeger.

Tryon, W. W. (1996). Yes—neural network learning theory can resolve the behavioral cognitive controversy. *The Behavior Therapist, 19*, 70, 72–73.

Tryon, W. W. (1998a). A neural network explanation of posttraumatic stress disorder. *Journal of Anxiety Disorders, 12*, 373–385.

Tryon, W. W. (1998b). Behavioral observation. In M. Hersen & A. S. Bellack (Eds.), *Behavioral assessment: A practical handbook*, 4th ed. (pp. 79–103). Boston: Allyn & Bacon.

Tryon, W. W. (1999). A bidirectional associative memory explanation of posttraumatic stress disorder. *Clinical Psychology Review, 19*, 789–818.

Wasserman, P. D. (1989). *Neural computing: Theory and practice*. New York: Van Nostrand-Reinhold.

Watson, J. B. (1913). Psychology as the behaviorist views it. *Psychological Review, 20*, 158–177.

Watson, J. B. (1930). *Behaviorism*, rev. ed. Chicago: University of Chicago Press.

Watson, J. B., & Raynor, R. (1920). Conditioned emotional reactions. *Journal of Experimental Psychology, 3*, 1–14.

Whitehurst, G. J., Fischel, J. E., DeBaryshe, B., Caulfield, M. R., & Falco, F. L. (1986). Analyzing sequential relations in observational data: A practical guide. *Journal of Psychopathology and Behavioral Assessment, 8*, 129–148.

Williams, J. M. G., Watts, F. N., MacLeod, C., & Mathews, A. (1988). *Cognitive psychology and emotional disorders*. New York: Wiley.

Wolpe, J. W. (1958). *Psychotherapy by reciprocal inhibition*. Stanford, CA: Stanford University Press.

Woods, P. J. (1974). A taxonomy of instrumental conditioning. *American Psychologist, 29*, 584–597.

6

Biological Model

Doil D. Montgomery and Pamela M. Planthara

Introduction

Within the biological models of behavior, there are various major themes about what determines or underlies both normal and abnormal behavior. The most widely accepted premise is that the nervous system is the center of control for all behavior. Therein lies the content of this chapter. What controls the development of the nervous system, and what elements combine to determine its state and function at any given time? To answer these questions, the following must be considered: (1) genetic determinants of the development of the nervous system, (2) how environmental factors interact with genetics to influence neural development; and (3) the dynamics of change in the developed nervous system.

We now know that the nervous system is a dynamic structure whose anatomy and chemical and electrical states are constantly changing. It is known that these changes are due to an interactive combination of neural activity determining behavior and behavior changing neural activity. This two-way interaction between the nerves initiating behavior and behavior changing neural connections and chemistry determines how the nervous system will perceive and respond to the world. Some of the most well-documented models are discussed in this chapter.

Major Models

There are three major biological models postulated to account for dysfunctional behavior: the anatomical model, the neuronal model, and the learned model. The anatomical model postulates that the brain and spinal cord are topographically organized. This means that specific areas of the brain and the spinal cord control or sense certain processes. As examples, the occipital area of the cortex processes visual information, and the motor strip on the cortex controls skeletal muscles. Therefore, when the anatomy is altered by various events, specific behaviors will change.

Doil D. Montgomery and Pamela M. Planthara • Center for Psychological Studies, Nova Southeastern University, Fort Lauderdale, Florida 33314.

Advanced Abnormal Psychology, Second Edition, edited by Hersen and Van Hasselt. Kluwer Academic / Plenum Publishers, New York, 2001.

The next model, the neuronal model, postulates that individual nerve cells function normally within their structural and chemical parameters. When the structure or chemistry is altered outside normal limits, behavior is changed. The last model, the learned model postulates that the anatomy and/or neural functioning is altered by experience. This model assumes that behavior previously learned and adaptive at that time and situation is now no longer appropriate and therefore is dysfunctional. The learning model does not postulate a dysfunctional nervous system but implies that the nervous system is functioning normally and is responding to events based on previous experience, but that the response is not appropriate in the present situation. These three models are not incompatible in that behaviors, once functional but now dysfunctional, may have changed neuronal structure and/or chemistry leading to further dysfunctional behaviors.

Our chapter is organized into the major dysfunctional types of behavior that has been the focus of most of the research into biological explanations of dysfunctional behavior. These areas will be schizophrenia, depression, anxiety, and Alzheimer's disease. There are many other specific disorders such as Parkinson's disease, Huntington's disease, obsessive compulsive disorder, and more global disorders such as obesity, and sexual disorders, which it has been shown, have a biological basis, but due to the limitation of space these and other dysfunctions are not discussed.

SCHIZOPHRENIA

Anatomical and Neurochemical Influences

For many years, this disorder has been the focus of attempts to understand the physiological basis of abnormal behavior. It has a prevalence of approximately 1% in the general population and is equally distributed worldwide (Jablensky et al., 1992). It is a public disorder that manifests itself in easily observed bizarre behavior. Many of the those suffering from it appear on our streets and comprise a large portion of the homeless. There have been several biological markers of this affliction, and although much research has been generated in this area, there are still many unknowns associated with its conditions of onset, manifestations, treatment, and instances of its sudden and unexplained termination. Features of the varied forms of this disorder include disturbance of thought, paranoid and/or grandiose delusions of self and others, extreme lability or flat affect, and auditory and visual hallucinations. The disorder usually has its onset during adolescence and is known to have a genetic propensity, but is certainly influenced by stress and coping styles. The key symptoms are a dissociative thinking style accompanied by hallucinations, delusional interpretations, and unusual affect.

Gross Anatomy

Because symptoms of this disorder are so bizarre and persistent, investigators have looked to structural changes in the brain to account for the behavior. One area of investigation is the gross structure of the brain. Early studies using postmortem evidence were inconclusive. Recent studies using advances in brain imaging techniques such as computerized axial tomograms (CAT) and magnetic resonance imaging (MRI) have revealed structural abnormalities that may be primary to the disorder. Enlarged cerebral ventricles, especially the lateral ventricles have been shown to be associated with schizophrenia (Hyde & Weinberger, 1990;

Torrey, Bowler, Taylor, & Gottesman, 1994). Andreasen (1994) found that enlarged ventricles are a static trait that remain years after the initial breakdown. Based on research by Gooding and Iacono (1995), these structural changes may be related to subgroupings of this disorder. One example of this subgrouping is that those who have larger ventricles have been shown to have a higher degree of cognitive impairment and social maladjustment (Kemali et al., 1985). These types of findings prompted some researchers such as Gottesman (1995) to call for more clearly delineated classifications to better differentiate among outcomes, which seem confusing due to lack of separating results along probable subcategories of this disorder.

The finding of larger ventricles combined with the results of the study by Mednick, Huttunen, and Machon (1994), which noted that the affected discordant, identical twin has a smaller hippocampus and amygdala, suggests that enlarged ventricles may be due to atrophy of neural tissue located near the ventricle. In addition to the smaller hippocampus, there is also histological evidence that nerve cells in this nucleus are not structurally organized in schizophrenics as they are in non-diagnosed individuals (Kovelman & Scheibel, 1984; Conrad, Abebe, Austin, Forsythe, & Scheibel, 1991). Additional evidence from a study by Machon, Mednick, and Huttenen (1994) suggests that this disarray of neural circuits could arise from maternal viral exposure during the second trimester of pregnancy.

Specific Structures

On the basis of postmortem studies, it is apparent that there are structural and neurochemical differences in the frontal cortex and the limbic system in schizophrenics (Benes, 1993; Akbarian et al., 1995; Wible et al., 1995). This is known as the corticolimbic hypothesis of schizophrenia (Benes, 1993). The corticolimbic system is comprised of the cortex, primarily the frontal cortex, the limbic system, and interconnecting fibers. The limbic system is a loosely defined, subcortical, widespread group of nuclei comprised of the septum, fornix, cingulate cortex, thalamus, hippocampus, amygdala, and mammillary bodies. The limbic system is implicated in controlling emotion, learning, and memory (Rosenzweig, Leiman, & Breedlove, 1999). It is further speculated that the structural and neurochemical changes in this part of the brain are likely to be a result of altered neural development of the fetus (Watson, 1996). Both increases and decreases in neurotransmitters, such as aspartate and GABA, have been found in the corticolimbic system nuclei of schizophrenic individuals (Watson, 1996). There is also evidence that schizophrenics have reduced blood flow in the frontal cortex during cognitive demanding tasks (Berman & Weinberger, 1990; Andreason et al., 1992; Weinberger et al., 1994).

Structures in the basal ganglion have also been implicated in schizophrenia because it has been found that nuclei in the basal ganglion of schizophrenics have higher concentrations of dopamine D2 receptors than normals (Seeman, Guan, & Van Tol, 1993). The basal ganglia are another group of subcortical nuclei comprised of the caudate, putamen, and the globus pallidus. The basal ganglia are important in controlling skeletal motor activity (Rosenzweig, Leiman, & Breedlove, 1999).

Neurotransmitters

Another major hypothesis for brain abnormalities in schizophrenics is the dopamine hypothesis. This is due, in part, to the findings that high levels of amphetamines induce conditions that mimic schizophrenia. Amphetamines promote the release of catecholomines, especially dopamine, and prolong the action of the neural transmitter by blocking its re-uptake.

Rapid relief from psychotic symptoms is often observed from the use of a dopamine antagonist. There are numerous well-controlled studies that demonstrate the effectiveness of blocking the psychotic effects in schizophrenics with dopamine blocking agents (see Rosenzweig, Leiman, & Breedlove, 1999). What is still unclear is whether this relationship to dopamine involvement is due to over production of dopamine in certain neural tissue, over sensitivity of post-synaptic membranes, or failure to re-uptake the neural transmitter after release (Davis et al., 1991; Brier et al., 1997; Rosenzweig, Leiman, & Breedlove, 1999). The related discovery that dopamine levels vary in different parts of the brain and that abnormal levels may be specifically related to aspects of the disorder raises intriguing questions about the complications of treatments. By using dopamine-related medications, abnormal levels in specific brain regions may be brought to normal levels while changing other brain site levels to a dysfunctional level (Watson, 1996).

It is becoming increasingly clear that schizophrenia involves both generalized changes in the brain, as well as regionally specific alterations in key components of the corticolimbic system and basal ganglia. Because the onset for most individuals occurs during adolescence or early adulthood, these findings highlight the importance of discovering the relationship to pre- and postnatal development of the brain and the way maturational changes interact with genetic and environmental factors. The challenge now facing the understanding of the biological mechanisms proposed is detailing the genetically determined structural architecture of specific brain regions during both prenatal and perinatal disturbance of the normal ontogeny of neural tissue. Understanding these mechanisms still may not help explain why the manifestation of schizophrenic symptoms typically occurs in late adolescence long after most neural tissue has been structurally formed.

Genetics

The role genetics plays in determining schizophrenia has been an area of interest for some time. The first evidence was provided by noting the familial relationship of schizophrenia in twin studies, where concordance rates for monozygotic twins were higher than those of dizygotic twins, and those adopted by normal parents, but had a schizophrenic biological parent, had a higher incidence of the disorder (see Slater & Roth, 1960) than those born to nonschizophrenic parents. Recent studies of families that have the disorder show a mean incidence of 46.1% for monozygous twins and only 13.5% for dizygous twins (Trimble, 1996). In the general population, the incidence rate is 0.9%, for half sibs it is 7.1%, full sibs 14.2%, children of one schizophrenic parent 16.4%, and for children of two schizophrenic parents 39.2% (Trimble, 1996). This ever increasing relationship with increased genetic similarity provides strong support for the idea that a major factor is some genetic determinant. Tsaung (1993) has provided evidence that when specific symptoms are considered, even stronger genetic relationships are found. Even though specific genetic markers have been postulated, to date none has been proven (Cichon et al., 1995). However, Crow (1991) has implicated a possible sex-related relationship on the Y chromosome as a source of the disorder. Some support is provided by evidence of a higher occurrence of child schizophrenia when the mother is schizophrenic than when the father is (Crow et al., 1994). However, environmental factors must play a significant role in that adopted children of schizophrenic mothers have a higher incidence of schizophrenia than those adopted by nonschizophrenic mothers (Kety, 1983; Kety et al., 1994).

In summary, the answer to the way the knowledge of dysfunctional neural tissue translates into schizophrenic behavior is presently explained as follows. Because the frontal cortex directs behavior based on perceived elements of the situation compared with memory through a complex network of informational pathways, such as the limbic system, the dysfunction of these abnormal pathways may prevent effective conversion of long-term memory into "working" memory to determine appropriate behavior (Goldman-Rabic, 1996).

DEPRESSION

No one is a stranger to feeling down or depressed, especially if the sadness is associated with loss. However, clinical depression is quite different from feeling down at certain times in your life. It is more debilitating and dangerous, and the overwhelming sadness combines with a number of symptoms. The DSM-IV characterizes depression as the following: an unhappy mood; diminished interests; disturbance in sleep and appetite, loss of energy; difficulty in concentration; feelings of worthlessness; restless agitation; and recurrent thoughts of death or suicidal ideation. It is estimated that 13–20% of the population suffers from depression (Cassens et al., 1990). Nemeroff (1996) estimates that 5 to 12% of men and 10 to 20% of women in the United States will suffer from a major depressive episode at some time in their life. Clinical studies of depression also estimate that individuals who have been depressed in the past will become depressed more than once and that up to 10% of these depressed individuals (about 1.0 to 1.5% of Americans) will experience manic phases in addition to depressive ones, a condition known as manic depressive illness or bipolar disorder (Mann & Kupfer, 1993). Individuals who experience bipolar disorder go from the top of the world to an abyss of despair, or vice versa. From not being able to get out of bed or talk to anyone, they become loquacious. This period of euphoria is known as mania. Mania is marked by a decreased need for sleep, hyperverbal or pressured speech, delusions of grandeur, racing thoughts, hyperactivity, and propensity to engage in potentially self-destructive activities (DSM-IV). Examples of some potentially self-destructive activities are promiscuous sex, spending sprees, or reckless driving. Not everyone is at equal risk of developing depression. It appears that those who are more prone to depression are individuals who may have inherited a vulnerability to this disorder. They are especially sensitive to the effects of environmental stress or lack of social support (Selye, 1978).

Genetic Hypothesis

Researchers have found that depression and manic depression frequently run in families (Cardoret & Winokur, 1975). In fact, research on depression in twins reveals a higher concordance rate for monozygotic twins than dizygotic twins (Moldin et al., 1991). These concordance rates are the same whether the twins are reared apart or together. In the same way, adoption studies show higher rates of affective illness in the biological parents than foster parents. These findings suggest that close blood relatives of individuals who have severe depression or bipolar disorder are much more likely to suffer from those conditions than members of the general population. During the past 20 years, genetic research has begun to focus on specific chromosomes implicated in depression. Much of this research has focused on chromosome 11 (Egeland et al., 1987; Baron et al., 1987). More recently, chromosome 18 and a site on chromosome 21 have been the focus of attention. The chromosomes have been implicated by contributing to a vulnerability to bipolar illness, but these findings await replication (Nemeroff, 1996).

Neurotransmitter Hypotheses

Other researchers are concentrating on neurotransmitters. In 1967, Joseph Schildkraut and Seymour Kety presented the monoamine hypothesis of depression. They postulated that depression is associated with a deficit of the monoamine transmitters norepinephrine and serotonin. The evidence for this hypothesis was supported by empirical findings of drug clinical efficacy of two forms: antidepressant drugs and electroconvulsive shock therapy. Antidepressant drugs inhibit monoamine oxidase, the enzyme that inactivates norepinephrine, dopamine, and serotonin, thereby increasing the availability of monoamines. Further support for the hypothesis came from a study using reserpine, an antihypertensive that depleted norepinephrine and serotonin in the brain. Fifteen percent of patients treated with reserpine developed significant depressive symptoms (Schildkraut, 1965; Bunney & Davis, 1965). It is also postulated that norepinephrine, dopamine, serotonin, and histamine are impacted by electroconvulsive shock treatment (ECT). Electroconvulsive treatment apparently increases postsynaptic responsiveness to norepinephrine, serotonin, and particularly dopamine, possibly by increasing receptor sensitivity (Grahame-Smith, Green, & Costain, 1978). Because feeding and locomotion are thought to be regulated by the dopaminergic systems this effect would explain ECT's effectiveness in patients who exhibit psychomotor retardation and weight loss (Ungerstedt, 1979). Another explanation is based on the observation that repeated convulsions in animals result in decreased synthesis and concentration of Gamma-aminobutryic acid (GABA) in certain regions of the brain. Consequently, ECT may act to switch off the inhibitory effects of GABA function (Green, 1978).

The most recent antidepressants are the serotonin re-uptake inhibitors (SSRIs) such as fluoxetine. There is evidence that decreased serotonin (5-HT) activity can either increase vulnerability to or cause depression (Dalack et al., 1995). Serotonin activity has been associated with numerous processes that are dysregulated in depression, including negative mood, sleep disturbance, shortened rapid eye movement (REM) latency, disturbed circadian rhythms, abnormal neuroendocrine functions, and sexual abnormalities. 5-HT and its major metabolite, 5-hydroxyindoleactic acid (5-HIAA), have been found to be depleted in both the brains of suicide victims and in the cerebrospinal fluid of depressed patients (Mann & Stanley, 1986).

Neuroreceptor Regulation Hypothesis

An alternative hypothesis proposed by Siever and Davis (1985) suggests that depression may be the result of diminished functioning of the neuroreceptor on the postsynaptic neuron, rather than depletion of a neurotransmitter. Here, impaired postsynaptic neurons result in down-regulation of neuronal transmitting activities. This suggests that stress and the release of glucocorticoids reduce brain production of neurotrophic factors, specifically brain-derived neurotropic factor (BDNF). Neurotropic factors have been implicated in the survival and growth of neurons (Ockel et al., 1996). A reduction in BDNF leads to neuronal atrophy at certain sites and therefore depression (Duman, 1998). According to this, drugs that increase stimulation of serotonin and norepinephrine lead to an increase in BDNF release. The BDNF then maintains other brain neurons to alleviate depression. Serotonin-producing neurons project from the raphe nuclei in the brain stem to neurons in diverse regions of the central nervous system, including those that secrete or control the release of norepinephrine. Serotonin-producing cells extend into many brain regions thought to participate in depressive symptoms—including the amygdala (an area involved in emotions), the hypothalamus (involved in appetite, libido, and sleep), and cortical areas that participate in cognition and other higher processes. Failure of this regulating mechanism that governs transmitting operations results in inappropriate response to external and internal stimuli. Because serotonin is depleted, other neurons are affected and depressive symptoms are thought to occur.

Neuroendocrine Hypothesis

CORTISOL ABNORMALITIES

Selye (1978) explored the effects of life stress on psychophysiological functioning. The hypothalamic–pituitary–adrenal (HPA) axis is the system that mediates the generalized stress response. Patients who have major depression have been observed to have hyperactivity of the hypothalamus–pituitary adrenal. Hypercortisolemia has long been recognized as an essential part of abnormal adaptation process to stress and, it has been shown, alters mood, cognition, and behavior (Stokes, 1995). This well-studied neuroendocrine abnormality occurs in 30 to 50% of depressed patients (Rubin, 1989). This finding has been elaborated in many studies of depression that have employed the dexamethasone suppression test (DST). Dexamethasone is a potent synthetic corticoid that ordinarily suppresses a rise in adrenocorticotropic hormone (ACTH). When given, dexamethasone seems to "trick" the hypothalamus into believing that there is a high level of circulating corticol. In nondepressed individuals, dexamethasone clearly suppresses cortisol levels, but in depressed individuals it fails to suppress circulating levels of cortisol, possibly due to the hyperactivity of the hypothalamus. As depression is relieved, dexamethasone again suppresses cortisol.

The following structures in the CNS have been implicated in depression. The basal forebrain has been implicated in behavioral arousal, motivated behavior, attention, learning, and memory. The projections of the basal forebrain complex to the amygdala (involved in emotions) and the hippocampus (involved in short-term memory) are important areas of stimulation and negative feedback of the HPA axis, respectively, and to the cortex, where metabolic changes have been noted in depression (Wainer, Steininger, Roback, Burke-Watson, Mufson, & Kordower, 1993). These structures provide a unifying framework for the hypothesis of dysregulated CNS cholinergic transmission influences the HPA axis in major depression (Dilsaver, 1986).

THYROID ABNORMALITIES

In recent years, studies have demonstrated that "subclinical" hypo- and hyperthyroid conditions can also produce depression. This can occur in patients whose traditional thyroid function tests are considered normal but who demonstrate increases in production of thyroid stimulating hormone (TSH) or an abnormally blunted TSH response to thyrotropin-releasing hormone (TRH) (Loosen, 1985; Loosen & Prange, 1982). This latter finding is the basis of the TRH test, developed with the hope that it would be a specific diagnostic tool for depression. Like the dexamethasone suppression test, the TRH test has proven to be another nonspecific measure of HPA axis dysregulation. In many cases, thyroid supplementation can enhance the responsiveness of patients to antidepressant drugs (Kalin et al., 1987). However, additional studies are needed to determine whether any components of the hypothalamic–pituitary–thyroid axis are sensitive and reliable markers of depression.

MELATONIN ABNORMALITIES

Another area of neuroendocrinology of depression focuses on the pineal gland's production of the hormone melatonin. This hormone is of particular interest, because its synthesis is almost exclusively controlled by noradrenergic neurotransmission, and thus it has become a marker for norepinephrine activity. The pineal gland synthesizes melatonin at night, and this nocturnal synthesis has been found diminished in depressed patients (Brown et al., 1985).

REPRODUCTIVE ENDOCRINOLOGY

Physicians have long been aware of the association between reproductive functions in women and specific depressive syndromes. These include postpartum depression, premenstrual dysphoric disorder, and menopause-related depression. Endocrinological changes are clearly associated with postpartum and menopausally precipitated depression. Average estrogen, progesterone, prolactin, and β-endorphin (opioid peptides) levels have been known to drop after delivery (Smith et al., 1990). As for premenstrual syndrome (PMS), numerous clinical studies have shown that hormonal and endocrine changes cause associated symptoms. However, studies indicate that different endocrine events may be involved at different levels, so that further research is needed.

Sleep Disturbance Hypothesis

Circadian (daily) rhythms are responsible for the normal regulation of sleep-wake cycles, patterns of arousal, and corresponding patterns of hormonal secretions. However, patterns of arousal are constantly changing because an individuals emotional state, vigilance, and attentional processes are constantly changing (Lang, 1995). Interestingly, there is evidence that there is a subset of depressed patients whose disorder may reflect a dysregulation in their circadian rhythm. There is much evidence that (1) emotional disturbances frequently result in changes in sleep regulation; (2) disrupted or insufficient sleep can cause changes in the control of affect and attention; and (3) the neurobiology underlying the regulation of sleep overlaps to a large extent with neurobehavioral systems involved in regulating arousal, attention, and emotions.

It is evident in both clinical and nonclinical populations that there is a close relationship between emotional level and sleep regulation. Cartwright and Wood (1991) and Hall, Dahl, Dew, and Reynolds (1987) found that most people who report emotional distress-trauma, separation, personal loss, anxiety provoking events, etc. experience at least transient disruptions in sleep. Even positive emotions can interfere with sleep. The early stages of an intense romantic relationship or the anticipation of an exciting trip is also often associated with disrupted sleep. This link between emotional regulation and sleep regulation is even more apparent in clinical disorders. Disturbed sleep is characteristic of affective disorders. A similar relationship can be shown in the opposite direction as well. Inadequate sleep results in alterations in affect, attention, mood deterioration, decreased arousal, difficulties with focused attention, and "tiredness." A third line of evidence to link the regulation of sleep, affect, and attention comes from neurobiology. The neurobehavioral systems involved in regulating sleep overlap with, and are closely linked to, neural systems involved in regulating affect and attention.

EEG sleep changes are among the most common psychobiologic correlates of depression that demonstrate abnormalities in 90% of adult subjects who have major depressive disorder

(Reynolds & Kupfer, 1987). Normally, an individual goes through four stages of sleep (stages 1 and 2 are lighter; stages 3 and 4 are deeper) before entering REM. Patients who have major depression have been found to have a reduction in stages 3 and 4 and an increase in 1 and 2. REM sleep is misplaced and extended in the sleep of depressives. Depressed patients describe having less sleep, more disrupted sleep, and more intense frequent dreaming. The brain regions and pathways critical for wakefulness, slow-wave sleep, REM sleep, and cycling between states involve a complex interplay among multiple cortical and subcortical systems. For example, it has been found that human sleep deprivation impairs the prefrontal cortical functioning which results in less executive control. This translates into decreased goal-directed behaviors and diminished cognitive modulation of drives, impulses, and emotions. There is a complex relationship between the control of sleep and affective disorders.

Understanding the psychophysiological aspects of depression is critically important. Exciting trends and core issues have been discussed regarding the biological factors that may underlie depression. However, it is important to remember that interaction does exist between behavior and biology. Understanding normal and abnormal behavior needs to take into account social, cultural, personal, and historical factors. Biology affects behavior, and the environment and behavior have important effects on biology. The challenge lies in integrating both biological and environmental factors to provide optimal understanding and treatment. It seems prudent to propose that the role of biological influences in mental disorder may be best understood in terms of the vulnerabilities or strengths of an organism that directly interact and influence the environment and behavioral factors. However, what is clear is that by distinguishing the biological markers and understanding the integration of environmental influences, health-care providers can improve methods of diagnosing, treating, and preventing depression.

ANXIETY

Anxiety is a normal reaction to many of life's stressors, and none of us is completely free from it. In fact, anxiety is undoubtedly useful in causing us to be more alert and to take important things seriously. However, the anxiousness that we may feel from time to time is different from overwhelming feelings of dread, apprehension, uncertainty, nervousness, impatience, irritability, concentration difficulties, and sleep disturbance (DSM-IV, 1994). Among some of the mental symptoms of anxiety, there are many physical symptoms of anxiety which can include increased blood pressure, difficulties in breathing, faintness, dizziness, chest pain, cramps, nausea, constipation, diarrhea, trembling, chills, sweating, frequent urination, muscle aches, and dry mouth. All of these symptoms can range from mild to severe. In the United States, about 13.1 million people suffer from anxiety disorders (Wilson, 1988). There are 14 categories of anxiety disorders listed in the DSM-IV. Each category has it own unique biological underpinnings; however, for the purposes of this chapter the major biological components of anxiety will be elaborated. Evidence from anatomical and physiological research, which include neural pathways, brain structures, and endocrine functions have been identified as being involved in anxiety disorders.

Autonomic Nervous System

Physiological symptoms are central to the assessment process as seen through the DSM-IV for specific anxiety disorders. A subject who is experiencing anxiety is undergoing many visceral changes such as changes in the heart rate, blood pressure, stomach contractions, dilations or constriction of blood vessels, skin resistance, or sweating of the palm or soles. The autonomic nervous system (ANS) is concerned with regulating these physiological variables. On account of the strong physiological component of anxiety, the debate over the cognitive and noncognitive aspects of anxiety was started as early as the first third of the twentieth century by William James and Walter Cannon. James (1884) proposed that "reflex currents" initiate visceral reactions and overt muscle activity that are interpreted by the cortex as the experience of emotion (Bindra, 1970). Cannon (1920) responded with the observation that activation of the autonomic nervous system and thus the physiological arousal may lead to feeling as if one is anxious. He demonstrated that cats exposed to barking dogs exhibited behavioral and physiological signs of fear that are associated with adrenal release of epinephrine. Other studies have activated the autonomic nervous system with chemical agents. Several different substances such as yohimbine, isoprenaline, adrenaline, lactate, caffeine, beta-carboline, and CO_2 induce anxiety (Ehlers et al., 1986; Barlow, 1988).

In 1970, John and Beatrice Lacey reported a longitudinal study that monitored individual response patterns by provoking the ANS. Under stress conditions, such as immersing hands in cold water, they found that there is an individual profile of response that starts from infancy. For example, some newborns responded with blood pressure changes, others with heart rate changes, and still others with gastric changes. Later, Jerome Kagan and colleagues investigated newborns' behavioral responses to cues such as alcohol-soaked cotton swabs. He measured the newborns' behavioral responses from not reacting very strongly to reacting strongly. Many of the newborns who reacted strongly in Kagan's study (1997) later were described as shy, and a third of them developed phobias by the time they were old enough to go to school. A literature review by Barlow (1988) concludes that anxious patients are hyperaroused and slow to habituate. Such a slower habituation rate correlates with higher anxiety. Therefore, these studies suggest inborn biological differences.

Genetic Studies

Research does indicate that genetic components contribute to the development of anxiety disorder. In fact, according to Slater and Shields (1969), more than 50% of first-degree relatives suffer from the same disorder. Shields (1962) reported that there is a higher concordance rate with anxiety between monozygotic twins than dizygotic twins.

Brain-Imaging Studies

Structural studies using (CT) and (MRI) have found increases in the size of cerebral ventricles in individuals who suffer from anxiety disorders. Functional brain-imaging studies such as positron emission tomography (PET), single photon emission tomography (SPECTS), and electroencephalography (EEG) of anxiety disorder patients have found abnormalities in the frontal cortex, the occipital and temporal areas, and the parahippocampal gyrus (Swedo et al., 1992; Rubin et al., 1995; Schwartz et al., 1996). Other researchers, such as Breiter et al. (1996), found increased activity of the anterior cingulate cortex, the basal ganglia, and the amygdala. Several regions of the prefrontal cortex showed increased activity in a functional MRI.

Neurotransmitters

The three major neurotransmitters associated with anxiety on the basis of animal studies and responses to drug treatment are norepinephrine, γ-amino butyric acid (GABA), and serotonin.

NOREPINEPHRINE

The theory of norepinephrine activity and its role in anxiety disorders is that affected patients may have a poorly regulated noradrenergic system that has occasional bursts of activity. The cell bodies of the noradrenergic system are primarily localized in the locus coeruleus (LC) of the rostral pons, and they project their axons to the cerebral cortex, the limbic system, the brain stem, and the spinal cord. The axon terminals contain inhibitory and excitatory amino acids, monamines, and neuropeptides, many of which exert differential physiological effects on LC activity (Van Bockstaele, 1998). Research studies have shown that stimulation of the locus coeruleus produces a fear response in the animal and that ablation of the same area inhibits or completely blocks the ability of the animals to form a fear response (Redmond, 1979). Clinical drug studies have found that clonidine inhibits locus coeruleus activity (Seiver & Uhde, 1984). Other evidence indicates that inhibitory neurochemicals, which arise from extrinsic sources, include γ-aminobutryic acid (GABA) and epinephrine, as well as the neuropeptides, methionine-5-enkephalin, and leucine-5-enkephaline (Van Bockstaele, 1998).

GABA

The implication of (GABA) neurons is that slowed activity increases anxiety by loss of inhibitory action on anxiety-producing brain sites. γ-Aminobutryic acid type A (GABA(A))-receptor agonist decreases anxiety by facilitating the neuronal influx of chloride. GABA is the most common inhibitory transmitter in the brain and blocks anxiety. Yet, the exact locus of anxiolytic action of GABA in the brain is not clearly delineated (Imamura & Prasad, 1998). Nevertheless, clinical drug studies have found that the GABA receptors of some patients with anxiety disorder function abnormally and their GABA receptors fail to release inhibitory transmitters. Benzodiazepenes have a potentiating effect on the GABA neurotransmitter and facilitate its release at the synapses. The ultimate function of the benzodiazepene–GABA receptor complex is to regulate permeability of neural membranes to chloride ions. The neuron is inhibited from firing by chloride ions moving into the nerve cell (Marx, 1985).

SEROTONIN

Due to the therapeutic effects of serotonergic antidepressants such as buspirone and clomipramine in alleviating symptoms of anxiety, serotonin has received attention in the pathogenesis of anxiety. Most of the serotonergic neuron-cell bodies are located in the raphe nuclei in the rostral brain stem and project to the cerebral cortex, the limbic system, particularly the amygdala and the hippocampus, and the hypothalamus. Clinical studies show that blocking the re-uptake of serotonin improves symptoms of anxiety (Owens & Nemeroff, 1994).

HYPOTHALAMIC–PITUITARY–ADRENOCORTICAL SYSTEM

The hypothalamic–pituitary–adrenocortical (HPA) system controls a variety of neuro-hormones that may be implicated in anxiety. Specific hormonal products of HPA such as cortisol, prolactin, and thyroid-stimulating growth hormone increase under stressful conditions (Curtis, Nesse, Buxto, & Lippman, 1979).

By investigating anatomical hypotheses and synaptic communication hypotheses, we achieve a better understanding of the biological components of anxiety. We now know that there is a strong genetic factor involved in developing anxiety. However, integrating environmental influences with biological markers will be the key to understanding anxiety fully.

ALZHEIMER'S DISEASE

The loss of cognitive ability from aging, not from injury, has been of interest for some time. One particular type of loss was identified by Alois Alzheimer in publications in 1906, 1907, and 1911 (see Forstl & Levy, 1991). This disorder is now known by his name: Alzheimer's disease (AD). He was the first to identify the neural changes of plaques and neurofibrillary tangles which are the major markers of this disorder. This disorder is found worldwide, and the frequency of occurrence increases exponentially with age (Rocca et al., 1991). The other major markers of this disorder are cerebral atrophy, enlarged sulci and narrow convolutions, reduced white matter, and ventricular enlargement. There is also evidence of reduced subcortical tissue in areas such as the hippocampus. One study by Saeb et al. (1988) found an average reduction of 40% in hippocampal volume compared to nondemented controls. In another study, Golomb (1994) reported evidence from a study of normals 55 to 87 years of age and found that reduction in the size of the hippocampus was more closely correlated with memory loss than was generalized shrinkage of the brain. These two studies emphasize the role of the hippocampus in memory loss of both normals and ADs.

Neurological Features

Neuritic plaques (Sps) are the prominent feature of AD. These plaques consist of an amyloid core surrounded by argyrophilic axonal and dendritic processes (Morris, 1996). The amyloid fibers are composed of residues of amyloid beta-protein. Amyloid is a generic description of a class of tissue protein. This tissue may be deposited throughout the body or may be confined to a particular organ. The amyloid associated with AD is deposited around meningeal and cerebral vessels and in gray matter. However, because it has been determined that amyloid beta-protein is found in several species and in body fluids, the exact role it plays in AD is unclear (Haass et al., 1992; Thinakaran et al., 1998).

Sps are present in various numbers in elderly nondemented individuals, but they are more uniformly distributed in demented patients (Mirra et al., 1991). Although widely distributed in the brain, greater concentrations are often observed in the cerebral cortex, hippocampus, and subcortical areas primarily in those that are part of the limbic system. However, recent studies have shown little or no correlation between the concentration of Sps and cognitive decline (Dickson et al., 1992). What has been correlated with cognitive decline is the neurofibrillary tangles (NFT). NFTs are abnormal helically wound filaments of a microtubule associated with glycoprotein (Goedert et al., 1988). Increased density of NFTs in the cortex and some subcortical areas, again primarily those in the limbic system, has been associated with cognitive and memory decline (Arriagada et al., 1992; Bierer et al., 1995).

Genetics

The two most prominent risk factors for Alzheimer are age and a family history of the disorder (Bird, Lampe, Wijsman, & Schellenberg, 1998). Early linkage between Down's syndrome and AD has implicated chromosome 21 (St. George-Hyslop et al., 1987; St. George-Hyslop, 1993). However, some cases of AD have also linked AD with abnormalities of chromosome 19. Chromosome 19 has been implicated with the age of onset of AD (Roses, 1994). Lampe, Bird, Nochlin et al. (1994) presented strong, detailed evidence of pathological findings on chromosome 14 and AD. Other chromosomes have also been associated with the onset of AD (Levy-Lahad et al., 1995). Although research on AD and chromosomal abnormalities is still in its infancy, a growing body of evidence points toward a strong linkage between chromosomal abnormalities and the onset of AD.

SUMMARY

The conclusion which may be drawn from the research indicates that certain specific pathologies have underlying biological mechanisms associated with them. What seems to be the most parsimonious explanation is that genetics provides a general template for neural development which is modified by the experiences of the individual. We inherit propensities which place limits on behavior, yet the constraints may be altered by impoverished or enriched environments or by intense or sustained interventions. Recent information about neural development indicates that only approximately half of the neurons produced during embryonic development will survive the development of the nervous system (Oppenheim, 1991). These findings combined with evidence from animal studies indicate that the major determinant as to which nerve cells die and which survive depends on which neurons are activated by experiences. The cells that are activated by experience survive and form connections with other neurons, and those that are not activated die. This provides powerful support for the role early experiences have on neural development and subsequent behavior.

There is also a growing body of evidence that chemical states of neural tissue underlie some pathological behavior. However, what is not clear is the cause and effect relationship between behavior and neural activity. For instance, although unusual dopamine levels are related to schizophrenia, the reason that specific levels are present in certain neural sites is not clear. Whether these unusual levels are a result of atypical experiences combined with genetic propensities or just result from genetic influences alone is unknown. So the reason that these levels are unusual in one or more neural site and not others is still a mystery. Another puzzle is why atypical levels of some neurotransmitters such as dopamine are associated with different disorders such as schizophrenia and depression.

By necessity, research on the biological basis of behavior is reductionistic. This approach is used when research that focuses on specific factors such as the nature of genetic determinants of behavior must look at specific disorders and specific biological factors to observe whether there is a relationship between well-defined aspects of the study. This type of research discovers the absence or presence of relationships in most instances, but it does not rule out the likelihood of other influences upon the relationship. These influences may be dietary, early learning experiences, cultural factors, and trauma, to mention just a few. Therefore, although research has clearly demonstrated that relationships exist among such factors as chromosomal abnormalities, neural tissue disorganization, gross anatomical brain changes, synaptic changes, and pathological behavior, there is no research on humans that unequivocally demonstrates a cause and effect relationship between biological factors and behavior. This does not mean they do not exist, just that it has yet to be demonstrated with present day techniques and technologies. The type of interventions needed to demonstrate such relationships are unethical because they would require manipulations that would change the course of the individual's life experiences. Perhaps with further advancement of techniques such as imaging with devices such as functional MRI, interventions which would provide cause and effect relationships could be conducted on humans with acceptable risks and outcomes. An example of this could be providing the individual with intense sensory stimuli while observing neural changes in particular areas of the nervous system.

In summary, this is an exciting time for individuals interested in the biological basis of behavior because new information is increasing rapidly. Through new assay techniques of tissue chemistry and new imaging techniques of neural and chromosomal tissue, new discoveries are being reported. There is great promise for better understanding of the biology of behavior which is likely to help direct early optimum experiences and specific interventions at multiple levels to facilitate the individual's development.

REFERENCES

Akbarian, S., Kim, J. J., Potkin, S. G., Hagman, J. O., Tafazzoli, A., Bunney, W. E., Jr., & Jones, E. G. (1995). Gene expression for glutamic acid decarboxylase is reduced without loss of neurons in prefrontal cortex of schizophrenics. *Archives of General Psychiatry, 52*, 267–278.

American Psychiatric Association. (1994). *Diagnostic and statistical manual of mental disorders*, 4th ed. Washington, DC: Author.

Andreasen, N. C., Rezai, K., Alliger, R., Swayze, V. W., II, Flaum, M., Kirchner, P., Cohen, G., & O'Leary, D. S. (1992). Hypofrontality in neuroleptic-naive patients and in patients with chronic schizophrenia. Assessment with xenon 133 single-photon emission computed tomography and the Tower of London. *Archives of General Psychiatry, 49*, 943–958.

Andreason, N. C. (1994). Changing concepts of schizophrenia and the ahistorical fallacy. *American Journal of Psychiatry, 151*, 1405–1407.

Arriagada, P. V., Growdon, J. H., Hedley-Whyte, T., and Human, B. T. (1992). Neurofibrillary tangles but not senile plaques parallel duration and severity of Alzheimer's disease. *Neurology, 42*, 631–639.

Barlow, D. H. (1988). *Anxiety and its disorders: The nature and treatment of anxiety and panic.* New York: Guilford.

Baron, M., Risch, N., Hamburger, R., Mandel, B., Kushner, S., Newman, M., Drumer, D., Belmaker, R. H. (1987). Genetic linkage between X-chromosome markers and bipolar affective illness. *Nature, 326*, 289–292.

Benes, F. M. (1993). The relationship between structural brain imaging and histopathologic findings in schizophrenia research. *Harvard Review of Psychiatry, 1*, 100–109.

Berman, K. F., & Weinberger, D. R. (1990). The prefrontal cortex in schizophrenia and other neuropsychiatric diseases: *In vivo* physiological correlates of cognitive deficits. *Progress in Brain Research, 85*, 521–536.

Bierer, L. M., Hof, P. R., Purohi, D. P., Carlin, L., Schmeider, J., Davis, K. L., Perl, D. P. (1995). Neocortical neurofibrillary tangle correlate with dementia severity in Alzheimer's disease. *Archives of Neurology, 52*, 81–88.

Bindra, D. A. (1970). Emotion and behavior theory: Current research in historical perspective. In P. Black (Ed.), *Physiological correlates of emotion* (pp. 3–20). New York: Academic.

Bird, T. D., Lampe, T. H., Wijsman, E. M., & Schellenberg, G. D. (1998). Familial Alzheimer's disease: genetic studies. In M. F. Folstein (Ed.), *Neurobiology of primary dementia.* Washington, DC: American Psychiatric Press.

Breier, A., Su, T. P., Saunders, R., Carson, R. E., Kolachana, B. S., DeBartolomeis, A., Weinberger, D. R., Weisenfeld, N., Malhotra, A. K., Eckelman, W. C., & Pickar, D. (1997). Schizophrenia is associated with elevated amphetamine-induced synaptic dopamine concentrations: Evidence from a novel positron emission method. *Proceedings of the National Academy of Sciences USA, 94*, 2569–2574.

Breiter, H. C., Rauch, S. L., Kwong, K. K., Baker, J. R., Weisskoff, R. M., Kennedy, D. N., Kendrick, A. D., Davis, T. L., Jiang, A. P., Cohen, M. S., Stern, C. E., Belliveau, J. W., Baer, L., O'Sullivan, R. L., Savage, C. R., Jenike, M. A., & Rosen, B. R. (1996). Functional magnetic resonance imaging of symptom provocation in obsessive–compulsive disorder. *Archives of General Psychiatry, 53*, 595–606.

Brown, R. P., Kocsis, J. H., & Frazer A. (1985). Serum melatonin in affective disorders. *American Journal of Psychiatry, 142*, 811–816.

Bunney, W. E., Jr., & Davis, J. M. (1965). Norepinephrine in depressive reactions: A review. *Archives of General Psychiatry, 13*, 483–494.

Cannon, W. B. (1920). *Bodily changes in pain, fear, and rage.* New York: Appleton.

Cardoret, R. J., & Winokur, G. (1975). X-linkage in manic-depressive illness. *Annual Review of Medicine, 26*, 21–25.

Cartwright, R. D., & Wood, E. (1991). Adjustment disorders of sleep: The sleep effects of a major stressful event and its resolution. *Psychiatry Research, 39*, 199–209.

Cassens, G., Wolfe, L., & Zola, M. (1990). The neuropsychology of depression. *Journal of Neuropsychiatry and Clinical Neurosciences, 2*, 202–213.

Cichon, S., Noethen, N. M., Catalano, M., Di Bella, D., et al. (1995). Identification of two novel polymorphisms and a rare deletion variant in the human dopamine D4 receptor gene. *Psychiatric Genetics, 5*(3), 97–103.

Conrad, A. J., Abebe, T., Austin, R., Forsythe, S., & Scheibel, A. B. (1991). Hippocampal pyramidal cell disarray in schizophrenia as a bilateral phenomenon. *Archives of General Psychiatry, 48*, 413–417.

Crow, T. J. (1991). The search of the psychosis gene. *British Journal of Psychiatry, 158*, 611–614.

Crow, T. J., Delisi, L. E., Lofthouse, R., Poulter, M., Lehner, T., Bass, N., Shah, T., Walsh, C., Boccio-Smith, A., & Shields, G. (1994). An examination of linkage of schizophrenia and schizoaffective disorder to the pseudoautosomal region (Xp22.3). *British Journal of Psychiatry, 164*, 159–164.

Curtis, G. C., Nesse, R., Buxton, M., & Lippman, D. (1979). Plasma growth hormone: Effect of anxiety during flooding in vivo. *American Journal of Psychiatry, 136*(4-A), 410–414.

Curtis, G. C., Nesse, R. M., Buxton, M., & Lippman, D. (1979). Plasma growth hormone: Effect of anxiety during flooding in vivo. *American Journal of Psychiatry, 136*, 410–414.

Dalack, G. W., Glassman, A. H., Rivelli S., Covey, L., & Stetner, F. (1995). Mood, major depression, and fluoxetine response in cigarette smokers. *American Journal of Psychiatry, 152*(3), 398–403.

Davis, K. L., Kahn, R. S., Ko, G., & Davidson, M. (1991). Dopamine in schizophrenia: A review and reconceptualization. *American Journal of Psychiatry, 148*, 1474–1486.

Dickson, D. W., Crystal, H. A., Mattiace, L. A., Masur, D. M., Blau, A. D, Davies, P., Yen, S. H., & Arson, M. K. (1992). Identification of normal and pathological aging in prospectively studied nondemented elderly humans. *Neurobiology of Aging, 13*, 179–189.

Dilsaver, S. C. (1986). Cholinergic mechanisms in depression. *Brain Research Reviews, 11*(3), 285–316.

Duman, R. S. (1998). Novel therapeutic approaches beyond the serotonin receptor. *Biological Psychiatry, 44*(5), 324–335.

Egeland, J. A., Gerhard, D. S., Pauls, D. L., Sussex, J. N., et. al. (1987). Bipolar affective disorder linked to DNA markers on chromosome 11. *Nature, 325*(6107), 783–787.

Ehlers, A., Margraf, J., Roth, W. T., Taylor, C. B., Maddock, R. J., Sheik, J., Kobell, M. L., McClenahan, K. L., Gossard, D., Blowers, G. H., Agras, W. S., & Kopell, B. S. (1986). Lactate infusions and panic attacks: Do patients and controls respond differently? *Psychiatry Research, 17*, 295–308.

Forstl, H., & Levy, R. (1991). Foreword to the translation of "On certain peculiar diseases of old age" (by Alois Alzheimer). *History of Psychiatry, ii*, 71–74.

Goedert, M., Wischik, C. M., Crowther, R. A., Walker, J. E., & Klug, A. (1988). Cloning and sequencing of the cDNA encoding a core protein of the paired helical filament of Alzheimer's disease: Identification as the microtubule-associated protein tau. *Proceedings of the National Academy of Sciences USA, 85*, 4051–4055.

Goldman-Rakic, P. S. (1996). Dissolution of cerebral cortical mechanisms in subjects with schizophrenia. In S. J. Watson (Ed.), *Biology of schizophrenia and affective disease* (pp. 113–128). Washington, DC: American Psychiatric Press.

Golomb, J., deLeon, M. J., George, A. E., Kluger, A., Convit, A., Rusinek, H., deSanti, S., Litt, A., Foo, S. H., & Ferris, S. H. (1994). Hippocampal atrophy correlates with severe cognitive impairment in elderly patients with suspected normal pressure hydrocephalus. *Journal of Neurology, Neurosurgery and Psychiatry, 57*, 590–593.

Gooding, D., & Iacono, W. (1995). Schizophrenia through the lens of a developmental psychopathology perspective. In *Developmental psychopathology*, Vol. 2: *Risk, disorder, and adaptation*. Wiley Series on Personality Processes (pp. 535–580). New York: Wiley.

Gottesman, I. L. (1995). *Schizophrenia genes: The origins of madness*. New York: Freeman.

Grahme-Smith, D. G., Green, A. R., & Costain, D. W. (1978). Mechanism of the anti-depressant action of electroconvulsive therapy. *Lancet, 1*, 254–256.

Green, A. R. (1978). ECT—How does it work? *Trends in Neuroscience, 1*, 53–54.

Haass, C., Schlossmacher, M. G., Hung, A. Y., Vigo-Pelfrey, C., Mellon, A., Ostaszewski, B. L., Lieberburg, I., Koo, E. H., Schenk, D., Teplow, D. B., & Selkoe, D. (1992). Amyloid beta peptide is produced by cultured cells during abnormal metabolism. *Nature, 359*, 322–325.

Hall, M. H., Dahl, R. E., Dew, M. A., & Reynolds, C. F. (1995). Sleep patterns following major negative life events. *Directions in Psychiatry, 15*, 1–10.

Hyde, T. M., & Weinberger, D. R. (1990). The brain in schizophrenia. *Seminars in Neurology, 10*, 276–286.

Imamura, M., & Prasad, C. (1998). Increased GABA-gated chloride ion influx in the hypothalamus of low anxiety rats. *Physiological Behavior, 64*(3), 415–417.

Jablensky, A., Sartorius, N., Ernberg, G., Anker, M., Korten, A., Cooper, J. E., Day, R., & Bertelsen, A. (1992). Schizophrenia: Manifestations, incidence, and course in different cultures. *Psychological Medicine, Monograph Supplement, 20.*

James, W. (1884). What is emotion? *Mind, 9*(Series I), 188–204.

Kagan, J. (1997). Temperament and the reactions to unfamiliarity. *Child Development, 68,* 139–143.

Kalin, N. H., Dawson, G., Traiot, P., Shelton, S., Barksdale, C., Weiler, S., & Thienemann, M. (1987). Function of the adrenal cortex in patients with major depression. *Psychiatry Research, 22,* 117–125.

Kemali, D., Galderisi, M. S., Ariano, M. G., Cesarelli, M., Milici, N., Salvati, A., Valente, A., & Volpe, M. (1985). Clinical and neuropsychological correlates of cerebral ventricular enlargement in schizophrenia. *Journal of Psychiatric Research, 19,* 587–596.

Kety, S. S. (1983). Mental illness in the biological and adoptive families of schizophrenic adoptees: Findings relevant to genetic and environmental factors in etiology. *American Journal of Psychiatry, 140,* 720–727.

Kety, S. S., Wender, P. H., Jacobsen, B., Ingraham, L. J., Jansson, L., Faber, B., & Kinney, D. K. (1994). Mental illness in the biological and adoptive relatives of schizophrenic adoptees. Replication of the Copenhagen study in the rest of Denmark. *Archives of General Psychiatry, 51,* 442–455.

Kovelman, J. A., & Scheibel, A. B. (1984). A neurohistological correlate of schizophrenia. *Biological Psychiatry, 19,* 1601.

Lacey, J. I., & Lacey, B. C. (1970). Some autonomic-central nervous system interrelationships. In P. Black (Ed.), *Physiological correlates of emotion.* New York: Academic.

Lampe, T. H., Bird, T. D., Nochlin, D., Nemens, E., Risse, S. C., Sumi, S. M., Koerker, R., Leaird, B., Wier, M., & Raskind, M. A. (1994). Phenotype of chromosome 14-linked familial Alzheimer's disease in a large kindred. *Annals of Neurology, 36,* 368–378.

Lang, P. J. (1995). The emotion probe: Studies of motivation and attention. *American Psychologist, 50*(5), 372–385.

Levy-Lahad, E., Wijsman, E. M., Nemens, E., Anderson, L., Goddard, K. A., Weber, J. L., Bird, T. D., & Schellenberg, G. D. (1995). A familial Alzheimer's disease locus on chromosome 1. *Science, 269,* 970–973.

Loosen, P. T. (1985). The TRH-induced TSH response in psychiatric patients: A possible neuroendocrine marker. *Psychoneuroendocrinology, 10,* 237–260.

Loosen, P. T., & Prange A. J., Jr. (1982). Serum thyrotropin response to thyrotropin-releasing hormone in psychiatric patients: A review. *American Journal of Psychiatry, 139,* 405–416.

Machon, R. A., Mednick, S. A., & Huttunen, M. O. (1997). Adult major affective disorder after prenatal exposure to an influenza epidemic. *Archives of General Psychiatry, 54,* 322–328.

Mann, J. J., & Stanley, M. (Eds.). (1986). Psychobiology of suicidal behavior. *Annals of the New York Academy of Science, 487,* 1–357.

Mann, J. J., & Kupfer, D. J. (Eds.). (1993). Biology of depressive disorders, Part A: A systems perspective. In *The depressive illness* (p. 272). New York: Plenum.

Marx, J. L. (1985). "Anxiety peptide" found in brain. *Science, 227,* 934.

Mednick, S. A., Huttunen, M. O., & Machon, R. A. (1994). Prenatal influenza infections and adult schizophrenia. *Schizophrenia Bulletin, 20,* 263–267.

Mirra, S. S., Heyman, A., McKeel, D., Sumi, S. M., Crain, B. J., Brownlee, L. M., Vogel, F. S., Hughes, J. P., vanBelle, G., & Berg, L. (1991). The consortium to establish a registry for Alzheimer's disease. *Neurology, 41,* 479–486.

Moldin, S. O., Reich, T., & Rice, J. P. (1991). Current perspectives on the genetics of unipolar depression. *Behavior Genetics, 21,* 211–242.

Morris, R. G. (1996). *The cognitive neuropsychology of Alzheimer-type dementia.* Oxford, England: Oxford University Press.

Nemeroff, C. B. (1996). The corticotropin-releasing factor (CRF) hypothesis of depression: New findings and new directions. *Molecular Psychiatry, 1*(4), 336–342.

Ockel, M., Lewin, G. R., & Barde, Y.A. (1996). In vivo effects of neurotrophin-3 during sensory neurogenesis. *Development, 122*(1), 301–307.

Oppenheim, R. W. (1991). Cell death during development of the nervous system. *Annual Review of Neuroscience, 14,* 453–501.

Owens, M. J., & Nemeroff, C. B. (1994). The role of serotonin in the pathophysiology of depression: Focus on the serotonin transporter. *Clinical Chemistry, 40,* 288–295.

Redmond, D. E. (1979). New and old evidence for the involvement of a brain norepinephrine system in anxiety. In W. E. Fann, I. Karacan, & A. Pokorny (Eds.), *Phenomenology and the treatment of anxiety* (pp. 152–203). New York: SP Medical and Scientific Books.

Reynolds, C. F., & Kupfer, D. J. (1987). Sleep research in affective illness: State of the art circa. *Sleep, 10*(3), 199–215.

Rocca, W. A., Hofman, A., Brayne, C., Breteler, M. M., Clarke, M., Copeland, J. R., Dartigues, J. F., Engedal, K.,

Hagnell, O., Heeren, T. J., et al. (1991). The prevalence of vascular dementia in Europe: Facts and fragments from 1980–1990 studies. *Annals of Neurology, 30,* 817–824.

Rosenzweig, M. R., Leiman, A. L., & Breedlove, S. M. (1999). *Biological psychology: An introduction to behavioral, cognitive, and clinical neuroscience.* Sunderland, MA: Sinaur Associates.

Roses, A. D. (1994). Apolipoprotein E affects the rate of Alzheimer disease expression: J-Amyloid burden is a secondary consequence dependent on APOE genotype and duration of disease. *Journal of Neuropathology and Experimental Neurology, 53,* 429–437.

Rubin, R. T. (1989). Pharmacoendocrinology of major depression. *European Archives of Psychiatry and Neurological Sciences, 238*(5–6), 259–267.

Rubin, R. T., Ananth, J., Villanueva-Meyer, J., Trajmar, P. G., & Mena, I. (1995). Regional 133 Xenon cerebral blood flow and cerebral 99m Tc-HM-PAO uptake in patients with obsessive–compulsive disorder before and during treatment. *Biological Psychiatry, 38,* 429–437.

Rubin, R. T., Poland, R. E., Lesser, I. M., & Martin, D. J. (1989). Neuroendocrine aspects of primary endogenous depression: V. Serum prolactin measures in patients and matched control subjects. *Biological Psychiatry, 25*(1), 4–21.

Saeb, J. P., Jagust, W. J., Wong, S. T. S., et al. (1988). Quantitative NMR measurements of hippocampal atrophy in Alzheimer's disease. *Magnetic Resonance Imaging, 8,* 200–208.

Schildkraut, J. J. (1965). The catecholamine hypothesis of affective disorders: A review of supporting evidence. *American Journal of Psychiatry, 139,* 471–475.

Schildkraut, J. J., & Kety, S. S. (1967). Biogenic amines and emotion. *Science, 156,* 21–30.

Schwartz, M. W., Peskind, E., Raskind, M., Boyoko, E. J., & Porte, D. (1996). Cerebrospinal fluid leptin levels: Relationship to plasma levels and to adiposity in humans. *Nature Medicine, 2,* 589–593.

Seeman, P., Guan, H. C., & Van Tol, H. H. (1993). Dopamine D4 receptors elevated in schizophrenia. *Nature, 365,* 441–445.

Selye, H. (1978). *The stress of life.* New York: McGraw-Hill.

Siever, L. J., & Uhde, T. W. (1984). New studies and perspectives on the noradrenergic receptor system in depression: Effects of the alpha-2 adrenergic agonist clonidine. *Biological Psychiatry, 142,* 184–187.

Shields, J. (1962). *Monozygotic twins brought up apart and brought up together.* London: Oxford University Press.

Siever, L. J., & Davis, K. L. (1985). Overview: Toward a dysregulation hypothesis of depression. *American Journal of Psychiatry, 142*(9), 1017–1031.

Slater, B., & Shields, J. (1969). Genetical aspects of anxiety. In *British Journal of Psychiatry Special Publication No. 3: Studies of Anxiety.* Ashford, Kent: Headly Bros.

Slater, E., & Roth, M. (1960). *Clinical Psychiatry,* 1st ed. London: Bailliere, Tindall, and Cassel.

Smith, R., Cubis J., Brinsmead, M., Lewin, T., Singh, B., Ownes, P., Chan, E. C., Hall, C., Adler, R., Lovelock, M., Hurt, D., Rowley, M., & Nolan, M. (1990). Mood changes, obstetric experiences and alterations in plasma cortisol, beta-endorphin and corticotrophin releasing hormone during pregnancy and the puerperium. *Journal of Psychosomatic Research, 34*(1), 53–69.

St. George-Hyslop, P. H. (1993). Recent advances in the molecular genetics of Alzheimer's disease. *Neuroscience, 1,* 171–175.

St. George-Hyslop, P. H., Tanzi, R. E., Polinsky, R. J., Haines, J. L., Nee, L., Watkins, P. C., Meyers, R. H., Feldman, R. G., Pollen, D., Drachman, D., Growdon, J., Bruni, A., Jean-Francois, F., Salmon, D., Frommelt, P., Amaducci, L., Sorbi, S., Piacentini, S., Stewart, G. D., Hobbs, W. J., Conneally, M., & Gusella, J. F. (1987). The genetic defect causing familial Alzheimer's disease maps on chromosome 21. *Science, 235,* 885–890.

Stokes, P. E. (1995). The potential role of excessive cortisol induced by HPA hyperfunction in the pathogenesis of depression. *European Neuropsychopharmacology, 5*(Suppl.), 77–82.

Swedo, S. E., Leonard, H. L., Kraesi, M. J. P., Rettew, D. C., Listwak, S. J., Berrettini, W., Stipetic, M., Hamburger, S., Gold, P. W., Potter, W. Z., & Rapoport, J. L. (1992). CSF neurochemistry in children and adolescents with obsessive–compulsive disorder. *Archives of General Psychiatry, 49,* 29–36.

Thinakaran, G., Regard, J. B., Bouton, C. M., Harris, C. L., Price, D. L., Borchelt, D. R., & Sisodia, S. S. (1998). Stable association of presenilin derivatives and absence of presenilin interactions with APP. *Neurobiology of Disease, 4,* 438–453.

Torrey, E. F., Bowler, A. E., Taylor, E. H., & Gottesman, I. I. (1994). *Schizophrenia and manic depressive disorder.* New York: Basic Books.

Trimble, M. R. (1996). Schizophrenia. In *Biological psychiatry* (pp. 183–225). New York: Wiley.

Tsuang, M. T. (1993). Genotypes, phenotypes, and the brain. *British Journal of Psychiatry, 163,* 299–307.

Ungerstedt, U. (1979). Central dopamine mechanisms and unconditioned behaviour. In A. S. Horn, J. Korf, & B. H. C. Westerink (Eds.), *The neurobiology of dopamine* (pp. 577–596). New York: Academic.

Van Bockstaele, E. J. (1998). Morphological substrates underlying opoiod, epinephrine and gamma-aminobutyric acid inhibitory actions in rat locus coeruleus. *Brain Research Bulletin, 47,* 1–15.

Wainer, B. H., Steininger, T. L., Roback, J. D., Burke-Watson, M. A., Mufson, E. J., & Kordower, J. (1993). Ascending cholinergic pathways: Functional organization and implications for disease models. *Progress in Brain Research, 98,* 9–30.

Watson, S. J. (1996). *Biology of schizophrenia and affective disease.* Washington, D.C.: American Psychiatric Press.

Weinberger, D. R., Aloia, M. S., Goldberg, T. E., & Berman, K. F. (1994). The frontal lobes and schizophrenia. *Journal of Neuropsychiatry and Clinical Neurosciences, 6,* 419–427.

Wible, C. C., Shenton, M. E., Hokama, H., Kikinis, R., Jolesz, F. A., Metcalf, D., & McCarley, R. W. (1995). Prefrontal cortex and schizophrenia. A quantitative magnetic resonance imaging study. *Archives of General Psychiatry, 52,* 279–288.

Wilson, J. (1988). Anxiety disorders: Current treatments and controversies. Paper presented at *Annual Convention of the American Psychological Association,* Atlanta, GA, August, 1988.

II

Childhood and Adolescent Disorders: Introductory Comments

Early writings on child and adolescent psychopathology described the parallels between disorders in these groups and adult populations. Clinical research conducted over the past quarter of the twentieth century, however, has revealed the unique and complex developmental characteristics of children and youth that led to disparate manifestations of numerous disorders at early stages of the life span. Further, investigative efforts are underscoring the multiple pathways to many of these difficulties. This is reflected by the wide range of symptoms and behavioral disorders observed in children and adolescents within diagnostic categories. Such problems now appear to be a function of the interaction of a variety of psychosocial and biological factors that influence development. The chapters in Part II provide an overview of current findings on each of the major disorders of childhood and adolescence.

In Chapter 7, Cynthia Miller-Loncar, Jamie M. Winter, and Thomas L. Whitman describe the contemporary approaches to mental retardation. They underscore that current perspectives are more holistic and emphasize the reciprocal influences among cognitive, behavioral, emotional, and physical functioning of persons who are mentally retarded. Definitions and classifications have become more cohesive across national organizations. Advances in identification and prevention have occurred as the roles of environmental and biological contributors have become better understood and systematically evaluated. In particular, the impact of poverty on child development continues to add new questions about the causes and treatment of mental retardation. Information on this disorder continues to expand as research and educational programs consider more dynamic aspects of development, such as motivation.

Similarly, in Chapter 8, Lynn Kern Koegel, Marta Valdez-Menchaca, Robert L. Koegel, and Joshua K. Harrower examine the role of behavioral, environmental, neurological, and physical processes in autism. These authors also describe the three general areas of autism (impaired social interaction, communication deficits, and decreased activities and interests), as well as heuristic approaches to evaluation and intervention for each. The current movement toward inclusion, early intervention, peer involvement in intervention, functional behaviors, creating stable and meaningful social relationships, and decreasing family stress is definitely a step toward meeting the need to significantly improve the quality of life for those who are autistic.

Strategies and issues pertaining to what is perhaps the most serious and recalcitrant of childhood disorders, attention-deficit/hyperactivity disorder, are covered by Mark D. Rapport (Chapter 9). Mounting evidence suggests that ADHD is significantly more common in certain families and inherited through some yet unknown mechanism and that underactivity of the prefrontal-striatal-limbic regions of the brain results. Differences in the neurophysiological functioning of the brain may help explain why these children experience profound difficulties in maintaining attention, regulating their arousal, inhibiting themselves in accordance with environmental demands, and getting along with others—yet only at specific times and under certain conditions. Research that focuses on executive and regulatory functioning and particularly working memory and subcomponents, such as the visuospatial control system, may help elucidate specific processes involved in the pathophysiology of ADHD.

In Chapter 10, Marc S. Atkins and Mary M. McKay point out how childhood conduct disorder—characterized by chronic patterns of social norm violations—represents a serious and seemingly intractable mental health problem. In recent years, there has been a growing awareness of the importance of an ecological perspective for understanding the onset and maintenance of children's conduct problems. School, family, and community contexts have been shown to provide powerful contexts for the emergence of children's conduct problems. As a result, new and promising interventions have been developed that offer renewed hope for the early and effective remediation of children's conduct problems. Only by considering both ecological and developmental perspectives will conduct problems be understood in the context of real-world concerns that impact children's relationships with family, teachers, and peers.

In Chapter 11, Thomas H. Ollendick and Devin A. Byrd show how DSM-IV diagnostic criteria have prompted the intricate examination of anxiety disorders in children and adolescents according to a specified set of characteristics, course, and prognosis. They argue that a global dimensional approach to anxiety and its disorders has afforded us the opportunity to explore physiology, effect, and cognition and their respective roles in the onset, expression, and course of these disorders. In epidemiological studies, research methodologies using structured and semistructured clinical interviews reveal high prevalence rates for the anxiety disorders that approach between 12 and 15% of the youth studies. Although genetic influences must be acknowledged in the course of these disorders, the contributions and influence of psychological and psychosocial factors (including attachment relationships, temperament, social support, life events, self-concept, and acculturation) cannot be ignored. With respect to treatment, behavioral and cognitive-behavioral strategies have been shown to be effective with anxious children and adolescents. But it is evident that these treatments have not been systematically examined in children who vary widely in age and ethnicity.

Chandra M. Grabill, Jeana R. Griffith, and Nadine J. Kaslow, in Chapter 12, state that depression in childhood can be a serious condition that interferes with the child's development and functioning, even upon remission from a depressive episode. Depression in children and adolescents tend to persist over time and to recur and thus necessitate treatment. The limited systematic treatment interventions conducted to date reveal that some form of psychosocial or pharmacological treatment is better than no treatment at all in ameliorating depressive symptoms and improving the course of the disorder. However, insufficient data exist to support the superiority of any given treatment. Further research needs to attend to development and implementation of effective interventions for depressed youth, as well as prevention programs for youth at risk of depression.

In Chapter 13 on eating disorders, Linda Krug Porzelius, Britta D. Dinsmore, and Darlene Staffelbach note that eating disorders are complex and chronic. Diagnostic criteria have changed dramatically, yet many questions remain. The complexity of the disorders is evidenced by high rates of comorbidity with anxiety disorders, depression, personality disorders, and substance abuse. Multiple etiological factors have been identified—including psychological, familial, biological, and sociocultural contributors—that combine in different ways for each individual. Sociocultural factors contribute to the development of eating disorders through their impact on dieting, body dissatisfaction, and fear of fat. However, etiological models must identify additional vulnerability factors because chronic dieting and body dissatisfaction do not always lead to eating disorders. Environmental factors implicated in the development of eating disorders include family relationships, family's attitudes toward weight and appearance, and sexual trauma. Individual characteristics are also implicated, including personality characteristics, interpersonal and social difficulties, coping skills, and mood regulation. Increasingly complex and sophisticated etiological models are being developed and tested.

7

Mental Retardation

Cynthia L. Miller-Loncar, Jamie M. Winter, and Thomas L. Whitman

Description of the Disorder

Individuals who are mentally retarded have been viewed in a variety of ways over the centuries. In Greek writings, mental retardation was mentioned as early as 1500 B.C. Later, in 500 B.C., Hippocrates wrote about skull deformities associated with retardation. During the Middle Ages, persons who were mentally retarded were viewed as fools, favored as "innocents of God," persecuted as witches, or considered possessed. In the sixteenth and seventeenth centuries, legal definitions were offered, and in the nineteenth century more sophisticated attempts were made to differentiate mental retardation from mental illness (Scheerenberger, 1987).

The development of intelligence tests in the early twentieth century, as well as the focus on both the environmental and genetic-organic causes of mental retardation, brought about considerable changes in views of this disorder. Intelligence tests provided a measure for assessing subaverage functioning and for distinguishing among different levels of retardation. The terms idiot, imbecile, and moron were introduced to identify those individuals whose test scores respectively fell below IQs of 25, 50, and 75 (Levine & Marks, 1928; Scheerenberger, 1987). As discussed in Scheerenberger (1987), Dugdale and Goddard proposed the term "familial retardation" to describe those individuals who did not have any obvious physical signs of mental retardation, thus recognizing that subgroups of mental retardation existed.

Researchers also acknowledged the variability of functioning in individuals who are mentally retarded and are of the same mental age. Recognizing the limitations of using intelligence tests as the sole means for classifying mental retardation, Porteus developed a test of "planfulness," and Doll proposed a measure of "social maturity," both of which today would be considered tests of adaptive behavior (Grossman, 1983). Intellectual functioning and adaptive behavior evolved as the key elements in definitions and classification systems of

Cynthia L. Miller-Loncar • Department of Pediatrics, Infant Development Center, Women & Infants' Hospital, Providence, Rhode Island 02903. **Jamie M. Winter and Thomas L. Whitman** • Department of Psychology, University of Notre Dame, Notre Dame, Indiana 46556.

Advanced Abnormal Psychology, Second Edition, edited by Hersen and Van Hasselt. Kluwer Academic/Plenum Publishers, New York, 2001.

mental retardation. More recently, theorists have emphasized the importance of considering motivational factors, as well as developmental issues (Hodapp, Burack, & Zigler, 1990; Hupp, 1995).

In the present chapter, definitional, classification, and epidemiological issues relating to mental retardation are discussed. Then, clinical pictures of persons who had different courses of development and prognoses associated with this complex disorder are presented. Finally, the diverse causes of mental retardation and issues relating to assessment and diagnosis are examined.

Definition and Classification of Mental Retardation

Several professional organizations provide formal criteria for defining and classifying mental retardation. There is general agreement among these organizations, but the definitions differ in the purposes for which they were developed, in the aspects of mental retardation that are emphasized, and in the audience toward which they are directed. Several current definitions are presented here, including those of the American Association on Mental Retardation (AAMR) (1992), the American Psychiatric Association in its *Diagnostic and Statistical Manual of Mental Disorders*, Fourth Edition (DSM-IV) (1994), and the international medical community as part of its International Classification of Diseases-10 (ICD-10) (1992). Finally, a more encompassing developmental disabilities definition adopted by Congress is also discussed.

DEFINITIONS

American Association on Mental Retardation.   The definition and classification schema proposed by the AAMR is the most widely recognized and used system in the United States. The AAMR first published a definition and classification system in 1921. This system has undergone several major revisions since that time. The current definition (American Association on Mental Retardation, 1992) characterizes the disorder of mental retardation as consisting of substantial limitations in present functioning, including significantly subaverage intellectual skills and coexisting limitations in two or more adaptive skill areas, which are manifested before 18 years of age. Under this definition, limitations in intellectual functioning refer to a fundamental restriction in a person's conceptual, practical, and social intelligence that impairs one's ability to learn and perform daily life skills. Significantly subaverage intellectual skills are defined by IQ scores of 70 to 75 or less. Limitations in adaptive skill areas are judged by standards of personal independence and social responsibility as defined by an individual's age and cultural group.

Despite specific criteria for diagnosing mental retardation, there is flexibility in making this diagnosis. For example, an IQ of 70, or two standard deviations less than the mean on standardized intelligence tests, is given as the cutoff score for mental retardation; however, this limit is intended as a general guideline. It may be extended up through an IQ of 75, depending on the reliability of the intelligence test. Such flexibility is important in schools or similar settings where it is necessary to formally identify individuals who need special educational services. Although there are standardized tests of adaptive behavior, there is also some flexibility in applying the criterion of adaptive behavior deficits, in part because of variability in cultural expectations.

The AAMR emphasis on a multidimensional approach to classifying and diagnosing mental retardation broadens the conceptualization of the disorder and avoids a reliance on IQ scores for classification. Its current definition stipulates that a comprehensive diagnosis must include evaluation in four domains. The first domain relates to the core conceptual definition and developmental period (birth to 18) that emphasizes both intellectual and adaptive behavioral deficiencies. Within the adaptive skill domain, the following areas of personal competence are specified: communication, self-care, home living, social skills, community use, self-direction, health and safety, functional academics, leisure, and work. Although deficiencies in at least two of these areas must be present, these deficits may coexist with strengths in other areas of personal competence. This domain is used to make the formal diagnosis of mental retardation.

After the diagnosis has been made, the individual is evaluated in the other three domains that include psychological/emotional, physical/health, and environmental dimensions. Assessment of the psychological/emotional and physical/health domains involves listing specific disorders that exist in these areas. The individual's current living situation is also evaluated to consider the extent to which the environment facilitates or restricts the individual's life satisfaction and to specify the optimal environment that would maximize the person's independence, productivity, and community integration. This proposed system stresses that mental retardation is not necessarily a lifelong condition and that the functioning of individuals with mental retardation can generally be expected to improve with appropriate services.

Diagnostic and Statistical Manual of Mental Disorders (DSM).   The DSM provides another classification system commonly employed by mental health clinicians and researchers. In the latest revision (DSM-IV, 1994), the definition of mental retardation has been modified to be more compatible with the AAMR definition. The definition of mental retardation, according to the DSM-IV, first requires a significant deficit in intellectual functioning. For a diagnosis of mental retardation, the individual must have an IQ of 70 or lower on an individually administered IQ test.

A DSM diagnosis of mental retardation also specifies that there must be significant deficits in adaptive behavior. The DSM-IV identifies the same adaptive skill areas as those in the AAMR definition and requires deficits in at least two of these areas. Unlike the IQ criterion, no specific score on a measure of adaptive functioning is required for the diagnosis of mental retardation. The final DSM definitional criterion is that mental retardation be manifest by age 18. This criterion differentiates mental retardation from deficits in intelligence and adaptive behavior that occur later in life as a consequence of illnesses or organic insult.

International Classification of Diseases.   The International Classification of Diseases (ICD) system was developed by the World Health Organization to provide the international medical community with a standard guide for gathering mortality and morbidity data. The tenth and most recent revision of this system, the ICD-10 (1992), characterizes mental retardation in terms of impairments in an individual's overall level of intelligence, which includes cognitive, language, motor, and social abilities. The criteria further specify that these impairments must occur during the developmental period. Assessment methods that are recommended include the use of standardized intelligence tests, as well as measures of social adaptation. The ICD-10 definition is complementary to the criteria found in the AAMR and DSM-IV definitions. This tenth revision departs from earlier ICD definitions that characterized mental retardation primarily in terms of subnormal intelligence.

Developmental Disabilities.   Mental retardation can also be subsumed under the more general definition of "developmental disabilities." Under this definition, developmental disabilities consist of severe, chronic conditions that are the result of mental and/or physical impairments. These conditions must be present before 22 years of age, are not transient, and require lifelong or extended individually based services. A developmental disability impacts three or more areas of life activity including self-care, language, learning, mobility, self-direction, independent living, and economic sufficiency. Within this definition, mental retardation is only one condition among a number of disorders that are collectively labeled developmental disabilities. Other disorders include learning disabilities, pervasive developmental disorders (e.g., autism), cerebral palsy, epilepsy, and other neurological impairments. This definition was adopted in 1978 by Congress and included in Section 102 (7) of Public Law 95-602, the Developmental Disabilities Assistance and Bill of Rights Act (often referred to as the DD act). It was intended to provide a guideline for identifying individuals who were eligible for government services and funding and not as a clinical criterion.

CLASSIFICATION

The population of persons with mental retardation is very heterogeneous. There are vast individual differences in the severity of the deficits, associated physical handicaps, and concurrent psychological disorders manifested, as well as the degree of dependence on environmental supports (Grossman, 1983). For this reason, attempts have also been made to divide mental retardation into more homogeneous subgroups. The most common subcategorizations of mental retardation have been based on etiology and level of functioning and include the following examples.

Etiological Classification.   The American Association of Mental Retardation system divides mental retardation into two distinct subgroups on the basis of general etiology. One subgroup, which accounts for approximately 25% of individuals with mental retardation, consists of individuals whose condition has organic causes, such as a central nervous system pathology, genetic disorder, and/or metabolic deficit. These individuals typically fall in moderate to severe ranges of intellectual deficiency, have associated physical handicaps or stigmata, and are usually diagnosed at birth or in early childhood. The second group, which accounts for the majority of cases of mental retardation, consists of individuals who have no apparent neurological damage or obvious physical signs of retardation, function in the mild range of mental retardation, and are found in disproportionate numbers in lower socioeconomic groups. Diagnosis of this latter group of individuals, typically, occurs during the school years. Although it is possible to distinguish between these two groups (organic versus nonorganic), there is no complete professional consensus concerning the utility of this type of dichotomous categorization.

Severity Classifications.   Another common method of categorizing mental retardation is by degree of severity of retardation. All of the previously mentioned classification systems (AAMR, DSM-IV, ICD-10) provide guidelines for distinguishing among four levels of severity. These categorizations, which are made solely on the basis of IQ scores, are as follows:

Mild Mental Retardation	50–55 to 70–75 IQ
Moderate Mental Retardation	35–40 to 50–55 IQ
Severe Mental Retardation	20–25 to 35–40 IQ
Profound Mental Retardation	less than 20 or 25 IQ

The overlap in IQ score cutoffs allows for some discretion in classifying "borderline" cases. A fifth category, unspecified mental retardation, is used when there is reason to suspect mental retardation, but the individual is untestable using a standardized IQ test.

Epidemiology

Epidemiology involves the scientific study of diseases and disorders in populations. Epidemiological research plays an important role in the study of the distribution, causes, treatment, and prevention of mental retardation and more generally influences the design of public health policies and programs.

Prevalence

Prevalence is the total number of persons with mental retardation who are present in a population at a given time. Prevalence data are used to project the type and amount of services needed for a given population. Based on the theoretical distribution of the normal curve, roughly 2.5% of the population are estimated to have intelligence scores lower than 2 standard deviations below the mean (one of the criteria for mental retardation). Recent population-based studies have estimated that prevalence rates range from 1% to 2% (Murphy, Yeargin-Allsopp, Decoufle, & Drews, 1995; Yeargin-Allsopp, Murphy, Oakley, & Sikes, 1992). The range observed in prevalence rate estimates may be due to differences in ascertainment methods, definition systems, and social and demographic compositions of populations. To obtain a more refined epidemiological picture of mental retardation, it is useful to look at the prevalence of mental retardation in relation to specific demographic characteristic such as age, sex, and socioeconomic status, all of which have been found to be related to prevalence.

Age

Prevalence of mental retardation varies across age groups. The prevalence rate is lowest for children under four years of age. This finding is probably related to the fact that identification of mental retardation during infancy and early childhood is difficult for all but the most severely retarded individuals. For several reasons, the prevalence figures for this disorder, especially mild and moderate retardation, increase during school years. As children enter the school system, widespread testing and identification is available. Moreover, increasing academic and social demands in the classroom environment reveal problems not likely to be manifested by the children in their homes and neighborhood environments. The President's Committee on Mental Retardation (1969) coined the phrase "the six hour retarded child" to describe children who were considered retarded during the school day, but who could function effectively in their neighborhood environments.

A similar explanation accounts for the decline in the identifiable prevalence of mental retardation with increasing age. Many mildly retarded persons who have had trouble in academic settings can, upon leaving these settings, function at least marginally well in vocational and community environments, and thus are no longer identified as mentally retarded. In addition, historically, the prevalence of mental retardation among older adults has been relatively low because these individuals had shorter life spans. This figure, however, has increased as improved medical care has become available.

Sex

Researchers report a higher prevalence of mental retardation among males than females. The reported male-to-female ratio is 1.6 to 1. Some suggest that this gender difference is most pronounced among the mildly retarded population (Katusic et al., 1996). Sex differences in prevalence rates among the mildly retarded have been attributed to the greater vulnerability of males to biological insult, the higher demands placed by society on males, and the greater proportion of behavioral problems among males. Higher prevalence rates of more severe retardation among males may be accounted for by the fact that biological defects associated with the X chromosome are more likely to be manifested by males than females.

SOCIOECONOMIC STATUS

Moderate, severe, and profound retardation have fairly similar prevalence rates across socioeconomic groups, although there tend to be slightly higher rates of each of these levels of mental retardation among low-income families. Mild retardation, however, has been estimated to be considerably more prevalent within the lower socioeconomic strata. Epidemiological studies suggest that individuals from lower socioeconomic classifications and who have minority status are overrepresented within the mild range of mental retardation (Drews, Yeargin-Allsopp, Decoufle, & Murphy, 1995). Some individuals attribute this finding to the use of intelligence tests that are culturally biased against minority groups (Mercer, 1973). Additional factors, such as poor nutrition, inadequate health care, impoverished environments, greater life stress, and unstable family situations are also likely to contribute to this greater estimated prevalence. Environmental causes of mental retardation are discussed in greater detail later in this chapter.

Epidemiology

A number of forces are currently acting to change the prevalence of mental retardation, including genetic screening, prenatal diagnostic procedures, elective abortions, newborn screenings for inborn errors of metabolism, early intervention and initiatives such as Healthy People 2000. Identification of problems during infancy should result in a reduction in some types of mental retardation, particularly if this assessment leads to earlier placement in prevention and treatment programs. The Infant Health and Development Program (1990) is an example of an early intervention program aimed at improving the functioning of low birth weight premature infants who are at risk for developmental delays. This program provided a combination of early educational programming, family support services, and pediatric care. Children who received the intervention displayed significantly higher cognitive development and fewer behavioral difficulties at three years of age, compared to children who did not receive the intervention. In addition to direct treatment programs, the U.S. Department of Health and Human Services designed Healthy People 2000 as a 10-year plan to reduce preventable disabilities and diseases in children and adults. Examples of objectives of this program aimed at reducing mental retardation include improving immunization levels, reducing unsafe blood lead levels in children, and increasing the proportion of newborns who are screened for genetic disorders (U.S. Dept. of Health and Human Services, 1990).

Although such programs were created to reduce developmental disabilities, advances in medicine have increased prevalence rates in specific populations. For example, there is a high rate of mental retardation among very low birth weight infants, who previously would not have lived, but are being saved by medical technology. Medical advances also have increased the life span of individuals who are retarded, thus increasing the prevalence rates of the disorder among the elderly population.

CLINICAL PICTURE

Clinical descriptions of individuals who are mentally retarded vary widely because of the range of functioning that encompasses this diagnosis. Individuals also vary because of the types of programming they receive, as well as the amount of developmental growth that results from this programming. To illustrate this diversity, two case descriptions of children with varying developmental levels are provided.

Case Description 1

Henry was a 5-year-old male, the younger of two children. He was the product of a full-term pregnancy. Although his prenatal, birth, and early childhood histories were unremarkable for any significant complications, Henry displayed significant delays in his language skills. He did not say his first word until he was 2½ years old and did not speak in simple phrases until 4½ years of age. Because of his language delays, Henry was sent for extensive hearing examinations, all of which indicated that his hearing was within normal limits.

In addition to his significant expressive language problems, Henry's parents reported that he was unable to grasp basic concepts such as colors, letters, and numbers and had significant difficulties with independent problem solving. Socially, he was a friendly child who liked to engage others in simple games. At 4 years of age, Henry was referred by his pediatrician for speech services and began receiving speech therapy from his school district.

As a consequence of concerns raised by Henry's speech therapist regarding his cognitive abilities, he was referred for extensive neurodevelopmental testing. Because of Henry's limited language skills, he was evaluated using both verbal and nonverbal tests of intelligence. Henry was assessed as having an overall IQ score of 65 on verbal tests and displayed nonverbal intelligence skills that were at a 2½ year age level. His language skills were at a 2 year age level. Henry was also found to be delayed in the adaptive behavior areas of daily living, socialization, and communication. Based on this evaluation, Henry received a formal diagnosis of mild mental retardation.

Henry's Individualized Education Program (IEP) at 5 years of age specified that he be placed in an early childhood classroom that focused on basic skill development. It further specified that he receive speech and language services three times each week. It was recommended that Henry's speech program combine spoken language with sign language to increase his expressive language skills. Henry's IEP also specified that he be integrated into a regular kindergarten class for part of his week to foster social skills. Based on his developmental levels, it was anticipated that Henry would continue to require placement in a special education classroom throughout his schooling. His educational instruction would include extensive resource support for subjects, such as reading and math, as well as integration with same age peers in other subject areas (e.g., art, gym).

Case Description 2

Alexis was a 4-year-old female, born at 26 weeks gestational age and weighing 770 grams at birth. During her hospitalization, Alexis required ventilator support for the first 37 days of life. Her perinatal course included a mild, bilateral intraventricular hemorrhage and multiple infections in the brain. She was discharged from the hospital at 94 days of life. Alexis's developmental progress was monitored by a neonatal follow-up clinic until she was 2 years of age. All of her major developmental milestones were delayed. She sat independently at 13 months, walked at 25 months, and said her first word at 30 months.

Alexis's treatment course included enrollment in an early intervention program, starting at her discharge from the hospital, as well as ongoing follow-up at the hospital clinic to monitor her medical and developmental progress. During the first three years of life, she received weekly visits from an early intervention specialist who worked with Alexis on her cognitive, motor, and language skills. This specialist also provided specific developmental activities for Alexis's family. At 3 years of age, Alexis's early intervention program assisted with her transition into the early childhood program in her school district. She attended school five half days a week and received both speech therapy as well as occupational therapy for fine motor delays.

At 4 years of age, the Bayley Scales of Infant Development-II were used to examine her progress. The Bayley Scales are normed for children up to 42 months of age, but this exam was used because of Alexis's limited cognitive, language, and attentional skills. Her overall performance revealed that she was functioning at approximately a 12-month age level in most areas. It was recommended that Alexis remain in a self-contained early childhood classroom and that programs focus on improving her self-help skills (e.g., using the bathroom, eating), behavioral cooperation, and communication of functional needs. Based on her skill levels, it was anticipated that Alexis would require extensive school supports for all areas of her functioning throughout her educational experience.

COURSE AND PROGNOSIS

As depicted in these case descriptions, Henry and Alexis were identified as being at risk for developmental delay at different points in their lives. Henry was identified when he reached school age, and Alexis was identified shortly after birth. The two children also varied in their early developmental trajectories. Henry displayed relatively normal development except in language and problem-solving areas, whereas Alexis displayed global delays beginning in infancy. Based on formal testing, Henry was assessed as having mild mental retardation whereas Alexis was evaluated as having severe mental retardation.

Although intelligence is a fairly stable trait, the development of adaptive behavioral skills continues during the life span. The course of development for an individual who is mentally retarded is reflected in the acquisition of daily-living, language, socialization, academic, and vocational skills. Each of these domains is briefly described here and are related to what Henry and Alexis might achieve.

Daily-Living Skills

Daily-living skills are areas of functioning often thought of as self-help skills. The development of these skills begins with self-feeding and also includes bathing, dressing, teeth brushing, and toileting. Persons who have profound delays may require considerable assistance before learning to perform these activities. It can be anticipated that Alexis would attain basic skills in this area. In contrast to persons who are profoundly mentally retarded, persons who have severe delays like Alexis generally require only minimal supervision to complete self-help behaviors, once they are taught. In the domestic arena, individuals who are severely mentally retarded typically learn such skills as putting household items away and wiping a tabletop, whereas the individual who is moderately mentally retarded will likely learn more complex skills, such as setting a table, making a sandwich, and making a bed. Persons who are mildly mentally retarded typically acquire independence in even more complex activities, such as meal preparation, house cleaning, and doing laundry. These individuals can also develop basic skills in money management, but may need assistance in learning to budget. As a person like Henry develops, he would be expected to reach this level of independence.

Language

Both receptive and expressive language deficiencies are common across all individuals who are mentally retarded. As indicated in the case studies, Alexis had only begun to imitate a few words by age 2½, whereas Henry had developed some functional communication skills. Upon reaching adulthood, individuals who have profound delays may use gestures to indicate needs and, if verbal, may possess a very limited vocabulary and follow only simple instructions. Individuals who are severely mentally retarded like Alexis may learn to speak in short sentences and recognize written symbols but probably will not read with comprehension. Persons who are moderately mentally retarded can generally carry on simple conversations and learn to read simple materials, whereas individuals who are mildly impaired can carry on everyday conversations and receive formal instruction in reading and writing. In Henry's case, although his overall functioning falls in mild ranges, his ability to obtain functional academic skills in reading and writing may be more limited as the result of his significant language difficulties.

Socialization

Individuals who are profoundly mentally retarded commonly engage in isolated, simple play activities but may also learn to participate in highly structured group games. Persons whose functioning falls in severely retarded ranges may spontaneously participate in group activities and show a preference for friends, a level which a person like Alexis could reasonably achieve. Individuals who have moderate delays are more likely to interact both cooperatively and competitively with others but may need assistance in initiating appropriate social activities. In contrast, persons who are mildly mentally retarded can more readily plan and carry out social activities and develop lasting friendships, including intimate sexual relationships. A person such as Henry may have a girlfriend and even eventually get married.

Academic Achievement

The focus of educational programming for persons who are severely and profoundly mentally retarded is typically on basic skill training in communication, daily living, and socialization. Although they may not develop extensive communication skills, they may learn to use alternative communication systems, such as sign language, picture boards, or computerized communication boards. Individuals like Alexis may learn to recognize "survival" signs, such as "stop," "walk," and "poison" but will not learn to read with any proficiency. Persons who are severely mentally retarded may also learn to identify coins and use them functionally for daily purchases but do not typically develop basic addition or subtraction skills. Individuals who are moderately mentally retarded can learn skills, such as adding coins, printing their names, and reading simple instructions. They may also develop more formal, albeit only rudimentary, skills in arithmetic and reading. Persons who are mildly mentally retarded, like Henry, may eventually achieve a fourth or fifth grade level in reading, writing, and arithmetic.

Vocational Training

Individuals who are profoundly and severely mentally retarded do not possess the attentional and specific job skills necessary for independent employment. When a person like Alexis completes her school years, she might receive limited vocational training in a sheltered setting. In contrast, individuals who have moderate delays may enter into supportive employment programs within a community setting, support that is eventually phased out. Through this type of program, adults who are mentally retarded can be prepared to handle maintenance and food service jobs in places such as motels and restaurants. A person who is mildly mentally retarded, like Henry, will probably receive vocational training as part of his education and then is ready for regular employment upon completing school.

ORGANIC AND PSYCHOSOCIAL PATTERNS

Although more than 200 types of mental retardation have been described in the literature, etiology is specified in less than 50% of the cases. The causes of mental retardation can be divided into two primary categories: organic and psychosocial. An organic cause is a physiological and/or anatomical defect that may have a genetic basis. In contrast, psychosocial causes have roots in the environment in which the individual lives. Both types of causes may have environmental origins. In this section, both types of causes are briefly described. For a more extensive discussion of the etiology of mental retardation, refer to Grossman (1983) and Moser (1995).

Organic Causes

Organic etiologies account for 15 to 25% of the cases of mental retardation. The major organic causes of mental retardation involve central nervous system impairments. Generally, the organic etiologies are associated with more severe levels of mental retardation and only infrequently with mild retardation. The onset of organic pathology can be in the prenatal, perinatal, or postnatal periods of development; however, organic problems have their inception during the prenatal period.

PRENATAL CAUSES

Organic impairments in the developing fetus during the prenatal period may result from single gene defects, chromosomal anomalies, chemical hazards, maternal infections, and other teratogens. Each of these etiological categories is briefly discussed.

Single Gene Defects.   It has been estimated that there are approximately 210 single-gene disorders that have a phenotype that leads to mental retardation. In 1990, Wahlstroem reported that 69 disorders had been mapped to an autosome and 73 to the X chromosome (cited in Thapar, Gottesman, Owen, O'Donovan, & McGuffin, 1994).

The most common of these is phenylketonuria (PKU), an autosomal recessive condition. Although rare, it occurs in about one in 10,000 to 14,000 live births, and it is estimated that one person in 70 is a carrier of the recessive gene. The infant who has PKU suffers from a deficiency of the liver enzyme phenylalanine hydroxylase that is needed to convert the amino acid phenylalanine to tyrosine. Tyrosine is an amino acid necessary for the development of certain hormones, including epinephrine. Due to this deficiency, phenylalanine is not broken down. Bodily fluids build up as a consequence which interferes with the process of myelination, thus damaging the central nervous system. If untreated, severe or profound mental retardation may result. However, newborn screening and subsequent dietary management have resulted in the successful control of PKU. Other recessive gene disorders include maple syrup urine disease, Tay–Sachs disease, and Niemann–Pick disease. In contrast to recessive gene disorders, dominant gene disorders account for a small proportion of cases of mental retardation.

Chromosomal Abnormalities.   Abnormalities of the chromosomes account for 10 to 20% of mild mental retardation and for up to 40% of cases of severe mental retardation (Goestason, Wahlstroem, Johannisson, & Holmqvist, 1991; Hagberg & Hagberg, 1984). In many cases, these disorders are associated with increased maternal age.

Down's syndrome is the most common genetic cause of mental retardation and is diagnosed in approximately one in 1000 live births. It is an autosomal disorder, most commonly associated with a third copy of the twenty-first chromosome, that results in mild to severe mental impairment. Clinical features also include a large tongue, epicanthic folds, and increased rates of congenital heart defects. Other autosomal chromosomal abnormalities that result in mental retardation include Edwards' syndrome, Patau's syndrome, and cri-du-chat syndrome.

Other chromosomal anomalies, such as fragile X syndrome, occur due to abnormalities of the sex chromosomes. Fragile X has an estimated rate of occurrence of one in 1250 male births and one in 2000 female births (Thapar et al., 1994). Affected individuals have a fragile site or constriction on the long arm of the X chromosome. Those diagnosed with this condition often have mild to moderate mental retardation; some individuals have profound deficits, whereas others possess normal intelligence.

Other abnormalities of the sex chromosomes often associated with mental retardation include Turner's syndrome and Klinefelter's syndrome. Turner's syndrome, a condition in which only one X chromosome is present, affects one in 2500 female births. Although affected individuals usually have normal IQs, females who have this condition characteristically possess a visual-spatial deficit. The incidence of Klinefelter's syndrome, which occurs among newborn males, is estimated to be one in 1000 and results from pairing two or more X chromosomes with a single Y chromosome. Most XXY individuals have normal intelligence; however, they have mean IQs below the general population, and many experience speech and language disorders.

Maternal Teratogens.   A third set of factors causally linked to mental retardation in the prenatal period are maternal teratogens. Teratogens are developmental toxins, such as chemical hazards and infectious agents, that can adversely impact fetal development (Kohlberg, 1999). Risks to the unborn child are typically greatest during the first trimester of pregnancy. Fetal exposure to chemical teratogens results from maternal exposure to a toxic substance. Alcohol is one substance that can have a substantial impact on the developing fetus. Fetal alcohol syndrome (FAS) results from maternal alcohol consumption during pregnancy, and the risk to the fetus is greatest during the first trimester. FAS occurs in one to two of every 1000 births. Mental retardation is accompanied by physical abnormalities, such as a small head, wide-spaced eyes, a flat nose, and a deep upper lip. Other common toxic hazards include drugs, radiation, and lead poisoning.

In addition to chemical teratogens, the child is also at risk prenatally from exposure to maternal infections. Although less common in recent decades, rubella is a viral infection that historically has been associated with mental retardation. Research indicates that fetal infection occurs 50% of the time when the mother has rubella during early pregnancy and that intellectual impairment occurs in half of the infected children. Toxoplasmosis, a protozoan infection carried and transferred to the mother from raw meat and fecal material, is another condition that can affect the developing fetus by damaging the central nervous system. Mental retardation from this infection results in 85% of live births. Other common maternal infections associated with mental retardation include cytomegalovirus, syphilis, and AIDS.

PERINATAL CAUSES

Organic causes of mental retardation also operate during the perinatal period. For example, cerebral trauma may result from an abnormal labor or delivery. Difficulties may occur as a result of the position of the baby during birth or the length of labor. Abnormal fetal positions can create critical pressure on the skull, and other complications, such as anoxia, can cause severe tissue damage to the brain. During prolonged labor, the child is at risk of oxygen deprivation if the umbilical cord becomes wrapped around its neck or if the placenta detaches from the uterine wall. The severity of impairment manifested in these situations is related to the degree of cerebral trauma. Because of improved medical procedures, these types of perinatal factors account for only a small number of cases of mental retardation.

Prematurity and low birth weight are the most common perinatal risk factors for mental retardation. Both are associated with a variety of maternal factors including poor nutrition, infections, substance abuse, and medical conditions, such as a thyroid deficiency, chronic diabetes, and anemia. Medical advances have dramatically increased the survival of children born prematurely. Unfortunately, the increased rate of survival, particularly among extremely premature ($<$ 28 weeks) and very low birth weight babies (1500 grams), is associated with a wide variety of perinatal insults, postnatal medical complications, and developmental sequelae. Medical complications include hydrocephalus, intraventricular hemorrhages, hypoglycemia, hypoxia, and respiratory distress, and the prevalence increases as birth weight decreases. Very low birth weight children also have significantly higher rates of cognitive deficiencies compared to sociodemographically matched control groups. The occurrence of cognitive delays among children who weigh less than 1,000 grams at birth ranges from 8 to 15% and increases to 20% for those children born at 750 grams or less (Hack, Klein, & Taylor, 1995).

POSTNATAL CAUSES

In addition to prenatal and perinatal manifestations, mental retardation can also be caused postnatally, most frequently during the early developmental period by an array of biological factors, including: (1) cerebral trauma associated with head injury and seizure disorders; (2) toxic poisoning, such as from lead and mercury; and (3) infectious diseases, such as meningitis and encephalitis. Conditions such as meningitis and encephalitis have debilitating effects primarily in infancy. Despite the numerous postnatal agents that can produce neurological insult, relatively few cases of mental impairment are associated with damage to the central nervous system during this period.

Psychosocial Causes

Although research has traditionally focused on biological causes of mental retardation, the majority of individuals who are mentally retarded (approximately 75%) do not manifest an identifiable organic etiology (Weisz, 1990). Typically, these individuals are mildly impaired and are commonly considered disabled as a result of psychosocial disadvantage. However, Zigler and Balla (1982) also suggested that this form of mental retardation may be polygenetic in origin and a normal expression of the population gene pool. This type of retardation most often occurs in families in which more than one member is mentally handicapped.

Psychosocially produced mental retardation likely has a complex etiology that results from a combination of biological and environmental influences. For example, Weisz (1990), discussing the importance of social influences on an individual's personal attributes (expectancy of success, outer directedness, and self-concept), suggests that a person's motivational orientation can be reduced as a consequence of inadequate social stimulation and a history of failure experiences. This, in turn, may adversely influence cognitive and behavioral functioning. It is important also to note that the vast majority of individuals who have psychosocially caused mental retardation are found in lower socioeconomic strata (Zigler, 1995). Recent research points to the strong role that poverty plays in negatively impacting cognitive and behavioral development in young children (Duncan, Brooks-Gunn, & Klebanov, 1994). Baumeister, Kupstas, and Klindworth (1991), discussing a phenomenon they refer to as the "New Morbidity," emphasize how factors associated with poverty (e.g., low birth weight, prematurity, alcohol use, AIDS, and adolescent parenting) combine to result in mental retardation. For example, children from low socioeconomic families are more likely to be born prematurely and consequently are more vulnerable to early biological insult. Limited economic, physical, or social resources may subsequently exacerbate developmental difficulties initially caused by such biological problems. In discussing the correlates and determinants of mental retardation in the children of adolescent mothers, Borkowski et al. (1992) similarly emphasize the influence that an array of socioeconomic and individual factors can have on a child's development. These factors include family, community social supports, maternal health, maternal nutritional status, maternal cognitive readiness, maternal personal adjustment, parental education, and parental learning ability.

DIAGNOSTIC CONSIDERATIONS

The diagnostic process, guided by the established criteria for defining mental retardation, facilitates the identification and description of mental retardation, establishes an individual's eligibility for services, and may identify causes of a developmental problem. Through this process, the individual's current level of functioning and developmental rate are evaluated, and information about remediation and educational planning is provided. In schools, one outcome of the diagnostic process is the creation of an Individualized Educational Program (IEP) for a child. Through repeated evaluations, this IEP changes as the child develops.

Major Assessment Tools

Historically, intelligence tests have been a central diagnostic tool for identifying mental retardation. Some of the more widely used assessments include the Stanford–Binet, the Wechsler Preschool and Primary Scale of Intelligence-Revised (WPPSI-R), the Wechsler Intelligence Scale for children-III (WISC-III), and the Wechsler Adult Intelligence Scale-Revised (WAIS-R). The use of IQ tests as a legitimate diagnostic tool has, however, been questioned since the Civil Rights movement of the 1960s, specifically because of the disproportionate number of minority children diagnosed as mildly mentally retarded. Mercer (1973) suggested that intelligence tests were culturally biased and discriminated against minority children who failed to meet the dominant culture's expectations for performance in school.

To address this problem, Mercer and Lewis (1978) developed the System of Multicultural Pluralistic Assessment (SOMPA). The SOMPA attempts to address IQ biases by taking into account social and cultural characteristics in calculating an IQ score. The SOMPA also examines factors such as the child's health history, physical impairments, and social milieu before making educational placement decisions. Validation research on the SOMPA indicates that it is similar to standardized intelligence tests in its predictive validity for measures of school achievement (Figueroa & Sassenrath, 1989). Constructors of standardized intelligence tests have attempted to address concerns related to cultural biases by establishing norms based on samples that reflect the current U.S. population and by validating the use of measures for diverse populations. Despite these changes, disproportionate numbers of minorities who live in poverty continue to be identified as mildly retarded.

Because of concerns regarding the narrow focus of intelligence tests and their use as an exclusive vehicle for defining mental retardation, the American Association of Mental Deficiency (AAMD) since 1959 has emphasized the importance of adaptive behavior in addition to cognitive ability in its definition of mental retardation. The most widely used assessment for examining adaptive behavior is the Vineland Adaptive Behavior Scales (Sparrow, Ballo, & Cicchetti, 1984). In addition to standardized measures, several sources (Gelfand, Jenson, & Drew, 1988; Sattler, 1990) published tables of representative behavior for different ages and degrees of mental retardation. These measures are useful to the extent that the informant who evaluates an individual's adaptive capabilities is an informed, accurate, and reliable observer.

Traditional methods of examining cognitive and adaptive abilities have also been supplemented by an examination of the child's developmental history and social environment. One environmental assessment tool used for this purpose is the Home Observation for Measurement of the Environment scale (HOME) (Caldwell & Bradley, 1984). The HOME is a semistructured observation-interview instrument. This device focuses on the types of physical environments and parental stimulation employed in the home to promote the child's cognitive development. The HOME assesses factors such as the appropriateness of play materials, language facilitation, encouragement of social maturity, and stimulation of academic behavior. A supplement to the HOME has been developed to address environmental issues specific to young children who live in impoverished urban households (Ertem, Forsyth, Avni-Singer, Damour, & Cicchetti, 1997). The Supplement to the HOME for Impoverished Families (SHIF) examines environmental and biological stressors specific to poverty (e.g., adequate nutrition) that may place children at further risk of developmental difficulties.

Assessment Emphases

Increasingly, the evaluation of mental retardation is taking place within an interdisciplinary, multivariate, and social-developmental framework. Particular attention is being given to early diagnosis and screening. Early assessment has been emphasized because of its implication for early intervention and prevention. Assessment can occur at a number of stages. Before conception, genetic screening can be used to provide families with information regarding their carrier status for transmitting genetic defects to their offspring. The process includes a review of the family history, as well as chromosomal and biochemical profiles of family members. Currently, a project to map the human genome is being coordinated by the National Center for Human Genome Research. The Human Genome Project (HGP) began in 1990 and one of the goals was to identify and assess the way genes act to produce mental retardation and the way early genetic manipulation might influence healthy development (Wingerson, 1990). Specific genes have already been discovered for a number of single gene conditions including fragile X syndrome, PKU, and Prader Willi syndrome. The HGP holds great potential for treating single gene disorders that cause severe mental retardation (Moser, 1995). However, it is less likely to provide treatment for mild mental retardation that may be polygenic or psychosocial in origin. Overall, this project will undoubtedly have profound influence on the information provided to families in genetic counseling programs. In the light of this, the HGP is also attempting to address ethical, legal, and social issues that may arise as a consequence of its findings.

In addition to preconception genetic screening, prenatal assessments, such as amniocentesis, ultrasonography, amniography, and fetoscopy, can be employed to identify the presence of a fetal defect. Typically, because these procedures are costly and sometimes risky, they are used selectively, for example, when the mother is 35 years or older, it is suspected that a parent is a carrier of a chromosomal defect, or there has been a previous birth of a chromosomally abnormal infant. Screening at this stage enables families to make decisions concerning continuance of the pregnancy, allows for implementing early prenatal medical intervention, and may help the family to prepare emotionally, physically, and medically for a child who has special needs.

Further assessment can also take place at birth. Newborns are now routinely screened for metabolic disorders that can produce mental retardation and other disabilities. Chromosomal and genetic disorders (e.g., PKU) can be identified and sometimes treated in the neonatal period.

Although early diagnosis can identify a child's specific needs, lead to the provision of necessary services, and facilitate interdisciplinary communication among professionals, this process can also stigmatize the child if it creates unrealistic perceptions and unwarranted negative projections by professionals and parents about a child's potential. Professionals in particular need to be sensitive to the effects of labels, candid about their inability to make specific predictions about long-term developmental outcome, and recognize that a handicap is only one defining characteristic of an individual's personality. Zigler and Balla (1982) emphasize the continuing need for flexibility in the diagnostic process due to the fact that individuals with similar psychometric profiles often respond in quite diverse ways to intervention.

In addition to early screening, a comprehensive assessment program examines the individual throughout the developmental period. Current social and behavioral theories emphasize the need for repeated assessments to evaluate the child's changing developmental status and needs, the effectiveness of educational programs, and the appropriateness of class placements. Rather than viewing mental retardation as a fixed trait, this approach to assessment captures the dynamic and changing quality of development, along with its social nature. For example, Vygotsky's (1978) theory of zone of proximal development views intelligence in terms of the individual's present developmental level and also in relation to the individual's capacity for new learning and the social contexts that support learning. This approach to dynamic assessment emphasizes a view of mental retardation as remediable and has direct implications for designing instructional programs.

Current assessment efforts are also increasingly emphasizing the view that persons who are mentally retarded vary in their cognitive functioning and also in their motivational, physical, and emotional characteristics and that assessment of these latter domains is critical for the development of effective educational programs. Motivational skills such as persistence and goal-directed behavior vary in individuals who are mentally retarded (for discussion see Hupp, 1995). Such abilities are critical for independent functioning and attaining cognitive skills. For this reason, educational interventions are beginning to focus on motivational factors in learning and on designing educational plans that match the individual's motivational orientation (Hauser-Cram & Shonkoff, 1995).

SUMMARY

During the past three decades, conceptualizations of mental retardation have undergone profound changes. Current perspectives are more holistic and emphasize the reciprocal influences among cognitive, behavioral, emotional, and physical functioning of persons who are mentally retarded. Definitions and classifications have become more cohesive across national organizations. Advances in identification and prevention have occurred as the role of environmental and biological contributors have become better understood and systematically evaluated. In particular, the impact of poverty on child development continues to add new questions about the causes and treatment of mental retardation. Information on this disorder continues to expand as research and educational programs consider more dynamic aspects of development such as motivation. The challenge faced by professionals in the field of mental retardation involves incorporating these advances into assessment and treatment models.

REFERENCES

American Association on Mental Retardation (1992). *Mental retardation: Definition, classification, and systems of supports*, 9th ed. Washington, DC: Author.

American Psychiatric Association. (1994). *Diagnostic and statistical manual of mental disorders*, 4th ed. Washington, DC: Author.

Baumeister, A. A., Kupstas, F. D., & Klindworth, L. M. (1991). *The new morbidity: A national plan of action*. Newbury Park, CA: Sage.

Borkowski, J. G., Whitman, T. L., Passino, A. W., Rellinger, E., Sommer, K., Keogh, D., & Weed, K. (1992). Unraveling the "new morbidity": Adolescent parenting and developmental delays. *International Review of Research in Mental Retardation 8*, 159–196.

Caldwell, B. M., & Bradley, R. H. (1984). *Home observation for measurement of the environment*. Little Rock: University of Arkansas at Little Rock.

Drews, C. D., Yeargin-Allsopp, M., Decoufle, P., & Murphy, C. C. (1995). Variation in the influence of selected sociodemographic risk factors for mental retardation. *American Journal of Public Health, 85*, 329–334.

Duncan, G. J., Brooks-Gunn, J., & Klebanov, P. K. (1994). Economic deprivation and early childhood development. *Child Development, 65*, 296–318.

Ertem, I. O., Forsyth, B. W., Avini-Singer, A. J., Damour, L. K., & Cicchetti, D. V. (1997). Development of a supplement to the HOME scale for children living in impoverished urban environments. *Developmental and Behavioral Pediatrics, 18*, 322–328.

Figueroa, R. A., & Sassenrath, J. M. (1989). A longitudinal study of the predictive validity of the System of Multicultural Pluralistic Assessment (SOMPA). *Psychology in the Schools, 26*, 5–19.

Gelfand, D. M., Jenson, W. R., & Drew, C. J. (1988). *Understanding child behavior disorders*, 2nd ed. New York: Harcourt Brace Jovanovich.

Goestason, R., Wahlstroem, J., Johannisson, T., & Holmqvist, D. (1991). Chromosomal aberrations in the mildly mentally retarded. *Journal of Mental Deficiency Research, 35*, 240–246.

Grossman, H. J. (1983). *Classification in mental retardation*. Washington, DC: American Association of Mental Deficiency.

Hack, M., Klein, N. K., & Taylor, H. G. (1995). Long-term developmental outcomes of low birth weight infants. *The Future of Children, 5*, 176–196.

Hagberg, B., & Hagberg, G. (1984). Aspects of prevention of pre-, peri- and postnatal brain pathology in severe and mild mental retardation. In J. Dobbing, A. D. Clarke, & J. A. Corbett (Eds.), *Scientific studies in mental retardation* (pp. 43–64). London: Royal Society of Medicine/Macmillan.

Hauser-Cram, P., & Shonkoff, J. P. (1995). Mastery motivation: Implications for intervention. In R. H. MacTurk &

G. A. Morgan (Eds.), *Mastery motivation: Origins, conceptualizations, and applications* (pp. 257–273). Norwood, NJ: Ablex.

Hodapp, R. M., Burack, J. A., & Zigler, E. (1990). *Issues in the developmental approach to mental retardation.* New York: Cambridge University Press.

Hupp, S. C. (1995). The impact of mental retardation on motivated behavior. In R. H. MacTurk & G. A. Morgan (Eds.), *Mastery motivation: Origins, conceptualizations, and applications* (pp. 221–236). Norwood, NJ: Ablex.

Infant Health and Development Program. (1990). Enhancing the outcomes of low birth weight, premature infants: A multisite randomized trial. *Journal of the American Medical Association, 263,* 3035–3042.

Katusic, S. K., Colligan, R. C., Beard, C. M., O'Fallon, W. M., Bergstralh, E. J., Jacobsen, S. J., & Kurland, L. T. (1996). Mental retardation in a birth cohort, 1976–1980, Rochester, Minnesota. *American Journal of Mental Retardation, 100,* 335–344.

Kohlberg, K. J. S. (1999). Environmental influences on prenatal development and health. In T. L. Whitman, T. V. Merluzzi, & R. D. White (Eds.), *Life-span perspectives on health and illness* (pp. 87–103). Mahwah, NJ: Erlbaum.

Levine, A. J., & Marks, L. (1928). *Testing intelligence and achievement.* New York: Macmillan.

Mercer, J. R. (1973). The myth of 3% prevalence. In R. K. Eyman, C. E. Meyers, & G. Tarjan (Eds.), *Sociobehavioral studies in mental retardation.* Monographs of the American Association on Mental Deficiency, *1,* 1–18.

Mercer, J. R., & Lewis, J. (1978). *SOMPA: Student assessment manual.* New York: Psychological Corporation.

Mitchell, J. V. (Ed.). (1985). *The ninth mental measurements yearbook.* Lincoln: University of Nebraska Press.

Moser, H. W. (1995). A role of gene therapy and mental retardation. *Mental Retardation and Developmental Disabilities Research Reviews: Gene Therapy, 1,* 4–6.

Murphy, C. C., Yeargin-Allsopp, M., Decoufle, P., & Drews, C. D. (1995). The administrative prevalence of mental retardation in 10-year-old children in metropolitan Atlanta, 1985 through 1987. *American Journal of Public Health, 85,* 319–323.

Nihira, K., Foster, R., Shellhaas, M., & Leland, H. (1974). *AAMD adaptive behavior scale, revised.* Washington, DC: American Association on Mental Deficiency.

Sattler, J. M. (1990). *Assessment of children,* 3rd ed. San Diego, CA: Author.

Scheerenberger, R. C. (1987). *A history of mental retardation: A quarter century of promise.* Baltimore: Paul H. Brookes.

Sparrow, S. S., Ballo, D. A., & Cicchetti, D. V. (1984). *Vineland adaptive behavior scales.* Circle Pines, MN: American Guidance Service.

Thapar, A., Gottesman, I. I., Owen, M. J., O'Donovan, M. C., & McGuffin, P. (1994). The genetics of mental retardation. *British Journal of Psychiatry, 164,* 747–758.

U.S. Department of Health and Human Services, Public Health Service (1990). Healthy people 2000: National health promotion and disease prevention objectives. DHHS Publication No. (PHS) 91-50212. Washington, DC: U.S. Government Printing Office.

Vygotsky, L. S. (1978). *Mind in society: The development of higher psychological processes.* Cambridge, MA: Harvard University Press.

Wahlstroem, J. (1990). Gene map of mental retardation. *Journal of Mental Deficiency Research, 34,* 11–27.

Weisz, J. R. (1990). Cultural-familial mental retardation: A developmental perspective on cognitive performance and "helpless" behavior. In R. M. Hodapp, J. A. Burack, & E. Zigler (Eds.), *Issues in the developmental approach to mental retardation* (pp. 137–168). Cambridge, England: Cambridge University Press.

Wingerson, L. (1990). *Mapping our genes: The genome project and the future of medicine.* New York: Penguin Books.

World Health Organization. (1992). International statistical classification of diseases, and related health problems, 10th revision. Geneva, Switzerland: Office of Publications, World Health Organization.

Yeargin-Allsopp, M., Murphy, C. C., Oakley, G. P., & Sikes, K. (1992). A multiple source method for studying prevalence of developmental disabilities in children. *Pediatrics, 89,* 624–630.

Zigler, E. (1995). Can we "cure" mild mental retardation among individuals in the lower socioeconomic stratum? *American Journal of Public Health, 85,* 302–304.

Zigler, E., & Balla, D. (Eds.). (1982). *Mental retardation: The developmental-difference controversy.* Hillsdale, NJ: Erlbaum.

8

Autism

Lynn Kern Koegel, Marta Valdez-Menchaca, Robert L. Koegel, and Joshua K. Harrower

There has been considerable progress and development in the diagnosis and intervention for children with autism during the past several decades. This chapter provides an account of the major findings that have led to our increased understanding of the behavioral manifestations of autism and the development of intervention techniques. Evidence on the etiology and intervention is reviewed within a framework that explores the possibility that neurological or physiological processes may result in an inappropriate level of social interaction which, in turn, leads to disabilities in communication and other problem behaviors that characterize autism. Understanding this atypical developmental track can lead directly to the understanding, intervention in, and prevention of many of the severe aspects of autism that are so stigmatizing and disabling to children, adolescents, and adults.

Description of the Disorder

In 1943, Kanner first categorized a perplexing group of eleven children who could be differentiated from other children who had disabilities in terms of their particular combination of idiosyncratic characteristics. To be diagnosed as autistic according to the DSM-IV (APA, 1994), children must behave abnormally in three general areas, including: (1) qualitative impairment in social interaction; (2) qualitative impairment in communication; and (3) restricted, repetitive and stereotyped patterns of behavior, interests, and activities. In addition, delays or abnormal functioning in social interaction, social communication, or symbolic or imaginative play occurs before three years of age. Because autism comprises such a diversity of behavioral characteristics, individuals with autism may appear vastly different based on the extent or degree of involvement within and across the symptoms.

For example, individuals with autism may be divided in three major subgroups in relation to their cognitive skills. One subgroup is formed by individuals who have intellectual func-

Lynn Kern Koegel, Marta Valdez-Menchaca, Robert L. Koegel, and Joshua K. Harrower • University of California at Santa Barbara, Santa Barbara, California 93106.

Advanced Abnormal Psychology, Second Edition, edited by Hersen and Van Hasselt. Kluwer Academic/Plenum Publishers, New York, 2001.

tioning in the range of mental retardation, as measured by standardized IQ tests. It has been estimated that approximately 60% of children with autism have IQs less than 50 (Schopler, 1978). However, some have suggested that these individuals actually may be more competent than can be measured by standardized testing (Koegel, Koegel, & Smith, 1997).

Another subgroup of individuals with autism, made popular in the movie *Rain Man*, can be characterized by isolated skill areas. These individuals have also been called "savant," "autistic savant," and "idiot savant." Savant skills often surprise people because they appear to be intelligence-independent, which is why the paradoxical term "idiot savant" was coined (Ho, Tsang, & Ho, 1992). Often, this profile can be seen at a fairly young age in preschoolers with autism who seem to solve difficult puzzles effortlessly. Two of the most common areas in which these individuals excel are music and mathematical calculations. Yet, in spite of remarkable accomplishments in these areas, it is typical for the children to have little appreciation of any social recognition for their accomplishments. When these individuals who have subjectively reported musical skills are tested systematically by experts, their skills often exceed even the best nondisabled musicians (Applebaum, Egel, Koegel, & Imhoff, 1979). Yet, they appear to have no special awareness of this superiority, or even any desire to excel above other individuals. Although this group of children receives considerable public attention, probably due to their uniqueness, they actually comprise a small percentage of the children diagnosed as having autism.

The remaining group of individuals with autism can be characterized by relatively high abilities in areas that require minimal language use. They function relatively well in daily living skills and nonverbal tasks but are challenged by situations that require social language use. Unfortunately, without intervention, this deficit can severely limit their ability to integrate into work responsibilities or other activities that require socialization. In spite of vastly different intellectual profiles, individuals in these subgroups, typically, reportedly have similar and profound social deficits (Frea, 1995; Koegel, Frea, & Surratt, 1994). However, the interaction between the degree of social impairment and other abilities (e.g., IQ) and skills, through a series of social transactions and developmental processes, will result in the wide diversity of profiles that characterize individuals labeled as having autism.

In most descriptions of autism, each of the aforementioned behavioral characteristics has been described, and often treated, as a separate entity. However, a recent shift in the field emphasizes the interrelationships among these areas (e.g., Koegel, Camarata, & Koegel, 1994; Koegel, Koegel, & Carter, in press; Mundy, Sigman, & Kasari, 1990). This has led to the hypothesis that autism may involve primary (causal) and secondary (manifestation) behaviors. From this perspective, a primary crux of autism may be the lack of appropriate social behavior. The individual with autism may develop secondary maladaptive behaviors, such as stereotypical behavior, lack of appropriate language development, and tantrums (Koegel, 1995). A number of studies (Carr & Durand, 1985; L. Koegel, Koegel, Hurly, & Frea, 1992; R. Koegel, Koegel, & Surratt, 1992; Todd, Horner, & Sugai, 1999) support this hypothesis by demonstrating the interrelationship of these patterns of behavior that show concomitant changes in untreated disruptive behaviors during intervention into communicative/social behaviors. While reading the following sections, describing the three general areas of autism, the reader is encouraged to contemplate how these areas may be related.

Social Interaction

Qualitative impairment in social interaction, which may play a central role in the disorder, is discussed throughout the life span of individuals with autism. As early as infancy, many parents report that their children "stiffen up" when they attempt to hold and cuddle them. During their first 5 years, children with autism may not form attachments or "bond" in the way typical children do. For example, they may not follow their parents about the house, run to greet them, seek comfort when hurt or upset, or develop routines such as the bedtime kiss-and-cuddle. Further, the lack of eye-to-eye gaze is characteristic of children with autism. Although many avoid eye contact, particularly when repeated efforts are made to gain their attention, others do not use eye gaze in a discriminatory way when in need (e.g., wanting attention or wanting to be picked up, etc.) (Rutter, 1978).

Some of these characteristics may be evident early, even before the child has been diagnosed or suspected of having autism. For example, in a preliminary study, Adrien et al. (1991) reviewed home videotapes of 12 children before the age of 2 and before they were diagnosed as having autism. Evaluation of these children's behavior, compared with control participants, revealed early difficulties in: (1) social interaction (tendency toward isolation, no eye contact, lack of postural adjustment, bad positioning of the head, lack of anticipatory movements, and lack of initiative); (2) emotional differences (deficit of facial expressions, absence of smiles, anxiety in new situations, and major emotional lability); (3) visual and auditory behaviors [inappropriate gaze and slow or delayed reactions (hypo- or hyperreactive)]; (4) disorders of tone and motor behavior (hypotonia, hand flapping, and lack of protective movements); and (5) atypical, socially stigmatizing behaviors (such as self-stimulatory and obsessive behavior).

As the child with autism develops, patterns of social difficulties continue and tend to become more problematic when greater levels of social competence are expected. Children with autism typically do not engage in appropriate spontaneous play with other children (Bednersh & Peck, 1986; Koegel, Dyer, & Bell, 1987; Libby, Powell, Messer, & Jordan, 1998; Wetherby & Prutting, 1984) and, without intervention, often fail to develop meaningful friendships in adolescence (Haring & Breen, 1992; Hurley-Geffner, 1995; Koegel, Frea, & Surratt, 1994; Meyer et al., 1998). This limited social network is particularly troubling to parents and others close to the child. In addition, it has important implications for their integration in society because the range of social experiences to which the child or adult is exposed will be significantly limited. Without being actively involved in reciprocal social communicative interactions, the child is unlikely to learn the important social and contextual rules that govern our behavior throughout life.

Communication Deficits

Children with autism are often classified into three groups by their language skills: nonverbal, verbal with language delays or difficulties, and echolalic. Early figures estimated that about 50% of children with autism never developed functional expressive language (Prizant, 1983); however, now that improved language teaching procedures are available, the outlook is considerably brighter. Some of the verbal children exhibit "echolalia," which is the repetition by the child of something heard in the speech of others. Echoic utterances are often rigidly reproduced and typically lack clear evidence of communicative intent (Koegel, 1995; Prizant & Rydell, 1984).

According to parent report, some of those in the nonverbal group use some words during the second year of life, but then cease to continue to use any words. Other nonverbal children reportedly never produce intelligible words. These children can produce noises, but it is difficult to get these noises under imitative control or to teach them to use the sounds in a socially meaningful way. Another group of children with autism appears nonverbal in early years but eventually develops some language that follows developmental language stages and parallels typically developing children (Tager-Flusberg et al., 1990).

Echolalic children may produce two forms of echolalic responses. "Immediate echolalia" is repetition(s) of all or part of an utterance, which is produced either following immediately or a brief time after the production of a model utterance. "Delayed echolalia" refers to utterances repeated at a significantly later time (Koegel, 1995; Prizant & Rydell, 1984). It has been speculated that much of immediate echolalia occurs when the child lacks understanding. Carr, Shreibman, and Lovaas (1975) demonstrated that such children echoed utterances that they did not understand and answered utterances that they understood. Delayed echolalia still continues to puzzle researchers. It has been theorized that much of delayed echolalia may produce some type of sensory rather than social input for the child (Lovaas, Varni, Koegel, & Lorsch, 1977). This was considered while it was observed that children with autism engaged in repetitive delayed echolalic responses without extinguishing, even when they were alone. In contrast, it has also been suggested that some forms of delayed echolalia (but not all) that occur when children are in the company of familiar people may serve a communicative intent, such as labeling, protesting, or requesting (Prizant & Rydell, 1984; Rydell & Mirenda, 1994).

Numerous barriers and obstacles are encountered by an individual who lacks social communication. Typically, developing infants meet their needs through crying, but they soon learn that verbalizations are more efficient and more desirable to a parent and are able to engage in communicative verbal exchanges that will foster their language development. However, when verbal skills fail to develop appropriately, failures in communication result in extreme frustration, which may lead the child to revert to early effective forms of communication, such as crying. As children with autism grow up, impairment in linguistic communication results in more restricted social environments and the use of elaborate forms of disruptive behavior to accomplish goals.

Poor social communication skills can be evidenced throughout life, even with adolescents whose language skills are somewhat delayed but sufficient for conversational interaction. This limited involvement in language interactions results in other inappropriate pragmatic behaviors, such as failure to initiate conversation and respond to the conversation of others (Koegel, Camarata, Valdez-Menchaca, & Koegel, 1998; Koegel et al., 1992), lack of appropriate turn-taking, dysprosody, inappropriate speech detail, perseveration, and preoccupations during conversation (Frea, 1995; Koegel & Frea, 1993). When one considers the fact that most individuals do not go through a day without using communicative and associated pragmatic skills, it is obvious that difficulties in this area are especially disabling in developing personal friendships and relationships. These difficulties are further disabling to an individual's functioning in social settings, such as school or work, which in turn hinders the flow of the interaction and may precipitate its termination.

Restricted Repertoire of Activities and Interests

The last area of behaviors characteristic to autism is the restricted repertoire of activities and interests. It is likely that the extremely restricted repertoire of activities of these children exacerbates their social relationships and also interferes with the very neurological development that may be necessary to overcome the problem. One of the most frequently exhibited behaviors is stereotypical behavior (also described as ritualistic behavior, stereotypy, self-stimulatory behavior, etc.). Stereotypical behavior occurs when an individual engages in a repetitive behavior that appears to serve no observable social function. It can be with an object, such as incessantly flipping a twig round and round between the fingers, or repetitively spinning the wheels of a toy truck, or with one's own body parts such as flipping the fingers in front of the eyes, hand-flapping, or body-rocking.

It has been theorized that these behaviors provide sensory input to the individual, and though all individuals need sensory input, those who have autism obtain it inappropriately, from a social perspective. It is very likely that this need for sensory stimulation is provided for in typical children through social communicative interactions. Very young children seem to seek attention constantly from their parents and greatly enjoy games, songs, stories, and other types of social communicative activities, but most children with autism do not actively seek such interactions. Without intervention, many can engage in stereotypical behavior for the entire day.

Aside from the socially stigmatizing effects of these behaviors, it has been shown that learning does not take place when certain types of stereotypical behaviors occur because stereotypical behavior is incompatible with appropriate response. However, when certain types of stereotypical behavior are suppressed, appropriate play increases spontaneously (Kern, Koegel, & Dunlap, 1984; Kern et al., 1982). It has also been shown that stereotypical behavior decreases when children are taught to orient to and comment upon their environment (Frea, 1997). Thus, providing antecedent intervention or engaging the child in incompatible behaviors can be effective in reducing stereotypical behaviors.

Another behavior seen in some children with autism is self-injury. Some have theorized that self-injury may be a type of stereotypical behavior taken to the extreme (Carr, 1982; Carr, Reeve, & Magito-McLaughlin, 1996). In other cases, these behaviors appear to have a communicative function (Carr & Durand, 1985; Carr et al., 1996). For example, when a teacher instructs a child to engage in a task s/he does not want to do, it might bang the head with a closed fist as a means of avoiding the task. Similarly, if a child does not want to engage in social interaction s/he may pick the skin intensely to the point of drawing blood, which would likely drive the communicative partner away, thus reinforcing the child's inappropriate behavior. While these forms of disruptive behavior may be performed to carry out a social function, they are not perceived by most members of society as forms of social behavior and may be particularly harmful to the ability of individuals with autism to be accepted in socially integrated settings. Assessing the motivation for these behaviors becomes critical in the intervention into these severe excess behavior problems so that intervention plans may be developed where the children are taught socially appropriate behaviors that will serve these same functions.

Another characteristic of autism is the tendency to prefer "sameness" in the environment. An example of this is a child who wears the same shirt daily and who cries and throws tantrums if the parent tries to put a different shirt on the child. Similarly, some children with autism may react when an item of furniture is rearranged in the house. This type of preoccupation also can be seen in types of ritualistic behavior and irrational fears occasionally exhibited by children with autism. As a whole, these inappropriate behaviors occur in varying degrees but, when present, interfere with common socially acceptable activities in a person's repertoire. Thus, it appears as though the person with autism is exhibiting a very limited and restricted repertoire of activities and that few of these activities contain social components.

CLINICAL PICTURE

Jacob

Jacob is a 3½-year-old boy who was brought to a pediatrician who specialized in developmental disabilities. His parents were concerned about his "inability to focus and pay attention." They were also concerned with his sleep difficulties and picky eating. Although his mother had some vaginal bleeding during the second trimester of pregnancy due to partial placenta previa, this problem cleared spontaneously and delivery was normal. His parents reported that Jacob's early motor milestones were age-appropriate. He sat up, crawled, and walked at expected times. They were concerned, however, that he did not like to be constrained or confined by adults. For example, he resisted contacts such as holding an adult's hand when crossing the street.

Communicatively, Jacob spoke single words during his first year of life and combined words by two and a half years. However, beginning his first year, his parents reported that he cried easily, became frustrated easily, and often had difficulty keeping to a schedule. They also reported that he was upset by new people and new situations, was withdrawn, and avoided playing with other children. In regard to play activities, they reported that he tended to take his toys apart, break them down into component parts, and then throw the parts. They also observed that he was preoccupied with smelling objects, spinning objects, and twisting his fingers in front of his eyes. Jacob's pediatrician recommended that he be put in a preschool; however, a first visit to a preschool was upsetting to his mother because he did not participate in any activity but appeared overaroused and ran about the classroom without focus. At this point, Jacob's parents sought further evaluation by a pediatrician who specialized in developmental difficulties.

Jacob's new pediatrician immediately recognized the symptoms of autism, which included frequent stereotypical behavior, lack of appropriate social behavior, lack of appropriate play, and delayed and inappropriate language skills. Although he was combining words, it was observed that he used rudimentary sentences in a delayed echoic manner and rarely directed utterances toward others except when requesting. After an extensive evaluation, including testing and observations, she diagnosed him as having autism and referred him to our clinic for intervention.

When Jacob's parents first brought him to our clinic, they felt deeply stressed and concerned that he was diagnosed as having autism. No matter how gently and sympathetically the diagnosis is presented to a parent, it is shocking and unsettling news. Sullivan (1978) eloquently discusses the fact that parents of children with autism find themselves, without warning, faced with a very personal, devastating problem, utterly alone, unprepared, and too often actually excluded from the very institutions established to help. During Jacob's first visit, his parents were in disbelief. While Jacob sat on the floor spinning Tinkertoys in front of his eyes, they pointed out that children with autism do not usually play with toys—and he was playing with the Tinkertoys. We had to explain to them that the way in which he was playing with the toys was stereotypical. They wanted to know if Jacob would ever become "normal." We could not answer this question, but we were able to assure them that there were many effective interventions available for autism and that with intervention they could expect to see progress throughout his life.

Three years later, after intensive intervention to increase appropriate social and language skills and concomitant decreases in inappropriate disruptive behavior, Jacob was placed in a regular education kindergarten class. By implementing special programs such as self-management, functional communication, and prepractice on tasks to be presented in the near future, Jacob advanced both socially and academically.

Currently, Jacob is receiving mostly A's and B's on his work in a regular education elementary classroom. Jacob is preparing for the transition from elementary to junior high school, where he will continue to participate fully in regular education classes. During the last few years, he has had best friends, gone to sleepovers, and attended friends' birthday parties. He engages in a variety of social activities with peers outside of school, including competing in races, rock climbing, and going to classes at the zoo. He also can play the violin at the adult level. In sum, Jacob currently engages in activities that are typical for children his age and displays similarly typical social communicative interactions with his peers.

Perry

Perry is three years old. During infancy, he enjoyed being held and was easily soothed. However, it was not clear that the social aspect of being held was as important to him as the physical aspect. His mother reported that although the quality of his babble seemed similar to that of his older sister, the quantity was much less. Instead of exhibiting these pre-linguistic types of behaviors, he was more interested in listening to music, which she used frequently to soothe him, particularly at bedtime.

All motor milestones, such as sitting up, crawling, and walking were age-appropriate. However, at the end of his first year, when most children have regularized their nighttime sleep patterns, Perry was awakening frequently throughout the night. He was also beginning to be upset when taken out of the house. He would cry and lie down on the floor as the family was leaving, and he had to be carried. Perry's mother expressed these concerns to her family pediatrician, but he reassured her that all children develop differently and she should not worry.

At 18 months, Perry's mother reported that he was using a small lexicon. When distressed, he was reported to say "mama." His parents reported that he could also say "dada," "car," "truck," "bottle," "milk," "plane," and "more." Although he rarely interacted or played with his older sister, he seemed to enjoy playing with small toys, especially little cars and trucks.

By two years of age, Perry stopped using any expressive language, and his only vocalizations were frequent humming sounds at various pitches. His mother, greatly concerned, returned to the pediatrician. The pediatrician reassured her that he seemed to be developing appropriately and she was probably being overly concerned about his language development. Approaching his third birthday, Perry was still not using any words and instead cried and threw tantrums whenever in need or in distress. At this point, his mother suspected he might be hearing-impaired and took him to an otorhinolaryngologist. Because of his frequent and intense tantrums, he was unable to take any type of behavioral hearing test. Thus, he was sedated and brain stem audiometry was performed. From the test results, they did not suspect hearing loss as a reason for Perry's language delay or for his failure to respond to initiations from others.

When Perry reached three years, four months, and his mother was nearly panicked over his failure to develop language, she pleaded with Perry's regular pediatrician for a referral to a pediatrician who specialized in developmental disabilities. After a lengthy evaluation, the new pediatrician noted numerous symptoms of autism, including a striking absence of social interaction. Although he frequently sat in his mother's lap voluntarily, he never acknowledged the pediatrician's presence. Additionally, although he played with toys somewhat appropriately, he never attempted any interactional play, even when coaxed by his mother. He had no expressive language skills and very limited receptive language skills. His most common mode of communication was crying and throwing tantrums whenever the smallest demand was made on him or when his mother attempted to have him change tasks. The pediatrician diagnosed him as having autism, and she referred him to our clinic for intervention.

When Perry came to our clinic, he interacted only with his mother. This interaction consisted of sitting on her lap, holding her cheeks with both hands while positioning his face directly in front of hers, and touching her nose with his. He appeared uninterested in any other adults. Further, he appeared interested in a limited number of toys, primarily small cars.

Whenever an adult tried to interact with him or engage him in any social way, he began crying and frequently lay on the floor face down. Occasionally, if an adult continued to press him to interact, he hit the side of his head with a closed fist or bit the skin on the top of his hand. He also attempted to kick and bite when we tried to get him to sit in a small chair. His mother reported numerous tantrums whenever she took him out in public. She complained that he appeared to have excessive preoccupations with specific objects, exhibited peculiar mannerisms, engaged in self-injurious behavior at home when frustrated, occasionally rocked back and forth, and appeared to be unaware of his immediate surroundings. Additionally, he was not toilet trained and was unable to dress himself.

Perry's mother was under extreme stress when she came to our clinic. She had recently divorced and felt unknowledgeable as to how to control her son. We recommended she begin by participating in our parent education program. She was delighted at the idea that she might be able to learn techniques to help her son. In later sections of this chapter, we will discuss interventions and the life-span needs and implications for adulthood.

Intensive intervention programs that incorporated the parent as an intervention agent were implemented to decrease Perry's aggressive, self-injurious behavior and tantrums, and to develop some speech, social behavior, and self-help skills. As a result of the intervention, Perry learned how to assist with setting the table and cooking, to play appropriately with his sister, to attempt to verbally communicate with consonant-vowel word approximations, and was toilet-trained. He learned to shake his head indicating "no" when he did not want something, a feeling previously expressed through tantrums and/or aggression. Nine years later, he is never aggressive with his mother and rarely (less than once per month) demonstrates self-injurious behavior. Occasionally, he and his sister fight, but he never shows aggression unless provoked. At first, these gains did not spontaneously generalize to the school. Reports began to be sent to his mother indicating that he was demonstrating aggressive behavior toward fellow classmates or his teacher in his classroom. However, a coordinated intervention plan implemented by his classroom teacher, school psychologist, and a consulting behavior analyst has begun to effectively reduce his problem behavior in the classroom. Further, Perry can now engage in a number of academic activities, including reading, math, and typing.

EPIDEMIOLOGY

For decades, the incidence of autism had been estimated at 4 or 5 per 10,000 births (Ritvo & Freeman, 1978; Wing, 1976). However, recent estimates indicate that the incidence rates are increasing (Wing, 1997). For example, researchers have reported the prevalence of children given labels within the autism spectrum (e.g., autism, pervasive developmental disorder) as ranging from 1 in 1,000 to 1 in 500 births (Rapin, 1997). There is recent evidence that the incidence rates are increasing even further. In a recent annual report to Congress on the implementation of the Individuals with Disabilities Act, the U.S. Department of Education reported an increase among children in the public schools diagnosed with autism of 178% from 1993 to 1997 (U.S. Department of Education, 1999). In California, for example, the number of children with a diagnosis of autism who received services has increased by more than 200% in the past 11 years (Department of Developmental Services, 1999). This increase was more than four times that of any other disability group for that period (Department of Developmental Services, 1999). Attempts to explain this increase have included: (1) the advent of explicit behavioral criteria for diagnosis in the DSM-IV that resulted in identifying many less severely affected children (Rapin, 1997); (2) improved diagnostic assessment devices (e.g., Lord et al., 1997); (3) changes in referral patterns; (4) wider diagnostic criteria; (5) greater awareness; and (6) genuine change (Wing, 1996, 1997). Autism has been found in all parts of the world and is four to five times more common in males than females (Ritvo & Freeman, 1978). The exact age of onset is unknown, but it is suspected that it is present at birth. Early diagnosis of autism is infrequent, most likely because all the individual symptoms of autism can be evidenced in typically developing children; thus, early signs may be unnoticed by families or physicians. For example, at a very young age, all children lack social play, demonstrate repetitive behaviors, cry or have tantrums to have their needs met, and "echo" adults' sounds and words.

Lack of social communication may be a first sign to many professionals and family members that a problem exists (DeGiacomo & Fombonne, 1998). Some nonverbal pragmatic behaviors characteristic of autism that may be evident early are lack of eye contact, inappropriate facial expression and gestures, and inappropriate emotion (Koegel, Frea, & Surratt, 1994). However, they may go unnoticed before expressive language in a social context is required at around the second year of life. Autism has attracted a lot of attention, most likely because of the large number and wide range of atypical behaviors demonstrated, the debilitating effect they can have on the individuals and their families, and the recent increase in the number of individuals diagnosed with this disability.

The etiology of autism is still unknown, but causal theories have changed considerably over the years. The first theories of causality were developed when psychodynamic theory was prevalent and many were based on descriptions of families, which led to the hypothesis that parents were part or all of the problem. Early, Kanner (1943) described many of the parents as highly intelligent, well educated, and usually professionals, who had cold, bookish, formal personalities, although he felt that these types of environmental circumstances interacted with organic, congenital characteristics (Eisenberg & Kanner, 1956). The most notable proponent of the parent-causation hypothesis was Bruno Bettelheim (1967), who authored *The Empty Fortress*. In this popular book, Bettelheim proposed that mothers of children with autism had a psychopathology that caused them to react abnormally to their children's normal behaviors. This, in turn, caused the children to withdraw. The parents' response to this withdrawal was extreme negative feelings and rejection, which in turn caused more withdrawal by the child. Thus, this pattern of negative interactions eventually caused the child to avoid adult interactions by exhibiting overt symptoms such as stereotypical behaviors and social withdrawal.

The parental-causation theory prevailed for several decades and, as one might imagine, caused many well intended families who were already burdened with the stress of having a child with a severe disability, to fall further into the depths of despair upon finding that they may be the cause. However, following an emphasis on scientifically based methodologies, rather than a previous tendency to rely on individual case histories, researchers subsequently have demonstrated that parents of children with autism do *not* significantly differ from parents of typically developing children (e.g., Egel, Koegel, & Schreibman, 1980; Hughes, Leboyer, & Bouvard, 1997; Koegel, Schreibman, O'Neill, & Burke, 1983; Wing, 1997). In addition, transactional views of parent–child interaction are likely to demonstrate that particular behaviors displayed by the parents of a child with autism may be appropriate adjustments to their child's behavior or style of interaction (Curcio & Paccia, 1987; Mahoney, 1988; Valdez-Menchaca, 1991).

Current theories regarding causation focus on organic factors. Organic research has revolved around some general areas including pre- and perinatal complications, genetic factors, neurochemical differences, and neurological and neuroanatomical differences. Because there have been no studies that show a single organic cause for autism among all individuals, we only briefly mention the wide variety of areas that have been or are currently being studied.

Prenatal, Perinatal, and Neonatal Complications

Increased incidence of pre-, peri-, and neonatal complications have been reported in a number of studies. Some signs of reduced optimality that have been found in autism are clinical dysmaturity, significant midtrimester bleeding, pre-/postmaturity, severe infection in pregnancy, generalized edema, medication for more than one week, in utero insults such as thalidomide embryopathy, and reduced Apgar scores (Coleman, 1994; Gillberg & Gillberg, 1983; Trottier, Srivastava, & Walker, 1999). Congenital rubella also reportedly occurred at a high rate in children who have autism or exhibit similar behaviors (Chess, 1971, 1977; DeLong, 1999).

Neuroanatomical, Neurological, and Neurochemical Research

Researchers have found patterns of cerebral lateralization and lack of left hemisphere specialization, as measured by EEGs and auditory cortical evoked responses. Reduced EEG power has been identified in the frontal and temporal regions of the left hemisphere for some children with autism (Dawson et al., 1995). These reversed asymmetries seem to be particularly likely to occur when more severe language impairment exists, and may subside as language improves (Dawson, Finley, Phillips, & Galpert, 1986; Dawson, Finley, Phillips, & Lewy, 1989; Dawson, Warrenburg, & Fuller, 1982). Dichotic listening tests that traditionally involve presenting the subject with two simultaneous signals (one in each ear) and asking the subject to recall what was heard, theoretically yield information related to the dominant hemisphere, so that cerebral asymmetry can be assessed. Although these tests have yielded mixed results, some reports show no right ear bias, as would occur with most nondisabled individuals (Arnold & Schwartz, 1983). This suggests that for at least a subgroup of children with autism, some important language functions appear to develop predominately in the right hemisphere (Prior & Bradshaw, 1979; Wetherby, Koegel, & Mendel, 1981).

It has also been hypothesized that the limbic system, which is associated with emotion, subconscious motor and sensory functions, intrinsic feelings of pain and pleasure, and which controls reward and punishment in learning-habituation and reinforcement, is related to autism. Because this part of the midbrain plays a major role in many interconnections and integration of large areas of functioning, its dysfunction could account for the multitude of disabilities in individuals with autism (Damasio & Maurer, 1978; Hetzler & Griffin, 1981; Ornitz, 1985). A positive correlation has recently been found between the severity of symptoms associated with autism and performance on neuropsychological tasks relating to the medial temporal lobe and related limbic structures (Dawson, Meltzoff, Osterling, & Rinaldi, 1998).

Similarly, subcortical dysfunction can cause impairments in social, emotional, and language functioning, hemispheric imbalance (relative right-hemisphere overactivation), difficulties in processing novel information, and overarousal. Some researchers have observed differences in auditory brain stem responses in individuals with autism (Fein, Skoff, & Mirsky, 1981; Gillberg, Rosenhall, & Johansson, 1983). It is noteworthy that all of these researchers have found only a subset of the children who have subcortical abnormalities. Other have found no consistent differences in auditorially evoked potentials with subjects diagnosed as having autism without mental retardation (Grillon, Courchesne, & Akshoomoff, 1989). Together, these results suggest the possibility that a subpopulation of individuals diagnosed as having autism may have subcortical neuroanatomical differences.

More recently, a number of researchers have suggested cerebellar involvement (Bauman & Kemper, 1985; Courchesne, 1987; Courchesne, Hesselink, Jernigan, & Yeung-Courchesne, 1987; Ritvo et al., 1986; Lincoln, Courchesne, Allen, Hanson, & Ene, 1998). Courchesne et al. (1987) used magnetic resonance imaging (MRI), a technique that yields considerable anatomical detail. Their work focused on adults and children whose brains are not likely to be complicated by mental retardation, epilepsy, drug use, postnatal trauma, or disease. Presently, they are pursuing work based on early findings of size differences between the hemispheres of the cerebellum and decreased or arrested development of specific areas in the cerebellum and parietal cortex in some cases (Townsend, Courchesne, & Egaas, 1996). In a recent postmortem study on the brain weights of individuals with autism, Courchesne, Mueller, and Saitoh (1999) found that, in the majority of cases, brain weight was normal, and only a small proportion of cases showed megalencephaly. However, the cases of megalencephaly that were observed were all beyond even the highest reports of brain weight in a sample of the literature among adults without disabilities (Courchesne et al., 1999). These findings suggest that cerebellar hypoplasia can be associated with enlarged regional cerebral volume in some cases among children with autism.

Neurological studies, particularly looking at nystagmus, found abnormalities (Ornitz, 1985; Ornitz, Brown, Mason, & Putnam, 1974; Ritvo et al., 1969) and differences in event-related brain potentials with individuals (Courchesne et al., 1989; Dawson et al., 1988). Such perceptual inconsistency could result in disturbances of relating, language, and communication as a consequence of inconstancy of perception due to faulty modulation of sensory input (Ornitz, 1985).

Neurochemical Factors

Differences in blood serotonin levels, particularly a tendency toward higher levels, have been found in a subgroup of individuals with autism (Campbell et al., 1974; McBride et al., 1998; Ritvo et al., 1984). Serotonergic activity in the brain exerts modulatory effects on many neuronal systems and, it has been asserted, affects various physiological functions and behaviors, such as sleep, body temperature, pain, sensory perception, sexual behavior, motor function, neuroendocrine regulation, appetite, learning and memory, and immune response.

Chromosomal and Genetic Patterns

A number of researchers have suggested that there may be some type of chromosomal or genetic factors that are etiologically significant in at least a subgroup of autism. These theories have been based on the greater prevalence of this disability in males than in females, maternal age (Gillberg & Gillberg, 1983; Tsai & Stewart, 1983), the identification of a "fragile" site on the X chromosome (fragile-X syndrome) (see August & Lockhart, 1984), a higher than expected incidence of families that had multiple cases of autism, and the far greater incidence of autism in monozygotic than in dizygotic twins (Ritvo, Ritvo, & Brothers, 1982; Szatmari, 1999). Recently, research has shown that the disorder is genetically heterogeneous, which could make the detection of genetic linkages more difficult (Szatmari, 1999). Finally, some researchers have found an increased incidence of minor physical anomaly compared to a control group. Some of these differences include low seating of the ears, hypertelorism, syndactylia, high palate, and abnormal head circumference (Walker, 1987). These congenital features also suggest a deviant intrauterine experience.

Conclusion

There are a number of likely reasons for such disparity and contradiction both within and across these organic-based studies. First, children with autism represent an extremely heterogeneous group in terms of their behavioral, cognitive, and linguistic abilities, which may be related to different areas or processes of neurological dysfunction. Second, some may have delayed brain and neural development, rather than abnormal development, in which case chronologically aged control groups would be irrelevant. Third, many have a history of medically prescribed drug use, anoxia, epilepsy, disease, postnatal trauma, or seizure activity that may result in permanent physiological cerebral damage and may be misinterpreted in tests as true congenital abnormalities. Fourth, some of the equipment used in the research lacks adequate sophistication to detect microscopic defects or metabolic processes and therefore has focused on gross anatomical correlates. Finally, there may be exogenous artifacts, particularly in research that requires behavioral responses because children with autism are classically inconsistent in their responses, and even getting them to attend for the presentation of stimuli may be difficult. In summary, although organic research is most likely to reveal the cause of autism in the future, it is very difficult and costly to conduct and may even yield a multitude of possible causes. However, it seems that because studies yield such variable and conflicting results, careful and precise behavioral descriptions and measurements of the presenting symptoms would allow researchers to search for possible subtypes when analyzing organic factors.

COURSE AND PROGNOSIS

Without intervention, prognosis is poor and individuals with autism are not likely to improve much throughout life (Demeyer et al., 1973; Howlin & Goode, 1998). In contrast, individuals who receive intervention can be expected to improve significantly throughout their lives.

Intervention approaches and theoretical perspectives are closely linked. The recent shift toward the conceptualization of autism that emphasizes the interrelationships among symptoms has significant implications for treating this disorder. For example, social deficits in autism may result in avoidance of, or inappropriate engagement in social interactions that may be associated with communication difficulties. Recent studies have documented this interrelationship between these characteristics of "autistic behavior." Specifically, when exposed to positive and responsive social contexts, attempts for communication may be enhanced, and when communication skills improve, untreated disruptive and stereotypical behaviors decrease (Carr, 1977; Carr & Durand, 1985; Koegel, Koegel, Hurley, & Frea, 1992; Koegel, Steibel, & Koegel, 1998). This integrative view emphasizes three major advances in the intervention into autism that have resulted in significant gains in the quality of life for these individuals. One major breakthrough in the treatment of autism and other severely challenging behaviors has been an attempt to examine the antecedents to, or consequences of, disruptive behaviors to assess the variables that maintain the disruptive behaviors. Such intervention programs replace these disruptive behaviors with appropriate "functionally equivalent" behaviors (Horner & Carr, 1997; O'Neill, Horner, Albin, Storey, & Sprague, 1990; Scott & Nelson, in press). For example, Carr and Durand (1985) identified students who were exhibiting self-injurious behavior, tantrums, and aggression to escape difficult tasks or to seek adult attention. These students were taught to use an appropriate and communicatively equivalent phrase of "Am I doing good work?" or "I don't understand." These communicatively equivalent phrases resulted in reducing or eliminating the disruptive behavior that served the same communicative function. Thus, these and other authors have shown that behavior problems can be reduced or eliminated by teaching communicative phrases that are effective in altering the stimulus conditions that control problems (Carr et al., 1999). Further, such programs can be effectively developed and implemented by parents of children with autism (Frea & Hepburn, 1999; Steibel, 1999).

Second, the focus of intervention for children with autism has shifted from considering individual target behaviors to a more global approach that focuses on target behaviors that result in more widespread gains. Such "pivotal intervention" approaches are conceptually important because it is essential to identify target behaviors for intervention that will produce simultaneous changes in many other behaviors, instead of treating each behavior individually— a task that would be prohibitively time-consuming and expensive and may not allow the person to make socially significant gains. Therefore, researchers have begun to define pivotal behaviors, such as motivation, responding to multiple cues, self-management and self-initiations, that are central to wide areas of functioning. Positive changes in pivotal behaviors should have widespread positive effects on many other behaviors and therefore constitute an efficient way to produce generalized behavioral improvements (Koegel, Koegel, Harrower, & Carter, 1999; Koegel, Koegel, & Carter, 1999).

Third, an increased awareness of the critical role that social context plays in the development of children who have autism and other disabilities has propelled a strong movement for including them in regular education classrooms (see Harrower, 1999) and other community settings (Koegel, Koegel, & Dunlap, 1996). Inclusive placements provide opportunities for social and intellectual development that could not occur when children with autism participated in segregated settings with other socially isolated children. In inclusive settings, children who have autism and other disabilities have more able peers available to assist them and serve as role models and they are also required to exhibit appropriate behavior and are challenged to participate in all or part of the regular education curriculum. We are only beginning to experience the social, communicative, and academic benefits that result from fully including children with disabilities in their own community and school environments.

Across the spectrum of autism, regardless of severity, communication is marked by numerous and often severe linguistic and pragmatic skill deficits that affect and limit the ability to integrate and socialize. This can affect interactions with family (Koegel et al., 1992; Koegel, Bimbela, & Schreibman, 1996), adults (Curcio & Paccia, 1987), peers (Haring, 1993), and the development of friendships (Hurley-Geffner, 1995; Meyer et al., 1998) in school, work sites, and other community settings. Adding to the difficulty of developing intervention programs for social communication is the issue that, taken as a whole, the literature shows that there is no one "autistic" pattern of communication. To the contrary, communicative acts that are topographically similar may have different communicative functions for different people and in different social contexts (Horner & Carr, 1997; Olley, 1986). Such individual, situational, and contextual differences make intervention and generalization a challenging area of study. However, one common deficit among individuals with autism is the lack of language used to communicate or the highly limited pragmatic functions of verbal responses. If one considers that much of language development is prompted by the child's motivation to communicate with the outside world, then the inherent difficulties one faces when attempting to communicate with children who are often unmotivated are considerable.

Such a severe lack of attempts to communicate has led some researchers to focus on the general area of *motivating* children with autism to communicate, as a pivotal target behavior (Koegel, Koegel, & Carter, 1999). One language development package that has focused on variables shown to improve motivation in other areas is the "Natural Language Intervention" paradigm (Koegel, O'Dell, & Koegel, 1987). This intervention package involves: (1) using stimulus items that are chosen by the individual rather than arbitrarily chosen by the language specialist, varying the stimulus items frequently, and using age-appropriate items found in the person's natural environment; (2) using less intrusive prompts when necessary, such as repeating the stimulus item rather than manual (physical) prompts; (3) allowing the person to use the stimulus item within a functional interaction, rather than unrelated stimulus materials such as picture cards, etc.; (4) rewarding any attempt to communicate, rather than rewarding only approximations or correct responses; and (5) using natural reinforcers (e.g., an opportunity to use the stimulus item), paired with social reinforcers, rather than unrelated extrinsic reinforcers.

These types of techniques have been very effective in developing an initial lexicon in nonverbal children (Koegel, O'Dell, & Koegel, 1987), and have also been expanded to include more complex language skills to assist more communicatively competent individuals (Koegel et al., 1989). It has been shown that parents can readily use them with their children (Laski, Charlop, & Schreibman, 1988) and thus can expand the language development activities throughout the day and in the child's natural environment. Similar to other intervention techniques that show an inverse relationship to other behaviors, significant decreases in disruptive behavior were observed by Koegel, Koegel, and Surratt (1992) when Natural Language Paradigm techniques were implemented.

Even when individuals become more competent with language and can produce sentences, they may still appear unmotivated or unwilling to use such skills in social communicative contexts where the intervention provider has very little or no control. Children with autism may use language to meet their needs or desires, but they may still exhibit disruptive behavior to avoid social interactions with others in certain community settings. *Self-management* is a technique that has recently been used to improve communication and related social skills in such cases. Because concomitant changes in untreated inappropriate behaviors also occur during self-management, it can be viewed as a pivotal skill. Most people tend to evaluate their own behavior constantly, but people with autism often do not exhibit that skill, and learning competent social interactions and other behaviors requires constant self-regulation.

In a study designed to increase social competence, L. Koegel and her colleagues (1992) taught students with autism (who typically became disruptive when others attempted to communicate with them) to self-monitor appropriate answers to questions. An advantage of this technique is that it can be used in community settings without the constant vigilance of an adult or intervention provider because it relies on the disabled individuals serving as their own intervention providers. The students monitored and significantly increased their appropriate responding to questions at home and in other community settings without the presence of their intervention providers. Again all of these students had relatively competent basic communication skills (i.e., good articulation, ability to formulate sentences, and good receptive language skills) but actively avoided social communication.

One possibility for this phenomenon is that social interactions may become punishing if they lack a minimum level of fluid or consistent responding and may result in disruptive behavior. However, by implementing programs that increase the probability of consistent responding, conversational interactions are more coherent and less aversive and, therefore, less likely to be associated with escape or avoidance-driven disruptive behavior. Further, increased responding allows the nondisabled communicative partner to adjust to the competency level of the disabled person, making the entire interaction more reinforcing to the dyad. Although not yet scientifically documented, this possibility is given credence by anecdotal observations of increases in untreated spontaneous utterances while students were self-managing their responses to questions. Other research studies have hypothesized that social skills directly involved in conversation may be part of a relatively large response class, so that positive changes in some social skills result in positive changes in other untreated social skills. Further adding to the practical utility of self-management techniques, recent studies have demonstrated that these procedures can be effectively implemented entirely within the context of full inclusion classrooms (Koegel, Harrower, & Koegel, 1999; Todd, Horner, & Sugai, 1999).

Another type of self-regulated response, child-initiations, may also be an important pivotal behavior if children are to achieve particularly favorable outcomes. L. Koegel, Koegel, Shoshan, and McNerney (1999) began conducting preliminary assessments to determine whether self-initiations might be associated with highly favorable postintervention outcomes. As Koegel et al. describe, in a first phase of this study, archival data were analyzed for six children who, at intake, appeared to have especially good prognoses according to traditional variables, but had extremely different outcomes (either exceptionally good or exceptionally poor) after years of intensive intervention. Results from this initial phase of the study indicated that the children who had highly favorable outcomes exhibited greater numbers of spontaneous self-initiations at preintervention. Given these results, the authors set out to assess whether a series of self-initiations could be taught to children with autism who demonstrated few or no spontaneous self-initiations at preintervention, and whether children who received this intervention would have highly favorable postintervention outcomes. First, the children were taught to initiate the early developing question "What's that?" in response to items they were unable to label (see Koegel, Camarata, Valdez-Menchaca, & Koegel, 1998). Similarly, the children were taught to initiate the questions, "Where is it?" and "Whose is it?" In addition to the child-initiated questions, the children were taught a variety of other types of verbal initiations such as those designed to elicit attention, to request assistance, and to seek play partners. Results indicated that the children learned and generalized a variety of self-initiations and that these children also had extremely favorable outcomes. Thus, these findings suggest that teaching self-initiations may be a key pivotal target behavior and an important prognostic indicator for increasing the likelihood of highly favorable postintervention outcomes for children with autism.

Both sign language and augmentative communication have been effective for students with autism who are failing to develop any expressive language skills. The advantage of sign representations for children or adults who are severely cognitively impaired is that such symbols are often easier to understand and thus more meaningful than the auditory symbol (word or phrase). And having some type of communicative system, rather than none, allows more opportunities for academic, vocational, and social development. Nonverbal individuals with autism have been taught sign language and have been able to create new sign combinations that had not been specifically taught to them, thus exhibiting some generative language skills (Carr, Binkoff, Kologinsky, & Eddy, 1978). Other types of augmentative communication devices have included pictorial representations, keyboards or other communication aids with letters so that disabled individuals can learn to express their communicative intent nonverbally (Lancoini, 1983; Light, Binger, Agate, & Ramsay, 1999; Schepis, Reid, Behrmann, & Sutton, 1998). Alternative communication systems are particularly effective and critical in the replacing communicatively motivated challenging behavior (e.g., aggression and throwing tantrums), and have been used effectively to increase social interactions in the classroom (Carter & Maxwell, 1998). Recently, these procedures have been effectively designed and implemented by parents of children with autism (Steibel, 1999). However, the bulk of assessment and intervention studies have focused on immediate establishment of systems. Because the study of augmentative and alternative communication is still in its infancy, there are questions yet to be answered (Sigafoos, 1998). Specifically, these questions concern the relationship between comprehension and production, the design selection techniques to accommodate the user's level of progress, and the inverse relationship between alternative communication and challenging behavior (Reichle et al., 1992). Further, questions that involve acquiring and maintaining motivation to use alternative communication, particularly with adults who may lack repeated exposure and thus reinforcement for its use, still need to be studied (Datillio & Camarata, 1991). Considering using such systems to prevent challenging behavior and for longitudinal planing for life-span needs is necessary (Reichle et al., 1992) and is an important area for future research (Koegel, Frea, & Surratt, 1994; Sigafoos, 1998).

Social interaction is closely related to communication. Social deficits have been a hallmark of autism since Kanner's first description. Even the label autism, an extension of the Greek derivative aut(os) meaning "self," connotes the antithesis of social competence. As discussed earlier, the prevailing social philosophy in our country has been gradually shifting from segregating individuals who have disabilities such as autism from school and community settings toward including all of the nation's citizens, regardless of ability level. Therefore, it has become clear that social skills need to be an integral component of any intervention program for individuals with autism to integrate them successfully into the community.

A number of researchers have successfully improved play interactions with children with autism and their peers in integrated settings. Haring and Lovinger (1989) taught young children to play appropriately and initiate social interactions (e.g., seeking a willing peer, offering toys, sharing, taking turns, etc.) with several different age-appropriate activities. This study took into consideration the play preferences of the disabled student and of his peers by having the former seek a child to offer a toy to, who was already playing with a toy that matched his own. Other researchers have found that child-preferred activities correlate with the amount of social avoidance behaviors exhibited by individuals with autism and that such children can be taught to initiate a shift to preferred activities. This, in turn, results in maintained reductions in social avoidance behaviors (Koegel, Dyer, & Bell, 1987). These studies focused on the disabled child, but other studies (Strain, 1983) have taught peer confederates to initiate social interactions by using verbal prompts (e.g., "Come play"), sharing of play items, and offering verbal assistance related to play (e.g., pulling a playmate who is seated in a wagon). Through role-play, peers were also taught to initiate and persevere if their attempts were ignored by the disabled child (Strain, Shores, & Timm, 1977). Some teacher prompting may be necessary for very young children to maintain high levels of social interaction (Odom, Hoyson, Jamieson, & Strain, 1985), but such prompting can be systematically faded, and continued social interactions will remain at high levels (Odom et al., 1992).

As individuals with autism and their peers mature, recruiting a peer "clique" to interact during recreational and leisure activities has been successful (Haring & Breen, 1992). Recruiting peers can easily be incorporated into existing school schedules and results in significant increases in nondisabled teens' social interactions with peers with autism (Shukla, Kennedy, & Cushing, 1998). It is hypothesized that recruiting the entire clique decreases the probability of stigma that may be attached to one peer who would break away from the clique to associate with a disabled peer (DuPaul, McGoey, & Yugar, 1997). Further, many commitments (e.g., eating lunch with a specific peer, peer mediation for social skills, etc.) can be rotated (Pierce &

Schreibman, 1997), and meeting as a group for discussion sessions can be highly motivating if the entire clique is included.

When those who have autism reach adulthood, social integration and social support are critical elements in determining their quality of life and are critical components of community integration (Risley, 1996). Kennedy, Horner, and Newton (1989) described patterns of social contact between persons with severe disabilities who live in community-based residential programs and typical members of local communities, who were not fellow residents or not paid to provide services. These longitudinal data, collected over a 2½-year period, showed that such individuals had a limited number of companions who remained part of their social spheres for more than a few months. In fact, the participants were rarely observed in having prolonged contact with anyone other than family members. The authors discuss the possibility that disabled individuals may be perceived as contributing less to people in their social networks. They suggest the need for strategies that increase or equalize the reciprocity in relationships between persons with and without disabilities to increase the likelihood of maintaining durable relationships.

To conclude, pivotal behaviors that lead to social communicative competence are important for ease of integration. Indeed, researchers, families, professionals, teachers, and others are becoming increasingly aware that intervention should begin at the earliest possible time. Evidence has begun to indicate that children are apt to make significantly more progress if specialized services are initiated well before they reach school age (Dunlap, Robbins, Dollman, & Plienis, 1988; Durand, 1999; Guralnick et al., 1996). It is likely that future research will focus more closely on prelinguistic behaviors that may be precursors to language development (Mundy et al., 1990) that are not developing typically in very young children. Early intervention is critical when one considers the life development of a child who is rejected by society and peers. Peer acceptance and friendships are critical for healthy development (Hurley-Geffner, 1995; Koegel, Frea, & Surratt, 1994), and children who are stigmatized tend to carry the role of the outcast into adulthood (Dodge, 1983). Further, the social awareness gained by typically developing children and the willingness of peers to assist with intervention programs have widespread implications in encouraging a more sympathetic and empathetic response from society as well.

An area of concern frequently overlooked when dealing with a disabled individual is familial stress related to certain specific subareas of the prognosis. R. Koegel et al. (1992) found higher stress on a number of measures among parents of children with autism than among parents in typical families, particularly as to their concern for the well-being of their child after they can no longer provide care for him or her. Other areas of parental stress included the level of cognitive impairment, the child's ability to function independently, and the child's ability to be accepted in the community. These and other familial needs are of critical importance in the diagnostic and intervention process (Moes, 1995; Schreibman, Kaneko, & Koegel, 1991) as social integration in regular communities has become the ultimate goal of intervention.

DIAGNOSTIC CONSIDERATIONS

Autism has many behavioral symptoms in common with other disabilities, but three features exhibited in combination by children with autism are unique to the diagnosis of this disability: difficulties in developing social relationships; language deficits and impaired comprehension, echolalia, and pronominal reversal; and restricted areas of interest that may present as perseverative, ritualistic behavior (APA, 1994; Volkmar & Lord, 1998). Autism can be differentiated from mental retardation by "splinter skills." Though children with mental retardation often exhibit a flat pattern of slower learning and reduced scores in all areas, children with autism typically exhibit some areas of higher functioning relative to other areas. Autism can be differentiated from childhood schizophrenia by age of onset. There is typically a bipolar distribution for children whose disorders begin before the age of three and a second large peak for those in whom disorders are first evident in early adolescence or just before (Rutter, 1978). Autism is most likely congenital and diagnosable before 30 months of age (Schreibman & Charlop, 1987).

Finally, although autism may involve an impairment of social/language skills, it can be differentiated from other language disabilities. For example, language delays in typically developing children often can be associated with chronic otitis media or other hearing loss. Many parents of children with autism initially suspect hearing loss, but actual documented evidence of hearing loss is not highly correlated with autism. Some children who have language delays and late onset of language (late talkers) also show higher receptive than expressive language skills, whereas individuals with autism have difficulties in both areas. Other language skills that differ greatly in the early language development of children with autism are pronominal reversal, lack of semantic intent in utterances, and echolalic responses. Finally, the numerous differences in pragmatic, social, and other associated behaviors are not as symptomatic in other central language disabilities (see also Bartak, Rutter, & Cox, 1975). For example, stereotypical behavior occurs in infancy but not often in young typically developing children, unlike stereotypical behavior in autism, which can persist throughout life at high levels.

Finally, it is important to note that because of a large degree of heterogeneity in individuals diagnosed with autism, a functional approach to the diagnosis is to behaviorally define the type and amount of each behavior exhibited by a particular individual. As such, communication with other professionals is clearer and more specific intervention plans can then be designed.

SUMMARY

Throughout this chapter we have attempted to point out the significant contributions that the integrative view that autism has interrelated symptoms has brought to the conceptualization of and intervention in this disorder.

Although there is a high probability that autism has an organic cause or causes, the specific etiology has yet to be clearly understood. We speculate that the social communicative and motivational problems prevalent in autism are both a cause and an effect of the neurological substrate. We are optimistic that the future holds exciting revelations, but the possibility of multiple causes emphasizes the importance of interdisciplinary approaches that carefully and specifically define behavioral characteristics and organic findings, so that subtypes can be classified. Those who interact with children with autism are well aware of the vast differences and abilities that are evident within the diagnosis.

The large number of behavioral differences exhibited by children with autism can be greatly stigmatizing in community settings. However, as more efficient and comprehensive intervention techniques are developed and as opportunities for integration are available, more widespread improvements are occurring. Integration of the very young and participation of typical peers in the intervention process increase our understanding of disabled individuals and improve the likelihood of their acceptance into society.

Finally, implementing programs that have both social significance and implications for life-span needs are important considerations. Specific behaviors, such as decreasing stereotypic behaviors and tantrums, and increasing play, cooperation, and self-initiations, are important in subjective observers' global impressions of persons with autism and may have important implications for long-term development (Koegel, Koegel, Shoshan, & McNerney, 1999). Determining key pivotal behaviors that result in more favorable prognosis will certainly be an important area of future research.

Many individuals with autism are still segregated from their peers, but researchers are gradually accumulating evidence that demonstrates improved functioning in integrated settings (Anderson & Won, 1990; Harrower, 1999; Kennedy, Cushing, & Itkonen, 1997; Shukla, Kennedy, & Cushing, 1999). The development of models designed to create and support stable relationships and to teach social and communicative behaviors so that people wtih disabilities can interact in vocational, home, neighborhood, community, and school settings and function independently with a high quality of life throughout the life span is still a critical need, which is likely to receive continued attention in the future (Haring, 1993; Risley, 1996). The current movement toward inclusion, early intervention, peer involvement in intervention, functional behaviors, creating stable and meaningful social relationships, and decreasing family stress is definitely a step toward meeting the need to improve the quality of life significantly for those who have autism.

ACKNOWLEDGMENTS. Preparation of this manuscript was supported in part by PHS Research Grant MH28210 from the National Institute of Mental Health and by U.S. Department of Education Grant 5830-257-LO-B. The authors thank Tom Haring, Ph.D., and Merith A. Cosden, Ph.D., for their comments and feedback on earlier drafts of this chapter. We also express appreciation to Karen Davidson, M.D., for her assistance with the clinical case descriptions and for her dedication to children with disabilities.

REFERENCES

Adrien, J. L., Faure, M., Perrot, A., Hameury, L., Garreau, B., Barthelemy, C., & Sauvage, D. (1991). Autism and family home movies: Preliminary findings. *Journal of Autism and Developmental Disorders, 21*, 43–49.

American Psychiatric Association. (1994). *Diagnostic and statistical manual of mental disorders*, 4th ed. Washington, DC: Author.

Anderson, J., & Won, K. (1990). The influence of participation in regular versus "special" education settings on students with challenging behaviors. Unpublished master's thesis. California State University, Hayward.

Applebaum, E., Egel, A. L., Koegel, R. L., & Imhoff, B. (1979). Measuring musical abilities of autistic children. *Journal of Autism and Developmental Disorders, 3*, 279–285.

Arnold, G., & Schwartz, S. (1983). Hemispheric lateralization of language in autistic and aphasic children. *Journal of Autism and Developmental Disorders, 13*, 129–139.

August, G. J., & Lockhart, L. H. (1984). Familial autism and the fragile-X chromosome. *Journal of Autism and Developmental Disorders, 14*, 197–204.

Bartak, L., Rutter, M., & Cox, A. (1975). A comparative study of infantile autism and specific developmental receptive language disorder: I. The children. *British Journal of Psychiatry, 126*, 127–145.

Bauman, M. L., & Kemper, T. L. (1985). Histo-anatomic observations of the brain in early infantile autism. *Neurology, 35*, 866–874.

Bednersh, F., & Peck, C. A. (1986). Assessing social environments: Effects of peer characteristics on the social behavior of children with severe handicaps. *Child Study Journal, 16*, 315–329.

Bettelheim, B. (1967). *The empty fortress*. New York: Free Press.

Campbell, M., Freidman, E., DeVito, E., Greenspan, L., & Collins, P. J. (1974). Blood serotonin in psychotic and brain damaged children. *Journal of Autism and Developmental Disorders, 4*, 33–41.

Carr, E. G. (1977). The motivation of self-injurious behavior: A review of some hypotheses. *Psychological Bulletin*, *84*, 800–816.

Carr, E. G. (1982). Sign language. In R. L. Koegel, A. Rincover, & A. L. Egel (Eds.), *Educating and understanding autistic children* (pp. 142–158). San Diego, CA: College-Hill Press.

Carr, E. G., Binkoff, J. A., Kologinsky, E., & Eddy, M. (1978). Acquisition of sign language by autistic children. I: Expressive labeling. *Journal of Applied Behavior Analysis*, *11*, 489–501.

Carr, E. G., & Durand, V. M. (1985). Reducing behavior problems through functional communication training. *Journal of Applied Behavior Analysis*, *18*, 111–126.

Carr, E. G., Levin, L., McConnachie, G., Carlson, J. I., Kemp, D. C., Smith, C. E., & Magito McLaughlin, D. (1999). Comprehensive multisituational intervention for problem behavior in the community: Long-term maintenance and social validation. *Journal of Positive Behavior Interventions*, *1*, 5–25.

Carr, E. G., Reeve, C. E., & Magito-McLaughlin, D. (1996). Contextual influences on problem behavior in people with developmental disabilities. In L. K. Koegel, R. L. Koegel, & G. Dunlap (Eds.), *Positive behavioral support: Including people with difficult behavior in the community* (pp. 403–423). Baltimore: Paul H. Brookes.

Carr, E. G., Schreibman, L., & Lovaas, O. I. (1975). Control of echolalic speech in psychotic children. *Journal of Abnormal Child Psychology*, *3*, 331–351.

Carter, M., & Maxwell, K. (1998). Promoting interaction with children using augmentative communication through a peer-directed intervention. *International Journal of Disability, Development and Education*, *45*, 75–96.

Chess, S. (1971). Autism in children with congenital rubella. *Journal of Autism and Childhood Schizophrenia*, *1*, 33–47.

Chess, S. (1977). Follow-up report on autism in congenital rubella. *Journal of Autism and Childhood Schizophrenia*, *7*, 69–81.

Coleman, M. (1994). Second trimester of gestation: A time of risk for classical autism? *Developmental Brain Dysfunction*, *7*, 104–109.

Courchesne, E. (1987). A neurophysiological view of autism. In E. Schopler & G. Mesibov (Eds.), *Neurobiological issues in autism*. New York: Plenum.

Courchesne, E., Hesselink, J. R., Jernigan, T. L., & Yeung-Courchesne, R. (1987). Abnormal neuroanatomy in a non-retarded person with autism: Unusual findings using magnetic resonance imaging. *Archives of Neurology*, *44*, 335–341.

Courchesne, E., Lincoln, A. J., Yeung-Courchesne, R., Elmasian, R., & Grillon, C. (1989). Pathophysiologic findings in nonretarded autism and receptive developmental language disorder. *Journal of Autism and Developmental Disorders*, *19*, 1–17.

Courchesne, E., Mueller, R., & Saitoh, O. (1999). Brain weight in autism: Normal in the majority of cases, megalencephalic in rare cases. *Neurology*, *52*(5), 1057–1059.

Curcio, E., & Paccia, J. (1987). Conversations with autistic children: Contingent relationships between features of adult input and children's response adequacy. *Journal of Autism and Developmental Disorders*, *17*, 81–93.

Damasio, A., & Maurer, R. (1978). A neurological model for childhood autism. *Archives of Neurology*, *35*, 777–786.

Datillio, J., & Camarata, S. (1991). Facilitating conversation through self-initiated augmentative communication treatment. *Journal of Applied Behavior Analysis*, *24*, 369–378.

Dawson, G., Finley, C., Phillips, S., & Galpert, L. (1986). Hemispheric specialization and the language abilities of autistic children. *Child Development*, *57*, 1440–1453.

Dawson, G., Finley, C., Phillips, S., Galpert, L., & Lewy, A. (1988). Reduced P3 amplitude of the event-related brain potential: Its relationship to language ability in autism. *Journal of Autism and Developmental Disorders*, *18*, 493–504.

Dawson, G., Finley, C., Phillips, S., & Lewy, A. (1989). A comparison of hemispheric asymmetries in speech-related brain potentials of autistic and dysphasic children. *Brain and Language*, *37*, 26–41.

Dawson, G., Klinger, L. G., Panagiotides, H., & Lewy, A. (1995). Subgroups of autistic children based on social behavior display distinct patterns of brain activity. *Journal of Abnormal Child Psychology*, *23*, 569–583.

Dawson, G., Meltzoff, A. N., Osterling, J., & Rinaldi, J. (1998). Neuropsychological correlates of early symptoms of autism. *Child Development*, *69*, 1276–1285.

Dawson, G., Warrenburg, S., & Fuller, P. (1982). Cerebral lateralization in individuals diagnosed as autistic in early childhood. *Brain and Cognition*, *2*, 346–354.

DeGiacomo, A., & Fombonne, E. (1998). Parental recognition of developmental abnormalities in autism. *European Child and Adolescent Psychiatry*, *7*(3), 131–136.

DeLong, G. R. (1999). Autism: New data suggest a new hypothesis. *Neurology*, *52*(5), 911–916.

DeMeyer, M. K., Barton, S., DeMeyer, W. E., Norton, J. A., Allen, J., & Steele, R. (1973). Prognosis in autism: A follow-up study. *Journal of Autism and Childhood Schizophrenia*, *3*, 199–246.

Department of Developmental Services. (1999, March). Changes in the population of persons with autism and pervasive developmental disorders in California's developmental services system: 1987 through 1998. *A Report to the Legislature.* Sacramento, CA: California State Health and Human Services Agency.

Dodge, K. A. (1983). Behavioral antecedents of peer social status. *Child Development, 54,* 1386–1399.

Dunlap, G., Robbins, F. R., Dollman, C., & Plienis, A. J. (1988). *Early intervention for young children with autism: A regional training approach.* Huntington, WV: Marshall University.

DuPaul, G. J., McGoey, K. E., & Yugar, J. M. (1997). Mainstreaming students with behavior disorders: The use of classroom peers as facilitators of generalization. *School Psychology Review, 26,* 634–650.

Durand, V. M. (1999). New directions in educational programming for students with autism. In D. B. Zager et al. (Eds.), *Autism: Identification, education, and treatment* (2nd ed., pp. 323–343). Mahwah, NJ: Erlbaum.

Egel, A. L., Koegel, R. L., & Schreibman, L. (1980). Review of educational-treatment procedures for autistic children. In L. Mann & D. Sabatino (Eds.), *Fourth review of special education* (pp. 109–150). New York: Grune & Stratton.

Eisenberg, L., & Kanner, L. (1956). Early infantile autism: 1943–1955. *American Journal of Orthopsychiatry, 26,* 55–65.

Fein, D., Skoff, B., & Mirsky, A. F. (1981). Clinical correlates of brain stem dysfunction in autistic children. *Journal of Autism and Developmental Disorders, 11,* 303–315.

Frea, W. D. (1995). Social-communicative skills in higher-functioning children with autism. In R. L. Koegel & L. K. Koegel (Eds.), *Teaching children with autism: Strategies for initiating positive interactions and improving learning opportunities* (pp. 53–66). Baltimore: Paul H. Brookes.

Frea, W. D. (1997). Reducing stereotypic behavior by teaching orienting responses to environmental stimuli. *Journal of the Association for Persons with Severe Handicaps, 22,* 28–35.

Frea, W. D., & Hepburn, S. L. (1999). A demonstration of teaching parents of children with autism how to perform functional assessments to plan interventions for extremely disruptive behaviors. *Journal of Positive Behavior Interventions, 1,* 112–116.

Gillberg, C., & Gillberg, I. C. (1983). Infantile autism: A total population study of reduced optimality in the pre-, peri-, and neonatal period. *Journal of Autism and Developmental Disorders, 13,* 153–166.

Gillberg, C., Rosenhall, U., & Johansson, E. (1983). Auditory brain stem responses in childhood psychosis. *Journal of Autism and Developmental Disorders, 13,* 181–195.

Grillon, C., Courchesne, E., & Akshoomoff, N. (1989). Brain stem and middle latency auditory evoked potentials in autism and developmental language disorder. *Journal of Autism and Developmental Disorders, 19,* 255–269.

Guralnick, M. J., Connor, R. T., Hammond, M., Gottman, J. M., & Kinnish, K. (1996). Immediate effects of mainstreamed settings on the social interactions and social integration of preschool children. *American Journal of Mental Retardation, 100,* 359–377.

Haring, T. G. (1993). Research basis of instructional procedures to promote social interaction and integration. In S. R. Warren (Ed.), *Advances in mental retardation and developmental disabilities.* Vol. 5: *Research basis of instruction* (pp. 129–164). Baltimore: Paul H. Brookes.

Haring, T. G., & Breen, C. G. (1992). A peer mediated social network intervention to enhance the social integration of persons with moderate and severe disabilities. *Journal of Applied Behavior Analysis, 25,* 319–334.

Haring, T. G., & Lovinger, L. (1989). Promoting social interaction through teaching generalized play initiation responses to preschool children with autism. *Journal of the Association for Persons with Severe Handicaps, 14,* 58–67.

Harrower, J. K. (1999). Issues concerning the educational inclusion of children with severe disabilities. *Journal of Positive Behavior Interventions, 1*(4), 215–230.

Hetzler, B., & Griffin, J. (1981). Infantile autism and the temporal lobe of the brain. *Journal of Autism and Developmental Disorders, 11,* 317–330.

Ho, E. D. E., Tsang, A. K. T., & Ho, D. Y. F. (1992). An investigation of the calendar calculation ability of a Chinese calendar savant. *Journal of Autism and Developmental Disorders, 21,* 315–327.

Horner, R. H., & Carr, E. G. (1997). Behavioral support for students with severe disabilities: Functional assessment and comprehensive intervention. *The Journal of Special Education, 31,* 84–104.

Howlin, P., & Goode, S. (1998). Outcome in adult life for people with autism and Asperger's syndrome. In Fred R. Volkmer et al. (Eds.), *Autism and pervasive developmental disorders* (pp. 209–241). New York: Cambridge University Press.

Hughes, C., Leboyer, M., & Bouvard, M. (1997). Executive function in parents of children with autism. *Psychological Medicine, 27,* 209–220.

Hurley-Geffner, C. M. (1995). Friendships between children with and without developmental disabilities. In R. L. Koegel & L. K. Koegel (Eds.), *Teaching children with autism: Strategies for initiating positive interactions and improving learning opportunities* (pp. 105–125). Baltimore: Paul H. Brookes.

Kanner, L. (1943). Autistic disturbances of affective contact. *Nervous Child, 2,* 217–250.

Kennedy, C. H., Cushing, L. S., & Itkonen, T. (1997). General education participation improves the social contacts and friendship networks of students with severe disabilities. *Journal of Behavioral Education, 7,* 167–189.

Kennedy, C. H., Horner, R. H., & Newton, J. S. (1989). Social contacts of adults with severe disabilities living in the community: A descriptive analysis of relationship patterns. *Journal of the Association for Persons with Severe Handicaps, 14,* 190–196.

Kern, L., Koegel, R. L., & Dunlap, G. (1984). The influence of vigorous vs. mild exercise on autistic stereotyped responding. *Journal of Autism and Developmental Disorders, 14,* 57–67.

Kern, L., Koegel, R. L., Dyer, K., Blew, P. A., & Fenton, L. R. (1982). The effects of physical exercise on self-stimulation and appropriate responding in autistic children. *Journal of Autism and Developmental Disorders, 4,* 399–419.

Koegel, L. K. (1995). Communication and language intervention. In R. L. Koegel & L. K. Koegel (Eds.), *Teaching children with autism: Strategies for initiating positive interactions and improving learning opportunities* (pp. 17–32). Baltimore: Paul H. Brookes.

Koegel, L. K., Camarata, S. M., Valdez-Menchaca, M., & Koegel, R. L. (1998). Setting generalization of question-asking by children with autism. *American Journal on Mental Retardation, 102,* 346–357.

Koegel, L. K., Harrower, J. K., & Koegel, R. L. (1999). Support for children with developmental disabilities in full inclusion classrooms through self-management. *Journal of Positive Behavior Interventions, 1,* 26–34.

Koegel, L. K., Koegel, R. L., & Dunlap, G. (Eds.). (1996). *Positive behavioral support: Supporting people with difficult behavior in the community.* Baltimore: Paul H. Brookes.

Koegel, L. K., Koegel, R. L., Harrower, J. K., & Carter, C. M. (1999). Pivotal response intervention. I: Overview of approach. *Journal of the Association for Persons with Severe Handicaps, 24*(3), 174–185.

Koegel, L. K., Koegel, R. L., Hurley, C., & Frea, W. D. (1992). Improving pragmatic skills and disruptive behavior in children with autism through self-management. *Journal of Applied Behavior Analysis, 25,* 341–354.

Koegel, L. K., Koegel, R. L., Shoshan, Y., & McNerney, E. (1999). Pivotal response intervention. II: Preliminary long-term outcome data on self-initiations. *Journal of the Association for Persons with Severe Handicaps, 24*(3), 186–198.

Koegel, L. K., Koegel, R. L., & Smith, A. (1997). Variables related to differences in standardized test outcomes for children with autism. *Journal of Autism and Developmental Disorders, 27,* 233–243.

Koegel, L. K., Steibel, D., & Koegel, R. L. (1998). Reducing aggression in children with autism toward infant or toddler siblings. *Journal of the Association for Persons with Severe Handicaps, 23,* 111–118.

Koegel, R. L., Bimbela, A., & Schreibman, L. (1996). Collateral effects of parent training on family interactions. *Journal of Autism and Developmental Disorders, 26,* 347–359.

Koegel, R. L., Camarata, S., & Koegel, L. K. (1994). Aggression and noncompliance: Behavior modification through naturalistic language remediation. In J. L. Matson (Ed.), *Autism in children and adults: Etiology, assessment and intervention* (pp. 165–180). Pacific Grove, CA: Brookes/Cole.

Koegel, R. L., Dyer, K., & Bell, L. K. (1987). The influence of child-preferred activities on autistic children's social behavior. *Journal of Applied Behavior Analysis, 20,* 243–252.

Koegel, R. L., & Frea, W. D. (1993). Treatment of social behavior in autism through the modification of pivotal social skills. *Journal of Applied Behavior Analysis, 26,* 369–377.

Koegel, R. L., Frea, W. D., & Surratt, A. (1994). Self-management of problematic social behavior. In E. Schopler & G. Mesibov (Eds.), *Behavioral issues in autism* (pp. 81–97). New York: Plenum.

Koegel, R. L., Koegel, L. K., & Carter, C. M. (1999). Pivotal teaching interactions for children with autism. *School Psychology Review, 28,* 576–594.

Koegel, R. L., Koegel, L. K., & Surratt, A. V. (1992). Language intervention and disruptive behavior in preschool children with autism. *Journal of Autism and Developmental Disorders, 22,* 141–154.

Koegel, R. L., O'Dell, M. C., & Koegel, L. K. (1987). A natural language paradigm for teaching non-verbal autistic children. *Journal of Autism and Developmental Disorders, 17,* 187–199.

Koegel, R. L., Schreibman, L., Good, A., Cerniglia, L., Murphy, C., & Koegel, L. K. (1989). *How to teach pivotal behaviors to children with autism: A training manual.* University of California: Santa Barbara.

Koegel, R. L., Schreibman, L., Loos, L. M., Dirlich-Wilhelm, H., Dunlap, G., Robbins, F. R., & Plienis, A. (1992). Consistent stress profiles in mothers of children with autism. *Journal of Autism and Developmental Disorders, 22,* 205–216.

Koegel, R. L., Schreibman, L., O'Neill, R. E., & Burke, J. C. (1983). Personality and family interaction characteristics of parents of autistic children. *Journal of Consulting and Clinical Psychology, 16,* 683–692.

Lancoini, G. E. (1983). Using pictorial representations as communication means with low-functioning children. *Journal of Autism and Developmental Disorders, 13,* 87–105.

Laski, K. E., Charlop, M. H., & Schreibman, L. (1988). Training parents to use the natural language paradigm to increase their autistic children's speech. *Journal of Applied Behavior Analysis, 21,* 391–400.

Libby, S., Powell, S., Messer, D., & Jordan, R. (1998). Spontaneous play in children with autism: A reappraisal. *Journal of Autism and Developmental Disorders*, 28, 487–497.

Light, J. C., Binger, C., Agate, T. L., & Ramsay, K. N. (1999). Teaching partner-focused questions to individuals who use augmentative and alternative communication to enhance their communicative competence. *Journal of Speech, Language, and Hearing Research*, 42, 241–255.

Lincoln, A., Courchesne, E., Allen, M., Hanson, E., & Ene, M. (1998). Neurobiology of Asperger syndrome: Seven case studies and quantitative magnetic resonance imaging findings. In E. Schopler & G. B. Mesibov (Eds.), *Asperger syndrome or high-functioning autism?* (pp. 145–163). New York: Plenum.

Lord, C., Pickles, A., McLennan, J., Rutter, M., Bergman, J., Folstein, S., Fombonne, E., Leboyer, M., & Minshew, N. (1997). Diagnosing autism: Analyses of data from the Autism Diagnostic Interview. *Journal of Autism and Developmental Disorders*, 27, 501–517.

Lovaas, O. I., Varni, J., Koegel, R. L., & Lorsch, N. (1977). Some observations on the non-extinguishability of children's speech. *Child Development*, 48, 1121–1127.

Mahoney, G. (1988). Communication patterns—mothers and mentally retarded infants. *First Language*, 8, 157–172.

McBride, P. A., Anderson, G. M., Hertzig, M. E., Snow, M. E., Thompson, S. M., Khait, V. D., Shapiro, T., & Cohen, D. J. (1998). Effects of diagnosis, race, and puberty on platelet serotonin levels in autism and mental retardation. *Journal of the American Academy of Child and Adolescent Psychiatry*, 37, 767–776.

Meyer, L. H., Monondo, S., Fisher, M., Larson, M. J., Dunmore, S., Black, J. W., & D'Aquanni, M. (1998). Frames of friendship: Social relationships among adolescents with diverse abilities. In L. H. Meyer, H. S. Park, M. Gernot-Scheyer, I. S. Schwartz, & B. Harry (Eds.), *Making friends: Influences of culture and development*. Baltimore: Paul H. Brookes.

Moes, D. (1995). Parent education and parenting stress. In R. L. Koegel & L. K. Koegel (Eds.), *Teaching children with autism: Strategies for initiating positive interactions and improving learning opportunities* (pp. 79–93). Baltimore: Paul H. Brookes.

Mundy, P., Sigman, M., & Kasari, C. (1990). A longitudinal study of joint attention and language development in autistic children. *Journal of Autism and Developmental Disorders*, 20, 115–128.

Odom, S. L., Chandler, L. K., Ostrosky, M., McConnell, S. R., & Reaney, S. (1992). Fading teacher prompts from peer-initiation interventions for young children with disabilities. *Journal of Applied Behavior Analysis*, 25, 307–318.

Odom, S. L., Hoyson, M., Jamieson, B., & Strain, P. S. (1985). Increasing handicapped preschoolers' peer interactions: Cross-setting and component analysis. *Journal of Applied Behavior Analysis*, 18, 3–16.

Olley, J. G. (1986). The TEACCH curriculum for teaching social behavior to children with autism. In E. Schopler & G. B. Mesibov (Eds.), *Social behavior and autism* (pp. 351–373). New York: Plenum.

O'Neill, R. E., Horner, R. H., Albin, R. W., Storey, K., & Sprague, J. R. (1990). *Functional analysis: A practical assessment guide*. Sycamore, IL: Sycamore Press.

Ornitz, E. M. (1985). Neurophysiology of infantile autism. *Journal of the American Academy of Child Psychiatry*, 24, 251–262.

Ornitz, E. M., Brown, M. B., Mason, A., & Putnam, N. H. (1974). Effect of visual input on vestibular nystagmus in autistic children. *Archives of General Psychiatry*, 31, 369–375.

Pierce, K., & Schreibman, L. (1997). Multiple peer use of pivotal response training to increase social behaviors of classmates with autism: Results from trained and untrained peers. *Journal of Applied Behavior Analysis*, 30, 157–160.

Prior, M., & Bradshaw, J. L. (1979). Hemispheric functioning in autistic children. *Cortex*, 15, 73–81.

Prizant, B. M. (1983). Echolalia in autism: Assessment and intervention. *Seminars in Speech and Language*, 4, 63–77.

Prizant, B. M., & Rydell, P. J. (1984). Analysis of functions of delayed echolalia in autistic children. *Journal of Speech and Hearing Research*, 27, 183–192.

Rapin, L. (1997). Autism. *New England Journal of Medicine*, 337, 97–104.

Reichle, J., Mirenda, P., Locke, P., Piche, L., & Johnston, S. (1992). Beginning augmentative communication systems. In S. F. Warren & J. Reichle (Eds.), *Causes and effects in communication and language intervention* (pp. 131–156). Baltimore: Paul H. Brookes.

Risley, T. (1996). Get a life!: Positive behavioral intervention for challenging behavior through life arrangement and life coaching. In L. K. Koegel, R. L. Koegel, & G. Dunlap (Eds.), *Positive behavioral support: Including people with difficult behavior in the community* (pp. 425–438). Baltimore: Paul H. Brookes.

Ritvo, E. R., & Freeman, B. J. (1978). National society for autistic children definition of the syndrome of autism. *Journal of Autism and Childhood Schizophrenia*, 8, 162–169.

Ritvo, E. R., Freeman, B. J., Scheibel, A. B., Duong, T., Robinson, H., Guthrie, D., & Ritvo, A. M. (1986). Lower Purkinje cell counts in the cerebella of four autistic subjects: Initial findings of the UCLA-NSAC autopsy research report. *American Journal of Psychiatry*, 143, 862–866.

Ritvo, E. R., Freeman, B. J., Yuwiler, A., Geller, E., Yokota, A., Schroth, P., & Novak, P. (1984). Study of fenfluramine in outpatients with the syndrome of autism. *Journal of Pediatrics, 105*, 823–828.

Ritvo, E. R., Ornitz, E. M., Eviatar, A., Markham, C. H., Brown, M. B., & Mason, A. (1989). Decreased postrotatory nystagmus in early infantile autism. *Neurology, 19*, 653–658.

Ritvo, E. R., Ritvo, E. C., & Brothers, A. M. (1982). Genetic and immunohematologic factors in autism. *Journal of Autism and Developmental Disorders, 12*, 109–114.

Rutter, M. (1978). Diagnosis and definition of childhood autism. *Journal of Autism and Childhood Schizophrenia, 8*, 139–167.

Rydell, P. J., & Mirenda, P. (1994). Effects of high and low constraint utterances on the production of immediate and delayed echolalia in young children with autism. *Journal of Autism and Developmental Disorders, 24*, 719–735.

Schepis, M. M., Reid, D. H., Behrmann, M. M., & Sutton, K. A. (1998). Increasing communicative interactions of young children with autism using a voice output communication aid and naturalistic teaching. *Journal of Applied Behavior Analysis, 31*, 561–578.

Schopler, E. (1978). On confusion in the diagnosis of autism. *Journal of Autism and Childhood Schizophrenia, 8*, 137–138.

Schreibman, L., & Charlop, M. H. (1987). Autism. In V. B. Van Hasselt & M. Hersen (Eds.), *Psychological evaluation of the developmentally and physically disabled* (pp. 155–174). New York: Plenum.

Schreibman, L., Kaneko, W., & Koegel, R. L. (1991). Positive affect of parents of autistic children: A comparison across two teaching techniques. *Behavior Therapy, 22*, 479–490.

Schreibman, L., Koegel, R. L., Mills, J. I., & Burke, J. C. (1981). Social validation of behavior therapy with autistic children. *Behavior Therapy, 12*, 610–624.

Scott, T. M., & Nelson, C. M. (in press). Using functional behavioral assessment to develop effective intervention plans: Practical classroom application. *Journal of Positive Behavior Interventions*.

Shukla, S., Kennedy, C. H., & Cushing, L. S. (1998). Adult influence on the participation of peers without disabilities in peer support programs. *Journal of Behavioral Education, 8*, 397–413.

Shukla, S., Kennedy, C. H., & Cushing, L. S. (1999). Supporting the social participation of intermediate school students with severe disabilities in general education classrooms. *Journal of Positive Behavior Intervention, 1*(3), 130–140.

Sigafoos, J. (1998). Assessing conditional use of graphic mode requesting in a young boy with autism. *Journal of Developmental and Physical Disabilities, 10*, 133–151.

Steibel, D. (1999). Using a parent problem-solving intervention to promote augmentative communication during daily routines. *Journal of Positive Behavior Interventions, 1*(3), 159–169.

Strain, P. S. (1983). Generalization of autistic children's social behavior change: Effects of developmentally integrated and segregated settings. *Analysis and Intervention in Developmental Disabilities, 3*, 23–24.

Strain, P. S., Shores, R. E., & Timm, M. A. (1977). Effects of peer social initiations on the behavior of withdrawn preschool children. *Journal of Applied Behavior Analysis, 10*, 289–298.

Sullivan, R. C. (1978). The hostage parent. *Journal of Autism and Childhood Schizophrenia, 8*, 233–248.

Szatmari, P. (1999). Heterogeneity and the genetics of autism. *Journal of Psychiatry and Neuroscience, 24*, 159–165.

Tager-Flusberg, H. (1990). Psycholinguistic approaches to language and communication in autism. In E. Schopler & G. B. Mesibov (Eds.), *Communication problems in autism* (pp. 69–87). New York: Plenum.

Todd, A. W., Horner, R. H., & Sugai, G. (1999). Effects of self-monitoring and self-recruited praise on problem behavior, academic engagement, and work completion in a typical classroom. *Journal of Positive Behavior Interventions, 1*, 66–76.

Townsend, J., Courchesne, E., & Egaas, B. (1996). Slowed orienting of the covert visual-spatial attention in autism: Specific deficits associated with cerebellar and parietal abnormality. *Development and Psychopathology, 8*, 563–584.

Trottier, G., Srivastava, L., & Walker, C. (1999). Etiology of infantile autism: A review of recent advances in genetic and neurobiological research. *Journal of Psychiatry and Neuroscience, 24*, 103–115.

Tsai, L. Y., & Stewart, M. A. (1983). Etiological implication of maternal age and birth order in infantile autism. *Journal of Autism and Developmental Disorders, 13*, 57–65.

United States Department of Education. (1999). Comparison of the 16th and 20th annual report to Congress on the implementation of the Individuals with Disabilities Education Act, number and change in number of children ages 6–21 served under IDEA, Part B, Autism.

Valdez-Menchaca, M. C. (1991). Child effects on maternal speech: Their implications for long-term maintenance of early intervention gains. State University of New York, Stony Brook. *Dissertation Abstracts International, 51*(11-A), 3681–3682.

Volkmar, F. R., & Lord, C. (1998). Diagnosis and definition of autism and other pervasive developmental disorders. In F. R. Volkmar et al. (Eds.), *Autism and pervasive developmental disorders*. New York: Cambridge University Press.

Walker, L. J. (1987). Procedural rights in the wrong system: Special education is not enough. In A. Gartner & T. Joe (Eds.), *Images of the disabled, disabling images* (pp. 97–115). New York: Praeger.

Wetherby, A., Koegel, R. L., & Mendel, M. (1981). Central auditory nervous system dysfunction in echolalic autistic individuals *Journal of Speech and Hearing Research, 24,* 420–429.

Wetherby, A. M., & Prutting, C. A. (1984). Profiles of communicative and cognitive-social abilities in autistic children. *Journal of Speech and Hearing Research, 27,* 364–377.

Wing, L. (1976). *Early childhood autism: Clinical, educational and social aspects,* 2nd ed. Oxford, England: Pergamon.

Wing, L. (1996). Autism spectrum disorders. *British Medical Journal, 312,* 327–328.

Wing, L. (1997). The autistic spectrum. *Lancet, 350,* 1761–1766.

9

Attention-Deficit/Hyperactivity Disorder

Mark D. Rapport

Description of the Disorder

Attention-deficit/hyperactivity disorder (ADHD) (American Psychiatric Association, 1994) is a complex and chronic disorder of brain, behavior, and development whose behavioral and cognitive consequences affect multiple areas of functioning. Historically, children who have ADHD were referred to as having "minimal brain damage" (1947 to early 1950s). The association between brain damage and behavioral deviance was logical and was introduced following the pandemic of encephalitis in the 1920s. Many of the postencephalitic children, it was observed, were motorically overactive, inattentive, and aggressive, in addition to displaying a wide variety of emotional and learning difficulties. Subsequent attempts to validate the concept of minimal brain damage, however, were unsuccessful. Neither "soft neurological signs," that is, objective physical evidence that is perceptible to the examining physician as opposed to the subjective sensations or symptoms of the patient, nor a positive history of brain damage or birth difficulties were evidenced in a majority of children who had histories of behavioral problems.

The concept of a clinical disorder resulting from brain damage was gradually discarded and replaced with the subtler but nebulous concept, "minimal brain dysfunction," or MBD (late 1950s to mid-1960s). The distinction between brain damage and brain dysfunction was important. It implied a *hypothesis* of brain dysfunction resulting from manifestations of central nervous system dysfunction, as opposed to brain damage as an assumed *fact* in affected children. It also suggested that a wide range of learning and behavioral disabilities could accompany the hypothesized deviations of the central nervous system. These symptoms could be inferred from various combinations of impairment in attention, impulse control, gross motor activity, perception, language, and memory, among others.

The concept of minimal brain dysfunction was eventually replaced with the moniker, "hyperkinetic reaction of childhood," in the American Psychiatric Association's second

Mark D. Rapport • Department of Psychology, University of Central Florida, Orlando, Florida 32816.

Advanced Abnormal Psychology, Second Edition, edited by Hersen and Van Hasselt. Kluwer Academic/Plenum Publishers, New York, 2001.

edition of its *Diagnostic and Statistical Manual* (American Psychiatric Association, 1968). The change in diagnostic labels reflected a general dissatisfaction with the untestable notion of brain dysfunction and concomitantly suggested that an excessive degree of and difficulties in regulating gross motor activity best represented the core symptoms of the disorder. The term "reaction" reflected prevailing psychoanalytic influences concerning causes of mental disorders during the 1960's.

The concept of an independent syndrome of *hyperactivity* prevailed between 1968 and 1979, during which time considerable effort was spent trying to validate the notion of a hyperactive child syndrome. An upsurge in child psychopathology research directly affected the evolution of thinking during this period and resulted in a focus on *attentional difficulties* or deficits as the core disturbance of the disorder. Excessive gross motor activity was subsequently relegated to an associative feature in defining the disorder, which in turn, was considered neither sufficient nor necessary to establish a formal diagnosis. This rather dramatic shift in diagnostic emphasis was reflected in the third edition of the *Diagnostic and Statistical Manual* (American Psychiatric Association, 1980), wherein the disorder was renamed "attention deficit disorder" (ADD) and could occur with hyperactivity (ADDH) or without hyperactivity (ADD).

A second important change in the DSM-III nomenclature involved conceptualizing the disorder itself. Earlier diagnostic conceptualizations of the disorder required, among other clinical criteria, that a child meet a specified number of symptoms from a prepared list to qualify for a diagnosis (e.g., any eight criteria on the list). This type of diagnostic conceptualization, in which no single behavioral characteristic is essential or sufficient for group membership and members that have a number of shared characteristics or clinical features are grouped together, is referred to as a *polythetic* schema. The DSM-III nomenclature, however, incorporated a *monothetic* schema for the first time, wherein an individual was now required to present with a specified number of symptoms from *each* of three independent behavioral categories to establish a diagnosis: inattention, impulsivity, and overactivity. The difference may appear subtle, but it has important implications for diagnostic categorization and defining what constitutes a particular clinical disorder. In the case of ADDH, for example, it would be much more difficult to meet multiple criteria in three distinct behavioral domains (versus from a single list of symptoms), which in turn, would have the effect of refining the disorder to a more homogeneous (similar) grouping of children.

As a consequence of this conceptual shift, researchers began focusing their efforts on establishing whether or not inattention, impulsivity, and hyperactivity were in fact independent behavioral domains—primarily by conducting factor analytic studies on child behavior rating scales obtained from classroom teachers. In factor analytic studies, researchers use statistical techniques to discern whether certain rating scale items or descriptions of specific types of behavior covary or "go together" to form one or more independent domains of behavior. If all items correlate highly with one another (i.e., they are significantly related to one another), then a single factor (e.g., "inattention") is thought to account for the different rating scale items. A two-factor solution suggests that some items or behavioral descriptions of behavior covary with one another but not with the remaining behavioral descriptions entered into the equation. It might subsequently be found that these remaining items covary or go together in a statistical sense to form a second behavioral domain, such as "impulsivity."

What emerged from factor analytic studies was a mixed and often confusing picture. Most studies failed to find evidence of independent factors or behavioral domains to support the three dimensions associated with ADDH. Several of the studies found evidence for a separate "attentional disturbance" domain, whereas impulsivity and hyperactivity loaded together on a second factor. That is, items comprising these latter two domains were frequently inseparable from one another, suggesting that impulsivity and hyperactivity were probably different but related behaviors of a single dimension of behavior.

The evolution from the DSM-III to the revised DSM-III-R edition (American Psychiatric Association, 1987) was much quicker than was the case with earlier evolutions. The disorder was renamed in the DSM-III revised edition, and hyperactivity reemerged as a central feature of the disorder. Several other important changes were adopted in the revised 1987 nomenclature. The modified monothetic classification schema that required the presence of behavior problems in three different dimensions (inattention, impulsivity, and hyperactivity) was discarded, and the new classification schema reverted back to a polythetic dimensional approach, that is, a diagnosis now required that eight out of 14 behaviors from a single list be present in a child for a minimum of 6 months duration, and onset of difficulties occurred before age seven. ADD without hyperactivity was abandoned as a distinct subtype of the disorder, and a secondary category termed "undifferentiated attention deficit disorder" was added to subsume those children who had attentional problems without hyperactivity. Finally, the "residual ADDH" category, which was used in the earlier edition to describe older individuals (usually adolescents) who no longer presented with the full complement of ADDH symptoms, was discarded.

The most recent version (4th edition) of the *Diagnostic and Statistical Manual* (DSM-IV; 1994) constitutes a modified classification schema, wherein three distinct subtypes of ADHD are possible. Diagnosis requires that a minimum of six symptoms be present for at least 6 months to a degree that is maladaptive and inconsistent with the child's developmental level in accord with two sets of criteria. Children who meet only the inattention criteria are thought to have a predominantly inattentive type of ADHD. Those who meet only the hyperactivity-impulsivity criteria are referred to as having a predominantly hyperactive-impulsive type of ADHD. And those who meet both sets of criteria have a combined type of ADHD.

EPIDEMIOLOGY

Epidemiology is concerned with the ways in which clinical disorders and diseases occur in human populations and with factors that influence these patterns of occurrence. Three interrelated components of epidemiological research involve (1) assessing the occurrence of new cases (incidence rate) or existing cases (prevalence rate) of the disorder at a given period of time or within a specific time period; (2) assessing how the disorder is distributed in the population, which may include information concerning geographic location, gender, socio-economic level, and ethnicity or culture; and (3) identifying factors associated with the variation and distribution of the disorder to generate etiological hypotheses.

Prevalence

Information concerning the incidence rate or number of new cases of ADHD in a given time frame is speculative at present because epidemiological studies have not been repeated over sufficiently long periods using identical populations. The limited information available suggest that the incidence of ADHD has increased somewhat during the past decade. This finding, however, may be due to improved detection and awareness of the disorder as opposed to any real increase in the number of affected individuals *per se*.

Studies that examined prevalence rates indicate that between 2% to 40% of the childhood population has ADHD. These estimates are highly unreliable because they are typically based on parent or teacher rating scale scores in the absence of a clinical interview or knowledge of the onset, course, and developmental history of symptoms. At best, they indicate that attentional and behavioral problems are highly prevalent in classrooms and at home. Better-controlled, epidemiological studies that incorporate diagnostic interviews and careful review of symptoms, however, are relatively consistent in showing that between 3% and 5% of the child population meets diagnostic criteria for ADHD.

Sex Ratio

Prevalence estimates suggest that more males than females are affected with the disorder and ratios range from 3:1 to 10:1 in nonreferred and clinic-referred samples, respectively. The clinic-referred sample estimates may be somewhat inflated, however, due to referral bias. For example, greater numbers of boys are typically referred to outpatient clinics because of obstreperous and particularly truculent behavior. Moreover, most of the rating scales upon which prevalence estimates are based fail to include separate norms for gender. Given that girls differ from boys in many aspects of behavior at various stages of their development, it seems plausible that they also manifest an altogether different pattern of behavioral disturbance and thus represent an underdiagnosed population of affected children. Recent evidence supports this supposition. Girls who have ADHD are reportedly more socially withdrawn, exhibit more internalizing symptoms (anxiety and depression), fewer behavioral and conduct problems, and more pronounced intellectual deficits than boys.

Culture and Socioeconomic Status

The prevalence of ADHD across cultures is relatively consistent when similar diagnostic criteria are employed in defining the disorder. Exceptions to this pattern occur in the United Kingdom and in the Hong Kong Chinese population, wherein lower and higher estimates are obtained, respectively. It is likely that the lower rates in the United Kingdom are due to differences in referral practices, whereas higher rates in Hong Kong appear to be associated with less tolerance by teachers and parents for relatively minor degrees of disruptive behavior. Prevalence estimates fluctuate moderately as a function of socioeconomic status (SES) and geographic area, and higher rates are associated with lower SES and with urban areas. Various explanations offered for these differences, such as social drift and poorer health care and nutrition, remain speculative.

CLINICAL PICTURES

Description and Distinguishing Features

The first distinction that should be noted in understanding children who have ADHD is that it is not the type or kind of behavior they exhibit that is particularly deviant but the quantity or degree and intensity of their behavior. They tend to exhibit higher rates of behavior and frequently with greater intensity in situations that demand lower rates or more subtle kinds of behavior (e.g., becoming disruptive and behaving inappropriately in school or while interacting with others). Lower rates of behavior are exhibited at other times when higher rates are demanded (e.g., not paying attention and completing academic assignments in the classroom). Overall, they appear to be out of sync with environmental demands and expectations, particularly in situations that require careful sustained attention and protracted effort in tasks that are not particularly interesting or stimulating to the child.

Children's behavior must also be viewed in an appropriate developmental context. For example, younger children typically are more active, cannot pay attention to a particular task for as long a time interval, and tend to spend less time in making decisions or analyzing problems compared to older children. Other factors, such as gender and cultural differences, may also play defining roles in determining what constitutes normality, and only when a child's behavior consistently and significantly exceeds these expectations is it considered deviant.

In ADHD, the developmental behavioral pattern typically observed is associated with an early onset, a gradual worsening of symptoms over time, and an unrelenting clinical course until late adolescence when the child is no longer in school. Most children who have ADHD continue to exhibit symptoms of the disorder as adults, whose severity depends upon a number of factors. As we see later in the chapter, many believe that the disorder is inherited and thus present from birth.

A third feature characteristic of children who have ADHD is that their behavioral difficulties tend to be pervasive across situations and settings. Most people are "hyper" at one time or another, experience difficulty concentrating, and act impulsively in particular situations. These occurrences tend to be isolated events, and one can usually point to particular environmental circumstances, situations, or contingencies that are responsible for or are contributing factors associated with the behavior (e.g., feeling ill or having to study for a particularly uninteresting class). Children who have ADHD, on the other hand, exhibit this constellation of behavior problems in most situations and settings, day after day, year after year. A gradual worsening of behavioral and academic difficulties is usually evident as the child grows older because the environment demands that one be able to pay attention, sit still, and control one's impulses for longer periods of time with increasing age. Difficulties are especially conspicuous upon entry into the fourth and seventh grades. Classroom demands and academic assignments are increasingly more complex, take longer to complete, and rely heavily on one's ability to work independently and organize information.

Children who have ADHD are also known for their "consistently inconsistent" behavior. They tend to behave rather erratically both within and across days, even when their home and school environments are relatively stable. Teachers frequently report, for example, that the child appears relatively settled and able to pay attention and complete academic assignments on some days, although most days are characterized by disruptiveness, inattention, and low work completion rates. Parents report a similar phenomenon at home, even among those who are highly skilled in managing their child's behavior. The reasons for the ADHD child's inconsistent pattern of behavior are varied, and as is discussed, may be related to a complex interaction between brain regulation mechanisms involved with working memory and prevailing environmental stimulation and contingencies.

Primary Symptoms and Diagnostic Criteria

The primary symptoms or clinical features of ADHD are developmentally inappropriate degrees of inattention, impulsivity, and gross motor overactivity. The current DSM-IV (American Psychiatric Association, 1994) diagnostic criteria for ADHD are presented in Table 1. The diagnosis requires that a child exhibit a minimum of six symptoms (or problem behaviors) listed under the A(1) criteria (attention-deficit/hyperactivity disorder, predominantly inattention type) but less than six symptoms from the "hyperactivity-impulsivity" list; a minimum of

TABLE 1. DSM-IV Diagnostic Criteria for Attention-Deficit/Hyperactivity Disorder[a]

A. Either (1) or (2)
  (1) six (or more) of the following symptoms of inattention have persisted for at least 6 months to a degree that is maladaptive and inconsistent with developmental level:
  Inattention
   (a) Often fails to give close attention to details or makes careless mistakes in schoolwork, work, or other activities
   (b) often has difficulty sustaining attention in tasks or play activities
   (c) often does not seem to listen when spoken to directly
   (d) often does not follow through on instructions and fails to finish schoolwork, chores, or duties in the workplace (not due to oppositional behavior or failure to understand instructions)
   (e) often has difficulty organizing tasks and activities
   (f) often avoids, dislikes, or is reluctant to engage in tasks that require sustained mental effort (such as schoolwork or homework)
   (g) often loses things necessary for tasks or activities (e.g., toys, school assignments, pencils, books, or tools)
   (h) is often easily distracted by extraneous stimuli
   (i) is often forgetful in daily activities
  (2) six (or more) of the following symptoms of hyperactivity-impulsivity have persisted for at least 6 months to a degree that is maladaptive and inconsistent with developmental level:
  Hyperactivity
   (a) often fidgets with hands or feet or squirms in seat
   (b) often leaves seat in classroom or in other situations in which remaining seated is expected
   (c) often runs about or climbs excessively in situations in which it is inappropriate (in adolescents or adults, may be limited to subjective feelings of restlessness)
   (d) often has difficulty playing or engaging in leisure activities quietly
   (e) is often "on the go" or often acts as if "driven by a motor"
   (f) often talks excessively
  Impulsivity
   (g) often blurts out answers before questions have been completed
   (h) often has difficulty awaiting turn
   (i) often interrupts or intrudes on others (e.g., butts into conversations or games)
B. Some hyperactive-impulsive or inattentive symptoms that cause impairment were present before age 7 years.
C. Some impairment from the symptoms is present in two or more settings (e.g., at school [or work] and at home).
D. There must be clear evidence of clinically significant impairment in social, academic, or occupational functioning.
E. The symptoms do not occur exclusively during the course of a Pervasive Developmental Disorder, Schizophrenia, or other Psychotic Disorder and are not better accounted for by another mental disorder (e.g., Mood Disorder, Anxiety Disorder, Dissociative Disorder, or a Personality Disorder).
Code based on type:
Attention-Deficit/Hyperactivity Disorder, Combined Type: if both Criteria A1 and A2 are met for the past 6 months.
Attention-Deficit/Hyperactivity Disorder, Predominantly Inattentive Type: if Criterion A1 is met but Criterion A2 is not met for the past 6 months.
Attention-Deficit/Hyperactivity Disorder, Predominantly Hyperactive-Impulsive Type: if Criterion A2 is met but Criterion A1 is not met for the past 6 months.
Note: For individuals (especially adolescents and adults) who currently have symptoms that no longer meet full criteria, "In Partial Remission" should be specified.

[a]Adapted from the *Diagnostic and Statistical Manual of Mental Disorders*, 4th ed. (pp. 83–85). Washington, DC: American Psychiatric Association, 1994. Reprinted by permission.

six symptoms listed under the A(2) criteria (attention-deficit/hyperactivity disorder, predominantly hyperactive-impulsive type) but less than six symptoms from the "inattentive" list; or a minimum of six symptoms from both lists (attention-deficit/hyperactivity disorder, combined type). It should be noted, however, that the DSM field trials contained large numbers of preschool children. As a result, many of the children who meet diagnostic criteria for the hyperactivity-impulsive subtype are likely to be reclassified as ADHD-combined subtype after entry into elementary school when prominent difficulties with attention emerge.

Additional changes in the DSM-IV are noteworthy. As shown in Table 1, symptoms of the disorder must cause some degree of impairment in multiple settings (e.g., both at home and at school). The intent of this criterion is to ensure that children show pervasive as opposed to situational based symptoms, the latter of which may suggest the presence of other clinical disorders or be due to a wide variety of environmental circumstances. A second criterion (see "E" in Table 1) was added to highlight the fact that many children display behaviors suggestive of ADHD that are better accounted for by another disorder. For example, some form of or disturbance in attention and concentration is central to nearly all disorders of childhood, ranging from depression and anxiety to mental retardation and autism. A diagnosis of ADHD is typically not warranted in these cases.

Individuals who have ADHD generally display some disturbance in each of the areas delineated in the DSM-IV and in most settings, but to varying degrees. Conversely, signs of the disorder may be minimal or even absent in novel settings (e.g., being examined in a doctor's office or clinical setting), when receiving individualized attention or under conditions in which stimulation or interest level is relatively high.

At home, inattention is commonly displayed by frequent shifts from one uncompleted activity to another and a failure to follow through and/or comply with instructions. The impulsivity component is often expressed by acting without considering either the immediate or delayed consequences of one's actions (e.g., running into the street, accident proneness), interrupting the conversation of other household members, and grabbing objects (not with malevolent intent) in the store while on shopping trips. Problems with overactivity are often expressed by difficulty remaining seated during meals, while completing homework or riding in the car, and excessive movement during sleep.

At school, inattention is usually evidenced by difficulty deploying and maintaining adequate attention (i.e., staying on-task), a failure to complete academic assignments and deficient organizational and informational processing skills. Impulsivity is expressed in a variety of ways, such as interrupting others, beginning assignments before receiving (or understanding) complete instructions, making careless mistakes while completing assignments, blurting out answers in class, and having difficulty waiting one's turn in both small group and organized sport activities. Hyperactivity is frequently manifested by fidgeting, twisting and wiggling in one's seat or changing seat positions, dropping objects on the floor, and emitting noises or playing with objects during quiet assignment periods. One should be careful to note, however, that all of these behaviors may be diminished or exacerbated by subtle changes in the environment. Teachers frequently comment, for example, that an identified child who has ADHD and is absorbed in a particular activity of high interest value or is working in a one-on-one situation with an adult can attend for normal time expectations and not move a muscle while doing so. Parents also report that their children who have ADHD can sit perfectly still while engaged in highly stimulating activities, such as watching movies (e.g., "Star Wars"), and while playing interactive computer or video games. This may have a direct bearing on the specific nature of the disorder.

Secondary Symptoms or Associated Features of ADHD

Secondary features are those behaviors and difficulties that occur at a greater than chance frequency in children who have a particular disorder but are neither necessary nor sufficient to serve as formal diagnostic criteria. Many of these symptoms or behaviors are reported early in the developmental course of the disorder and may thus represent less prominent features of the disorder. These include lability of mood, temper tantrums, low frustration tolerance, social disinhibition, cognitive impairment with associated learning disability, and perceptual motor difficulties (Barkley, 1998). Other aspects of disturbance or behavioral difficulties may be secondary to or may be direct and indirect consequences of the disorder. For example, disturbed peer and interpersonal relationships, academic underachievement, school failure, decreased self-esteem, depressed mood, and conduct problems are characteristic of many children who have ADHD. The presence or absence of attendant aggressive or conduct features is especially important and may be of both diagnostic and prognostic value.

Case Description

Kevin was an 8-year-old boy who had a chronic history of multiple behavioral and academic problems. His mother brought him to an outpatient mental health facility for evaluation following a school conference in which issues were raised concerning his ability to perform on grade level and "immature" behavior.

Assessment. A semistructured clinical interview was conducted with Kevin's mother, during which her son's developmental, medical, educational, and mental health history were reviewed. Age, onset, course, and duration of the symptoms or behaviors related to each of the clinical disorders described in the DSM-IV were reviewed for purposes of diagnostic formulation. Following the clinical interview, a battery of broad- (e.g., Child Behavior Checklist, Child Symptom Inventory) and narrowband (e.g., ADHD Rating Scale, Barkley's Home and School Questionnaires) teacher and parent rating scales was administered to help quantify the degree and pervasiveness of Kevin's difficulties. Finally, psychoeducational tests were administered to assess Kevin's intellectual and academic abilities and current level of functioning (see Rapport, 1998, for a review of appropriate instruments).

Diagnosis. The results obtained from the assessment workup indicated that Kevin met diagnostic criteria for attention-deficit/hyperactivity disorder (ADHD), combined type, as well as for a developmental arithmetic disorder (considered a "learning disability" in his state). Problems were also noted with peer relationships, compliance with adults, following oral and written directions, short-term memory, and self-esteem.

Treatment. A meeting was scheduled with Kevin's parents. Treatment recommendations were offered that specifically targeted their son's behavior and academic performance in school. It was felt that Kevin's academic problems, low self-esteem, and at least some interpersonal problems were directly related to his difficulties in paying attention and completing academic assignments correctly in school consistently. The parents consented to an alternating trial of methylphenidate (MPH) and attention training to determine their relative benefits. As with most parents, they were concerned about having their son on medication.

Pharmacological treatment consisted of a closely monitored trial of MPH (Ritalin) at each of four doses: 5-mg (0.23 mg/kg), 10-mg (0.46 mg/kg), 15-mg (0.64 mg/kg), and 20-mg (0.92 mg/kg) following baseline (no medication) assessment. Each dose was tried for a minimum of two weeks before the dosage was increased. The behavioral intervention component involved using the Attention Training System (ATS) during two of Kevin's most difficult morning academic periods (phonics and math) and instituted for a 3-week period initially, then a 4-week period during the last experimental condition (see Figures 1 and 2). Teacher ratings were obtained weekly with the teacher blind to medication conditions.

Treatment Outcome. An ABACBC (reversal) within-subject design was used to compare the effects of MPH at different doses with no-medication conditions (baseline) and

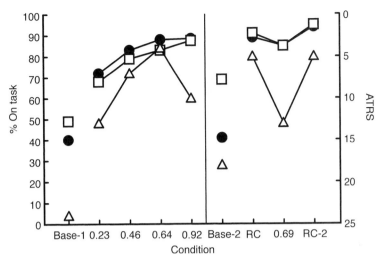

FIGURE 1. Mean percentage of daily observations in which Kevin was on-task (left-hand ordinate) during the two morning academic assignments periods (math = closed circles; phonics = open squares) during no-treatment (baseline), methylphenidate treatment (0.23-mg/kg through 0.92-mg/kg doses), and behavioral treatment (response cost) conditions. Weekly teacher ratings (ATRS) are shown as open triangles and are interpreted using the right-hand ordinate. Upward movement on the vertical axis indicates improvement in all measures.

then to contrast the most effective MPH dose with the behavioral intervention. Direct observation of Kevin's attention and completion of academic assignments were conducted daily and at the same time each morning—approximately 45 minutes after ingestion of the morning medication and at the same time on no-medication days (see Figures 1 and 2).

Before any intervention (see first baseline condition in Figure 1), Kevin experienced significant difficulty in paying attention, as evidenced by his 40% to 48% on-task rate during the two morning academic assignment periods. Consistent with this low rate of attention, he completed between 35% and 60% of his academic assignments on a daily basis during the initial 3-week baseline (no intervention) period (Figure 2). A clear and somewhat dramatic increase in attention was observed under each of the medication conditions, and there was a concomitant increase in the percentage of academic assignments completed (see 0.23- through 0.92-mg/kg MPH dose conditions in Figures 1 and 2). Academic assignment accuracy remained relatively high and stable throughout the course of both interventions, which is noteworthy given his increase in academic productivity. Teacher ratings using the Abbreviated Conners Teacher Rating Scale (ATRS) generally paralleled changes observed in attention and academic performance (see Figures 1 and 2).

A return to baseline (no intervention) conditions was initiated following the medication trial to ensure that observed changes were due to active drug as opposed to some other phenomenon (e.g., developmental maturity, so that improvement might be observed with the passage of time regardless of intervention). Clearly this was not the case. Kevin's attention and academic productivity returned to near pretreatment levels (see second baseline in Figures 1 and 2).

The second stage of the evaluation was established so that the MPH dose deemed most therapeutic during the initial titration trials could be compared directly with the attention training program. The 15-mg (0.69 mg/kg) dose was selected instead of the 20-mg dose because Kevin's academic performance declined under the higher dose condition, despite slightly higher levels of attention (see "% on-task" compared with "% completed" at the 0.92-mg/kg dose condition in Figures 1 and 2).

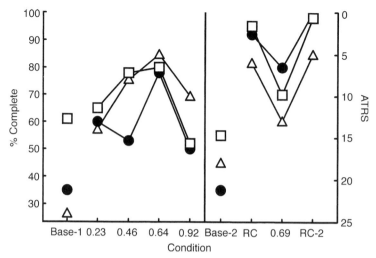

FIGURE 2. Mean percentage of academic assignments completed daily (left-hand ordinate) during the two morning academic assignments periods (math = closed circles; phonics = open squares) during no-treatment (baseline), methylphenidate treatment (0.23-mg/kg through 0.92-mg/kg doses), and behavioral treatment (response cost) conditions. Weekly teacher ratings (ATRS) are shown as open triangles and are interpreted using the right-hand ordinate. Upward movement on the vertical axis indicates improvement in all measures.

The Attention Training System (ATS) consists of a student and teacher module created specifically for use in classroom environments. The student module (see Figure 3) is placed on the child's desk before beginning an academic assignment, and automatically awards the child one point per minute on the cumulative counter (see front face of the ATS) throughout the assignment period. Thus, at the end of a 30-minute assignment period, the number "30" would show on Kevin's cumulative counter if he stayed focused throughout the period. The handheld teacher module controls the student module and can be used anywhere in the classroom, enabling the teacher to work with other children while visually monitoring Kevin's progress. As long as Kevin stays focused and in his seat, the teacher does nothing— as noted above, the ATS automatically awards Kevin one point per minute. When Kevin strays off-task, the teacher simply presses the button on her handheld device, which in turn, illuminates the red dome on top of Kevin's student module and simultaneously deducts one point from his cumulative total. At the end of the assignment period, Kevin is permitted to trade in his earned points for an equal amount of free time. Structured free time can be spent working on a variety of educational activities in the classroom (e.g., working at the computer, listening to taped stories by means of an audio headset).

The ATS stands in contrast to most standard behavioral interventions in which praise, tokens, or check marks are used for feedback, either during or immediately following an academic period. The reasons for this are twofold. First, applied research has clearly shown us that the delivery of tokens, checkmarks, and praise tend to interrupt ADHD children's academic productivity and require a disproportionate amount of teacher time (a primary reason that the programs are frequently abandoned by teachers). In other cases, feedback is delayed until the end of an assignment period, which is at odds with the impulsive nature and inadequate delays skills exhibited by most children who have ADHD. The ATS circumvents these shortcomings by providing immediate and continuous feedback (positive by accumulated points, and negative by point reductions) throughout the assignment period.

Introduction of the ATS resulted in clear and sustained increases in Kevin's attention and academic performance, as well as improved teacher ratings, during the ensuing 3-week

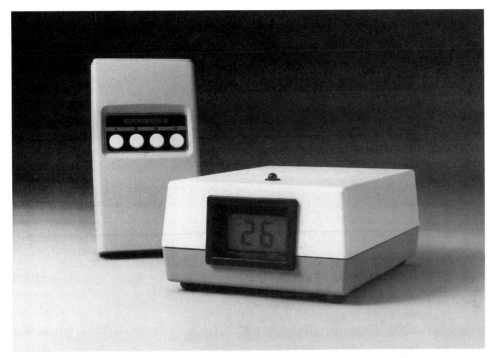

FIGURE 3. The Attentional Training System (ATS). Invented by M. D. Rapport, Ph.D. (see Rapport, Murphy, & Bailey, 1982) for treating children with ADHD. Manufactured and distributed for commercial use by Gordon Systems, DeWitt, NY.

period. These effects, when contrasted with the 15-mg (0.69-mg/kg) MPH condition, indicate that both interventions improved Kevin's attention to a similar degree and somewhat higher rates of academic performance were associated with the ATS. Discontinuation of MPH and a return to the ATS during the final 4-weeks of observation essentially replicated the effects observed previously (see Figures 1 and 2).

The results were shared with Kevin's parents and classroom teacher. It was agreed that he would continue with the ATS intervention for the remainder of the school year. The ATS was removed approximately 4 weeks later according to suggestions provided in the manual and was replaced with a free-time product completion contingency. Kevin was required to complete all of his academic work with at least 80% accuracy in exchange for 10-minutes of in-class structured free time following each academic period.

Follow-up at the end of the school year indicated that Kevin maintained the therapeutic gains made during the formal assessment period of the evaluation and was promoted to the fourth grade. His fourth grade teacher, however, was not interested in establishing an ongoing behavioral management system in the classroom. A 15-mg b.i.d. (twice a day) regimen of MPH was subsequently prescribed by his pediatrician, which proved relatively successful throughout the school year.

COMMENT

Several points are worth noting. First, combined behavioral and medication intervention are nearly always required for more severe cases of ADHD. Second, just as medication must be carefully titrated to achieve optimal results, behavioral interventions must be created using great care and attention to detail and nearly always require periodic adjustment to maintain their effectiveness. Finally, a host of parameters must be considered when creating a behavioral program. Questions concerning what will serve as an effective incentive for the child, how well the teacher will cooperate given the existing classroom demands, and how to intervene at other times during the day when the program is not operative, must be addressed.

COURSE AND PROGNOSIS

Early Childhood

Several well-controlled studies indicate that difficulties with attention and overactivity are relatively common among preschoolers. Only a small subset of these children continue to manifest symptoms characteristic of ADHD by the time they are 4 to 5 years of age. These symptoms strongly predict continued difficulties and a probable clinical diagnosis by ages 6 and 9 (Campbell, 1990). Thus, the necessity of considering both the degree and duration of behavioral disturbance cannot be overemphasized, particularly in very young children.

Parents describe children in this age group, who continue to exhibit a durable pattern of ADHD symptoms, as always on the go, fearless, restless, continually getting into things, disobeying parental commands, obstreperous, highly curious about their environment, and requiring high levels of adult supervision. Other problems, such as perceptual motor difficulties, sleep and eating difficulties, accident proneness, speech and language difficulties, and toilet training difficulties, are reported in a subset of these children. Those who have advanced intellectual and cognitive skills and who tend not to be aggressive are generally easier to manage both at home and in preschool. The parents of these children are under enormous daily stress in their caregiver roles, the reciprocal interaction of which not infrequently results in psychiatric disability, marital problems, alcoholism, and increased risk for child abuse.

Middle Childhood

Between the ages of 6 and 12 years, children who have ADHD continue to demonstrate difficulties with attention, impulsivity, overactivity, and compliance with adult requests. These difficulties are exacerbated after they enter elementary school. A subsequent increase in outpatient referral rates results from two primary factors. Classroom teachers are more familiar with age-appropriate norms for behavior. And children are expected to sit still, pay attention, and engage in more difficult academic tasks and organized activities for longer periods of time. In some cases, children are excused as "immature" by well-meaning school personnel and forced to repeat the grade or are passed marginally with the expectation that "maturation" will occur during the summer months.

Increasing social and academic demands impact their already handicapping condition to an even greater extent during these primary school years and cause greater stress to already overburdened parents and teachers. Homework assignments add an additional source of conflict to the familial environment because 25% or more of the children experience significant difficulties in reading and/or develop other academic skill disorders. Their inattention, impulsivity, and higher than normal activity level predestines them to develop poor peer and interpersonal relationships that results in a pattern of social isolation and low self-esteem in later years.

Adolescence

One of the prevailing myths about children who have ADHD is that they "outgrow" the disorder when they reach adolescence. Follow-up and long-term outcome studies, however, inform us that approximately 70% of children diagnosed as having ADHD in childhood continue to display symptoms of and meet diagnostic criteria for ADHD as adolescents. Primary difficulties with attention/concentration, impulsivity, and difficulty following directions remain, whereas the overactivity component of the disorder diminishes somewhat and transitions into fidgeting and restlessness with increasing age.

Perhaps more unsettling are the findings that between 40% and 60% of adolescents who have ADHD also meet diagnostic criteria for conduct disorder (CD)—a disorder characterized by serious and pervasive antisocial behavior. These comorbid adolescents, in turn, are also more likely to engage in substance use (e.g., cigarette smoking) and abuse (e.g., alcohol and marijuana).

One of the strongest predictors during early childhood of a well functioning, stable, successful adult is academic achievement. Follow-up studies of children who have ADHD during their adolescent years, particularly those comorbid for CD, have been alarmingly negative with regard to academic outcome. They are significantly more likely to have been suspended or expelled from school, three times more likely to have failed at least one grade, and their standardized achievement test scores are below normal in math, reading, and spelling. Of even greater concern is that 25% to 31% fail to complete high school. Overall, adolescents who have ADHD, and particularly those carrying a dual diagnosis of CD, represent a population at high risk for a variety of negative outcomes associated with psychiatric disability, social, and adult occupational functioning.

Adult Outcome and Long-Term Prognosis

Three trajectories have been postulated concerning the long-term outcome of children who have ADHD: developmental delay, developmental decay, and continuous display. The first trajectory presumes that ADHD is a neuromaturational problem and that associated difficulties will eventually diminish with age. The developmental decay trajectory holds that the primary symptom picture will worsen with increasing age, and that specific clinical features will be manifested somewhat differently in older children. The continuous display trajectory posits that the primary symptom picture will continue to be manifested with increasing age at a more or less similar degree of severity. But, similar to the decay model, the topography of clinical features (e.g., inattention, impulsivity) will change to reflect difficulties associated with adolescence and adulthood.

Each of the three outcome trajectories is supported in part by the existing, albeit scant, literature concerning adults diagnosed as having ADHD during childhood. Between 50% and 65% of diagnosed children continue to experience difficulties with core clinical symptoms and related behavioral problems as adults. It is estimated that only 11% are free of any psychiatric diagnosis and considered well-functioning adults. These rather bleak estimates are tempered somewhat, when one considers that only about a third of the "normal" population of children is free of psychiatric disability as adults.

Other areas of adult functioning are equally impaired. Relatively few adults who had a childhood diagnosis of ADHD go on to complete a university degree program (approximately 5% vs. 41% of control children). Significant minorities of them (20% to 25%) continue to display persistent patterns of antisocial behavior. Poor work records, lower job status, difficulties in getting along with supervisors, and overall lower socioeconomic status attainment are common, and greater difficulties with social skills, unstable marriages, and lower self-esteem prevail. Conversely, other adults who have ADHD function normally and even exceptionally well as adults. The limited evidence available indicates that a supportive, stable family environment, milder ADHD symptoms, higher intelligence, greater emotional stability, and no concomitant conduct disorder and especially aggression during childhood, are the best predictors of positive adult outcomes.

FAMILIAL AND GENETIC PATTERNS

Familial Contributions

Studies that examined the families of children who had ADHD represent an important avenue of inquiry concerning the heritability of the disorder. Although one cannot completely separate the role of genetics from that of deviant child rearing practices, family-genetic studies can nevertheless improve our understanding of the psychobiology of ADHD, and specifically address whether ADHD tends to run in families (i.e., by establishing familial risk).

In the most comprehensive and methodologically eloquent study conducted to date, Biederman, Faraone, Keenan, Knee, and Tsuang (1990) evaluated family-genetic and psychosocial risk factors for ADHD among 457 first-degree relatives of clinically referred children and adolescents who had ADHD and compared them with psychiatric and normal controls. Age-corrected rates of illness, termed *morbidity risks*, were used to adjust upward the degree to which an individual was counted as "healthy" as a function of increasing age. Use of this technique has been woefully absent in a majority of family-genetic studies, but it is necessary because many psychiatric disorders have a variable age of onset (e.g., major depression). Consequently, the fact that one may not have lived through the "risk period" must be taken into account and corrected for statistically.

Several important findings emerged from the Biederman et al. (1990) study. The first of these was that parents of children who had ADHD were significantly more likely to be separated or divorced relative to the psychiatric and normal comparison groups. This finding, however, must be interpreted cautiously. It could indicate a greater degree of psychopathology among the parents or alternatively, reflect the strain placed on couples raising a child who has ADHD. A second major finding of the study was that the probabilities or risks of having ADHD among relatives of ADHD children were 7.6 and 4.6 times the odds for having ADHD among the relatives of normal or psychiatric control groups, respectively. In examining these odds ratios, it was found that nearly 65% of the children who had ADHD had at least one relative who had ADHD compared with 24% and 15% of the psychiatric and normal control groups, respectively. Relatives of ADHD children were also at higher risk for both antisocial disorder and mood disorders. These disorders were significantly more prevalent in the families of children who had ADHD. Finally, both parents as well as brothers of children who had ADHD had a significantly higher risk for ADHD compared to relatives of control groups: 44% of the fathers, 19% of the mothers, and 39% of the brothers of ADHD children also had ADHD. Finally, all of the aforementioned findings remained significant after controlling for social class and intactness of families among the different groups.

The conclusion that can be drawn from this and other studies is that ADHD is a highly familial disorder that places affected individuals at significant risk for adult psychopathology and dysfunctional marriages.

Genetic Factors

The role of hereditary transmission of ADHD has been investigated in several studies during the past 30 years. Unfortunately, the bulk of this research is not interpretable because of numerous methodological problems and poorly defined diagnostic groups of children. Two recent twin studies, however, indicate significantly greater concordance (agreement) for hyperactive symptoms between identical than between fraternal twins, and heritability of ADHD is estimated at .73 to .91. Both studies (Gjone, Stevenson, & Sundet, 1996; Levy et al., 1997) included large cohorts of children (915 and 1938 subjects, respectively). Estimated heritability was based on the extent to which co-twins of identical probands had scores more similar to their deviant proband and more different from the mean for the total population than co-twins of fraternal probands. Of perhaps greater significance were the findings in both studies suggesting that ADHD is best viewed as the extreme of a behavior that varies genetically throughout the entire population rather than as a disorder that has discrete boundaries.

In summary, ADHD is an inheritable condition, whose symptomatology may be diminished or exacerbated by prevailing environmental conditions. There is also evidence to indicate that different etiological factors involving pregnancy, birth complications, exposure to lead or drugs, and a variety of central nervous system insults may be the primary culprit in a small subset of these children. The majority, however, inherit the disorder through some yet unknown mechanism, and underactivity of the prefrontal-striatal-limbic regions of the brain results. A different and admittedly speculative view of the disorder is that the brains of children who have ADHD are not abnormal. Rather, they operate differently under certain environmental conditions—primarily conditions that involve sustained concentration and working memory demanded by routine and nonstimulating tasks characteristic of classroom learning. From the perspective of biological evolution, it could be argued that many of the behavioral characteristics that typify children who have ADHD may have had high adaptive value in earlier societies and cultures that relied on acting and shifting attention quickly without undue reflection and placed limited demands on working memory.

Neurological, Neurophysiological, and Neuroanatomical Factors

Results of routine neurological examinations are usually normal in children who have ADHD. Research that investigated the presence of neuromaturational signs (i.e., signs that a person's brain represents a more immature form of development) has been equivocal but generally suggests either nonspecific or no increased frequency of soft signs in this population. Also, as noted previously, the overwhelming majority of children who have ADHD do not have a history of brain injury or damage. More recent studies using advanced brain scanning techniques, such as computed tomography (CT) scan analysis, have also failed to reveal differences in brain structure. Preliminary findings using the higher resolution magnetic resonance imaging (MRI), however, have been more promising but await replication.

Neurochemical abnormalities, particularly those involving the monoamines, comprising the catecholamines (dopamine and norepinephrine) and an indoleamine, (serotonin) have been implicated as potential contributing factors in the pathophysiology of ADHD. The evidence to date remains speculative but suggests a possible selective deficiency in the availability of dopamine and/or norepinephrine.

More promising results have emerged in three studies. Lou (1990), using single photon emission computed tomography (SPECT) to measure cerebral blood flow in the brain, reported hypoperfusion (reduced) and low neural activity in the striatal and orbital prefrontal regions of children who have ADHD compared with controls, whereas the primary sensory and sensorimotor regions were hyperperfused (overly active). Ongoing studies by Satterfield (1990), using EEG brain electrical activity mapping (BEAM) techniques, have been relatively consistent with Lou's findings in showing abnormality in information processing in the frontal lobes of children who have ADHD. Finally, Zametkin et al. (1990), in studying adults who had been hyperactive since childhood, reported reduced glucose metabolism in various areas of the brain, particularly the premotor and superior prefrontal regions—areas known to be associated with regulating attention, motor activity, and information processing.

Recent findings buttress those derived from earlier works in showing neurophysiological dysfunction in children who have ADHD, particularly within the cortical and subcortical structures that serve the frontal/striatal system. Quantitative electroencephalogram (QEEG) profile comparisons between 407 children with ADHD and 310 normal children reveal two major neurophysiological subtypes among children who have ADHD (Chabot & Serfontein, 1996). The first subtype evidences varying degrees of EEG slowing, whereas the second shows an increase in EEG activity. Both abnormalities are particular to the frontal regions. The subtypes are thought to reflect the interaction of the cortical and subcortical structures contained within the frontal/striatal system and affect the range of attention, hyperactivity, and learning problems evidenced by the children. Interhemispheric power asymmetry (i.e., imbalance in neuroactivity between the right and left hemispheres) was also common among the ADHD sample, indicating abnormal right hemisphere function, as well as interhemispheric communication between the two regions.

Results from the first comprehensive morphometric analysis are consistent with hypothesized dysfunction of right-sided prefrontal-striatal systems in ADHD. Castellanos et al. (1996) compared volumetric measures of both prefrontal (attention) and basal ganglia (motor control) structures in 57 boys who had ADHD and 55 healthy matched control children using magnetic resonance imaging (MRI) scans. Both the caudate nucleus and globus pallidus, but not the putamen, were reported to be significantly smaller (predominantly in the right hemisphere) in ADHD children. Response inhibition measures derived from three attentional tasks were correlated with anatomical measures of frontostriatal brain structures in a complementary study (Casey et al., 1997). The results suggest that the distractibility and impulsivity characteristic of children who have ADHD reflect deficits in response inhibition. A nontechnical explanation of these findings involves understanding that the prefrontal cortex, located in the frontal lobe just behind the forehead, serves as the brain's command center. Commands emanating from this area are translated into action by the caudate nucleus and globus pallidus, both of which are located near the middle of the brain. By analogy, the prefrontal cortex can be viewed as the steering wheel and the caudate and globus as the accelerator and brakes, respectively. It is the braking or inhibitory function that appears to be dysfunctional or different in children who have ADHD, according to recent reports.

Collectively, results from positron emission tomography (PET), magnetic resonance imaging (MRI), and regional cerebral blood flow studies provide compelling evidence that ADHD results from a developmental abnormality in the frontal/cortical, striatal and thalamic circuits, particularly with respect to the right hemisphere. The findings are also consistent with speculations concerning a possible selective deficiency in the availability of two of the brain's neurotransmitter systems: dopamine and norepinephrine. Prefrontal-limbic connections are known to contain relatively high amounts of these neurotransmitters. Psychostimulants (the primary pharmacological treatment for children who have ADHD) are known agonists (they increase neurotransmitter function) of these systems. And implicated brain areas underlie several aspects of inattention, executive function, and learning. Thus, findings to date highlight several possibilities concerning the pathogenesis of and treatment response observed in children who have ADHD.

The findings of striatal and frontal/prefrontal involvement particular to the right hemisphere in children who have ADHD implicate working memory systems as a logical candidate for investigation. Three components of working memory have been identified (Baddeley, 1986). These include the central executive, the phonological loop (and its two subsystems), and the visuospatial sketchpad. This latter component is mediated by parietal and prefrontal areas of the right hemisphere and is responsible for processing visual information both directly and indirectly (i.e., for stimuli such as printed words and pictures which can be recorded in phonological form but are nonauditory). Deficient functioning of this system, coupled with central executive dysfunction, is consistent with the constellation of symptoms observed in children who have ADHD and might help to explain why they can perform well on certain tasks, in specific settings, and at particular times, but not in others.

DIAGNOSTIC CONSIDERATIONS

Diagnosing ADHD represents one of the most difficult endeavors for mental health practitioners. A variety of clinic-based tests (e.g., the Continuous Performance Test, Matching Familiars Figures Test, subtest configurations of intelligence batteries) have been touted as useful diagnostic tools. But none has differentiated children who have ADHD from other common pathological conditions of childhood with an acceptable degree of accuracy (i.e., poor specificity). Detailed information concerning the child's pre-, peri-, and postnatal history, medical, developmental, and educational history, and family functioning must be obtained—preferably using one of the recently standardized structured or semistructured clinical interviews. Onset and course of symptomatology are also essential to the differential diagnostic process, as well as extensive consideration of alternative and/or other existing psychopathological and medical conditions. A variety of broad- and narrowband behavior rating scales have been standardized in recent years to help quantify the nature and severity of behavioral disability (see Rapport, 1998, for a comprehensive review of the assessment of ADHD). Finally, several clinic-based, computerized instruments and observational techniques are currently being evaluated for their sensitivity and specificity in diagnosing ADHD and differentiating it from other forms of childhood psychopathology, but these await empirical testing.

SUMMARY

Attention-deficit/hyperactivity disorder is considered one of the most serious and enigmatic childhood disorders for which there is no known cure. Our current understanding of ADHD suggests that it is a complex and chronic disorder of brain, behavior, and development and has behavioral and cognitive consequences that pervade multiple areas of functioning. Mounting evidence suggests that ADHD is significantly more common in certain families and inherited through some yet unknown mechanism and that underactivity of the prefrontal-striatal-limbic regions of the brain results. Differences in the neurophysiological functioning of the brain may help explain why these children experience profound difficulties in maintaining attention, regulating their arousal, inhibiting themselves in accordance with environmental demands, and getting along with others—yet, only at specific times and under certain conditions. Research that focuses on executive and regulatory functioning and particularly on working memory and sub-components such as the visuospatial control system may help elucidate specific processes involved in the pathophysiology of ADHD.

REFERENCES

American Psychiatric Association. (1968). *Diagnostic and statistical manual of mental disorders*, 2nd ed. Washington, DC: Author.

American Psychiatric Association. (1980). *Diagnostic and statistical manual of mental disorders*, 3rd ed. Washington, DC: Author.

American Psychiatric Association. (1987). *Diagnostic and statistical manual of mental disorders*, 3rd rev. ed. Washington, DC: Author.

American Psychiatric Association. (1994). *Diagnostic and statistical manual of mental disorders*, 4th ed. Washington, DC: Author.

Baddeley, A. (1986). *Working memory*. Oxford, England: Clarendon Press.

Barkley, R. A. (1998). *Attention deficit hyperactivity disorder: A handbook for diagnosis and treatment*. New York: Guilford.

Biederman, J., Faraone, S. V., Keenan, K., Knee, D., & Tsuang, M. T. (1990). Family-genetic and psychosocial risk factors in DSM-III attention deficit disorder. *Journal of the American Academy of Child and Adolescent Psychiatry, 29*, 526–533.

Campbell, S. B. (1990). *Behavior problems in preschoolers: Clinical and developmental issues*. New York: Guilford.

Casey, B. J., Castellanos, F. X., Giedd, J. N., Marsh, W. L., Hamburger, S. D., Schubert, A. B., Vauss, Y. C., Vaituzis, A. C., Dickstein, D. P., Sarfatti, S. E., & Rapoport, J. L. (1997). Implication of right frontostriatal circuitry in response inhibition and attention-deficit/hyperactivity disorder. *Journal of the American Academy of Child and Adolescent Psychiatry, 36*, 374–383.

Castellanos, F. X., Giedd, J. N., Marsh, W. L., Hamburger, S. D., Vaituzis, A. C., Dickstein, D. P., Sarfatti, S. E., Vauss, Y. C., Snell, J. W., Lange, N., Kaysen, D., Krain, A. L., Ritchie, G. F., Rajapakse, J. C., & Rapoport, J. L. (1996). Quantitative brain magnetic resonance imaging in attention-deficit hyperactivity disorder. *Archives of General Psychiatry, 53*, 607–616.

Chabot, R. J., & Serfontein, G. (1996). Quantitative electroencephalographic profiles of children with attention deficit disorder. *Biological Psychiatry, 40*, 951–963.

Gjone, H., Stevenson, J., & Sundet, J. M. (1996). Genetic influence on parent-reported attention-related problems in a Norwegian general population twin sample. *Journal of the American Academy of Child and Adolescent Psychiatry, 35*, 588–596.

Levy, F., Hay, D. A., McStephen, M., Wood, C., & Waldman, I. (1997). Attention-deficit hyperactivity disorder: A category or a continuum? Genetic analysis of a large-scale twin study. *Journal of the American Academy of Child and Adolescent Psychiatry, 36*, 737–744.

Lou, H. C. (1990). Methylphenidate reversible hypoperfusion of striatal regions in ADHD. In K. Conners & M. Kinsbourne (Eds.), *Attention deficit hyperactivity disorder: ADHD; clinical, experimental and demographic issues* (pp.137–148). Munich, Germany: Medizin Verlag.

Rapport, M. D. (1998). Treating children with attention-deficit/hyperactivity disorder (ADHD). In V. B. Van Hasselt & M. Hersen (Eds.), *Handbook of psychological treatment protocols for children and adolescents* (pp. 65–107). Mahwah, NJ: Erlbaum.

Rapport, M. D., Murphy, A., & Bailey, J. S. (1982). Ritalin versus response cost in the control of hyperactive children: A within-subject comparison. *Journal of Applied Behavior Analysis, 15*, 20–31.

Satterfield, J. H. (1990). BEAM studies in ADD boys. In C. K. Conners & M. Kinsbourne (Eds.), *Attention deficit hyperactivity disorder* (pp. 127–136). Munich, Germany: Medizin Verlag.

Zametkin, A. J., Nordahl, T. E., Gross, M., King, A. C., Semple, W. E., Rumsey, J., Hamburger, S., & Cohen, R. M. (1990). Cerebral glucose metabolism in adults with hyperactivity of childhood onset. *New England Journal of Medicine, 323*, 1361–1366.

10

Conduct Disorder

Marc S. Atkins and Mary M. McKay

Conduct problems, including aggression, lying, and stealing, interfere with a child's functioning within the family, school, and peer group. The emergence of childhood conduct problems can be best understood from an ecological perspective that acknowledges the importance of contextual factors, such as qualities of the home environment, relationships with parental figures, school and classroom organization, teacher style, and peer relationships (Dishion & Patterson, 1997; Tolan, Guerra, & Kendall, 1995). Interventions that target these contextual influences have demonstrated significant promise (Guerra, Tolan, & Hammond, 1995; Henggeler, Schoenwald, Borduin, Rowland, & Cunningham, 1998). Specifically, this chapter provides a description of childhood conduct disorder, its prevalence and course, and a summary of empirical findings that link factors within the child, family, peer group, and community with the emergence and progression of conduct difficulties.

DESCRIPTION OF THE DISORDER

Conduct Disorder (CD) is defined in the latest revision of the Diagnostic and Statistical Manual of Mental Disorders (DSM-IV; American Psychiatric Association, 1994) as a "repetitive and persistent pattern of behavior in which either the basic rights of others or major age-appropriate societal norms or rules are violated" (p. 85). The diagnosis is listed in the DSM-IV as one of three Attention Deficit and Disruptive Behavior Disorders; the others are Attention-Deficit Hyperactivity Disorder and Oppositional Defiant Disorder. The symptoms of CD are categorized into four main groupings: (1) aggression toward people and animals, (2) destruction of property, (3) deceitfulness or theft, and (4) serious violations of rules. Subtypes of CD are determined by age of onset: the Childhood Onset type in which at least one conduct problem has been evident before age 10, and the Adolescent Onset type in which no conduct problems have been evident before age 10. The severity of the disorder is noted as mild if there are relatively few conduct problems that cause only minor harm to others. Severe conduct problems are defined by an excess of behaviors necessary to make the diagnosis or which

Marc S. Atkins • Department of Psychiatry, University of Illinois at Chicago, Chicago, Illinois 60612.   Mary M. McKay • Columbia University School of Social Work, New York, New York 10025.

Advanced Abnormal Psychology, Second Edition, edited by Hersen and Van Hasselt. Kluwer Academic/Plenum Publishers, New York, 2001.

cause substantial harm to others. Moderate severity is defined by behaviors falling in the intermediate range. A diagnosis of ODD is not given if a child meets criteria for CD.

Subtypes of Childhood Aggression

An extensive literature has examined subtypes of childhood aggression to inform diagnosis and to enhance the development of deficit-specific interventions for antisocial youth. Loeber and Schmaling (1985a) summarized studies of childhood antisocial behavior on a dimension ranging from overt or confrontational aggression (e.g., fighting, temper tantrums) to covert antisocial behavior that occurs outside direct supervision (e.g., theft, truancy, drug use). In a separate study, Loeber and Schmaling (1985b) described three mutually exclusive subtypes: Excessive Fighter Group (those who fought, but did not steal), Exclusive Theft Group (those who stole, but did not fight), and Versatile Antisocial Group (those who stole and fought). This has proved to be an important model, which has led to further research on differential pathways to antisocial behavior (Loeber, Farrington, Stouthamer-Loeber, Moffitt, & Caspi, 1998).

Dodge and colleagues proposed a highly influential subtyping model based on children's social information processing skills (Dodge & Schwartz, 1997). Two types of aggression were identified. Proactive aggression was defined as aggression that is purposeful and rewarding (e.g., aggression for property or to enhance peer status). Reactive aggression was defined as aggression in response to actual or imagined aversive provocation unrelated to reward motivation, and with person-oriented aggression, agitation, and impulsivity. A considerable body of research has supported the distinction between proactive and reactive aggression, both in regard to different patterns in children's early developmental histories and differential pathways for adult outcomes (Dodge, Lochman, Harnish, Bates, & Pettit, 1997).

The third model for distinguishing aggression subtypes is based on the degree of impulse control associated with the disorder (Vitiello & Stoff, 1997). In studies of psychiatrically impaired youth, laboratory measures of impulsivity have been associated with an inability to inhibit aggression in the presence of cues for punishment (Atkins, Osborne, Bennett, Hess, & Halperin, 1999), and a history of initiating physical fights (Halperin, Newcorn, Matier, Bedi, Hall, & Sharma, 1995). Conduct-problem boys who have impulsive response styles were most likely to become adult psychopaths (Lyman, 1998), supportive of Lyman's (1996) theory that impulse control deficits are core features of juvenile chronic offender.

EPIDEMIOLOGY

Conduct disorder is the most common reason for referral to a child mental health clinic and accounts for one-third to one-half of all child and adolescent mental health referrals (Kazdin, 1995). The prevalence rate is estimated at between 2% and 6% (Institute of Medicine, 1989). Tremendous economic, social, and human costs are associated with the early display of antisocial behavior. Longitudinal studies show a dramatic rise in antisocial behavior in the early adolescent years (Moffitt, 1993). Surveys of youth indicate that approximately 50% of teens admit to theft, 35% to assault, 45% to property destruction, and as many as 60% admit to engaging in multiple antisocial acts (Kazdin, 1995). Males are three times more likely than females to display conduct difficulties (Robins, 1991). However, as discussed later, when girls experience conduct problems, the long-term prognosis is as bad as for boys, if not worse.

For urban, minority youth, the prevalence of antisocial behavior has particularly serious implications. Urban communities have violent crime rates 4 to 10 times higher than the national average (Fingerhut & Kleinman, 1990). Homicide is now the leading cause of death for African-American males between the ages of 15 and 24 (Center for Disease Control, 1991). These community-level factors contribute to high prevalence rates of conduct disorder in urban communities that are more than five times the national estimates (Tuma, 1989). In urban, low-income communities, rates of disruptive behavior were more than twice as high as in other urban communities (Tolan & Henry, 1996).

CLINICAL PICTURE

Suzanne is a 10-year-old, African-American female who was referred to an outpatient child mental health clinic by the school social worker. Her paternal grandmother, who was also her foster mother, brought her to the clinic. Suzanne was a tall, thin child who initially presented as quiet. She was easily engaged by play materials at the clinic, and, as she warmed up to the examiner, presented as verbal, energetic, and engaging.

Presenting difficulties included significant disruptive behavior at home and at school. At school, she was physically aggressive toward peers and, at times, teachers. When angered by others, she would frequently retaliate by destroying their personal property. In addition, she was described by her teachers as frequently lying, having substantial difficulty maintaining peer friendships, and consistently refusing to follow directions or classroom rules. She had also been accused of stealing supplies from her classmates. At home, Suzanne was also highly explosive. She displayed frequent outbursts of anger, which included shouting and destroying toys and furniture. Her grandmother admitted to having great difficulty setting limits with her and often actively tried "not to upset her."

Academically, Suzanne displayed average to above average abilities in all subjects. Her standardized reading and mathematics tests were at grade level, although her grades did not reflect her abilities. She frequently failed to complete in-class and homework assignments. In the classroom, Suzanne performed better in situations that were highly structured and engaging. For example, she was highly motivated in art and music and was well behaved during these activities. However, during activities that required independent work or in interaction with other students, Suzanne's behavior often escalated to the point that she was removed from the room to sit in the hallway or go to the principal's office. Socially, Suzanne was isolated from her peers and had few friends. On occasion, Suzanne would engage in organized games at recess. However, these interactions almost always led to conflict that resulted in Suzanne either leaving the game in frustration or being removed from the game by a supervising adult due to her negative behavior. Even though Suzanne had significant difficulty getting along with peers, she expressed strong desires for peer acceptance.

Suzanne's family history revealed numerous traumas and transitions in caregivers. For the first two years of her life, Suzanne was cared for by her mother, who was 18 at the time of her birth, and her maternal grandmother. Suzanne's father was largely uninvolved, but contributed financially to her support. At the age of 2½, Suzanne's mother was tragically killed in a car accident. Suzanne's maternal grandmother assumed responsibility for her care. However, her own health problems forced her to approach Suzanne's father after approximately eight months to solicit help in Suzanne's care. After Suzanne's third birthday, she went to live full-time with her father, who was then 21 years old, and his family that consisted of his mother, two younger brothers, and a sister. Her maternal grandmother died shortly thereafter due to complications from diabetes.

Over time, Suzanne developed a close relationship with her father. Initial behavioral difficulties at school were resolved by close cooperation between her father and her teacher.

At home, Suzanne was often left in the care of her adolescent aunt and uncles while her caretakers (father and grandmother) were at work. During her fourth and fifth year, Suzanne's behavioral difficulties increased at home. Her attitude was generally noncompliant away from her father, and soon other members of the household were refusing to watch her in his absence.

As Suzanne entered the first grade, her father was diagnosed with a debilitating illness that took his life a year later; the third death of a significant caregiver in three years. Suzanne initially responded to his death by withdrawing both at home and at school. By the beginning of the third grade, however, her behavior at home and at school was beginning to cause serious concern. Following the death of her father, Suzanne's paternal grandmother assumed responsibility for her care. In response to Suzanne's escalating behavioral difficulties, her grandmother decided to take an early retirement from her job to devote more time to Suzanne's care. Her grandmother was also deeply affected by the death of her son and admitted that she has been depressed as a result since then. Although Suzanne's grandmother expressed deep affection for Suzanne, as well as empathy for her multiple losses, she also questioned whether she would be able to continue to provide a stable home for Suzanne due to Suzanne's increasing behavioral difficulties. During the initial interview at the mental health clinic, Suzanne's grandmother inquired about possible foster care or residential placements.

Following her father's death, Suzanne began to spend more time outside the home with older children in the neighborhood. During the fourth grade, she had contact with the police for throwing rocks at cars, shoplifting, and being outside the home after curfew. While in the community, Suzanne was also victimized by older children on two occasions when her bicycle and her new roller skates were taken from her. She reported few peer friendships and an increasingly mistrustful approach towards peers and adults.

COURSE AND PROGNOSIS

There is considerable evidence for the stability of aggressive and antisocial behavior (Loeber & Stouthamer-Loeber, 1998). Nevertheless, most aggressive children do not grow up to be antisocial adults. Recent studies have revealed the importance of contextual factors on course and prognosis. Poverty is strongly related to preadolescent conduct disorder, whereas conduct disorder in adolescence occurs irrespective of family income (Loeber, Green, Keenan, & Lahey, 1995). Family and peer group influences in childhood are highly predictive of juvenile offending (Patterson, Forgatch, Yoerger, & Stoolmiller, 1998), although this varies by cultural groups, family context, and child gender (Deater-Decker, Dodge, Bates, & Pettit, 1998). These studies suggest that it is not the presence of conduct problems by themselves that is predictive of later problems, but rather the degree to which personal characteristics are affected by social and environmental factors (Dishion & Patterson, 1997).

Influences on Course and Prognosis

COMMUNITY INFLUENCES

There is an increasing awareness that characteristics of communities influence levels of children's conduct problems. For example, CD is more prevalent among African-American children and adolescents relative to nonminority children and adolescents, suggesting an ethnic bias in the diagnosis (Hudley & Graham, 1995). However, an extensive evaluation of psychopathology in urban poor children found that individual and community poverty had differing influences across ethnic groups (Guerra, Huesmann, Tolan, Van Acker, & Eron,

1995). All groups (White, African-American, and Hispanic) evidenced a significant association between neighborhood violence and aggression, whereas only White children evidenced a significant association between individual poverty and aggression. However, African-American children experienced the greatest economic hardship and also the highest rates of aggression, therefore, confounding poverty and ethnicity.

The confounding of race and economic hardship suggests that it is the stressors associated with urban living and poverty that have serious implications for children's adjustment. Greenberg et al. (1999) found that the quality of the neighborhood, but not ethnicity, predicted children's psychological and academic performance when followed from kindergarten through the end of first grade. For example, as many as two-thirds of school-age children who lived in low-income inner-city communities in Chicago reported witnessing a serious assault, and one-third had witnessed a homicide (Bell & Jenkins, 1991). Surveys in New Orleans and Washington, DC, indicated that 51% of New Orleans fifth graders and 32% of the Washington, DC children were victims of violence (Osofsky, Wewers, Hann, & Fick, 1993; Richters & Martinez, 1993). Inner-city children's exposure to violence predicted increases in aggression and depression at one-year follow-up, even controlling for prior levels of these problems (Gorman-Smith & Tolan, 1998). Exposure to violence was not related to measures of family relationship or parenting, indicating that community-level variables were predominant. The impact of community violence on children may also be mediated by its effects on parents. Violence and poverty affect parents' ability to monitor and discipline their children consistently and to provide needed support and nurturance (Gorman-Smith, Tolan, & Henry, in press). Not surprisingly, low-income urban communities were associated with decreased children's attachments to school and increased associations with delinquent peers (Fagan, Piper, & Moore, 1986).

SCHOOL INFLUENCES

Disruptive classroom behavior is associated with specific teachers' behavior management practices (Hawkins & Lam, 1987). Teachers' appropriate use of classroom management methods such as rewards for positive behavior, negative consequences for inappropriate behavior, and the establishment of clear rules and organized classroom routines are associated with reduced aggression and improved academic performance (Hawkins, 1997). Positive student-teacher relationships are associated with students' attachment to school (Hawkins, 1997) and achievement (Wang, Haertel, & Walberg, 1997) and may be especially important in urban, low-income schools where student–teacher interactions are often disrupted by daily stressors (Atkins et al., 1998; Boyd & Shouse, 1997).

PEER GROUP INFLUENCES

Peer group attitudes toward aggression and peer group social support are important influences on children's aggression (Huesmann, Guerra, Miller, & Zelli, 1992). Group social context (affective quality, level of tension, degree of playfulness) and peer group norms also influence both the level of aggression and children's attitudes towards aggression (DeRosier, Cillessen, Coie, & Dodge, 1994; Stromshak, Bierman, Bruschi, Coie, & Dodge, 1999). For aggressive children, group attitudes toward aggression appear to influence peer group acceptance. Highly aggressive boys are viewed more positively by other group members in groups that have higher levels of aggression (Wright, Giammarino, & Parad, 1986).

Peer social rejection is also strongly associated with aggression which often leads to deviant peer relationships, supportive of delinquency development (Dishion, 1990). Delinquent peer dyads respond more positively to discussions involving rule-breaking than do nondelinquent dyads, suggesting that these behaviors may be supported through positive peer interactions (Dishion, Spracklen, Andrews, & Patterson, 1996). Victimization by peers is common for aggressive children and is associated with poor adjustment and worse prognosis (Hess & Atkins, 1998; Schwartz, McFadyen-Ketchum, Dodge, Pettit, & Bates, 1998).

CHILD INFLUENCES

Social competence influences children's tendencies toward aggression (Lochman & Dodge, 1994). Boys rated as aggressive by teachers had deficits in social problem solving relative to nonaggressive boys and had a greater tendency toward planned aggression compared to violent offenders (Lochman, 1992). Children's use of emotion-focused coping strategies predicted disruptive behavior in a 3-year longitudinal study (Steele, Forehand, Armistead, Morse, Simon, & Clark, 1999). Improving children's social cognitive skills and improving anger control are key components of interventions for aggressive children (Kazdin, 1995; Lochman, 1992).

Children's attitudes toward aggression also predict levels of aggressive behavior (Huesmann et al., 1992), although, as noted previously, these attitudes are highly influenced by peer group norms. Inclination to endorse aggressive solutions to conflicts has been associated with bullying; distorted appraisals of mild provocations have been associated with overreactive, hostile forms of aggression (Dodge & Schwartz, 1997). Temperamental characteristics such as negative mood and resistance to adult control are predictive of poor outcome for aggressive children, especially if parental support and peer friendships are lacking (Bates, Pettit, Dodge, & Ridge, 1998; Hess & Atkins, 1998).

Gender Differences.   Conduct disorders are two to three times more prevalent among boys than girls but are second only to depression among psychiatric disorders experienced by girls (Zoccolillo, 1993). Longitudinal studies have found strong associations between female childhood conduct problems and a host of medical and mental health problems in early adulthood including poor physical health, alcohol or marijuana dependence, tobacco dependence, sexually transmitted disease, and early pregnancy (Bardone, Moffitt, Caspi, Diskson, Stanton, & Silva, 1998; Woodward & Fergusson, 1999).

There is evidence that girls' aggression does not display the same continuity as boys' over the life course. For example, peer or teacher ratings of girls' aggression at age 10 did not predict delinquent behavior at age 14 or in early adulthood (Stattin & Magnusson, 1989; Tremblay, Masse, Perron, Leblanc, Schwartzman, & Ledingham, 1992). Assessment of comorbid problems is also critical because conduct problems of girls often co-occur with anxiety disorders and depression (Loeber & Keenan, 1994). A gender difference in response to treatment is suggested by Webster-Stratton (1996), who found that parents' psychological states and parenting style predicted positive response to treatment for girls but not for boys.

Conduct problems in girls can no longer be easily characterized as nonconfrontational or self-directed. A small group of girls exhibit aggressive behavior that is as severe and persistent as boys', and a second, larger group of girls exhibits subtle social aggression, ostracism of others, and defiance during the transition of adolescence (Cairns & Cairns, 1994). Outcomes for these girls include teenage pregnancy, school dropout, and reliance on social services (Lewis et al., 1991). To date, early identification and accurate assessment of conduct problems in girls remains an underresearched area of critical importance.

Academic Underachievement. Academic deficits are common for children who have CD. It appears that co-occurring attention problems lead to academic problems for children who have CD (Frick et al., 1991), although by adolescence, conduct problems are strongly associated with school failure (Hinshaw, 1992a). Academic deficits may result from missed instruction due to disruptive and off-task classroom behavior or from discouraged teachers who are reluctant to insist that the students perform challenging tasks. Either way, aggressive youth may possess inadequate skills in basic areas and may continue to fall behind academically as adolescents (see Table 1).

Familial and Genetic Patterns

Heredity of Antisocial Behavior

The persistence of antisocial behavior suggests a genetic basis, although there is dispute as to the strength of this relationship. Several sources of information are used to support the heredity of antisocial behavior. *Family history* is a clear determinant of antisocial behavior in offspring; however, this may be confounded by the social learning in families (Patterson, 1997). A history of parental antisocial behavior may suggest genetic transmission of conduct problems, or the influence of aggressive modeling by parents, or the impact of adult psychopathy on family functioning. In fact, all three are plausible explanations that may operate concurrently.

A stronger test of the heredity of antisocial behavior is *twin studies* in which identical monozygotic (MZ) twins are compared to nonidentical dizygotic (DZ) twins. Several studies have indicated a higher concurrence of antisocial behavior among MZ than among DZ twins (e.g., Cloninger & Gottesman, 1987). However, MZ twins have a greater reciprocal influence on each other than DZ twins. This has been shown to account for much of the concurrence of later criminality, such that genetic influence appears significant but modest (Carey, 1992).

The third source of evidence for the genetic basis of antisocial behavior is *adoption studies*. In these investigations, the relationship between biological offspring is compared to the influence of the adopted family on the child to provide independent assessments of genetic

---

TABLE 1. Important and Key Points: Description, Epidemiology, Course, and Prognosis

---

1. *Childhood Onset type* and *Adolescent Onset type*, across three categories for severity: mild, moderate, or severe.
2. Three subtypes of childhood aggression have been identified: overt vs. covert antisocial behavior, proactive vs. reactive aggression, and impulsive vs. nonimpulsive aggression.
3. The prevalence of Conduct Disorder, estimated at 2% and 6%, accounts for one-half to one-third of all child and adolescent mental health referrals.
4. Urban, low-income communities have the highest rates of violent crime. This contributes to high rates of childhood conduct problems via exposure of children to aggressive and traumatic events, disrupting parenting practices, and children's decreased attachment to school.
5. Teachers' appropriate use of classroom management practices and positive relationships with students influence children's conduct problems. Peer group attitudes toward aggression and social support are also important influences in children's conduct problems, as are children's social competence and temperament.
6. Boys are more likely than girls to be aggressive, but longitudinal studies have found a host of medical and mental health problems associated with female childhood conduct problems.
7. Academic underachievement is common for children who have conduct problems and, when it continues into adolescence, is associated with poor long-term outcomes.

---

and social influences on behavior. A review of adoption studies of criminality indicated mixed support for a genetic explanation (Peter, Atkins, & McKay, 1999). In support of the genetic model, several studies have shown a substantial genetic loading for antisocial behavior by demonstrating higher associations for biological family history of antisocial behavior with adoptees' behavior than for nonrelative adoptive family history. However, there is a lack of consensus regarding the specific behaviors related to biological family history and, because the onset of criminality is often specific to factors such as social environment, sex, age, or type of criminality, it is often difficult to distinguish these factors from genetic factors. Therefore, results in one study are often highly specific to factors not measured in other studies.

Rutter and colleagues, in a review of genetic factors associated with childhood psychiatric disorders (Rutter, Macdonald, Le Couteur, Harrington, Bolton, & Bailey, 1990), noted that the genetic influence on conduct problems is stronger for the prediction of adult conduct problems than for juvenile offending. Further, even for predicting adult conduct problems, genetic influence was most pronounced when combined with environmental risk factors such as adverse adoptee home environment or multiple temporary placements. Thus, although there is consensus that some characteristics of childhood CD are inherited, it remains difficult to tease apart the psychosocial and genetic influences (Peters et al., 1999) (see Table 2).

Family Factors

Family factors have been consistently implicated in the onset and maintenance of childhood aggression and are among the most powerful predictors of risk (Loeber & Stouthamer-Loeber, 1998). Family characteristics, such as the extent of support within the family and family values, have been linked to the emergence of disruptive behavior in urban adolescents (Florsheim, Tolan, & Gorman-Smith, 1996). Parents' depression and social isolation is also associated with higher rates of children's aggression (Conger, Patterson, & Ge, 1995), especially in low-income communities (McLoyd, 1990). Parenting strategies associated with aggression in young children are inconsistent and harsh discipline (Chamberlain & Patterson, 1995), overly restrictive control (Bates et al., 1998), and poor parent–child communication and warmth (Gorman-Smith, Tolan, Zelli, & Huesmann, 1996). Other significant risk factors for childhood conduct disorder are marital adjustment of parents, social stress, and parental alcoholism and criminal activity (Florsheim et al., 1996; Pettit, Bates, & Dodge, 1997). As parents experience more of their own life crises, child rearing becomes more stressful and leads to greater parent–child conflict and impaired child–parent relationships (Wahler, 1990).

Parental involvement in their child's schooling is a critical component of children's

TABLE 2. Important and Key Points: Genetic Patterns

1. Family history is a clear determinant of antisocial behavior but is confounded by the social learning in families.
2. A higher concordance of antisocial behavior is found in identical twins compared to nonidentical twins. However, after controlling for greater reciprocal influence in identical twins, the genetic influence on antisocial behavior appears modest.
3. Adoption studies indicate higher associations for a biological family history of antisocial behavior on children's conduct than for an adoptive family history. However, methodological differences across studies make it difficult to distinguish genetic influences from influences of the social environment.
4. Genetic influence is clearer for adult conduct problems than for childhood conduct problems. Even for adult conduct problems, genetic influence is most evident when combined with environmental risk factors.

attachment to school and is highly related to positive outcome for children with conduct problems (Atkins et al., 1998). Higher grades are associated with parents' monitoring of homework and daily activities, frequent contact with schools, and high educational expectations (Henderson & Berla, 1994). Parents' use of home-based activities (e.g., checking homework, rewarding academic success) is associated with improved academic and social behavior, especially when paired with remedial academic programs (Bryk & Driscoll, 1988; Heller & Fantuzzo, 1993) (see Table 3).

DIAGNOSTIC CONSIDERATIONS

There is considerable support for aspects of the DSM-IV CD diagnosis. The validity of the CD diagnosis was evaluated in the DSM-IV field trials of 440 clinically referred youth and was cross-validated in a household sample of 1,285 nonreferred youth (Lahey et al., 1994, 1998). In both samples, there was a large decline in the incidence of aggression at age 10. The distinction between Childhood Onset CD and Adolescent Onset CD was confirmed in the referred sample. Adolescent-Onset CD was associated with being female, not having a corresponding diagnosis of Oppositional Defiant Disorder, and not having a family history of antisocial behavior, relative to Childhood-Onset CD. These results were consistent with studies that indicate differential predictors and pathways for early versus late onset CD (Hinshaw, Lahey, & Hart, 1993; Tolan & Thomas, 1995).

However, interrater reliability of these criteria was less impressive. Despite extensive refinement of diagnostic criteria, interrater reliability and test–retest reliability were not improved compared to prior criteria and remained moderately low by psychometric standards (Lahey et al., 1994). Apparently, further revisions are required to eliminate items that contribute to low agreement and low stability. In addition, additional efforts to train clinicians may be needed to reduce differences across diagnosticians.

Another feature of the CD diagnosis that has been studied extensively is the hierarchical relationship between ODD and CD in which ODD is assumed to be present if a CD diagnosis is warranted. This is supported by studies that found that most children who have CD have early histories of ODD and that there are similar family correlates for CD and ODD (Loeber, Lahey, & Thomas, 1991). For example, harsh discipline and poor supervision are related to both CD and ODD symptoms, although these relationships are stronger for CD than for ODD.

However, there are two issues which argue against the interdependence of CD and ODD. First, adolescent-onset CD showed little continuity with childhood ODD (Lahey, Loeber,

TABLE 3. Important and Key Points: Family Factors

---

1. Parental depression and social isolation are associated with high rates of children's conduct problems, especially in low-income communities.
2. Parenting strategies associated with children's conduct problems are the use of inconsistent and harsh discipline, overly restrictive control, and poor parent–child communication and warmth.
3. Lack of social support within the family and deviant family values are associated with adolescent conduct problems.
4. Other risk factors for children's conduct problems are marital adjustment, social stress, and parental alcoholism and criminal activity.
5. As parents experience more of their own life crises, child rearing can become more stressful and lead to impaired child–parent relationships.

Quay, Frick, & Grimm, 1992). Second, the unique relationship of ODD to CD has not been demonstrated. For example, ODD symptoms often overlap ADHD symptoms in normative and clinic samples (Reeves, Werry, Elkind, & Zametkin, 1987). This may indicate that ODD symptoms are global markers of maladjustment rather than a specific risk marker for CD (Lahey et al., 1992). Consideration of the co-occurrence of CD and ODD may be a more useful strategy to assess fully all aspects of a child's antisocial activities.

Psychiatric Comorbidity

Comorbidity, the co-occurrence of two or more psychiatric disorders, is an important consideration in children's mental health. In a sample of 961 young adults assessed since birth, comorbid cases experienced a wide range of physical, educational, and economic problems, relative to single disordered cases (Newman, Moffitt, Caspi, & Silva, 1998). This is illustrated clearly in the comorbid relation of ADHD with CD. There are estimates of 30% to 60% overlap, depending upon age, sex, and primary symptoms (Szatmari, Boyle, & Offord, 1989). The overlap is much lower in children referred for ADHD; however, about 10% of ADHD children receive a concurrent diagnosis of CD (Lalonde, Turgay, & Hudson, 1998).

There is considerable evidence that CD children who have ADHD are a distinct subgroup of behaviorally disordered children. Relative to children with one or the other disorder, these children have higher rates of family dysfunction, academic deficits, and poor peer relationships (Hinshaw, 1993). ADHD is associated with early onset CD (Loeber et al., 1995) and the core features of ADHD, impulsivity and hyperactivity, are two of the most prominent risk factors for long-term juvenile offending (Loeber et al., 1998). Not surprisingly, the co-occurrence of CD and ADHD is associated with poor long-term prognosis (Moffitt, 1990) (see Table 4).

SUMMARY

Childhood conduct disorder, characterized by chronic patterns of social norm violations, represents a serious and seemingly intractable mental health problem. In recent years, there has been a growing awareness of the importance of an ecological perspective for understanding the onset and maintenance of children's conduct problems. School, family, and community contexts provide powerful contexts for the emergence of children's conduct problems. As a

---

TABLE 4. Important and Key Points: Diagnostic Considerations

1. Studies of the validity of the DSM-IV CD diagnosis indicate strong support for the distinction of childhood vs. adolescent onset CD.
2. Interrater reliability and test-retest reliability were similar to earlier DSM CD criteria and low by psychometric standards. Additional training may be needed to reduce differences across interviewers.
3. The hierarchical relationship between ODD and CD is not empirically supported, especially for Adolescent Onset CD. Consideration of the co-occurrence of ODD and CD may be more useful to assess fully all aspects of a child's antisocial behavior.
4. The most common comorbid psychiatric condition with CD is ADHD. The combination of ADHD and CD is distinct from either disorder. It is more common in associated Childhood Onset CD than Adolescent Onset CD and, relative to either disorder, comorbid ADHD/CD is associated with higher rates of family dysfunction, academic deficits, poor peer relations, and worse long-term prognosis.

result, new and promising interventions have been developed that offer renewed hope for the early and effective remediation of children's conduct problems.

Nevertheless, much remains to be learned about children's conduct problems. It is clear that there are multiple pathways to conduct disorder, based on the complex interplay of ecological, biological, and psychosocial factors. Given the multiplicity of problems and factors that impact long-term outcome and the multiple pathways to antisocial behavior, it is clear that children's conduct problems must be understood from both an ecological framework, in which problems are understood as a function of the context in which they occur (Dishion & Patterson, 1997) and a developmental framework, in which the trajectory and presentation of problems is understood in regard to children's developmental tasks (Hinshaw et al., 1993). Only by considering both ecological and developmental perspectives will conduct problems be understood in the context of real-world concerns that impact children's relationships to family, teachers, and peers.

REFERENCES

American Psychiatric Association. (1994). *Diagnostic and statistical manual of mental disorders*, 4th ed. Washington, DC: Author.

Atkins, M. S., McKay, M., Arvanitis, P., London, L., Madison, S., Costigan, C., Haney, M., Zevenbergen, A., Hess, L., Bennett, D., & Webster, D. (1998). An ecological model for school-based mental health services for urban low income aggressive children. *The Journal of Behavioral Health Services and Research, 5*, 64–75.

Atkins, M. S., Osborne, M., Bennett, D., Hess, L., & Halperin, J. (submitted). Children's competitive peer aggression during reward and punishment.

Bardone, A., Moffitt, T., Caspi, A., Dickson, N., Stanton, W., & Silva, P. (1998). Adult physical health outcomes of adolescent girls with conduct disorder, depression, and anxiety. *Journal of the American Academy of Child and Adolescent Psychiatry, 37*, 594–601.

Bates, J. E., Pettit, G., Dodge, K., & Ridge, B. (1998). Interaction of temperamental resistance to control and restrictive parenting in the development of externalizing behavior. *Developmental Psychology, 34*, 982–995.

Bell, C. C., & Jenkins, E. J. (1991). Traumatic stress and children. *Journal of Health Care for the Poor and Underserved, 2*, 175–185.

Boyd, W. L., & Shouse, R. (1997). The problems and promise of urban schools. In H. Walberg, O. Reyes, & R. Weissberg (Eds.), *Children and youth: Interdisciplinary perspectives* (pp. 141–165). Thousand Oaks, CA: Sage.

Bryk, A. S., & Driscoll, M. (1988). *The school as community: Theoretical foundations, contextual influences, and consequences for students and teachers.* Chicago: University of Chicago, Benton Center for Curriculum and Instruction.

Cairns, R. B., & Cairns, B. D. (1994). *Lifelines and risks: Pathways of youth in our time.* New York: Cambridge University Press.

Carey, G. (1992). Twin imitation for antisocial behavior: Implications for genetic and family environment research. *Journal of Abnormal Psychology, 101*, 18–25.

Center for Disease Control. (1991). Weapon-varying among high school students—United States, 1990. *Morbidity and Morality Weekly Report, 40*, 681–684.

Chamberlain, P., & Patterson, G. (1995). Discipline and child compliance in parenting. In M. Bornstein (Ed.), *Handbook of parenting*, Vol. 4: *Applied and practical parenting* (pp. 205–225). Mahwah, NJ: Erlbaum.

Cloninger, C. R., & Gottesman, I. (1987). Genetic and environmental factors in antisocial behaviors disorders. In S. Mednick, T. Moffitt, & S. Stack (Eds.), *The causes of crime: New biological approaches* (pp. 92–109). New York: Cambridge University Press.

Conger, R., Patterson, G., & Ge, X. (1995). It takes two to replicate: A mediational model for the impact of parents' stress on adolescent adjustment. *Child Development, 66*, 80–97.

Deater-Deckard, K., Dodge, K., Bates, J., & Pettit, G. (1998). Multiple risk factors in the development of externalizing behavior problems: Group and individual differences. *Development and Psychopathology, 10*, 469–493.

DeRosier, M. E., Cillessen, A. H., Coie, J. D., & Dodge, K. A. (1994). Group social context and children's aggressive behavior. *Child Development, 65*, 1068–1079.

Dishion, T. J. (1990). The peer context of troublesome child and adolescent behavior. In P. Leone (Ed.), *Understanding the troubled and troublesome youth* (pp. 128–153). Newbury Park, CA: Sage.

Dishion, T. J., & Patterson, G. R. (1997). The timing and severity of antisocial behavior: Three hypotheses within an ecological framework. In D. Stoff, J. Breiling, & J. Maser (Eds.), *Handbook of antisocial behavior* (pp. 205–217). New York: Wiley.

Dishion, T. J., Spracklen, K., Andrews, D., & Patterson, G. (1997). Deviancy training in male adolescent friendships. *Behavior Therapy, 27,* 373–390.

Dodge, K. A., Lochman, J. E., Harnish, J. D., Bates, J. E., & Pettit, G. S. (1997). Reactive and proactive aggression in school children and psychiatrically impaired chronically assaultive youth. *Journal of Abnormal Psychology, 106,* 37–51.

Dodge, K. A., & Schwartz, D. (1997). Social information processing mechanisms in aggressive behavior. In D. Stoff, J. Breiling, & J. Maser (Eds.), *Handbook of antisocial behavior* (pp. 171–180). New York: Wiley.

Fagan, J. A., Piper, E., & Moore, M. (1986). Violent delinquents and urban youth. *Criminology, 24,* 439–471.

Fingerhut, L., & Kleinman, J. (1990). International and interstate comparisons of homicide among young males. *Journal of the American Medical Association, 263,* 3292–3295.

Florsheim, P., Tolan, P., & Gorman-Smith, D. (1996). Family processes and risk for externalizing behavior problems among African-American and Hispanic boys. *Journal of Consulting and Clinical Psychology, 64,* 1222–1230.

Frick, P. J., Kamphaus, R., Lahey, B., Loeber, R., Christ, M., Hart, E., & Tannenbaum, L. (1991). Academic underachievement and the disruptive behavior disorders. *Journal of Consulting and Clinical Psychology, 59,* 289–294.

Gorman-Smith, D., & Tolan, P. (1998). The role of exposure to community violence and developmental problems among inner-city youth. *Development and Psychopathology, 10,* 101–116.

Gorman-Smith, D., Tolan, P., & Henry, D. (in press). A developmental-ecological model of the relation of family functioning to patterns of delinquency. *Journal of Quantitative Criminology.*

Gorman-Smith, D., Tolan, T., Zelli, A., & Huesmann, L. (1996). The relation of family functioning to violence among inner-city minority youth. *Journal of Family Psychology, 10,* 115–129.

Greenberg, M. T., Lengua, L., Coie, F., Pinderhughes, E., Bierman, K., Dodge, K., Lockham, J., & McMahon, R. (1999). Predicting developmental outcomes at school entry using a multiple-risk model: Four American communities. *Developmental Psychology, 35,* 403–417.

Guerra, N. G., Huesmann, L., Tolan, P. , Van Acker, R., & Eron, L. (1995). Stressful events and individual beliefs as correlates of economic disadvantage and aggression among urban children. *Journal of Consulting and Clinical Psychology, 63,* 518–528.

Guerra, N. G., Tolan, P., & Hammond, R. (1995). Interventions for adolescent violence. In L. Eron, J. Gentry, & P. Schlagel (Eds.), *Reason to hope: A psychosocial perspective on violence and youth* (pp. 383–404). Washington, DC: American Psychological Association.

Halperin, J., Newcorn, J., Matier, K., Bedi, G., Hall, S., & Sharma, V. (1995). Impulsivity and the initiation of fights in children with disruptive behavior disorders. *Journal of Child Psychology and Psychiatry, 36,* 1199–1211.

Hawkins, J. D. (1997). Academic performance and school success: Sources and consequences. In R. Weissberg, T. Gullotta, R. Hampton, B. Ryan, & G. Adams (Eds.), *Enhancing children's wellness* (pp. 278–305). Thousand Oaks, CA: Sage.

Hawkins, J. D., & Lam, T. (1987). Teacher practices, social development, and delinquency. In J. Burchard & S. Burchard (Eds.), *Prevention of delinquent behavior* (pp. 241–274). Newbury Park, CA: Sage.

Heller, L. R., & Fantuzzo, J. (1993). Reciprocal peer tutoring and parent partnership: Does parent involvement make a difference? *School Psychology Review, 22,* 517–534.

Henderson, A., & Berla, N. (1994). *A new generation of evidence: The family is critical to student achievement.* Washington, DC: National Committee for Citizens in Education.

Henggeler, S. W., Schoenwald, S., Borduin, C., Rowland, M., & Cunningham, P. (1998). *Multisystemic treatment of antisocial behavior in children and adolescents.* New York: Guilford.

Hess, L. E., & Atkins, M. S. (1998). Victims and aggressors at school: Teacher, self, and peer perceptions of psychosocial functioning. *Applied Developmental Science, 2,* 75–89.

Hinshaw, S. P. (1992a). Externalizing behavior problems and academic underachievement in childhood and adolescence: Causal relationships and underlying mechanisms. *Psychological Bulletin, 111,* 127–155.

Hinshaw, S. P. (1992b). Academic underachievement, attention deficits, and aggression: Comorbidity and implications for intervention. *Journal of Consulting and Clinical Psychology, 60,* 893–903.

Hinshaw, S. P., Lahey, B., & Hart, E. (1993). Issues of taxonomy and comorbidity in the development of conduct disorder. *Development and Psychopathology, 5,* 31–49.

Hudley, C., & Graham, S. (1995). School-based interventions for aggressive African-American boys. *Applied and Preventive Psychology, 4,* 185–195.

Huesmann, L. R., Guerra, N. G., Miller, L. S., & Zelli, A. (1992). The role of social norms in the development of aggressive behavior. In H. Zumckly & A. Fraczek (Eds.), *Socialization and aggression* (pp. 139–152). New York: Springer-Verlag.

Institute of Medicine (1989). *Research on children and adolescents with mental, behavioral, and developmental disorders*. Washington, DC: National Academy Press.

Kazdin, A. E. (1995). *Conduct disorders in childhood and adolescence*, 2nd ed. Thousand Oaks, CA: Sage.

Lahey, B. B., Applegate, B., Barkley, R., Garfinkel, B., McBurnett, K., Kerdyk, L., Greenhill, L., Hynd, G., Frick, P., Newcorn, J., Biederman, J., Ollendick, T., Hart, E., Perez, D., Waldman, I., & Shaffer, D. (1994). DSM-IV field trails for oppositional defiant disorder and conduct disorder in children and adolescents. *American Journal of Psychiatry, 151*, 1163–1171.

Lahey, B. B., Loeber, R., Quay, H., Applegate, B., Shaffer, D., Waldman, I., Hart, E., McBurnett, K., Frick, P., Jensen, P., Dulcan, M., Cannino, G., & Bird, H. (1998). Validity of DSM-IV subtypes of conduct disorder based on age of onset. *Journal of the American Academy of Child and Adolescent Psychiatry, 37*, 435–442.

Lahey, B. B., Loeber, R., Quay, H. C., Frick, P. J., & Grimm, J. (1992). Oppositional defiant and conduct disorders: Issues to be resolved for DSM-IV. *Journal of the American Academy of Child and Adolescent Psychiatry, 31*, 539–546.

Lalonde, J., Turgay, A., & Hudson, J. (1998). Attention-deficit hyperactivity disorder subtypes and comorbid disruptive behavior disorders in a child and adolescent mental health clinic. *Canadian Journal of Psychiatry, 43*, 623–628.

Lewis, D. O., Yeager, C. A., Cogham-Portorreal, C. S., Klein, N., Showalter, C., & Anthony, A. (1991). A follow-up of female delinquents: Maternal contributions to the perpetuation of deviance. *Journal of the American Academy of Child and Adolescent Psychiatry, 30*, 197–201.

Lochman, J. E. (1992). Cognitive-behavioral intervention with aggressive boys: Three-year follow-up and preventive effects. *Journal of Consulting and Clinical Psychology, 60*, 426–432.

Lochman, J. E., & Dodge, K. A. (1994). Social-cognitive processes of severely violent, moderately aggressive, and nonaggressive boys. *Journal of Consulting and Clinical Psychology, 62*, 366–374.

Loeber, R., Farrington, D., Stouthamer-Loeber, M., Moffitt, T., & Caspi, A. (1998). The development of male offending: Key findings from the first decade of the Pittsburgh youth study. *Studies on Crime and Crime Prevention, 7*, 141–171.

Loeber, R., Green, S., Keenan, K., & Lahey, B. (1995). Which boys will fare worse? Early predictors of the onset of conduct disorder in a six-year longitudinal study. *Journal of the American Academy of Child and Adolescent Psychiatry, 34*, 499–509.

Loeber, R., & Keenan, K. (1994). Interaction between conduct disorder and its comorbid conditions: Effects of age and gender. *Clinical Psychology Review, 14*, 497–523.

Loeber, R., Lahey, B. B., & Thomas, C. (1991). Diagnostic conundrum of oppositional defiant disorders and conduct disorder. *Journal of Abnormal Psychology, 100*, 379–390.

Loeber, R., & Schmaling, K. (1985a). The utility of differentiating between mixed and pure forms of antisocial child behavior. *Journal of Abnormal Child Psychology, 13*, 315–335.

Loeber, R., & Schmaling, K. (1985b). Empirical evidence for overt and covert patterns of antisocial conduct problems: A meta-analysis. *Journal of Abnormal Child Psychology, 13*, 337–353.

Loeber, R., & Stouthamer-Loeber, M. (1998). Juvenile aggression at home and at school. In D. Elliott, B. Hamburg, & K. Williams (Eds.), *Violence in American schools: A new perspective* (pp. 94–126). New York: Cambridge University Press.

Lynam, D. R. (1996). The early identification of chronic offenders: Who is the fledgling psychopath. *Psychological Bulletin, 120*, 209–234.

Lynam, D. R. (1998). Early identification of the fledgling psychopath: Locating the psychopathic child in the current nomenclature. *Journal of Abnormal Psychology, 107*, 566–575.

McLoyd, V. C. (1990). The impact of economic hardship on black families and children: Psychological distress, parenting, and socioemotional development. *Child Development, 61*, 311–346.

Moffitt, T. E. (1990). Juvenile delinquency and attention-deficit disorder: Developmental trajectories from age 3 to 15. *Child Development, 61*, 893–910.

Moffitt, T. E. (1993). Adolescence-limited and life-course-persistent antisocial behavior: A developmental taxonomy. *Psychological Review, 100*, 674–701.

Newman, D. L., Moffitt, T., Caspi, A., & Silva, P. (1998). Comorbid mental disorders: Implications for treatment and sample selection. *Journal of Abnormal Psychology, 107*, 305–311.

Osofsky, J. D., Wewers, S., Hann, D., & Fick, A. C. (1993). Chronic community violence: What is happening to our children? *Psychiatry, 56*, 36–45.

Patterson, G. R. (1997). Performance models for parenting: A social interactional perspective. In J. Grusec & L.

Kuczynski (Eds.), *Parenting and children's internalization of values: A handbook of contemporary theory* (pp. 193–226). New York: Wiley.

Patterson, G. R., Forgatch, M., Yoerger, K., & Stoolmiller, M. (1998). Variables that initiate and maintain an early-onset trajectory for juvenile offending. *Development and Psychopathology, 10,* 531–547.

Peters, B. R., Atkins, M., & McKay, M. (1999). Adopted children's behavior problems: A review of five explanatory models. *Clinical Psychology Review, 19,* 297–328.

Pettit, G., Bates, J., & Dodge, K. (1997). Supportive parenting, ecological context, and children's adjustment: A seven-year longitudinal study. *Child Development, 68,* 908–923.

Reeves, J. C., Werry, J. S., Elkind, G. S., & Zametkin, A. (1987). Attention deficit, conduct, oppositional, and anxiety disorders in children: II. Clinical characteristics. *Journal of the American Academy of Child and Adolescent Psychiatry, 26,* 144–155.

Richters, J. E., & Martinez, P. (1993). The NIMH community violence project: Vol. 1. Children as victims of and witnesses to violence. *Psychiatry, 56,* 7–21.

Robins, L. N. (1991). Antisocial personality. In L. Robins & D. Regier (Eds.), *Psychiatric disorder in America.* New York: Macmillan.

Rutter, M., Macdonald, H., LeCouteur, A., Harrington, R., Bolton, P., & Bailey, A. (1990). Genetic factors in child psychiatric disorders—II: Empirical findings. *Journal of Child Psychology and Psychiatry, 31,* 39–83.

Schwartz, D., McFadyen-Ketchum, S., Dodge, K., Pettit, G., & Bates, J. (1998). Peer group victimization as a predictor of children's behavior problems at home and in school. *Development and Psychopathology, 10,* 87–99.

Simmons, R. G., & Blythe, D. A. (1987). *Moving into adolescence: The impact of pubertal change and school context.* New York: Aldine De Gruyter.

Stattin, H., & Magnusson, D. (1989). The role of early aggressive behavior in the frequency, seriousness, and types of later crime. *Journal of Consulting and Clinical Psychology, 57,* 710–718.

Steele, R. G., Forehand, R., Armistead, L., Morse, E., Simon, P., & Clark, L. (1999). Coping strategies and behavior problems of urban African-American children: Concurrent and longitudinal relationships. *American Journal of Orthopsychiatry, 69,* 182–193.

Stromshak, E. A., Bierman, K., Bruschi, C., Dodge, K., & Coie, J. (1999). The relation between behavior problems and peer preference in different classroom contexts. *Child Development, 70,* 169–182.

Szatmari, P., Boyle, M., & Offord, D. (1989). ADHD and conduct disorder: Degree of diagnostic overlap and differences among correlates. *Journal of the American Academy of Child and Adolescent Psychiatry, 28,* 865–872.

Tolan, P. H., Guerra, N., & Kendall, P. (1995). A developmental-ecological perspective on antisocial behavior in children and adolescents: Toward a unified risk and intervention framework. *Journal of Consulting and Clinical Psychology, 63,* 579–584.

Tolan, P. H., & Henry, D. (1996). Patterns of psychopathology among urban-poor children. II: Comorbidity and aggression effects. *Journal of Consulting and Clinical Psychology, 64,* 1094–1099.

Tolan, P. H., & Thomas, P. (1995). The implications of age of onset for delinquency risk II. *Journal of Abnormal Child Psychology, 23,* 157–181.

Tremblay, R. E., Masse, B., Perron, D., Leblanc, M., Schwartzman, A. E., & Ledingham, J. E. (1992). Early disruptive behavior, poor school achievement, delinquent behavior, and delinquent personality: Longitudinal analyses. *Journal of Consulting and Clinical Psychology, 60,* 64–72.

Tuma, J. (1989). Mental health services for children: The state of the art. *American Psychologist, 44,* 188–189.

Vitiello, B., & Stoff, D. M. (1997). Subtypes of aggression and their relevance to child psychiatry. *Journal of the American Academy of Child and Adolescent Psychiatry, 36,* 307–315.

Wahler, R. G. (1990). Some perceptual functions of social networks in coercive mother–child interactions. *Journal of Social and Clinical Psychology, 9,* 43–53.

Wang, M. C., Haertel, G. D., & Walberg, H. J. (1997). Fostering educational resilience in inner-city schools. In H. J. Walberg, O. Reyes, & R. P. Weissberg (Eds.), *Children and youth: Interdisciplinary perspectives* (pp. 119–140). Thousand Oaks, CA: Sage.

Webster-Stratton, C. (1996). Early onset conduct problems: Does gender make a difference? *Journal of Consulting and Clinical Psychology, 64,* 540–551.

Woodward, L., & Fergusson, D. (1999). Early conduct problems and later risk of teenage pregnancy in girls. *Development and Psychopathology, 11,* 127–141.

Wright, J. C., Giammarino, M., & Parad, H. W. (1986). Social status in small groups: Individual-group similarity and the social misfit. *Journal of Personality and Social Psychology, 50,* 523–536.

Zoccolillo, M. (1993). Gender and the development of conduct disorder. *Development and Psychopathology, 5,* 65–78.

11

Anxiety Disorders

Thomas H. Ollendick and Devin A. Byrd

Anxiety disorders are characterized by an *avoidance* of a variety of feared stimuli or situations that are often important for optimal development and/or by somatic or physiological *distress* in the presence of these stimuli or situations. Typically, disturbances in physiology, affect, and cognition are present in all anxiety disorders. For some children and adolescents, synchrony among these three response systems is evident; for others, however, desynchrony occurs. For example, they may experience high levels of cognitive worry but not elevated levels of physiological arousal. Although synchrony or desynchrony in physiology, affect and cognition may allow for an overall understanding of these disorders, and the basic psychopathological processes associated with them, categorical criteria such as those expressed in the DSM-IV provide a picture of their clinical presentation that frequently leads to specific assessment and treatment procedures. The specific features of each disorder and specific characteristics of these disorders as they occur in childhood are discussed briefly in the section that follows.

Description of the Disorders

Panic attacks are described as a specific moment of profound fright or displeasure accompanied by four of 13 cognitive and physical symptoms such as accelerated heart rate and thoughts of going crazy or dying. Individuals who experienced fewer than four symptoms and met all other criteria are stated to have experienced a "limited-symptom attack" (DSM-IV, 1994). Panic attacks occur unexpectedly, escalate in intensity in a brief period of time, and typically result in an overwhelming desire for the individual to leave the immediate surroundings and to retreat to a safer location. Variations in the initiation and impact of environmental circumstances lead to three distinct types of panic attacks: (1) *situationally bound panic attacks* that elicit an anxiety response when the individual encounters a feared situation; (2) *situationally predisposed panic attacks* that are more unpredictable and may or may not occur when the individual encounters the feared situation; and (3) *unexpected panic attacks*

Thomas H. Ollendick and Devin A. Byrd • Department of Psychology, Virginia Polytechnic Institute and State University, Blacksburg, Virginia 24061.

Advanced Abnormal Psychology, Second Edition, edited by Hersen and Van Hasselt. Kluwer Academic / Plenum Publishers, New York, 2001.

that happen "out of the blue," seemingly without warning or influence from the environment. Panic attacks can and do occur in all anxiety disorders.

The defining features of *panic disorder*, according to DSM-IV, are as follows: (1) the person has experienced repeated *and* unexpected episodes of panic; (2) in addition, at least one of the episodes is followed by persistent worries, often lasting a month or more, of having another attack or the possible consequences of the attack; and (3) at least four of the following feelings or sensations: shortness of breath, dizziness or faintness; increased or pounding heart rate; trembling or shaking; feeling of choking, sweating, stomach distress or nausea; feeling that one's surroundings or oneself are not quite real; feelings of numbness or tingling sensations; hot flashes or chills; chest pain or discomfort; a fear of dying; and a fear of losing control or of going crazy. In many cases of panic disorder, the episodes may occur daily or at least several times a week. After the first episode of unexpected, inexplicable panic, reassurance by a family doctor or psychologist is usually sufficient to provide temporary relief and a sense of calm. However, when the second or subsequent episodes occur, reassurance is of little value. The person begins to fear that more episodes will occur at unpredictable times and in unexpected settings. The person then becomes even more anxious and apprehensive and rarely achieves a sense of safety thereafter. Panic disorders are thought to be relatively rare in children but occur with some frequency in adolescents (Ollendick, Mattis, & King, 1994).

The presence of a distinct and incessant fear of objects and situations, along with an immediate anxiety response upon exposure to the feared object or situation, are the fundamental features of *specific phobia*. Moreover, unlike adolescents and adults, children may not recognize the illogical nature of their fear(s). Subtypes of specific phobia include the following: (1) situational type (e.g., airplanes, elevators), (2) natural environment type (e.g., storms, water), (3) animal type, (4) blood-injection-injury type, and (5) other type (e.g., vomiting, contracting an illness).

Social phobia is marked by the presence of chronic fear or avoidance of social events and/or performance situations in which the individual might be evaluated by others and result in potential embarrassment or disgrace. Children who experience symptoms of social phobia are likely to avoid social situations involving peers (e.g., playing games), classroom activities (e.g., volunteering to answer questions), and family interactions (e.g., not participating in group activities). In addition, children who have social phobia are likely to experience anxiety nearly every time exposure to the situation occurs and may evidence crying or withdrawing from others in such situations. The primary concern of socially phobic children derives from a desire to avoid embarrassment or humiliation in front of others. In fact, this fear may actually cause impairment in the daily functioning of the child in a number of areas. For example, social anxiety may preclude a child from wanting to speak to or in front of others, to eat in public, or to put on public recitals.

Obsessive–compulsive disorder (OCD) is comprised of both *obsessions* (chronic thoughts, impulses images or ideas that are irritating, unwarranted, and cause considerable anxiety) and *compulsions* (recurrent behaviors that reduce an individual's anxiety and anguish concerning certain thoughts or actions, and that result in a significant amount of time lost each day and marked distress). Criteria for obsessions consist of (1) repetitive and intrusive thoughts, impulses, or images that frequently cause a considerable amount of anxiety and turmoil; (2) an effort to discontinue these repetitive and intrusive thoughts by performing an additional thought or behavior; and (3) an awareness that the obsessions are a function of one's own mind. Criteria for compulsions consist of (1) recurrent behaviors (e.g., touching items in a certain manner, ordering) or mental actions (e.g., saying words over and over, counting) that are performed in response to an obsession, and (2) the function or purpose of the compulsion is to reduce any anxiety resulting from an obsession or to circumvent an anticipated scenario. Common compulsions in children are hand washing, counting, and other ritual-like behaviors.

The primary components of *separation anxiety disorder* (SAD) include significant anxiety upon anticipation of, or actual separation from, a parent or an important adult figure (i.e., individuals to whom the child is attached). In children, the expressed fear and anxiety must be considered inappropriate for the child's age. It is common for very young children to express a fear of separation. Criteria for SAD include the following: (1) repetitive, inordinate turmoil upon separation from attachment individuals; (2) repetitive, inordinate worry about losing or harm happening to attachment individuals; (3) repetitive, inordinate turmoil that an unexpected situation will result in the separation from attachment individuals; (4) repetitive hesitation or unwillingness to attend school due to worry about being separated from attachment individuals; (5) repetitive and inordinate worry and fear of being alone or without attachment figures at home or in other environments; (6) repetitive hesitation or unwillingness to go to sleep without being near attachment individuals; (7) repetitive nightmares focused on themes of separation; and (8) repetitive complaints of physical symptoms upon anticipation or actual separation from attachment individuals.

Generalized anxiety disorder (GAD, formerly known as overanxious disorder) is characterized by chronic and heightened anxiety or worry about numerous situations or events that occur at home, school, or in extracurricular activities. Along with these initial criteria, a child may find it difficult to stop worrying, especially in stressful situations. These children are known to worry about the past, the present, and the future. They are, in short, chronic worriers. Diagnostic features of GAD include (1) feeling uptight and tense, (2) weariness, (3) trouble concentrating, (4) grumpiness, (5) muscle strain, and (6) sleep difficulties.

Posttraumatic stress disorder (PTSD) involves experiencing a life event that is traumatic, life threatening, or out of the ordinary in normal life experiences. Life events such as witnessing a shooting, getting robbed, being sexually abused, experiencing a natural disaster (i.e., flood, earthquake) or a man-made disaster (i.e., fire), and being physically abused may qualify as traumatic events. Of course, these events are not necessarily traumatic to every child who experiences them; rather, the child's own understanding and his or her "meaning" of the event may qualify the type of response observed (Keppel-Benson & Ollendick, 1993). To meet criteria for PTSD, several symptoms must be expressed in three major areas: *intrusion*, *avoidance* and *overarousal*. Symptoms of intrusion include (1) repetitive, bothersome dreams of the event that may or may not have recognizable content; (2) a feeling as if the event were happening again; (3) repetitive and unavoidable thoughts, perceptions, or images of the event which may be evidenced in play activity; (4) extreme psychological torment when reminded of the event by internal or external sources that typify the traumatic event; and (5) extreme physiological responses when reminded of the event by internal or external sources that typify the traumatic event. Symptoms of avoidance include (1) a feeling that one's life is shortened; (2) an inability to have loving feelings; (3) feelings of being apart from or not in touch with others; (4) anhedonic feelings about activities that once were enjoyable; (5) lacking the ability to recall significant parts of the traumatic event; (6) avoidance of situations (i.e., people, places, or things) that remind the person of the traumatic event; and (7) avoidance of thoughts, feelings, or conversations referring to the traumatic event (DSM-IV, 1994). Overarousal symptoms include (1) an overemphasized startle response, (2) an increased reaction to stimuli, (3) trouble concentrating, (4) grumpiness or an inability to control anger, and (5) problems falling and staying asleep.

EPIDEMIOLOGY

Before the early 1980s, few epidemiological studies of childhood anxiety existed; however, since that time, a considerable amount of research has been done. Numerous studies have found that anxiety disorders are the most prevalent disorder in childhood and adolescence, even more so than conduct disorder, oppositional defiant disorder, attention-deficit hyperactivity disorder, depressive disorders, substance abuse, and eating disorders (Anderson, Williams, McGee, & Silva, 1987; Kashani & Orvaschel, 1990). Epidemiological studies continue to show the pervasiveness, severity, and duration of anxiety disorders in children and adolescents. Studies have been conducted in both clinical and nonclinical samples.

Studies conducted with nonclinical samples have revealed prevalence rates that range from 2.7 % to 7.3% for overanxious disorder, 0.7% to 12.9% for separation anxiety disorder, 2.4% to 9.2% for simple or specific phobia, and 1.0% to 1.1% for social phobia (Anderson et al., 1987; Bird et al., 1988; Costello et al., 1988b; Kashani & Orvaschel, 1990; Velez, Johnson, & Cohen, 1989). Overall, prevalence rates for anxiety disorders have been estimated at 12% in community samples (Anderson et al., 1987), perhaps as high as 17%.

Epidemiological studies conducted with boys and girls have often revealed that girls are more likely to evince higher levels of anxiety than boys (LaPouse & Monk, 1959). For instance, research studies have shown that girls have a higher prevalence rate than boys for simple phobia (Kashani et al., 1987), separation anxiety disorder (Kashani et al., 1987; Velez et al., 1989), and overanxious disorder (Velez et al., 1989). On the other hand, some researchers have reported that differences between boys and girls in fears and worries are negligible or nonexistent before age 5 (Anderson, 1994). Following entry into primary schools, however, girls tend to increase their self-reports of fears and worries more than boys (Werry & Quay, 1971). Marks (1987) notes that significant differences between boys and girls for fears are not usually evidenced until 10 or 11 years of age when boys evidence a drastic decline in self-reported levels of fears. However, Ollendick and colleagues (Ollendick, King, & Frary, 1989; Ollendick & Yule, 1990; Ollendick, Yang, King, Dong, & Akande, 1996) report differences in fear between boys and girls as early as 7 years of age that persist into adolescence and young adulthood.

During the early years of development, young children are likely to report *fears and worries* related to fear of animals, strangers, the dark, being alone, storms, going to see the doctor or dentist, or being separated from their parents or another important individual, as evidenced in separation anxiety disorder (Anderson, 1994; Graham, 1979). Conversely, adolescents usually report fewer fears and worries (Ollendick et al., 1989, 1994); however, the prevalence of *anxiety disorders* increases during this developmental period (Kashani et al., 1987; LaPouse & Monk, 1959). Although the occurrence of fears and worries does not end once a child becomes an adolescent, a change in the source of the anxiety may occur. Specifically, children have a tendency to fear objects and situations wherein they perceive themselves as having little or no control (i.e., storms, the dark). The source of fears and worries during the period of adolescence typically resides in social evaluative situations (i.e., test taking, speaking in front of others, and dating situations) and a general worry for numerous life situations, as evidenced in generalized anxiety disorder (Anderson, 1994).

Prevalence rates for anxiety disorders in multiethnic populations have received some limited attention. A study of Japanese adolescents conducted by Abe and Matsui (1981) revealed that girls were more likely to report symptoms of phobia than boys, whereas self-reported fears for social situations were equally reported by both boys and girls. Last and Perrin (1993) conducted a study involving 30 African-American and 139 Caucasian children.

Results of this study revealed that Caucasian children were more likely to report a higher lifetime prevalence rate for separation anxiety disorder, avoidant disorder, overanxious disorder, panic disorder, obsessive–compulsive disorder, and social phobia. Conversely, African-American children were more likely to report a higher lifetime prevalence rate for posttraumatic stress disorder and simple phobia. In addition, 53% of Caucasian children reported experiencing symptoms of school refusal, whereas 30% of African-American child participants reported experiencing such symptoms.

Overall, epidemiological studies conducted during the past 15 years have shown a rather clear and consistent picture of anxiety disorders in children and adolescents. According to this research, girls are more likely to experience and report fears and worries at an earlier age and for longer periods of time than boys. One possible explanation for the decline of self-reported fears by boys upon entering school may be related to the development of social desirability in boys or increased peer pressure to "not be afraid." Results of studies also reveal that younger children are more likely to experience fears and worries than their adolescent counterparts, who are more likely to experience anxiety disorders. Studies conducted of varying ethnic groups have provided suggestive, albeit scant, information. To date, adequate epidemiological information has been obtained for gender and age but not ethnicity. In sum, additional studies need to be conducted in all areas (i.e., gender, age, and ethnicity), as well as interactions among these characteristics, to provide a better understanding of the clinical presentation and correlates of anxiety disorders in children and adolescents.

CLINICAL PICTURE

Gaining a full understanding of each anxiety disorder often requires referral to specific criteria that differentiate one disorder from another (e.g., the specific features associated with each anxiety disorder discussed earlier in the chapter). On the other hand, it is also possible to understand anxiety disorders by examining the three features (i.e., physiology, affect, and cognition) that are common to all anxiety disorders.

The examination of biological factors in the development of childhood anxiety disorders has resulted in a wealth of information necessary to understand the role of *physiology* in the expression of anxiety. One researcher who has contributed to the advancement of theory in this field is Panksepp (1990). Specifically, work with the central nervous system as it relates to the amygdala, anterior lateral hypothalamus, and central gray area has led to the endorsement of this system as a biological substrate that signifies danger and identifies a "fundamental fear state in humans" (Kagan, 1998). More specifically, the main function of this system is to produce a primary fear state that results in freezing, flight, or a defensive aggressive response based upon the nature of the danger. Gray (1982) expanded on Panksepp's biological position to explain how human affective systems help account for human temperaments. Gray speculated that the behavioral inhibition system was "activated by conditioned stimuli associated with punishment; events linked to omission or termination of reward and novelty." Secondly, Gray stated that the flight-fight system (involving the amygdala, hypothalamus, and central gray) was activated by aversive events like pain that resulted in escape behavioral responses. Thirdly, the behavioral approach system (involving the basal ganglia, dopaminergic tracts, thalamus, and neocortical areas) is said to be associated with reward or termination of punishment that results in "approach behavior" (Kagan, 1998).

Research studies conducted on anxiety disorders and *cognition* have revealed that maladaptive thought patterns often result in maintaining and increasing the intensity of anxiety symptom expression. Automatic thoughts and/or cognitive schemas that are consistent with themes of anxiety play an important role in the progression and maintenance of anxiety disorders (Beck, Emery, & Greenberg, 1985). *Automatic thoughts* are cognitions that occur before and/or during an anxiety-provoking situation. These thoughts, considered maladaptive, impede the person's ability to deal effectively with an anxiety-provoking situation (Beck et al., 1985). Furthermore, if an individual's anxious thoughts persist, a pattern of responding to these anxious situations is created and the individual utilizes that pattern in future situations. This pattern of responding often includes (1) "hypervigilance and selective abstraction of possible danger cues, to the exclusion of other environmental cues; (2) magnification of the degree of threat; and (3) overgeneralization of environmental cues that represent danger." Thus, anxious children tend to have a maladaptive or distorted way of thinking about anxiety-provoking or dangerous situations in relation to normal children. Furthermore, *cognitive schemas* serve as "maps" (i.e., memories) of previously encountered anxiety-provoking experiences that are usually recalled when a child encounters similar situations in the future. Thus, the process of *cognitive rumination*, or the replay of a situation in which the child experienced the excessive anxiety, frequently aids in solidifying the cognitive schema. The repetitive process of engaging in cognitive rumination and cataloging "anxiety-provoking" cognitive schemas hinders a child's ability to perform well in subsequent situations of a similar nature.

Research studies conducted with "test-anxious children" provide a rather descriptive illustration of the interaction among automatic thoughts, cognitive schemas, cognitive rumination, and subsequent poor academic performance. The main factors that contribute to poor academic performance during test-taking have been outlined by Wine (1971) in a "cognitive-attentional model of anxiety." Specifically, the model states that test-anxious children often divide their cognitive efforts into two areas during the test-taking process: (1) task irrelevant thoughts (i.e., debilitating thoughts) and (2) task relevant thoughts (i.e., facilitative thoughts). In contrast, Wine states that children who are not test-anxious typically focus their cognitive efforts in the area of task-relevant thoughts (i.e., facilitative thoughts) and subsequently perform better on tests than their anxious counterparts during evaluative situations. Additional test-anxiety research by Zatz and Chassin (1983) revealed similar debilitating cognitive patterns for test-anxious children. In particular, results of a study conducted with fifth and sixth grade children revealed that test-anxious children reported more negative self-evaluation items, fewer positive self-evaluation items, and more off-task thoughts than low to moderately test-anxious children. Highly test-anxious children also reported more on-task and coping self-statements than their low to moderately test-anxious counterparts. These results suggest that test-anxious children were more likely to engage in task-debilitating and task-facilitating thoughts during the course of test-taking situations than their low to moderate test-anxious counterparts. Therefore, taking the previous concepts into consideration, the interaction of automatic thoughts (i.e., off-task thoughts), cognitive schemas (i.e., previous poor test performances), and cognitive rumination (i.e., repetitive thoughts) illustrates the process that can lead to increased levels of anxiety. Warren, Ollendick, and King (1996) demonstrated similar effects in early adolescent children.

As a child matures, its cognitive schemas and cognitive rumination develop into "cognitive thought-patterns" (i.e., attributional style) that are not just used occasionally but are accessed more frequently and usually on a daily basis. *Attributional Style* is described as an individual's explanation of, or way of understanding, daily life events (Seligman, Abramson, Semmel, & von Baeyer, 1979). The manner in which a child attributes causes of daily life events can positively or negatively affect how it views a single event, as well as others in the future. In particular, it is hypothesized that children make attributions for life events according to the following three dimensions: (1) internality versus externality, (2) stability versus instability, and (3) globality versus specificity. The first dimension examines whether the cause of the event was a result of the individual (i.e., internal), something or someone else (i.e., external), or both. The second dimension reveals whether the individual thinks the event will most likely occur again with high frequency (i.e., stable), will never happen again (i.e., unstable), or may occur again but not necessarily so. Finally, the third dimension deals with whether the event affected most areas of one's life (i.e., global), affected only a specified area of one's life (i.e., specific), or affected some areas of their life.

Attributional style has been categorized according to two types: *positive* and *negative*. A positive attributional style is viewed as an optimistic style of explaining life events, whereas a negative attributional style has been described as a pessimistic manner by which or through which individuals explain life events. Attributional style has typically been used to examine the nature of attributions in depressed children; however, most recently, attributional style has also been examined in anxiety disorders. The connection between anxiety and the negative attributional style might be explained by the fact that people who believe that failures are due to internal and stable causes may directly link those attributions to their fear and avoidance of certain situations (Bell-Dolan & Wessler, 1994). Initially, work in the area of anxiety and attributions for children led researchers to examine test-taking situations and children's levels of performance. However, more recent theories and research have expanded the study of anxiety and attributions to include interpersonal interactions (i.e., part of social-evaluative situations), which tend to elicit negative attributional styles. For example, in a study conducted by Bell-Dolan and Last (1990), the attributional styles of children and adolescents, who ranged in age from 7 to 17 years, were examined. The children and adolescents were categorized as normal controls, those who had attention-deficit hyperactivity disorder, and those who had an anxiety disorder. Results showed that anxious children made more negative attributions for bad life events than normal children; however, no differences were noted in attributions for positive life events. An examination of an anxious child's attributions may reveal valuable information concerning the presence, severity, and pattern of negativistic thinking that could be linked to the maintenance of anxious symptomatology over time.

The role of cognitions in the presentation of anxiety disorders can be considered paramount to the physical and affective components of anxiety, even though the contributions of the two latter components to the manifestation of anxiety should not be ignored. Frequently, the course and duration of anxiety disorders are governed by maladaptive cognitions that act as "triggers" for recalling cognitive schemas of previously experienced anxiety-provoking situations. This interactive process frequently activates the physical and affective components of the anxiety process. Moreover, investigation of factors such as the habitual explanation of life events (i.e., attributional style) provides a wealth of information. In fact, investigating the role of attributional style in anxiety disorders may, in time, reveal an even greater influence on the perpetuation of anxiety disorders than cognitive schemas and provide additional information concerning the course and prognosis for the specific anxiety disorders.

COURSE AND PROGNOSIS

Changes in the course (i.e., manifestation) of anxiety can occur across situations and over time. Studies of children who had anxiety disorders reveal that fluctuations between the development of new anxiety disorders and the attenuation of symptoms associated with others can occur over short and long periods of time (see Seligman & Ollendick, 1998). In one study, children between 6 and 19 years of age were diagnosed with overanxious disorder and separation anxiety disorder (Keller et al., 1992). Results of the study revealed that the average length of time for both disorders was 4 years, and that after an 8-year period, 46% of the children were likely to have retained anxiety symptoms from their original diagnosis. In addition, results revealed that 31% of children who recovered from an anxiety disorder experienced a subsequent anxiety episode. A cross-sectional, longitudinal study conducted with 151 children and adolescents between the ages of 2 and 15 years of age (Cantwell & Baker, 1989) also revealed similar findings. Children and adolescents were diagnosed with overanxious disorder, avoidant disorder, or separation anxiety disorder. During the follow-up evaluations, obtained 4–5 years later, 24% of the children and adolescents had the same diagnosis evidenced during the initial assessment. In addition, children diagnosed with avoidant disorder had the greatest stability rates during the 4–5 year period, whereas children diagnosed with separation anxiety disorder had the lowest stability rates and best recovery rates of the three anxiety disorders.

Developmentally, fears may evolve for a number of reasons. Frequently, young children develop fears due to the emergence of a *perception of danger*, although they may not understand how the situation may or may not affect them. For instance, children exposed to new environments (i.e., daycare) may develop certain fears due to a perception of threat or danger involving those new situations. An additional component that may affect the development of fears in childhood is *level of control*. A child who perceives that a situation is potentially dangerous and feels little or no control over it is more likely to develop subsequent fears than a child who perceives that a dangerous situation is controllable. As a child matures into an adolescent, it gains a greater understanding and ability to make decisions about dangerous situations and levels of controllability. Moreover, an ability to examine situations for danger and controllability enables the adolescent to establish the *rational* or *irrational* basis of a feared situation or subsequent danger.

During late childhood and adolescence, fear associated with encountering evaluative situations has a tendency to increase, often in situations involving academic testing and social evaluation. One study that examined test anxiety in 47 Australian adolescents (grades 9 and 10) revealed that 18 of the children identified as high-test-anxious were also diagnosed with an anxiety or phobic disorder. In comparison, only two of the children identified as low-test-anxious were also diagnosed with an anxiety or phobic disorder (King, Mietz, Tinney, & Ollendick, 1995). The most common diagnosis for test-anxious children was overanxious disorder, whereby a tendency for the child to engage in worry about numerous areas of its life predominated. Results of the King et al. study also revealed that the high-test-anxious adolescents endorsed significantly higher levels of self-reported fear on the Fear Survey Schedule for Children-Revised (Ollendick, 1983) and the Revised Children's Manifest Anxiety Scale (Reynolds & Richmond, 1978) than their low-test-anxious counterparts.

The role of *gender* in the manifestation of anxiety often reveals a clinical picture of differences between boys and girls; girls show heightened levels of fear or anxiety. Results of studies consistently reveal that girls are more likely to (1) experience symptoms of anxiety and (2) experience anxiety for longer periods of time than boys (Ollendick & King, 1991, 1994; Treadwell, Flannery-Schroeder, & Kendall, 1995). For instance, girls consistently report increased anxious symptomatology on self-report measures such as the Revised Children's Manifest Anxiety Scale and the State Trait Anxiety Inventory for Children (STAIC; Papay & Hedl, 1978) than their male counterparts. Similarly, girls have also reported elevated levels of fear on subscale scores of the Fear Survey Schedule for Children Revised and overall fear scores (Ollendick, Matson, & Helsel, 1985; Ollendick et al., 1989).

Studies reveal that the course of anxiety symptoms and the disorder itself is variable. Although remission of symptoms and disorders is common, relapse rates also indicate the potential for the same disorder to reappear or new anxiety disorders to appear following remittance of an anxiety disorder. In reference to prognosis, several factors such as attachment relationships, temperament, social support, life events, self-concept and acculturation can influence the course of anxiety.

In the clinical and research literature, it has been shown that a child's early *attachment relationships* are the basis for future relationships and are also the source of potential difficulties. In particular, Bowlby (1951) asserted that attachment behaviors are understandable within the realm of the greater environment because they relate to the child's ultimate goal of establishing a *sense of protection* in relation to the caregiver (Thompson, 1998). For instance, if a young child fails to feel protected and at ease in the family environment, it may be unable to feel secure in subsequent situations involving other individuals, and this may result in the development of anxious symptomatology at a very early age. Ainsworth (1973) was influential in classifying three specific attachment behaviors (insecure-avoidant, insecure-resistant, secure) according to Bowlby's theory of attachment (Thompson, 1998). In addition, other researchers, such as Main and Solomon (1990), suggested establishing the presence of a fourth classification of attachment in children, *disorganized*, children who are described as behaviorally inconsistent (Thompson, 1998).

Research has shown a developmental relationship between attachment and personality formation. More specifically, results reveal that the mastery, or failure thereof, of establishing secure attachment relationships subsequently affects the child's level of independence and ability to interact effectively in other relationships (Thompson, 1998). Therefore, it is possible that deficiencies acquired at an early age may influence in the future development of anxious symptomatology or full-blown disorders such as separation anxiety and social phobia.

Secondly, *temperament* can be defined as, "inherent, constitutionally-based characteristics in emotional, motor, attentional reactivity and self-regulation that constitute the core of personality and influence directions for development" (Rothbart & Bates, 1998, p. 106). The three temperament types are defined as (1) *easy* (i.e., regular in bodily activity), (2) *slow to warm up* (i.e., inhibited and tending to withdraw), and (3) *difficult* (i.e., children who have minimal regularity) (Thomas & Chess, 1977). Because frequent interactions between a child (with a slow to warm up or difficult temperament) and its parents (and other individuals), are less than optimal, negative interactions may result in a child developing feelings of anxiety when encountering social interactions.

Social support is a construct that has frequently been examined by researchers who seek to examine the protective factors and development of subsequent psychological distress such as anxiety. The basic premise is that social support can be a risk or protective factor against harmful psychological symptoms. Thus, if individuals can secure and/or access a number of resources from their social support networks (i.e., peers, siblings, parents), then they will be better able to counteract the effects of stressful life events (i.e., test taking, giving a speech, panic attacks). Results from studies have shown that social support can be conceptualized according to several classes of support such as nuclear family support, extended family support (i.e., kin networks), and peer support (i.e., non-kin networks).

Other researchers have indicated that stressful life events are significantly correlated with an increase in susceptibility to psychological distress such as anxiety. Specifically, repeated exposure to chronic, *daily hassles* increases the rate of psychological problems or distress (Burnham, Hough, Karno, Escobar, & Telles, 1987; Dressler, 1985), whereas *major stressful life events* moderate the effects of these daily life hassles. The impact of life events on subsequent psychological distress (i.e., anxiety, depression) has most often been examined in studies involving attributional style. Such studies reveal that positive attributions may insulate the person from the insidious effects of repeated stress.

Although not discussed as extensively in the literature, it can be postulated that a child's self-concept can impact the development and subsequent level of anxiety. Harter (1986) has emerged as a significant theoretician and contributor to the field of self-concept research on children and adolescents. She has partitioned the construct of self-concept into five distinct domains in children: *scholastic importance*, *athletic competence*, *physical attractiveness*, *social acceptance*, and *appropriate behavioral conduct*. Through numerous research studies (Harter, 1986; Harter & Jackson, 1993; Harter & Whitesell, 1996), Harter and her colleagues have determined that these distinct domains hold different levels of significance for parents (i.e., parent-salient) and peers (i.e., peer-salient) and can have positive and/or negative effects on the development of children and adolescents.

Utilizing James's (1892) theory of self-worth, researchers examined the construct of self-concept in terms of the dimensions of *competence* and *importance*. In particular, research determined that a child's level of competence (i.e., high or low) in domains of importance (according to self, parents or peers) has a significant impact on self-concept (Renouf & Harter, 1990). Renouf and Harter further assert that as a result of a child's success or failure in an identified domain of importance, differential affective responses ensue. Specifically, if a child achieves success in an identified domain of importance, its affective response will be one of cheerfulness and positive affect. Although not discussed in the literature heretofore, if a child fails or has considerable difficulty in succeeding in an identified domain of importance, it can be surmised that its affective response may result in anxious symptomatology. For example, a child who experiences test anxiety may believe that it is not competent in the academic domain of self-concept and expresses low self-concept accordingly. Similarly, a child who experiences social anxiety frequently may also report low self-concept for the social acceptance domain of self-concept.

Finally, level of *acculturation* may be related to the development of anxiety in children and adolescents. Acculturation can be defined as the extent to which ethnic-cultural minorities participate in the cultural traditions, values, beliefs, and practices of their own culture versus those of the majority culture (Landrine & Klonoff, 1996). Research studies have shown that a strong relationship exists between an individual's level of acculturation (i.e., traditional, bicultural, and highly acculturated) and the development of subsequent psychological disorders (Burnham, Hough, Karno, Escobar, & Telles, 1987; Montgomery & Orozco, 1985). For example, an African-American child's efforts to balance personal ethnic group needs with efforts to create and maintain positive interactions with the majority culture (i.e., Caucasian values and traditions) may result in a variety of psychological disorders, including anxiety. In one early study, Fordham and Ogbu (1986) investigated the relationship among acculturation, ethnicity, and achievement in highly acculturated African-American children. They observed that African-American children who desired to achieve success in the academic world often did so by embracing the attitudes, behaviors, and values normally associated with the majority culture. As a result, these highly acculturated students were often castigated by their African-American peers for not being "Black enough," though they were not totally accepted by their Caucasian counterparts either. As a result of being rejected by their African-American peers and not being totally accepted by their Caucasian peers, these highly acculturated children and adolescents were at increased risk of experiencing symptoms of psychological distress. Upon investigation of other ethnic groups, similar results may be revealed.

Treatment

To date, treatments for anxiety disorders in children and adolescents have included techniques such as *response prevention, modeling, systematic desensitization, flooding, contingency management*, and *cognitive-behavioral procedures*. Several well-controlled single-case design studies provide preliminary evidence for the utility of behavioral and cognitive-behavioral procedures with overanxious and separation-anxious youth (e.g., Eisen & Silverman, 1993; Hagopian, Weist, & Ollendick, 1990; Kane & Kendall, 1989; Ollendick, 1995; Ollendick, Hagopian, & Huntzinger, 1991). These early studies provided the foundation for the randomized clinical trials that followed. Three such studies were conducted.

In the first study, Kendall (1994) compared the outcome of a 16-session cognitive-behavioral treatment (CBT) protocol to a wait-list control condition. Forty-seven 9- to 13-year-old children who met diagnoses for an anxiety disorder (overanxious disorder, separation anxiety disorder, or avoidant disorder) were assigned randomly to treatment or the wait-list control condition. Treatment was conducted with a manual and was flexibly implemented. On a majority of the measures, treated children fared better than wait-list children. The most dramatic difference was the percentage of children *not* meeting diagnostic criteria for an anxiety disorder at the end of treatment: 5% of the wait-list group versus 64% of treated cases. One- and three-year follow-up revealed that treatment gains were maintained (Kendall & Southam-Gerow, 1996). More recently, Kendall and colleagues reaffirmed the efficacy of this treatment with 94 children (aged 9 to 13) randomly assigned to CBT and wait-list control conditions (Kendall et al., 1997). Seventy-one percent of the children did *not* meet diagnostic criteria at the end of treatment, compared to 5.8% of those in the wait-list condition.

Subsequent to Kendall's first randomized clinical trial, his CBT approach was evaluated independently by an investigatory team in Australia (Barrett, Dadds, & Rapee, 1996). In this study, 79 children ranging between 7 and 14 years of age were randomly assigned to one of three conditions: (1) Cognitive Behavioral Treatment (CBT), (2) CBT plus Family Anxiety Management Training (CBT + FAM), and (3) a wait-listing control condition (WL). Treatment was 12 weeks in duration. Results revealed that both CBT and CBT + FAM significantly decreased self-report measures of anxiety following the conclusion of treatment. Moreover, self-reports of the children reflected continued improvements and maintenance of treatment gains at 6- and 12-month follow-up sessions. In fact, participants from the CBT + FAM condition evidenced significant improvements over participants from the CBT condition in several of the dependent variables. In addition, at posttreatment, 26% of the wait-list children were diagnosis-free, compared to 57% of the CBT-only and 84% of the combined treatment conditions. At follow-up six months later, 71% of the CBT children were diagnosis-free versus 84% of the CBT + FAM children; at one-year follow-up, CBT + FAM still was superior to the CBT alone condition (96% compared to 71%). Results of this study indicate that the combination of both a cognitive behavioral treatment (CBT) and a family component (FAM) is more effective in treating anxiety than CBT alone (Ollendick & King, 1998).

Although results of these studies are favorable, most of them have been conducted and evaluated with Caucasian samples, and few ethnic minorities were represented. The absence of such youth in these studies is especially important inasmuch as research shows that African-American clients have a tendency to attend fewer sessions, are less likely to benefit from treatment (Sue, Fujino, Takeuchi, & Zane, 1991), and are more likely to terminate treatment than their Caucasian counterparts (Rosenheck, Fontana, & Cottrol, 1995). Consequently, the relative lack of ethnic minority youth in treatment studies raises questions concerning the validity of established treatment protocols for use with nonmajority children and adolescents. Solutions to the present difficulties have been offered by some researchers who advocate using ethnically sensitive treatment as an approach to therapy with African-American and other nonmajority youth (Byrd, Davis-Parker, Shenoy, Ollendick, & Jones, 1997).

CASE DESCRIPTION

Lacy, an 8-year-old Caucasian girl in the third grade of a local elementary school, was brought to our clinic by her parents for a psychological evaluation, presenting complaints centered on three problematic areas: (1) Lacy's concern that her mother might be injured and possibly die, (2) nighttime problems characterized by refusal to go to and sleep in her own bed, and (3) statements from Lacy that "Maybe I just don't belong on this earth." These problems were reported to have begun approximately seven months before her first appointment. At that time, Lacy's mother had back surgery. The surgery occurred in early July, and Lacy's fears about her mother's health preceded surgery by about three weeks. These worries continued to mount during the summer months but did not reach a point where they kept Lacy homebound or continually at her mother's side. In fact, she was able to attend a church summer camp (first week in August) and spend the night with friends periodically throughout the remainder of the summer. Her worries were expressed primarily through excessive questions about mother's health, statements about her own health, and seeking reassurance from her mother (and occasionally her father) that it was okay for her to be away from home.

When she began the third grade, her problems began to worsen, as she expressed continual concern about "being away from mother all day." Lacy reported that she was afraid something might happen to her mother and that no one would be there to help her. Lacy's father worked an early morning shift (6:00 a.m. to 2:00 p.m.), and her only sister (Tammy, age 19) worked during the day as well (8:00 a.m. to 3:00 p.m.). Due to travel requirements, her father left home about 5:00 a.m. and returned about 3:30 p.m. Her sister left home for work about 7:15 a.m., whereas Lacy left for school at 7:45 a.m. Lacy was the last member of her family to leave the home. Due to complications from the back surgery, her mother remained at home and was temporarily unemployed. Before the surgery, she worked as a receptionist at a local medical clinic.

Lacy never became school avoidant, possibly because both parents insisted that she go to school each day. The parents did report, however, that she frequently complained of headaches and stomachaches on school days and that on at least four occasions she had been allowed to stay home from school due to reported illness. Throughout this period, she continued to excel in school (A's and B's) and to have several friends. Teachers reported that she was well-liked, a class leader, hard working, and a good student.

Around the third week of the school term, she began to express increasing concern about sleeping in her own bedroom (her bedroom was upstairs, across the hall from her sister's; her parents' bedroom was downstairs on the first floor). She complained about having nightmares and being frightened by "zombies" who came into her room. During the next three months, the nightmares increased to the point where she was either sleeping in her parents' room or outside their door. In addition, she exhibited a number of avoidant behaviors, including arguing about bedtime, refusing to go to bed, getting out of bed, calling out once in bed, and making numerous requests (e.g., drink of water, go to the bathroom). Also, she became more "clingy" to her mother and wanted to be near her after school until bedtime. Further, she stopped spending weekend nights at her friends and did not invite any of her friends to stay with her. She continued to go to school, however, and did well academically. Her mother started back to work on a part-time basis at this time.

About four weeks before her first appointment (February), Lacy began to make disparaging statements about herself and seemed to be "sad and unhappy." At this time, her father reported first hearing the statement, "Maybe I just don't belong on this earth." Both parents reported similar depressive statements during the ensuing weeks. Although they felt that Lacy would "outgrow" her worries about her mother's health and the nighttime fears, they were greatly concerned by her verbal statements and sullen appearance. Referral was made at that time upon recommendation of the family physician.

During the initial interview conducted with her parents present, Lacy appeared more anxious than depressed. She fidgeted in her chair, clasped and unclasped her hands, swung her feet, bit her lips, and stammered as she spoke. She reported being "very afraid" that her mother "might get sick again," even though at this time her mother had returned to work part time. She wondered aloud, "Who will take care of her.... Daddy is always at work and Sissy is at work too, you know." As for her nighttime fears, she indicated that the zombies were real ("I really saw them! They were real!") and that they might kill her. She stated further that a boy had told her "nightmares can cause you to be frightened to death." Presumably, linking this thought with her overarching concerns about her mother's well-being, she was convinced that she would die and "no one would be there to help Mommy." As for her depressive and suicidal-like thoughts, she stated in a rather straightforward way, "I can't be happy ... I used to be ... but not now ... even my friends don't like me now."

Based on this initial interview and the reported chronology of events, it was hypothesized that Lacy's primary problem centered on separation anxiety. She had exaggerated and unrealistic worries that harm would come to her mother and/or herself and that she would be separated from her mother. She complained of physical distress upon leaving for school, was reluctant to have friends over or to stay with friends, and refused to sleep alone. Further, social withdrawal and depression were evident. In brief, she showed marked signs of the major criteria for SAD.

During the second session, the Anxiety Disorders Inventory for Children (Silverman & Nelles, 1988) was administered. It confirmed the impression of SAD, as well as accompanying major depression. Other anxiety disorders, such as avoidant disorder and overanxious disorders, were ruled out by the presence of good friendships at school and on weekends and the specific focus of the separation anxiety concerns. She did have additional phobias, but these all seemed related to nighttime fears and being left alone.

Results of psychometric assessment supported this picture. Lacy completed the Revised Children's Manifest Anxiety Scale (Reynolds & Richmond, 1979), the Fear Survey Schedule for Children-Revised (Ollendick, 1983), and the Children's Depression Inventory (Kovacs, 1978). On the RCMAS, she received a score of 18, well above the mean for her age. Among her endorsements were, "Often I feel sick in my stomach," "I have bad dreams," "I wake up scared some of the time," "I worry when I go to bed at night," and "It is hard for me to get to sleep at night." Similarly, she scored above age and gender norms on the FSSC-R. She obtained a total score of 168 and endorsed 26 fears ("a lot"). Among the specific fears were "ghosts or spooky things," "getting lost in a strange place," "a burglar breaking into our house," "the sight of blood," "cemeteries," "nightmares," "going to bed in the dark," "being alone," "dark places," and "having my parents argue." Similarly, on the CDI, she obtained an elevated score of 16; again, this score was well above the average for her age and gender. Items such as "I am sad many times," "I do not like myself," "I have trouble sleeping every night," and "I think about killing myself, but would not do it" were endorsed. Importantly, she also reported that "I have fun in many things," "I have fun at school many times," and "I have plenty of friends." Finally, on the Revised Behavior Problem Checklist (Quay & Peterson, 1983), both parents rated her high on the anxiety-withdrawal factor (scores of 15 and 12). Other factor scores, except the one for motor excess, were within normal limits. Clearly, these self-report and other report instruments confirmed the overall picture that Lacy had separation anxiety to a significant degree.

Based on our assessment, we decided to address her nighttime fears directly. This decision was based on the relationship of these fears to the separation problems and our previous experience that children generally respond favorably to the treatment procedures available for nighttime fears. A procedure based on the work of Graziano and Mooney (1980, 1982) was used. Initially, relaxation training and self-instruction training were implemented during six sessions. Response to these procedures was slow and only partially effective. Lacy continued to report considerable "state" anxiety about sleeping in her own bed and to average only two nights a week sleeping in her own room throughout this phase of treatment. Accordingly, a reinforcement component was added. Within three weeks, Lacy was sleeping in her own bed seven nights a week and reporting much less anxiety. Nightmares desisted and she started once again to have friends spend the night with her. In addition, four weekly sessions served to bolster these effects. A total of 13 weekly treatment sessions was conducted. Follow-up sessions at one month and six months posttreatment were provided to monitor these gains and to conduct post-treatment assessment. Significant reductions in anxiety, fear, and depression were noted. Further, although both mother and father continued to view Lacy as somewhat anxious (anxiety-withdrawal scores of 8 and 7, respectively), her scores were significantly below those reported at pretreatment. Finally, at follow-up, she was sleeping in her own bed seven nights a week, reporting no nightmares, no longer expressing concern about her mother's or her own well-being, and expressing positive statements about herself. Throughout treatment, her father and sister continued to work their regular schedules; as previously noted, her mother worked part time as well.

Overall, this case nicely illustrates the complexity of SAD, as well as its assessment and treatment. Multimodal assessment was undertaken, and treatment based on this assessment was implemented (Ollendick & Huntzinger, 1990).

FAMILIAL PATTERNS

Researchers and clinicians alike have frequently noted that children who present with symptoms of anxiety and/or fears also have parents (Rutter et al., 1990) and siblings who experience symptoms of anxiety. For instance, in one study conducted by Turner, Beidel, and Costello (1987), children who had anxious parents were seven times more likely to be diagnosed with an anxiety disorder than children of nonanxious parents. In addition, Biederman, Rosenbaum, Bolduc, Faraone, and Hirshfield (1991) examined children of parents diagnosed with major depression, panic disorder with agoraphobia, and panic disorder with agoraphobia *and* major depression. Results revealed that children who had PD with agoraphobic parents and PD with agoraphobia and depressed parents were at a significantly greater risk of developing an anxiety disorder versus children of parents who had major depression alone.

Some studies have revealed that first-degree relatives of individuals who had panic disorder have a four to seven times greater chance of developing panic disorder (DSM-IV, 1994, p. 400), and evidence also exists for the transmission of specific phobias, social phobia, and OCD among first-degree relatives. Data from studies involving monozygotic and dizygotic twins, family observations, and familial history also support the claim of familial transmission (Thapar & McGuffin, 1995). Overall, strong evidence for a familial component of anxiety rests in theories concerning genetic transmission, as well as specific learning histories of fear- or anxiety-inducing experiences. Such a conclusion is consistent with recent experimental evidence that affirms the role of family (especially parental) enhancement of avoidant responses in anxious children (see Barrett, Rapee, Dadds, & Ryan, 1996; Dadds, Barrett,

Rapee, & Ryan, 1996) and the need to involve family members more centrally in the therapeutic process with anxious children (see Ginsburg, Silverman, & Kurtines, 1995; Ollendick & Ollendick, 1997).

DIAGNOSTIC CONSIDERATIONS

In children, anxiety disorders are frequently observed along with other disorders such as conduct disorder (CD), oppositional defiant disorder (ODD), attention-deficit/hyperactivity disorder (ADHD), and major depressive disorder (MDD) (Anderson, 1994; Seligman & Ollendick, 1998). One difficulty that arises during the investigation of more than one disorder or set of symptoms deals with the construct validity of the diagnosis itself. This issue is most commonly observed and raised in making distinctions between anxiety and depression.

Norvell, Brophy, and Finch (1985) conducted a study of 30 inpatient children and found that children's self-reports of anxiety (RCMAS) and depression (CDI) were significantly correlated with one another ($r = .70$). A study of 107 adolescents conducted by Byrd and Ollendick (1996) revealed a significant correlation ($r = .79$) between measures of anxiety (RCMAS) and depression (CDI). In addition, results of a study conducted by Laurent and Stark (1993) revealed that children who were *comorbid* with both anxiety and depression reported significantly more negative statements than their anxious counterparts. Results from these and other studies provide support for the notion that considerable overlap exists between anxiety and depression (King, Ollendick, & Gullone, 1991). Consequently, the ability of instruments to discriminate effectively between anxiety and depression is called into question (Hodges, 1990; Ollendick et al., 1991). As a result, researchers have studied both differences and commonalities between these two disorders.

In 1984, Watson and Clark proposed the concept of *negative affectivity*, or the combination of both anxiety and depression, which is characterized by an overall "bad or negative mood." They describe negative affectivity as a predisposition to experience negative emotions that ultimately affect the person's cognition, self-concept, and world view. The major characteristics of negative affectivity are identified as (1) feelings of nervousness, tension, worry, anger, guilt, self-dissatisfaction, and sadness; (2) a pervasive disposition that can manifest itself in the absence of overt stress; and (3) a focus on the subjective experience as opposed to the objective condition (in which individuals focus more intently on themselves and their surroundings as opposed to how they perform in the outside world).

Negative affectivity is also described by Watson and Clark (1984) as the tendency to experience a wide range of negative and upsetting emotions. Emotions experienced by individuals who have high levels of negative affect include anxiety, tension, anger, worry, frustration, hostility, contempt, disgust, guilt, worthlessness, dissatisfaction, and irritability. High negative affect individuals have a tendency to possess a negative self-concept and to be self-critical, as well as to be dissatisfied with themselves. They also tend to be more introspective and to exhibit behavior withdrawal that reflects a feeling of helplessness, as also seen in depression (Watson et al., 1988). Thus, negative affectivity is seen as a construct that is common to both anxious and depressed individuals; however, Watson and Clark have proposed that positive affectivity differentiates anxiety from depression.

Positive affectivity is a dimension that involves pleasurable involvement in an activity. Furthermore, a high level of positive affectivity includes enthusiasm, energy level, mental alertness, interest, joy, well-being, social dominance, and determination, whereas low positive affectivity involves fatigue, lethargy, and poor functioning (Watson & Tellegen, 1985). Anxiety has been characterized by high negative affectivity, physiological arousal, and varying levels of positive affectivity; depression, on the other hand, has been depicted as a combination of high negative affectivity, low physiological arousal, *and* low positive affectivity (Watson et al., 1988). Studies suggest that positive affectivity is a critical factor in distinguishing between anxiety and depression (Watson & Tellegen, 1985); for example, results from a study conducted by Watson et al. (1988) showed that depressed subjects scored lower on positive affectivity than anxious subjects. These distinctions between negative and positive affectivity may have important implications in the assessment, diagnosis, and treatment of children who have varying levels of anxiety and depression.

SUMMARY

DSM-IV diagnostic criteria have prompted the intricate examination of anxiety disorders in children and adolescents according to a specified set of characteristics, course, and prognosis. In addition, a global dimensional approach to anxiety and its disorders has afforded us the opportunity to explore physiology, affect, and cognition and their respective roles in the onset, expression, and course of these disorders. In epidemiological studies, research methodologies using structured and semistructured clinical interviews have revealed high prevalence rates for the anxiety disorders that approach between 12 and 15% of the youth studied. Although genetic influences must be acknowledged in the course of these disorders, the contributions and influence of psychological/psychosocial factors, including attachment relationships, temperament, social support, life events, self-concept, and acculturation cannot be ignored. Inclusion of these variables in anxiety studies will allow for an even more comprehensive "picture" of anxiety disorders than is observed presently. Considering the potential impact of these variables on the manifestation of anxiety, it is possible that present diagnostic considerations for determining the presence and severity of anxiety disorders will be inadequate to capture differential manifestations in children and adolescents according to age, gender, and ethnicity. Moreover, although behavioral and cognitive-behavioral treatments are effective with anxious children and adolescents, it is evident that these treatments have not been systematically examined in children who vary widely in age and ethnicity. Such studies may need to develop age- and ethnicity-appropriate interventions to realize their maximum effectiveness. Inclusion of family members in treatment may also prove useful. Future studies should examine the effectiveness of these treatment processes in real-life clinical and school settings to determine their utility.

REFERENCES

Abe, K., & Matsui, T. (1981). Age-sex trends of phobic and anxiety symptoms in adolescence. *British Journal of Psychiatry, 138*, 297–302.

Achenbach, T. M., & Edelbrock, C. S. (1991). *Manual for the child behavior checklist and profile.* Burlington: University of Vermont.

Ainsworth, M. D. S. (1973). The development of infant–mother attachment. In B. Caldwell & H. Ricciuit (Eds.), *Review of child development research*, Vol. 3 (pp. 1–94). Chicago: University of Chicago Press.

American Psychiatric Association. (1994). *Diagnostic and statistical manual of mental disorders*, 4th ed. Washington, DC: Author.

Anderson, J. C. (1994). Epidemiological issues. In T. H. Ollendick, N. J. King, & W. Yule (Eds.), *International handbook of phobic and anxiety disorders in children and adolescents* (pp. 43–65). New York: Plenum.

Anderson, J. C., Williams, S. M., McGee, R., & Silva, P. (1987). DSM-III disorders in pre-adolescent children: Prevalence in a large sample from the general population. *Archives of General Psychiatry, 44,* 69–76.

Barrett, P. M., Dadds, M. R., & Rapee, R. M. (1996). Family treatment of childhood anxiety: A controlled trial. *Journal of Consulting and Clinical Psychology, 64,* 333–342.

Barrett, P. M., Rapee, R. M., Dadds, M. R., & Ryan, S. M. (1996). Family enhancement of cognitive style in anxious and aggressive children: Threat bias and the fear effect. *Journal of Abnormal Child Psychology, 24,* 187–203.

Beck, A. T., Emery, G., & Greenberg, R. L. (1985). *Anxiety disorders and phobias: A cognitive perspective.* New York: Basic Books.

Bell-Dolan, D. J., & Last, C. G. (1990). *Attributional style of anxious children.* Paper presented at the *24th Meeting of the Association for the Advancement of Behavior Therapy,* San Francisco.

Bell-Dolan, D. J., & Wessler, A. E. (1994). Attributional style of anxious children: Extensions from cognitive theory and research on adult anxiety. *Journal of Anxiety Disorders, 8,* 79–96.

Biederman, J., Rosenbaum, J. F., Bolduc, E. A., Faraone, S. V., & Hirshfield, D. R. (1991). A high risk study of young children of parents with panic disorder and agoraphobia with and without comorbid major depression. *Psychiatry Research, 37,* 333–348.

Bird, H., Canino, G., Rubio-Stipec, M., Gould, M. S., Ribera, J., Sesman, N., Woodbury, M., Huertas-Goldman, S., Pagan, A., Sanchez-Lacay, A., & Moscoso, M. (1988). Estimates of the prevalence of childhood maladjustment in a community survey in Puerto Rico: The use of combined measures. *Archives of General Psychiatry, 45,* 1120–1126.

Bowlby, J. (1951). *Maternal care and mental health.* Geneva: World Health Organization.

Burnham, M. A., Hough, R. L., Karno, M., Escobar, J. I., & Telles, C. A. (1987). Acculturation and lifetime prevalence of psychiatric disorders among Mexican-Americans in Los Angeles. *Journal of Health and Social Behavior, 28,* 89–102.

Byrd, D. A., Davis-Parker, M. N., Shenoy, U. A., Ollendick, T. H., & Jones, R. T. (1997). Culturally sensitive treatment for anxiety disorders in African-American children and adolescents. Unpublished manuscript. Department of Psychology, Virginia Polytechnic Institute and State University, Blacksburg, VA.

Byrd, D. A., & Ollendick, T. H. (1996). Anxiety and depression in children and adolescents: An examination of cognition and attributional style. Unpublished manuscript. Department of Psychology, Virginia Polytechnic Institute and State University, Blacksburg, VA.

Cantwell, D. P., & Baker, L. (1989). Stability and natural history of DSM-III childhood diagnoses. *Journal of the American Academy of Child and Adolescent Psychiatry, 28,* 691–700.

Cooley, C. H. (1902). *Human nature and the social order.* New York: Charles Scribner's Sons.

Costello, E. J., Costello, A. J., Edelbrock, C. S., Burns, B. J., Dulcan, M. J., Brent, D., & Janiszewski, S. (1988). DSM-III disorders in pediatric primary care: Prevalence and risk factors. *Archives of General Psychiatry, 45,* 1107–1116.

Dadds, M. R., Barrett, P. M., Rapee, R. M., & Ryan, S. (1996). Family process and child anxiety and aggression: An observational analysis. *Journal of Abnormal Child Psychology, 24,* 715–734.

Dressler, W. W. (1985). Extended family relationships, social support, and mental health in a southern Black community. *Journal of Health and Social Behavior, 26,* 39–48.

Eisen, A. R., & Silverman, W. K. (1993). Should I relax or change my thoughts? A preliminary examination of cognitive therapy, relaxation training, and their combination with overanxious children. *Journal of Cognitive Psychotherapy: An International Quarterly, 7,* 265–279.

Fordham, S., & Ogbu, J. U. (1986). Black students' school success: "Coping with the burden of 'acting white.'" *The Urban Review, 18,* 176–206.

Ginsburg, G. S., Silverman, W. K., & Kurtines, W. K. (1995). Family involvement in treating children with phobic and anxiety disorders: A look ahead. *Clinical Psychology Review, 15,* 457–473.

Graham, P. (1979). Epidemiological studies. In H. C. Quay & J. S. Werry (Eds.), *Psychopathological disorders of childhood,* 2nd ed. (pp. 185–209). New York: Wiley.

Gray, J. A. (1982). *The neuropsychology of anxiety.* New York: Cambridge University Press.

Graziano, A. M., & Mooney, K. C. (1980). Family self-control instruction for children's nighttime fear reduction. *Journal of Consulting and Clinical Psychology, 48,* 206–213.

Graziano, A. M., & Mooney, K. C. (1982). Behavioral treatment of "night-fears" in children: Maintenance of improvement at 2- to 3-year follow-up. *Journal of Consulting and Clinical Psychology, 50,* 598–599.

Hagopian, L. P., Weist, M. D., & Ollendick, T. H. (1990). Cognitive-behavior therapy with an 11-year-old girl fearful of AIDS infection, other diseases, and poisoning: Case study. *Journal of Anxiety Disorders, 4,* 257–265.

Harter, S. (1986). Processes underlying the construction, maintenance, and enhancement of the self-concept in children. In J. Suls & A. Greenwald (Eds.), *Psychological perspectives on the self* (pp. 137–181). Hillsdale, NJ: Erlbaum.

Harter, S., & Jackson, B. K. (1993). Young adolescents' perceptions of the link between low self-worth and depressed affect. *Journal of Early Adolescence, 13*, 383–407.

Harter, S., & Whitesell, N. R. (1996). Multiple pathways to self-reported depression and psychological adjustment among adolescents. *Development and Psychopathology, 8*, 761–777.

Hodges, K. (1990). Depression and anxiety in children: A comparison of self-report questionnaires to clinical interview. *Psychological Assessment: A Journal of Consulting and Clinical Psychology, 2*, 376–381.

James, W. (1892). *Psychology: The briefer course.* New York: Henry Holt.

Kagan, J. (1998). Biology and the child. In W. Damon (Series Ed.) & N. Eisenberg (Vol. Ed.), *Handbook of child psychology*: Vol. 3. *Social, emotional, and personality development.* 5th ed. (pp. 177–235). New York: Wiley.

Kane, M., & Kendall, P. C. (1989). Anxiety disorders in children: A multiple baseline evaluation of a cognitive-behavioral treatment. *Behavior Therapy, 20*, 499–508.

Kashani, J. H., & Orvaschel, H. (1990). A community study of anxiety in children and adolescents. *American Journal of Psychiatry, 144*, 584–589.

Keller, M. B., Lavori, P. W., Wunder, J., Beardslee, W. R., Schwartz, C. E., & Roth, J. (1992). Chronic course of anxiety disorders in children and adolescents. *Journal of the American Academy of Child and Adolescent Psychiatry, 31*, 595–599.

Kendall, P. C. (1994). Treating anxiety disorders in children: Results of a randomized clinical trial. *Journal of Consulting and Clinical Psychology, 62*, 100–110.

Kendall, P. C., Flannery-Schroeder, E., Panichelli-Mindel, S. M., Southam-Gerow, M., & Warman, M. (1997). Therapy for anxiety-disordered youth: A second randomized clinical trial. *Journal of Consulting and Clinical Psychology, 65*(3), 366–380.

Kendall, P. C., & Southam-Gerow, M. A. (1996). Long-term follow-up of a cognitive-behavior therapy for anxiety-disordered youth. *Journal of Consulting and Clinical Psychology, 64*, 724–730.

Keppel-Benson, J. M., & Ollendick, T. H. (1993). Posttraumatic stress disorder in children and adolescents. In C. F. Saylor (Ed.), *Children and disasters: Issues in clinical child psychology* (pp. 29–43). New York: Plenum.

King, N. J., Mietz, A., Tinney, L., & Ollendick, T. H. (1995). Psychopathology and cognition in adolescents experiencing severe test anxiety. *Journal of Clinical Child Psychology, 24*, 49–54.

King, N. J., Ollendick, T. H., & Gullone, E. (1991). Negative affectivity in children and adolescents: Relations between anxiety and depression. *Clinical Psychology Review, 11*, 441–459.

Kovacs, M. (1978). The interview schedule for children (ISC): Inter-rater and parent-child agreement. Unpublished manuscript, University of Pittsburgh.

Kovacs, M. (1981). Rating scales to assess depression in school aged children. *Acta Paedopsychiatrica, 46*, 305–315.

Landrine, H., & Klonoff, E. A. (1996). *African American acculturation: Deconstructing race and reviving culture.* London: Sage.

LaPouse, R., & Monk, M. (1959). Fears and worries in a representative sample of children. *American Journal of Orthopsychiatry, 29*, 803–818.

Last, C. G., & Perrin, S. (1993). Anxiety disorders in African-American and White children. *Journal of Abnormal Child Psychology, 21*(2), 153–164.

Laurent, J., & Stark, K. D. (1993). Testing the cognitive content-specificity hypothesis with anxious and depressed youngsters. *Journal of Abnormal Psychology, 102*, 226–237.

Main, M., & Solomon, J. (1990). Procedures for identifying infants as disorganized/disoriented during the Ainsworth Strange Situation. In M. T. Greenberg, D. Cicchetti, & E. M. Cummings (Eds.), *Attachment in the preschool years* (pp. 121–160). Chicago: University of Chicago Press.

Marks, I. (1987). The development of normal fear: A review. *Journal of Child Psychology and Psychiatry, 28*, 680–697.

Montgomery, G. T., & Orozco, S. (1985). Mexican-Americans' performance on the MMPI as a function of level of acculturation. *Journal of Clinical Psychology, 41*, 203–212.

Norvell, N., Brophy, C., & Finch, A. J. (1985). The relationship of anxiety to childhood depression. *Journal of Personality Assessment, 49*, 150–153.

Ollendick, T. H. (1983). Reliability and validity of the revised Fear Survey Schedule for Children (FSSC-R). *Behaviour Research and Therapy, 21*, 685–692.

Ollendick, T. H. (1995). Cognitive behavioral treatment for panic disorder with agoraphobia in adolescents: A multiple baseline design analysis. *Behavior Therapy, 26*, 517–531.

Ollendick, T. H., Hagopian, L. P., & Huntzinger, R. (1991). Cognitive-behavior therapy with nighttime fearful children. *Journal of Behavior Therapy and Experimental Psychiatry, 22*, 113–121.

Ollendick, T. H., & Huntzinger, R. M. (1990). Separation anxiety disorder in childhood. In M. Hersen & C. G. Last (Eds.), *Handbook of child and adult psychopathology: A longitudinal perspective* (pp. 133–149). New York: Pergamon.

Ollendick, T. H., & King, N. J. (1991). Origins of childhood fears: An evaluation of Rachman's theory of fear acquisition. *Behaviour Research and Therapy, 29,* 117–123.

Ollendick, T. H., & King, N. J. (1994). Diagnosis, assessment, and treatment of internalizing problems in children: The role of longitudinal data. *Journal of Consulting and Clinical Psychology, 62,* 918–927.

Ollendick, T. H., & King, N. J. (1998). Empirically supported treatments for children with phobic and anxiety disorders: Current status. *Journal of Clinical Child Psychology, 27*(2), 156–162.

Ollendick, T. H., King, N. J., & Frary, R. B. (1989). Fears in children and adolescents: Reliability and generalizability across gender, age, and nationality. *Behaviour Research and Therapy, 27,* 19–26.

Ollendick, T. H., Matson, J. L., & Helsel, W. J. (1985). Fears and worries in children: Normative data. *Behaviour Research and Therapy, 23,* 465–467.

Ollendick, T. H., Mattis, S., & King, N. J. (1994). Panic in children and adolescents: A critical review. *Journal of Child Psychology and Psychiatry, 35,* 113–134.

Ollendick, T. H., & Ollendick, D. G. (1997). Helping children handle stress and anxiety. *In Session: Psychotherapy in Practice, 3,* 89–102.

Ollendick, T. H., Yang, B., King, N. J., Dong, Q., & Akande, D. (1996). Fears in American, Australian, Chinese, and African children and adolescents: A cross-cultural study. *Journal of Child Psychology and Psychiatry and Allied Disciplines, 37,* 213–220.

Ollendick, T. H., & Yule, W. (1990). Depression in British and American children and its relation to anxiety and fear. *Journal of Consulting and Clinical Psychology, 58*(1), 126–129.

Panksepp, J. (1990). The psychoneurology of fear. In G. D. Burrows, M. Roth, & R. Noyes (Eds.), *The neurobiology of anxiety:* Vol. 3. *Handbook of anxiety* (pp. 3–58). New York: Elsevier.

Papay, J. P., & Hedl, J. J. (1978). Psychometric characteristics and norms for disadvantaged third and fourth grade children on the State-Trait Anxiety Inventory for Children. *Journal of Consulting and Clinical Psychology, 6,* 115–120.

Quay, H. C., & Peterson, D. R. (1983). Manual for the revised behavior problem checklist. Unpublished manuscript.

Renouf, A. G., & Harter, S. (1990). Low self-worth and anger as components of the depressive experience in young adolescents. *Development and Psychopathology, 2,* 293–310.

Reynolds, C. R., & Richmond, B. O. (1979). What I think and feel: A revised measure of children's manifest anxiety. *Journal of Abnormal Child Psychology, 6,* 271–280.

Rosenheck, R., Fontana, A., & Cottrol, C. (1995). Effect of clinician-veteran racial pairing in the treatment of posttraumatic stress disorder. *American Journal of Psychiatry, 152,* 555–563.

Rothbart, M. K., & Bates J. E. (1998). Temperament. In W. Damon (Series Ed.) & N. Eisenberg (Vol. Ed.), *Handbook of child psychology:* Vol. 3. *Social, emotional, and personality development,* 5th ed. (pp. 105–176). New York: Wiley.

Rutter, M., McDonald, H., LeCouteur, A., Harrington, R., Bolton, P., & Bailey, A. (1990). Genetic factors in child psychiatric disorders II. Empirical findings. *Journal of Child Psychology and Psychiatry, 31,* 39–83.

Seligman, M. E. P., Abramson, L. Y., Semmel, A., & von Baeyer, C. (1979). Depressive attributional style. *Journal of Abnormal Psychology, 88,* 242–247.

Seligman, L. D., & Ollendick, T. H. (1998). Comorbidity of anxiety and depression in children and adolescents: An integrative review. *Clinical Child and Family Psychology Review, 1*(2), 125–144.

Silverman, W. K., & Nelles, W. B. (1988). The Anxiety Disorders Interview Schedule for Children. *Journal of the American Academy of Child and Adolescent Psychiatry, 27,* 772–778.

Sue, S., Fujino, L. H., Takeuchi, D. T., & Zane, N. W. S. (1991). Community mental health services for ethnic minority groups: A test of the cultural responsiveness hypothesis. *Journal of Consulting and Clinical Psychology, 59,* 533–540.

Thapar, A., & McGuffin, P. (1995). Are anxiety symptoms in childhood heritable? *Journal for Child Psychology and Psychiatry, 36,* 439–447.

Thomas, A., & Chess, S. (1977). *Temperament and development.* New York: Brunner/Mazel.

Thompson, R. A. (1998). Early sociopersonality development. In W. Damon (Series Ed.) & N. Eisenberg (Vol. Ed.), *Handbook of child psychology:* Vol. 3. *Social, emotional, and personality development,* 5th ed. (pp. 25–104). New York: Wiley.

Treadwell, K. R. H., Flannery-Schroeder, E. C., & Kendall, P. C. (1995). Ethnicity and gender in relation to adaptive functioning, diagnostic status, and treatment outcome in children from and anxiety clinic. *Journal of Anxiety Disorders, 9*(5), 373–384.

Turner, S. M., Beidel, D. C., & Costello, A. (1987). Psychopathology in the offspring of anxiety disorders patients. *Journal of Consulting and Clinical Psychology, 55,* 229–235.

Velez, C. M., Johnson, J., & Cohen, P. A. (1989). A longitudinal analysis of selected risk factors for childhood psychopathology. *Journal of the American Academy of Child and Adolescent Psychiatry, 28,* 861–864.

Warren, M. K., Ollendick, T. H., & King, N. J. (1996). Test anxiety in girls and boys: A clinical-developmental analysis. *Behaviour Change, 13,* 157–170.

Watson, D., & Clark, L. A. (1984). Negative affectivity: The disposition to experience aversive emotional states. *Psychological Bulletin, 96,* 465–490.

Watson, D., Clark, L. A., & Carey, G. (1988). Positive and negative affectivity and their relation to anxiety and depressive disorders. *Journal of Abnormal Psychology, 97,* 346–353.

Watson, D., & Tellegen, A. (1985). Toward a consensual structure of mood. *Psychological Bulletin, 98,* 219–235.

Werry, J. S., & Quay, H. C. (1971). The prevalence of behavior symptoms in younger elementary school children. *American Journal of Orthopsychiatry, 41,* 136–143.

Wine, J. D. (1971). Test anxiety and directions of attention. *Psychological Bulletin, 76,* 92–104.

Zatz, S., & Chassin, L. (1983). Cognitions in test-anxious children under naturalistic test-taking conditions. *Journal of Consulting and Clinical Psychology, 53,* 393–401.

12

Depression

Chandra M. Grabill, Jeana R. Griffith, and Nadine J. Kaslow

Introduction

Cases of despondency and depression in children and adolescents were reported as early as the seventeenth century, and reports on melancholia in youth appeared by the mid-nineteenth century. Prior to the 1970s, however, little attention was paid to depression in youth. This paucity of interest can be attributed to suppositions of the era's prevailing classical psychoanalytic theory that precluded childhood depression due to children's immature superego development and lack of a stable self-concept. Other theorists postulated that children could not tolerate prolonged feelings of dysphoria and thus "masked" their depressive symptoms with myriad emotional and behavioral symptoms. The turning point occurred at the 1970 Fourth Congress of the Union of European Pedopsychiatrists in Stockholm that focused on childhood and adolescent depressive states. These European pedopsychiatrists concluded that depression was a mental disorder found in a significant percentage of troubled young people and as such deserved study. Increased attention to childhood and adolescent depression in the United States can be dated to Schulterbrandt and Raskin's (1977) book, *Depression in Childhood: Diagnosis, Treatment and Conceptual Models*, which detailed findings from a conference sponsored by the National Institute of Mental Health. This group of clinicians and researchers concurred with the European group's conclusion that depression in youth exists. Their work sparked research in the areas of diagnostic classification, assessment, biopsychosocial sequelae, and treatment. As a result, during the past 20 years there has been a proliferation of relevant theoretical, clinical, and empirical papers, and depression remains a major focus of child and adolescent psychopathology. This chapter summarizes pertinent literature regarding the description, epidemiology and course, clinical picture, familial and genetic patterns, and diagnostic considerations of depressive disorders in children and adolescents.

Chandra M. Grabill • Sexton Woods Psychoeducational Center, DeKalb County School System, Chamblee, Georgia 30341.   Jeana R. Griffith and Nadine J. Kaslow • Department of Psychiatry and Behavioral Sciences, Emory University School of Medicine at Grady Memorial Hospital, Atlanta, Georgia 30335.

Advanced Abnormal Psychology, Second Edition, edited by Hersen and Van Hasselt. Kluwer Academic/Plenum Publishers, New York, 2001.

DESCRIPTION OF THE DISORDER

The *Diagnostic and Statistical Manual of Mental Disorders*, 4th Ed. (DSM-IV; American Psychiatric Association [APA], 1994) provides the standard criteria for diagnosing depression in children and adolescents. These criteria are comparable to those of adult depressive disorders, although the DSM-IV acknowledges age-specific features that influence presentation across the life span. Although data exist supporting the utility of these diagnostic criteria for youth, reservations about the validity of these criteria for children and adolescents have been expressed by developmental psychopathologists (Carlson & Garber, 1986).

According to DSM-IV, a spectrum of depressive disorders can be diagnosed depending on the degree of severity and duration. First, major depressive disorder is diagnosed when a child or adolescent exhibits a change from previous functioning and at least five of the following nine symptoms during a single two-week period: depressed or irritable mood, diminished interest or loss of pleasure in almost all activities (anhedonia), weight change or appetite disturbance, sleep disturbance, psychomotor agitation or retardation, fatigue or loss of energy (anergia), feelings of worthlessness or inappropriate guilt, decreased concentration or indecisiveness, and recurrent thoughts of death or suicidal ideation. At least one of the symptoms must be either depressed or irritable mood, or anhedonia. In addition, the symptoms must cause significant impairment in daily functioning. This symptom picture cannot be attributable to a medical condition, reflect the normal reaction to the death of a loved one, or be due to the direct effects of a substance (e.g., drugs of abuse or medication).

A major depressive episode may be rated according to severity, the presence of psychotic features such as delusions or hallucinations, and remission status. It also is specified whether the episode is chronic (persisted for at least two consecutive years), catatonic (characterized by a psychomotor disturbance), melancholic (characterized by a loss of interest in pleasurable activities), or atypical (characterized by mood reactivity). Some depressive disorders may have a seasonal pattern and if so, this would be specified as part of the diagnosis. Although there has been increasing attention to a seasonal pattern in depressive disorder in adults, there has been a limited amount of research on a seasonal pattern in children and adolescents (Rosenthal et al., 1986; Swedo et al., 1995). Seasonal affective disorders may be difficult to diagnose because children experience a recurring universal stressor each fall as they begin a new school year, and due to their young age, many children fail to meet the diagnostic criteria because they have not experienced sufficient prior episodes of depression (Weller & Weller, 1991).

Youth who manifest chronic depressive symptoms may meet diagnostic criteria for the second DSM-IV depressive spectrum diagnosis, dysthymic disorder. Dysthymia is diagnosed when the youth exhibits a depressed or irritable mood that persists for a year or longer without a symptom-free period of more than two months. In addition to a chronic depressed or irritable mood, two of the following symptoms must be present: poor appetite or overeating, insomnia or hypersomnia, low energy or fatigue, low self-esteem, poor concentration or difficulty with decision making, or feelings of hopelessness. There must be no evidence of an unequivocal major depressive episode during the first year of the disturbance; no history for manic, mixed, or hypomanic episodes; and the disorder must not be superimposed on an underlying organic condition or chronic psychotic disorder. The symptoms must cause a clinically significant level of distress or interfere with daily functioning.

The third, least serious form of depressive disorder in youth is classified in DSM-IV as adjustment disorder with depressed mood. An individual receives this diagnosis when the depressive symptoms develop in reaction to an identifiable psychosocial stressor or multiple stressors; symptoms must develop within three months of the onset of the stressor(s). In such cases, the maladaptive nature of the depressive reaction is indicated by either impaired academic or social functioning or distress exceeding normal, expectable reactions to the stressor(s). The symptom picture is not consistent with any other specific mental disorder and may not represent an uncomplicated bereavement.

The DSM-IV also includes a diagnostic category entitled depressive disorder not otherwise specified (NOS). This category encompasses disorders with depressive features that do not meet the criteria for the aforementioned depressive disorders.

The presence of more than one diagnosis is termed psychiatric comorbidity. Between 40–70% of children and adolescents who receive a diagnosis of major depression or dysthymia also meet diagnostic criteria for at least one additional psychiatric disorder and 20–50% have two or more additional diagnoses (Birmaher et al., 1996a). Dysthymia and major depression often co-occur; 70% of dysthymic children also have a coexisting diagnosis of major depressive disorder (Birmaher et al., 1996a). The most prevalent comorbid conditions that occur with a depressive disorder include anxiety disorders, disruptive disorders, and substance abuse (Birmaher et al., 1996a). Additional comorbid conditions include eating disorders, obsessive–compulsive disorder, and specific developmental disorders (e.g., Alessi & Magen, 1988). Researchers have examined personality dysfunction in depressed adolescents (e.g., Marton et al., 1989) and have found that a significant percentage of these youth meet criteria for an Axis II personality disorder, most frequently borderline personality disorder. According to Kovacs (1985), these comorbid disorders complicate the diagnostic and treatment process and may differentially affect the course of the disorders.

Depressive disorders exist throughout the life span, but there are differences in symptom manifestation that depend on the developmental stage (Birmaher et al., 1996a). Although infants do not manifest depressive disorders in accordance with DSM-IV criteria, Spitz (1946) and Bowlby (1980) described institutionalized infants separated from their primary caretakers as listless, withdrawn, and weepy, refusing to eat, and having disturbed sleep patterns. These authors termed this syndrome "anaclitic depression," and similar symptom patterns can be observed today in infants separated from primary caretakers, infants who are chronically hospitalized for medical problems, and some infants whose primary caretakers are severely depressed. Age-specific features commonly manifested in depressed preschoolers include angry affect, uncooperativeness, apathy, and a lack of playfulness. These symptoms often occur in response to stressful life events. However, given that children do not use language to effectively communicate affective states before age seven, preschoolers are rarely diagnosed as depressed. To make this diagnosis, attention must be directed to their nonverbal communication. In elementary school children, common manifestations of depression include social withdrawal, depressed appearance, somatic complaints, agitation, separation anxiety, and phobias. Some severely depressed elementary school children also exhibit mood congruent auditory hallucinations. Depressed adolescents exhibit a more classic picture of depression that often is accompanied by affective lability (mood swings), irritability, inattention to personal appearance, extreme sensitivity to interpersonal rejection, and acting-out behaviors (negativism, aggression, antisocial behaviors, substance abuse, school problems) (Kutcher & Marton, 1989). It is not uncommon for depressed adolescents to express a dysphoric mood state via suicidal gestures or attempts; a significant percentage of adolescents who attempt suicide meet criteria for major depression (Lewinsohn, Rohde, & Seeley, 1993).

Epidemiology

The reported prevalence of depression in children and adolescents varies widely. This variation is a function of the heterogeneity of populations sampled (age, gender, setting), small sample sizes, inconsistencies in the types of instruments used, differences in the number and types of informants, shifting diagnostic criteria, and different methods of defining depression (symptom, syndrome, or disorder) (Fleming & Offord, 1990). To date, no large-scale epidemiological studies have been conducted with representative samples of children and adolescents for the explicit purpose of ascertaining the prevalence of depressive disorders in youth. Until more methodologically sophisticated studies are undertaken, the extant epidemiological data must be viewed as only a partial picture.

Kashani and Sherman (1988) reviewed the prevalence of depression across the life span. Depression in preschoolers is very rare and has been estimated at less than 1% in the general population. These studies used primarily adult criteria for diagnosing depression, and it is conceivable that if more developmentally sensitive criteria are used, the reported rates of depression in preschoolers may increase. Investigators have found a population prevalence of depression in children that ranged from 0.4% to 2.5% (Birmaher et al., 1996a). During adolescence, there is an increase in the prevalence rates of major depressive disorder that ranges from 0.4% to 8.3% (Birmaher et al., 1996a). Epidemiological studies have identified mid and late adolescence as peak risk periods for the development of depression (e.g., Burke, Burke, Reigier, & Rae, 1990; Lewinsohn, Rohde,& Seeley, 1998). There have been multiple explanations for the increased rates of depression in adolescents, including: biological changes associated with the onset of puberty; adolescents' increased self awareness of symptoms, making it easier for them to report symptoms to others; and a decrease in protective factors, such as spending time with family (Harrington, 1993).

Opposed to these estimates regarding the general population, the prevalence of depression found has been higher in special populations of children and adolescents (Stark, 1990). In clinical samples, it has been estimated that prevalence rates of depression in children and adolescents range from 10% to 50% (McCracken, 1992; Peterson et al., 1993). Higher rates of depression are also reported in children evaluated in an educational diagnostic center, children with chronic illnesses, and children whose parents are depressed.

Demographic factors, including age, gender, socioeconomic status (SES), and ethnicity influence prevalence rates of mood disorders in youth. The prevalence of depression increases with age (Angold, 1988; Moreau, 1996). Before adolescence, the literature suggests that the rate of depression in boys is either equal to or somewhat greater than the rate of depression in girls. In adolescence, however, depression is more prevalent in females than males (see review by Nolen-Hoeksema & Girgus, 1994). Female adolescents report more depressive symptoms, self-consciousness, stressful life events, negative body image, rumination, and low self-esteem than adolescent males (Allgood-Merten, Lewinsohn, & Hops, 1990; Gjerde, Block, & Block 1988). In contrast, dysthymic adolescent males evidence a more externalizing pattern of personality characteristics because they are often viewed as disagreeable and antagonistic (Gjerde et al., 1988). Although scant relevant literature precludes definitive conclusions, some data suggest that youth from lower socioeconomic backgrounds exhibit more depressive symptomatology than their counterparts from middle and upper class backgrounds (Schwartz, Gladstone, & Kaslow, 1998b). These differences may be due to the effects of poverty, poor education, and life stress. Some studies have found no differences in the prevalence of depressive symptoms across ethnic groups, but others have found higher rates among African-American and Mexican-American youth (see review by Roberts, Roberts, & Chen, 1997).

Some evidence suggests greater risk for depression among youth who reside in socially disadvantaged environments characterized by poverty, lack of adequate resources, and oppression of minorities.

CLINICAL PICTURE

Case Vignette

Ned (not his real name) is an 11-year-old, Caucasian male whose parents contacted one of the authors (NJK) regarding their concerns about Ned since the announcement of their marital separation and impending divorce eight months prior. At the initial interview, the parents reported that Ned had become socially withdrawn and less involved with music and scholastic activities. They reported that this was a significant change from his previous level of functioning because he had been a popular child who did extremely well in school and excelled in playing the violin. His parents also commented that he seemed unhappy nearly every day, regardless of daily events. His dysphoria appeared more profound when there was increased tension between his parents. Reports from Ned's teachers revealed that his academic performance continued to be above average, but he no longer evidenced enthusiasm about learning and was less active in class and with his peers. Upon initially meeting with Ned, he looked sad and at times tearful, made little eye contact, had dull eyes (lacked a gleam in his eyes), had shoulders hunched forward, spoke quietly and slowly without animation, and moved slowly. Although his parents and teachers reported that he used to have a good sense of humor and was quite playful interpersonally, during initial sessions he appeared to lack a sense of humor and rarely smiled or laughed. In addition to acknowledging feeling unhappy, Ned reported somatic complaints (e.g., headaches) and said that he never felt like he had the energy to do much. Unlike some other depressed children, he did not report stomachaches, or sleep or appetite disturbances. He described himself as bored with his friends and appeared to be apathetic about school and music endeavors. The content of his verbal communications revealed his lack of enjoyment in activities typically considered fun by his peers, his low self-esteem, and feelings of worthlessness. It was not uncommon to hear him say, "I'm not very smart. I'm ugly. Nobody really likes me. My parents are so wrapped up in their own problems, I'm not sure if they love me." His feelings of helplessness were evidenced both in his reluctance to take initiative and such verbalizations as, "Why should I bother trying, it doesn't matter what I do. I can never do it good enough." He often communicated his feelings of hopelessness in such statements as, "Things will never get better for our family." He denied, however, any suicidal ideation, attempts, or plans. When meeting with Ned, the therapist often found herself feeling sad, drained of energy, and, at times, helpless. Thus, although she felt considerable empathy for his distress, she often found herself feeling powerless to help him effect change in his life. Based on information gleaned from Ned's self-report, from other informants (e.g., parents, teachers), and from the therapist's observations, it appeared that Ned met DSM-IV criteria for major depression, single episode, of moderate severity, and without psychotic features. This diagnosis was based on the length of the episode, and the nature and severity of the symptoms. Concurrent cognitive-behaviorally oriented group therapy for depressed youth and interpersonal family therapy were recommended to enable Ned to discuss the aspects of the family situation that he found particularly upsetting and to help the family cope more effectively with the changes associated with the pending divorce.

Kaslow and Racusin (1990) and Racusin and Kaslow (1991) presented an organizational strategy that more systematically captures the domains of functioning affected by depressive disorders in children and adolescents. These domains include psychological symptomatology, cognitive, affective, interpersonal, family, adaptive behavior and neurobiological functioning. We will now briefly highlight depressed youths' functioning in the cognitive, affective, interpersonal, adaptive behavior, and neurobiological domains. Psychological symptomatology has already been discussed in detail in the section describing depressive disorders in youth. Family functioning will be covered later in the section on familial and genetic patterns.

In terms of their cognitive functioning (see reviews by Kaslow & Racusin, 1990; Kaslow, Brown, & Mee, 1994), depressed children and adolescents display deficits in instrumental responding manifested by a lack of motivation to complete tasks correctly and efficiently. They also believe that their behavior cannot control environmental events. These motivational deficits, behavioral problems, and associated cognitions are typically manifested in feelings of helplessness. Compared to their nondepressed counterparts, depressed youth also have lower self-esteem, feel more hopeless about their futures, and perceive that they are less competent. Further, these youth often evidence cognitive distortions, most notably a maladaptive attributional style. Specifically, they tend to blame themselves for negative events and see the causes of these events as stable over time and generalizable across situations (internal, stable, global attributions for negative events). Simultaneously, depressed youth tend to believe and give credit to other people or circumstances for good events and view the causes of these positive events as unstable over time and specific to the situation (external, unstable, specific attributions for positive events). For example, when a depressed child receives a poor grade on a test, it is not uncommon for that child to think, "I am really dumb." More adaptive attributions to this negative event typically held by nondepressed children may include: "I need to study more for the next test," "The teacher made a stupid test," or "I never was very good at math, but I'm good in other subjects." Further, depressed youth evidence deficits in self-monitoring, self-evaluation, and self-reinforcement. In particular, they are overly focused on negative events to the exclusion of positive events, more influenced by immediate rather than delayed consequences of their actions, set unrealistic expectations for their performance and feel badly about themselves when they fail to meet these standards, and engage in excessive self-punishment and insufficient self-reinforcement.

In the affective domain, depressed youth verbalize a pattern of emotional experiences similar to those reported by depressed adults. Specifically, depressed youth endorse high levels of sadness, anger, self-directed hostility, and shame (Blumberg & Izard, 1985). Nonverbally, as noted before, depressed youth, particularly those in an inpatient psychiatric service, show slow activity (latency, gestures, self movements), flat affect (intonation, facial expressiveness), and outward signs of sadness (e.g., tearfulness) (Kazdin, Sherick, Esveldt-Dawson, & Rancurello, 1985). However, investigators have noted less robust relationships between clinical diagnoses of depression and nonverbal behavior for children than those obtained for adults (Kazdin et al., 1985). Research also suggests that depressed youth exhibit affect regulation difficulties (see review by Garber, Braafladt, & Zeman, 1991). More specifically, depressed youth exhibit fewer and more maladaptive emotion-regulating strategies (e.g., withdrawal and aggression) than nondepressed youth.

In the interpersonal sphere, the literature suggests that depressed youth exhibit relationship deficits with peers, parents, and siblings (e.g., Altmann & Gotlib, 1988; Puig-Antich et al., 1993). Depressed elementary school children are often viewed negatively or are rejected by peers and teachers (Bell-Dolan, Reaven, & Peterson, 1993; Dalley, Bolocofsky, & Karlin, 1994; Rudolph, Hammen, & Burge, 1994). In addition, they are rated by peers and adults as less likeable and attractive, as engaging in fewer positive behaviors, and in greater need of therapy than their nondepressed peers (Mullins, Peterson, Wonderlich, & Reaven, 1986). Research also suggests a relationship between social competence and depression. Individuals who were rated by their teachers, peers, and self as less socially competent, had higher scores on a measure of depressive symptoms than those who were rated as more socially competent (Cole, 1990). Interpersonal deficits tend to persist, even after the child or adolescent has recovered from a depressive episode (Puig-Antich et al., 1993).

Some data suggest that depressed children and adolescents exhibit impairments in adaptive behavior, defined as deficits in communication, socialization, and daily living skills. Depressed youth have impaired communication because they are less verbal within the family system, with their peers, and with authority figures (Schwartz, Kaslow, Racusin, & Carton, 1998). They are also less assertive than their nondepressed counterparts (Kaslow, Deering, & Ash, 1996). More specifically, some research suggests that depressed youth exhibit deficits in social problem solving, although additional research is needed to substantiate these claims (Kaslow, Croft, & Hatcher, 1999). Depressed youth tend to be more socially withdrawn than nondepressed youth (Kaslow et al., 1996). In the area of daily living skills, depressed youth exhibit insufficient attention to self-care and personal hygiene (Schwartz et al., 1998a). However, it is interesting to note that psychiatrically hospitalized children who have comorbid mood/anxiety disorders and disruptive behavior disorders exhibit less impaired daily living skills than youth hospitalized for disruptive behavior disorders (Woolston et al., 1989). It has been hypothesized that the presence of a mood or anxiety disorder tempers the daily living skill impairments associated with disruptive behavior due to the children's desire to please others and the inhibition of acting-out behavior. These impairments are manifested across settings and relationships.

Finally, considerable strides have been made in the past decade in exploring psychobiological parameters of childhood depression (Burke & Puig-Antich, 1990; Emslie, Weinberg, Kennard, & Kowatch, 1994). Although depressed adults exhibit patterns of cortisol hypersecretion, research on depressed children has not consistently found this pattern. However, similar to adults, dexamethasone nonsuppression has also been found in children and adolescents who have depressive disorders (Birmaher et al., 1996a). Other biological markers that have been studied in adults, such as growth hormone secretion, have only recently been examined in children and adolescents. These initial studies suggest that depressed children have hyposecretion of growth hormone in response to an insulin challenge. Some studies suggest that there may be hypersecretion of growth hormone during sleep; however, more recent research has not found this hypersecretion (Birmaher et al., 1996a). Of particular interest is the finding that these irregularities in growth hormone secretion persist even upon recovery from the depressive episode. Neurotransmitters play a vital role in regulating mood. Although limited research has been conducted with children and adolescents, there are indications that neurotransmitter abnormalities (e.g., norepinephrine, acetylcholine, serotonin) are linked to depression in adults (Kaslow et al., 1999).

There is considerable evidence of EEG sleep abnormalities in depressed adults, and thus a number of polysomnography studies have been conducted with depressed youth. Early studies reveal virtually no abnormalities in EEG sleep parameters in depressed children before puberty, but more recent research suggests that there may be differences in REM sleep during depressive episodes and after recovery (Emslie et al., 1994). In adolescents, there is evidence of REM abnormalities similar to those found in depressed adults (Emslie et al., 1994). Overall, studies on sleep abnormalities in depressed youth have not found consistent sleep changes similar to adults (Birmaher et al., 1996a). It has been hypothesized that the lack of EEG sleep abnormalities in depressed youth may be attributable to maturational factors that modify the neuroregulation of the sleep cycle or the neurobiology of the initiation or maintenance of depressive episodes in individuals before puberty.

COURSE AND PROGNOSIS

Short-term follow-up and longitudinal studies reveal that depressed youth have chronic depressions that persist over time; experience recurrent episodes of depression; may exhibit social, educational, and neurobiological impairments even upon remission from a depressive episode; and are at increased risk of developing other psychiatric impairments (e.g., affective disorders, suicidal behavior). These impairments often necessitate intensive psychological and psychiatric intervention, including hospitalization and psychopharmacological treatments.

Typically, a major depressive episode lasts seven to nine months, whereas the length of dysthymia may exceed three years (Kovacs, 1989). Dysthymic children have episodes that last an average of four years (Birmaher et al., 1996a). Those youth who have a dysthymic disorder or a chronic depression are initially less responsive to psychosocial and pharmacological interventions than those youth who manifest acute depressive onset. Children who have adjustment disorder and depressed mood have episodes that last, on average, between three and six months (APA, 1994). Children and adolescents generally have a shorter period of time to recovery than adults, but their long-term prognosis is poor because they are likely to have recurrent episodes of depression throughout their lives (Kovacs, 1996).

Comorbid psychiatric conditions influence the course and prognosis of depressive disorders. Children who have coexisting cases of major depression and dysthymia or major depression and an anxiety disorder may have longer recovery periods (Kovacs, Gatsonis, Paulauskas, & Richards, 1989; Kovacs et al., 1997), whereas the presence of other nonaffective psychiatric conditions does not influence recovery periods (Kovacs et al., 1997). After recovery from a depressive episode, children who have comorbid conduct disorders or anxiety disorders often manifest continued conduct problems or anxiety symptoms (Kovacs et al., 1989). However, the presence of a comorbid psychiatric disorder does not increase one's risk of future depressive episodes. Several psychosocial variables are associated with a more positive prognosis, most notably, high levels of age-appropriate family closeness and cohesiveness, the availability of satisfactory social support networks, and positive aspects of self-esteem. In summary, the outcome of mood disorders in children and adolescents appears relatively poor.

FAMILIAL AND GENETIC PATTERNS

Genetics

Given the paucity of information regarding genetic patterns in depressed children and adolescents, a brief description of the major genetic studies of depressed adults will follow (Weller & Weller, 1991). Twin studies reveal that concordance for affective disorders in monozygotic twins is 76% compared to 19% in dizygotic twins. When monozygotic twins are reared apart, the concordance rate for affective disorders is only 67%, suggesting an interaction between genetic and environmental factors in the expression of affective disorders. Data from adoption studies also support the importance of both genetic and environmental factors in the development of depressive disorders.

Family Psychiatric History

Extant family history research on childhood depression can be grouped into two categories: (1) studies of lifetime psychiatric diagnoses of first- and second-degree relatives of youth who have major depression and (2) investigations of the offspring of depressed adult probands. Studies using the lifetime family history method reveal increased rates of affective disorders in families of children diagnosed with depression at an early age (Birmaher et al., 1996a). For example, in prepubertal depressed probands, the risk of depression in first-degree adult relatives was .53 (Puig-Antich et al., 1989), whereas the risk of depression among adult first-degree relatives of depressed adolescents was only .37 (Burke & Puig-Antich, 1990). Additionally, depressed children and adolescents have an increased family history of alcoholism, anxiety disorders, antisocial personality, and suicidality (Burke & Puig-Antich, 1990; Mitchell, McCauley, Burke, Calderon, & Schloredt, 1989; Todd, Geller, Neuman, Fox , & Hickok, 1996).

During the past decade, a plethora of studies has examined the offspring of depressed parents but the majority of research was on depressed women (see reviews by Birmaher et al., 1996a; Downey & Coyne, 1990; Hammen, 1991). Children of depressed parents are at significantly increased risk of clinical depression, as well as heightened rates of a range of internalizing and externalizing problems and social and academic adjustment difficulties. Parental concordance for diagnoses (i.e., both parents have a psychiatric diagnosis) results in a substantially increased risk of major depression and anxiety disorders in their children (Merikangas, Prusoff, & Weissman, 1988). A number of potential links have been offered to explain the association between parental depression and child adjustment, including genetic factors, maladaptive parenting patterns, interpersonal context of depression, and comorbid impairment of depressed persons (e.g., personality disorders). Indeed, the psychological adjustment of children of depressed parents is mediated by the severity and course of their parents' affective disorders and comorbid psychiatric conditions, level of expressed emotion, severity of marital discord, level of stressful life events, problematic parenting behaviors associated with depression, and adequacy of familial social supports (Hammen, 1991). Although children who have parents with affective disorders are at risk of depression, several psychosocial factors seem to serve a protective function. For example, children who have good physical health, high intelligence, good relationships with peers and family, involvement in extracurricular activities, high self-esteem, positive coping strategies, and an internal locus of control show more resilience against depression (Beardslee & Wheelock, 1994).

Family Dynamics

Recently, researchers have begun to examine family dynamics associated with the development and maintenance of depression in children and adolescents. According to this research, serious family dysfunction and negative life events are key family variables that apparently correlate with depressive symptoms in youth. The specific nature of this family dysfunction and negative life events have included the following: family conflict; parent–child conflict; marital conflict, particularly regarding child-rearing; parental death, divorce, or separation; and child maltreatment or physical abuse (Kaslow, Deering, & Racusin, 1994; Kaslow & Racusin, 1990). Additionally, youth who become depressed are more likely than their nondepressed counterparts to experience maternal rejection, low levels of parental support, and less secure attachment to their parents (Kaslow et al., 1994).

Depressed children and adolescents perceive their families more negatively than do their nondepressed peers (e.g., Kaslow, Rehm, Pollack, & Siegel, 1990; Stark, Humphrey, Crook, & Lewis, 1990), and depressed adolescents are less satisfied with their families' functioning than nondepressed adolescents (Cumsille & Epstein, 1994). Specifically, depressed children report their families are less cohesive, more conflict-ridden, less successful at conflict resolution, and less emotionally expressive (Kaslow et al., 1994). They indicate that their parents are autocratic, and thus these youth experience that they have minimal input into decision-making. These families tend to engage in fewer social, recreational, or cultural activities than characteristic of families without a depressed youth (Stark et al., 1990). Additionally, the mothers of depressed youth report less communication with their children than mothers of nondepressed youth and the affective tone of communication between the mother and depressed child is frequently hostile, tense, and punitive (Puig-Antich et al., 1985). Interestingly, these problematic communication patterns are no longer evident when the child's depression resolves.

Research on the interactional patterns between depressed children and their parents suggests a cycle that perpetuates the children's depression (e.g., Kaslow et al., 1996). In this cycle, the parent typically displays a parenting style that is hostile, critical, and vacillates between overcontrolling and rejecting. This leads the child to develop a sense of helplessness and inhibition. Next, this helpless and inhibited behavior on the part of the depressed child is frustrating for the parents, who often feel that their efforts in helping are rejected and respond angrily with increased hostility and aggression. In turn, this angry response serves to further exacerbate the child's depressive symptoms and associated cognitions, feelings, and behaviors.

DIAGNOSTIC CONSIDERATIONS

When diagnosing a mood disorder in children or adolescents, the clinician or clinical researcher must take a number of variables into account. To paint a comprehensive picture of depression, it is essential to use a multitrait, multimethod, multi-informant approach to assessment (Schwartz et al., 1998a). Multitrait refers to addressing psychological symptomatology; cognitive, affective, interpersonal, family, adaptive behavior; and neurobiological variables delineated in prior sections of this chapter. Multimethod assessment involves incorporating a variety of assessment techniques into the diagnostic battery. Specifically, the diagnosis of a depressive disorder in a child or adolescent may be based upon the child's self-report, structured interviews with the child and/or parent, ratings by others (clinicians, staff, parent, teacher), peer nominations, behavioral observations, and projective techniques. The type of instrument used influences the nature of the information obtained. For example, a child's self-report of depression on a questionnaire captures only the depressive symptoms of which the child is aware and willing to acknowledge. The use of projective techniques, though potentially most effective in examining underlying dynamics associated with depression, does not address the presence of actual depressive symptoms. Clinician ratings may represent information from a variety of perspectives and are often influenced by raters' clinical judgment. Observational data typically yield a rich portrait of the child's verbal and nonverbal behavior and interaction style, yet fail to provide information about specific DSM-IV symptoms. Each assessment type provides a different window into a child's depressive experience.

Multi-informant assessment is gathering information regarding the individual's functioning from the youth and also from others such as parents, teachers, peers, and clinicians (Kazdin, 1994). This topic has received considerable attention in the childhood psychopathology literature during the past 10 to 15 years (e.g., Achenbach, McConaughy, & Howell, 1987; Schwartz et al., 1998b), and underscores the need to garner information from multiple sources regarding multiple domains of functioning. Problematic interinformant agreement and contradictory findings regarding the assessment of depression in children and adolescents is an area of particular concern in the diagnostic process. Some researchers describe acceptable rates of agreement between parent and child reports of the child's depression, whereas others have found minimal correspondence in these reports (Kazdin, 1994). Many of these studies reveal that depressed youth portray themselves as more depressed than they are described by their parents, and the opposite trend has been found by other investigators. Kazdin (1988) speculated that children may deny their depressive symptoms more often than their parents and thus may be more likely to underreport their distress on self-report inventories. The child's age and gender, the varying item content of scales given to different reporters, the nature of the youth's disorder, and the degree and type of parental psychopathology are all factors that contribute to the discrepancy in parent and children's reports. It is important to note that it is not necessarily the case that one informant is "right" and the other informant "wrong" regarding the child's psychological status. Rather, the discrepancy in reports may be indicative of the fact that depressed children present differently across settings and with various informants (Kaslow & Racusin, 1990). Some research has suggested that children may be more accurate than their parents in reporting depressive symptoms; therefore, as a general rule, children's self-report should be given more credence assessing depression (Kolko & Kazdin, 1993). Low correlations between self- and informant reports across types of assessment measures employed, as well as moderate concurrence of symptoms across functional domains, have led investigators to utilize assessment batteries that measure a range of symptoms and multiple areas of functioning using various techniques and based on information from a variety of informants (Kazdin, 1994).

In addition to these questions regarding selection of assessment tools and how and from whom information is gathered, the diagnosis of mood disorders in youth must take into consideration the demographics and social characteristics of the individual assessed. In particular, it is essential to conduct assessments within a developmental framework. As noted earlier in this chapter, the age of the youth assessed significantly influences the expression of depressive symptoms and of the disorder (Schwartz et al., 1998b). For example, when a toddler cries relatively easily over a small incident, it may be considered an age-appropriate expression of distress, whereas this same behavior in an elementary school age child may indicate a dysphoric mood state. Age, however, is only one factor in considering a symptom potentially reflective of depression. The toddler who cries frequently may indeed be depressed if inconsolable or unable to play. Thus, labeling a given behavior as a symptom of depression must take into account developmental expressions of the behavior in both normal and depressed youth (Digdon & Gotlib, 1985).

Gender is another demographic variable that may influence the expression and subsequent diagnosis of a depressive disorder. For example, an early adolescent male who reports feeling helpless and behaves in a helpless manner may be characterized more quickly as depressed than an early adolescent female who reports similar cognitions and expresses similar behaviors. In the adolescent girl, these cognitions and behaviors may be considered reflective of socialization factors that need to be "teased out" from actual symptoms of depression, whereas in the adolescent male a helpless stance is more readily considered a depressive symptom and generally not reflective of socialization practices.

A third group of demographic characteristics that may influence the manifestation and diagnosis of depressive disorders relates to racial, ethnic, or cultural background. In the past few years, investigators have begun to examine depression cross-culturally (e.g., Canada, Israel, New Zealand, Spain, Sweden, United States). Due to the paucity of research that addresses this question, however, little is known regarding cross-cultural similarities or differences among children and adolescents. Extant data suggest that though there are similarities in the incidence of depressive symptoms cross-culturally, some salient differences in regard to symptom presentation have emerged. For example, Swedish adolescents who are depressed rate themselves as having more feelings of failure, unattractiveness, and self-accusation than their American counterparts assessed by the same instrument (Larsson & Melin, 1990). In a related vein, although the overall incidence of depression in African-American youth appears comparable to that of their Caucasian peers, some researchers (e.g., Politano, Nelson, Evans, Sorenson, & Zeman, 1986) have found that depressed African-American youth report less suicidality and dysphoric mood and more acting-out symptoms (e.g., oppositionality) than their Caucasian peers. There also are some data suggesting that Hispanic-American youth endorse significantly more depressive symptoms on a self-report measure (Worchel et al., 1990) and on diagnostic interviews (Roberts et al., 1997) than their non-Hispanic Caucasian peers.

Another variable that complicates a clear diagnosis of depressive disorders is physical illness. Some medically ill youth may present with neurovegetative difficulties (e.g., sleep and eating difficulties) and somatic complaints (e.g., stomachaches and headaches). For some of these individuals, these symptoms indicate the presence of a mood disorder, whereas for others the symptoms may reflect the disease process or the iatrogenic effects of medical treatments. Often, these symptoms signal the presence of both psychological and physical difficulties. To diagnose mood disorders appropriately in medically ill children, a careful and individualized assessment must be conducted (Waller & Rush, 1983). Children who have chronic medical conditions may be at increased risk of depression (Bennett, 1994), but it is not always the case that medically ill children endorse higher levels of symptoms associated with depression than their healthy peers. For example, children in whom cancer has been diagnosed often report less depression than psychiatric patients (Worchel et al., 1988) or normal controls (Bennett, 1994), possibly reflecting denial of disease and distress as a coping mechanism. A complete medical evaluation and consultation with medical providers may be essential for a thorough diagnosis of depression in youth who are concerned about medical illnesses.

As noted earlier, a high incidence of comorbid depressive and other psychiatric disorders in children and adolescents complicates the diagnostic process. For example, the strong association of depressive disorders with anorexia nervosa and bulimia nervosa has received considerable attention (Braun, Sunday, & Halmi, 1994; Swift, Andrews, & Barklage, 1986). Given that dysphoric mood, irritability, weight loss, sleep disturbance, diminished interest in sex, social withdrawal, and concentration difficulties are integral features of the starvation process and essential symptoms of a depressive syndrome, it is not surprising that the majority of anorexic patients meet diagnostic criteria for major depressive disorder. The presence of these symptoms, however, rather than indicating depression, may more accurately reflect evidence of semistarvation syndrome. This particularly may be the case in those anorexic individuals who do not express feelings of worthlessness or self-reproach and who are not preoccupied with suicidal ideation or recurrent thoughts of death. These latter thoughts, though typically observed in depressed patients, are not generally reported by women who suffer from anorexia nervosa. Thus, although these individuals might technically meet DSM-IV criteria for major depressive disorder, other factors such as the psychobiological effects of starvation and the absence of self-deprecatory thoughts and suicidal ideation call into question a diagnosis of depression.

TREATMENT OF CHILD AND ADOLESCENT DEPRESSION

Researchers have begun to examine the efficacy of psychosocial and psychopharmacological treatments in improving outcomes for depressed youth (see Johnston & Fruehling, 1994; Kaslow & Thompson, 1998; Lewinsohn & Clarke, 1999; Lewinsohn, Clarke, &

Rohde, 1994; Stark, Rouse, & Kurowski, 1994). Many types of interventions are used in treating depression in youth, and the treatments can be conducted in individual, family, and group formats. The most common psychosocial approaches to treatment, cognitive-behavioral and psychodynamic, are briefly discussed here. Then, pharmacological interventions are reviewed.

Cognitive-behavioral therapies (CBT) have been the most researched type of psychotherapy for depressed youth. The assumption underlying CBT is that depression is the result of maladaptive cognitions, and the goal of treatment is to change these cognitions and their resulting behaviors. Treatment components often include relaxation training, cognitive restructuring, attribution retraining, increasing pleasant activities, as well as problem solving, social skills, and communication training. In addition, parent training may also be included to enhance parenting skills. CBT has been found effective for both depressed children and adolescents (Kaslow & Thompson, 1998; Lewinsohn & Clarke, 1999; Reinecke, Ryan, & Dubois, 1998; Stark et al., 1994).

Psychodynamic psychotherapy is another approach to treating child and adolescent depression (Shaffi & Shaffi, 1992). The assumption of psychodynamic therapy is that depression results from the individual's unconscious conflicts; the goal of treatment is to increase the youth's awareness of unconscious processes to work through these conflicts. The relationship between the therapist and the depressed youth is central to treatment. In session, the therapist maintains an accepting and nonjudgmental stance to encourage the child's expression of emotional conflicts. The use of play is important to the treatment, particularly for younger children, because it enhances the relationship between the child and the therapist. Psychodynamic treatments tend to be less directive and of longer duration than CBT. In contrast to CBT, psychodynamic interventions have not received much research attention during the past decade.

Pharmacotherapy is the major alternative to psychotherapeutic approaches to improving youths' short- and long-term course of depressive disorders. The two most commonly used classes of antidepressant medications used in treating children and adolescents are tricyclic antidepressants (TCAs) and selective serotonin re-uptake inhibitors (SSRIs). Initial methodologically flawed studies suggested that tricyclic antidepressants (e.g., imipramine, nortriptyline, amitriptyline) were effective in ameliorating depressive symptoms in 60 to 80% of depressed children (Birmaher et al., 1996b). However, TCAs must be carefully monitored due to cardiac side effects and the potential for lethality in overdose. In contrast, SSRIs (fluoxetine, sertraline) have fewer side effects and have been effective in treating depression in children and adolescents (Emslie et al., 1997). Therefore, SSRIs are becoming more popular than the TCAs as a first-line pharmacological treatment for depression (American Academy of Child and Adolescent Psychiatry [AACP], 1998).

Results from treatment outcome studies suggest that psychosocial interventions are effective in treating depression in children and adolescents (Kaslow & Thompson, 1998; Lewinsohn & Clarke, 1999) and antidepressants may be helpful for some youth (Emslie et al., 1997). Recently, the American Academy of Child and Adolescent Psychiatry (AACP, 1998) adopted practice standards for treating depressed youth. They argued that psychotherapy should be the first-line of intervention in depression. Though pharmacological treatment has been effective, the AACP indicated that it should not be used as the only treatment for children and adolescents and it should be used for certain types of depression (e.g., bipolar disorder, severe depression, depression that does not respond to psychotherapy) (AACP, 1998).

Research over the past decade has indicated that psychological treatments are effective in ameliorating depressive symptoms in youth, but the research has not clearly indicated that a single approach or modality (individual, family, or group) is most effective. This may be due to the relative dearth of empirically supported treatment research on depression in children and adolescents (Kaslow & Thompson, 1998). As more empirically supported treatment research is conducted, a greater understanding may develop of the types of treatment that are most efficacious.

SUMMARY

Depression as a clinical syndrome can be observed in a significant percentage of children and adolescents in the general population and a high percentage of clinical samples. Depression "runs in families" (Hammen, 1991), and thus, many depressed children have depressed parents. Although there are many parallels between child/adolescent and adult depression, the unique developmental characteristics of youth result in varying manifestations of the disorder during the life span. When diagnosing a depressive disorder in a child or adolescent, it is essential to incorporate information obtained from a multitrait, multimethod, and multi-informant assessment. This enables the clinician to develop a comprehensive picture of the depressed child's functioning across varying domains. Domains that deserve particular attention include psychological symptomatology; cognitive, affective, interpersonal, family, adaptive behavior; and neurobiological functioning. It is in these domains in which depressed youth's functioning may be most impaired.

Depression in childhood can be a serious condition that interferes with the child's development and functioning, even upon remission from a depressive episode. Depressions in children and adolescents tend to persist over time and to recur and thus necessitate treatment. The limited systematic treatment interventions conducted to date reveal that some form of psychosocial or pharmacological treatment is better than no treatment at all in ameliorating depressive symptoms and improving the course of the disorder. However, insufficient data exist to support the superiority of any given treatment. Further research needs to attend to the development and implementation of effective interventions for depressed youth, as well as prevention programs for youth at risk of depression.

REFERENCES

Achenbach, T. M., McConaughy, S. H., & Howell, C. T. (1987). Child/adolescent behavioral and emotional problems: Implications of cross-informant correlations for situational specificity. *Psychological Bulletin, 101*, 213–232.

Alessi, N. E., & Magen, J. (1988). Comorbidity of other psychiatric disturbances in depressed, psychiatrically hospitalized children. *American Journal of Psychiatry, 145*, 1582–1584.

Allgood-Merten, B., Lewinsohn, P. M., & Hops, H. (1990). Sex differences and adolescent depression. *Journal of Abnormal Psychology, 99*, 55–63.

Altmann, E. O., & Gotlib, I. H. (1988). The social behavior of depressed children: An observational study. *Journal of Child Psychology, 16*, 29–44.

American Academy of Child and Adolescent Psychiatry. (1998). Practice parameters for the assessment and treatment of children and adolescents with depressive disorders. *Journal of the American Academy of Child and Adolescent Psychiatry, 37*(Supplement), 63S–83S.

American Psychiatric Association. (1994). *Diagnostic and statistical manual of mental disorders*, 4th ed. Washington, DC: Author.

Angold, A. (1988). Childhood and adolescent depression. I. Epidemiological and aetiological aspects. *British Journal of Psychiatry, 152*, 601–617.

Beardslee, W. R., & Wheelock, I. (1994). Children of parents with affective disorders: Empirical findings and clinical implications. In W. M. Reynolds & H. F. Johnston (Eds.), *Handbook of depression in children and adolescents* (pp. 463–479). New York: Plenum.

Bell-Dolan, D. J., Reaven, N. M., & Peterson, L. (1993). Depression and social functioning: A multidimensional study of the linkages. *Journal of Clinical Child Psychology, 22,* 306–315.

Bennett, D. S. (1994). Depression among children with chronic medical problems: A meta-analysis. *Journal of Pediatric Psychology, 19,* 149–169.

Birmaher, B., Ryan, N. D., Williamson, D. E., Brent, D. A., Kaufman, J., Dahl, R. E., Perel, J., & Nelson, B. (1996a). Childhood and adolescent depression: A review of the past 10 years. Part I. *Journal of the American Academy of Child and Adolescent Psychiatry, 35,* 1427–1439.

Birmaher, B., Ryan, N. D., Williamson, D. E., Brent, D. A., & Kaufman, J. (1996b). Childhood and adolescent depression: A review of the past 10 years. Part II. *Journal of the American Academy of Child and Adolescent Psychiatry, 35,* 1575–1583.

Blumberg, S. H., & Izard, C. E. (1985). Affective and cognitive characteristics of depression in 10- and 11-year-old children. *Journal of Personality and Social Psychology, 49,* 194–202.

Bowlby, J. (1980). *Attachment and loss*: Vol. 3. *Loss: Sadness and depression.* New York: Basic Books.

Braun, D. L., Sunday, S. R., & Halmi, K. A. (1994). Psychiatric comorbidity in patients with eating disorders. *Psychological Medicine, 24,* 859–867.

Burke, K. C., Burke, J. D., Reigler, D. A., & Rae, D. S. (1990). Age at onset of selected mental disorders in five community populations. *Archives of General Psychiatry, 47,* 511–518.

Burke, P., & Puig-Antich, J. (1990). Psychobiology of childhood depression. In M. Lewis & S. M. Miller (Eds.), *Handbook of developmental psychopathology* (pp. 327–339). New York: Plenum.

Carlson, G. A., & Garber, J. (1986). Developmental issues in the classification of depression in children. In M. Rutter, C. E. Izard & P. B. Read (Eds.), *Depression in young people* (pp. 399–434). New York: Guilford.

Cole, D. (1990). Relation of social and academic competence to depressive symptoms in childhood. *Journal of Abnormal Psychology, 99,* 42–429.

Cumsille, P. E., & Epstein, N. (1994). Family cohesion, family adaptability, social support, and adolescent depressive symptoms in outpatient clinical families. *Journal of Family Psychology, 8,* 202–214.

Dally, M. B., Bolocofsky, D. N., & Karlin, N. J. (1994). Teacher-ratings and self-ratings of social competency in adolescents with low- and high-depressive symptoms. *Journal of Abnormal Child Psychology, 22,* 477–485.

Digdon, N., & Gotlib, I. H. (1985). Developmental considerations in the study of childhood depression. *Developmental Reviews, 5,* 162–199.

Downey, G., & Coyne, J. C. (1990). Children of depressed parents: An integrative review. *Psychological Bulletin, 108,* 50–76.

Emslie, G. J., Weinberg, W. A., Kennard, B. D., & Kowatch, R. A. (1994). Neurobiological aspects of depression in children and adolescents. In W. M. Reynolds & H. F. Johnston (Eds.), *Handbook of depression in children and adolescents* (pp. 143–165). New York: Plenum.

Emslie, G. J., Rush, A. J., Weinberg, W. A., Kowatch, R. A., Hughes, C. W., Carmody, T., & Rintelmann, J. (1997). A double-blind, randomized, placebo-controlled trial of fluoxetine in children and adolescents with depression. *Archives of General Psychiatry, 54,* 1031–1038.

Fleming, J. E., & Offord, D. R. (1990). Epidemiology of childhood depressive disorders: A critical review. *Journal of American Academy of Child and Adolescent Psychiatry, 29,* 571–580.

Garber, J., Braafladt, N., & Zeman, J. (1991). The regulation of sad affect: An information-processing perspective. In J. Garber & K. A. Dodge (Eds.), *The development of emotion regulation and dysregulation* (pp. 208–240). New York: Cambridge University Press.

Gjerde, P. F., Block, J., & Block, J. H. (1988). Depressive symptoms and personality during late adolescence: Gender differences in the externalization-internalization of symptom expression. *Journal of Abnormal Psychology, 97,* 475–486.

Hammen, C. (1991). *Depression runs in families: The social context of risk and resilience in children of depressed mothers.* New York: Springer Verlag.

Harrington, R. (1993). *Depressive disorder in childhood and adolescence.* Chichester, England: Wiley.

Johnston, H. F., & Fruehling, J. J. (1994). Pharmacotherapy for depression in children and adolescents. In W. M. Reynolds & H. F. Johnston (Eds.), *Handbook of depression in children and adolescents* (pp. 365–397). New York: Plenum.

Kashani, J. H., & Sherman, D. D. (1988). Childhood depression: Epidemiology, etiological models, and treatment implications. *Integrative Psychiatry, 6,* 1–8.

Kaslow, N. J., Brown, R. T., & Mee, L. L. (1994). Cognitive and behavioral correlates of childhood depression: A developmental perspective. In W. M. Reynolds & H. F. Johnston (Eds.), *Handbook of depression in children and adolescents* (pp. 97–121). New York: Plenum.

Kaslow, N. J., Croft, S. S., & Hatcher, C. A. (1999). Depression an bipolar disorder in children and adolescents. In S. D. Netherton, D. Holmes, & C. E. Walker (Eds.), *Child and adolescent psychological disorders: A comprehensive textbook* (pp. 264–281). New York: Oxford University Press.

Kaslow, N. J., Deering, C. G., & Ash, P. (1996). Relational diagnosis of child and adolescent depression. In F. W. Kaslow (Ed.), *Handbook of relational diagnosis and dysfunctional family patterns* (pp. 171–185). New York: Wiley.

Kaslow, N. J., Deering, C. G., & Racusin, G. R. (1994). Depressed children and their families. *Clinical Psychology Review, 14*, 39–59.

Kaslow, N. J., & Racusin, G. R. (1990). Childhood depression: Current status and future directions. In A. S. Bellack, M. Hersen, & A. E. Kazdin (Eds.), *International handbook of behavior modification and therapy*, 2nd ed. (pp. 649–667). New York: Plenum.

Kaslow, N. J., Rehm, L. P., Pollack, S. L., & Siegel, A. W. (1990). Depression and perception of family functioning in children and their parents. *American Journal of Family Therapy, 18*, 227–235.

Kaslow, N. J., & Thompson, M. P. (1998). Applying the criteria for empirically supported treatments to studies of psychosocial interventions for child and adolescent depression. *Journal of Clinical Child Psychology, 27*, 146–155.

Kazdin, A. E. (1988). The diagnosis of childhood disorders: Assessment issues and strategies. *Behavioral Assessment, 10*, 67–94.

Kazdin, A. E., Sherick, R. B., Esveldt-Dawson, K., & Racurello, M. D. (1985). Nonverbal behavior and childhood depression. *Journal of American Academy of Child Psychiatry, 24*, 303–309.

Kazdin, A. E. (1994). Informant variability in the assessment of childhood depression. In W. M. Reynolds & H. F. Johnston (Eds.), *Handbook of depression in children and adolescents* (pp. 249–271). New York: Plenum.

Kolko, D. J., & Kazdin, A. E. (1993). Emotional/behavioral problems in clinic and nonclinic children: Correspondence among child, parent, and teacher reports. *Journal of Child Psychology and Psychiatry, 34*, 991–1006.

Kovacs, M. (1985). The natural history and course of depressive disorders in childhood. *Psychiatric Annals, 15*, 387–389.

Kovacs, M. (1989). Affective disorders in children and adolescents. *American Psychologist, 44*, 209–215.

Kovacs, M., Gatsonis, C., Paulauskas, S., & Richards, C. (1989). Depressive disorders in childhood: IV. A longitudinal study of comorbidity with and risk for anxiety disorders. *Archives of General Psychiatry, 46*, 776–782.

Kovacs, M. (1996). Presentation and course of major depressive disorder during childhood and later years of the life span. *Journal of the American Academy of Child and Adolescent Psychiatry, 35*, 705–715.

Kovacs, M., Obrosky, D. S., Gatsonis, C., & Richards, C. (1997). First-episode major depressive and dysthymic disorder in childhood: Clinical and sociodemographic factors in recovery. *Journal of the American Academy of Child and Adolescent Psychiatry, 36*, 777–784.

Kutcher, S. P., & Marton, P. (1989). Parameters of adolescent depression: A review. *Psychiatric Clinics of North America, 12*, 895–918.

Larsson, B., & Melin, L. (1990). Depressive symptoms in Swedish adolescents. *Journal of Abnormal Child Psychology, 18*, 91–103.

Lewinsohn, P. M., & Clarke, G. N. (1999). Psychosocial treatments for adolescent depression. *Clinical Psychology Review, 19*, 329–342.

Lewinsohn, P. M., Clarke, G. N., & Rohde, P. (1994). Psychological approaches to the treatment of depression in adolescents. In W. M. Reynolds & H. F. Johnston (Eds.), *Handbook of depression in children and adolescents* (pp. 309–344). New York: Plenum.

Lewinsohn, P. M., Rohde, P., & Seeley, J. R. (1993). Psychosocial characteristics of adolescents with a history of suicide attempt. *Journal of the American Academy of Child and Adolescent Psychiatry, 32*, 60–68.

Lewinsohn, P. M., Rohde, P., & Seeley, J. R. (1998). Major depressive disorder in older adolescents: Prevalence, risk factors, and clinical implications. *Clinical Psychology Review, 18*, 765–794.

Marton, P., Korenblum, M., Kutcher, S., Stein, B., Kennedy, B., & Pakes, J. (1989). Personality dysfunction in depressed adolescents. *Canadian Journal of Psychiatry, 34*, 810–813.

McCracken, J. T. (1992). The epidemiology of child and adolescent mood disorders. *Child and Adolescent Psychiatric Clinics of North America, 1*, 53–72.

Merikangas, K. R., Prusoff, B. A., & Weissman, M. M. (1988). Parental concordance for affective disorders: Psychopathology in offspring. *Journal of Affective Disorders, 15*, 279–290.

Mitchell, J., McCauley, E., Burke, P., Calderon, R., & Schloredt, K. (1989). Psychopathology in parents of depressed children and adolescents. *Journal of the American Academy of Child and Adolescent Psychiatry, 28*, 352–357.

Moreau, D. (1996). Depression in the young. In J. A. Sechzer, S. M. Pfafflin, et al. (Eds.), *Women in mental health. Annals of the New York Academy of Sciences, 789,* 31–44.

Mullins, L. L., Peterson, L., Wonderlich, S. A., & Reaven, N. M. (1986). The influence of depressive symptomatology in children on the social responses and perception of adults. *Journal of Clinical Child Psychology, 15,* 233–240.

Nolen-Hoeksema, S., & Girgus, J. (1994). The emergence of gender differences in depression during adolescence. *Psychological Bulletin, 115,* 424–443.

Peterson, A. C., Compas, B. E., Brooks-Gunn, J., Stemmler, M., Ey, S., & Grant, K. E. (1993). Depression in adolescence. *American Psychologist, 48,* 155–168.

Politano, P. M., Nelson, W. M., Evans, H., Sorenson, S., & Zeman, D. (1986). Factor analytic evaluation of differences between Black and Caucasian emotionally disturbed children on the Children's Depression Inventory. *Journal of Psychopathology and Behavioral Assessment, 8,* 1–7.

Puig-Antich, J., Goetz, D., Davies, M., Kaplan, T., Davies, S., Ostrow, L., Asnis, L., Twomey, J., Iyengar, S., & Ryan, N. D. (1989). A controlled family history study of prepubertal major depressive disorder. *Archives of General Psychiatry, 46,* 406–418.

Puig-Antich, J., Kaufman, J., Ryan, N. D., Williamson, D., Dahl, R. E., Lukens, E., Todak, G., Ambrosini, P., Rabinovich, H., & Nelson, B. (1993). The psychosocial functioning and family environment of depressed adolescents. *Journal of the American Academy of Child and Adolescent Psychiatry, 32,* 244–253.

Puig-Antich, J., Lukens, E., Davies, M., Goetz, D., Brennan-Quattrock, J., & Todak, G. (1985). Psychosocial functioning in prepubertal major depressive disorders. I. Interpersonal relationships during the depressive episode. *Archives of General Psychiatry, 42,* 500–507.

Racusin, G. R., & Kaslow, N. J. (1991). Assessment and treatment of childhood depression. In P. A. Keller & S. R. Heyman (Eds.), *Innovations in clinical practice: A sourcebook,* Vol. 10 (pp. 223–243). Sarasota, FL: Professional Resource Exchange.

Reinecke, M. A., Ryan, N. E., & DuBois, D. L. (1998). Cognitive-behavioral therapy of depression and depressive symptoms during adolescence: A review and meta-analysis. *Journal of the American Academy of Child and Adolescent Psychiatry, 37,* 26–34.

Roberts, R. E., Roberts, C. R., & Chen, Y. R. (1997). Ethnocultural differences in prevalence of adolescent depression. *American Journal of Community Psychology, 25,* 95–110.

Rosenthal, N. E., Carpenter, C. J., James, S. P., Parry, B. L., Rogers, S. L. B., & Wehr, T. A. (1986). Seasonal affective disorder in children and adolescents. *American Journal of Psychiatry, 143,* 356–358.

Rudolph, K. D., Hammen, C., & Burge, D. (1994). Interpersonal functioning and depressive symptoms in childhood: Addressing the issues of specificity and comorbidity. *Journal of Abnormal Child Psychology, 22,* 355–371.

Schulterbrandt, J. G., & Raskin, A. (Eds.). (1977). *Depression in childhood: Diagnosis, treatment, and conceptual models.* New York: Raven.

Schwartz, J. A. J., Gladstone, T. R. G., & Kaslow, N. J. (1998b). Depressive disorders. In T. H. Ollendick & M. Hersen (Eds.), *Handbook of child psychopathology,* 3rd ed. (pp. 269–289). New York: Plenum.

Schwartz, J. A. J., Kaslow, N. J., Racusin, G. R., & Carton, E. R. (1998a). Interpersonal family therapy for childhood depression. In V. B. Van Hasselt & M. Hersen (Eds.), *Handbook of psychological treatment protocols for children and adolescents* (pp. 109–151). Mahwah, NJ: Erlbaum.

Shafii, M., & Shafii, S. L. (1992). Dynamic psychotherapy of depression. In M. Shafii & S. L. Shafii (Eds.), *Clinical guide to depression in children and adolescents* (pp. 157–175). Washington, DC: American Psychiatric Press.

Spitz, R. (1946). Anaclitic depression. *Psychoanalytic Study of the Child, 5,* 113–117.

Stark, K. (1990). *Childhood depression: School-based intervention.* New York: Guilford.

Stark, K. D., Humphrey, L. L., Crook, K., & Lewis, K. (1990). Perceived family environments of depressed and anxious children: Child's and maternal figure's perspectives. *Journal of Abnormal Child Psychology, 18,* 527–547.

Stark, K. D., Rouse, L. W., & Kurowski, C. (1994). Psychological treatment approaches for depression in children. In W. M. Reynolds & H. F. Johnston (Eds.), *Handbook of depression in children and adolescents* (pp. 275–307). New York: Plenum.

Swedo, S. E., Pleeter, J. D., Richter, D. M., Hoffman, C. L., Allen, A. J., Hamburger, S. D., Turner, E. H., Yamada, E. M., & Rosenthal, N. E. (1995). Rates of seasonal affective disorder in children and adolescents. *American Journal of Psychiatry, 152,* 1016–1019.

Swift, W. J., Andrews, D., & Barklage, N. E. (1986). The relationship between affective disorder and eating disorders: A review of the literature. *American Journal of Psychiatry, 143,* 290–299.

Todd, R. D., Geller, B., Neuman, R., Fox, L. W., & Hickok, J. (1996). Increased prevalence of alcoholism in relatives of depressed and bipolar children. *Journal of the American Academy of Child and Adolescent Psychiatry, 35,* 716–724.

Waller, D. A., & Rush, J. (1983). Differentiating primary affective disease, organic affective syndromes, and situational depression on a pediatric service. *Journal of the American Academy of Child Psychiatry, 22*, 52–58.

Weller, E. B., & Weller, R. A. (1991). Mood disorders. In M. Lewis (Ed.), *Child and adolescent psychiatry: A comprehensive textbook* (pp. 646–664). Baltimore: Williams & Wilkins.

Woolston, J. L., Rosenthal, S. L., Riddle, M. A., Sparrow, S. S., Cicchetti, D., & Zimmerman, L. D. (1989). Childhood comorbidity of anxiety/affective disorders and behavior disorders. *Journal of the American Academy of Child and Adolescent Psychiatry, 28*, 707–713.

Worchel, F. F., Hughes, J. N., Hall, B. M., Stanton, S. B., Stanton, S., & Little, V. Z. (1990). Evaluation of subclinical depression in children using self-, peer-, and teacher-report measures. *Journal of Abnormal Child Psychology, 18*, 271–282.

Worchel, F. F., Nolan, B. F., Willson, V. L., Purser, J. S., Copeland, D. R., & Pfefferbaum, B. (1988). Assessment of depression in children with cancer. *Journal of Pediatric Psychology, 13*, 101–112.

13

Eating Disorders

Linda Krug Porzelius, Britta D. Dinsmore, and Darlene Staffelbach

The majority of women in Western industrialized countries experience some symptoms of eating disorder, including body dissatisfaction, excessive weight concerns, chronic dieting, and extreme weight control practices. Almost all women report some dissatisfaction with their bodies and appearance, and more than half report significant dissatisfaction (Cash & Henry, 1995). The term "normative discontent" highlights just how widespread weight concerns are among girls and women in our society (Striegel-Moore, Silberstein, & Rodin, 1986).

Sociocultural factors play an important casual role in "normative discontent" and in severe eating disorders (for reviews, see Gilbert & Thompson, 1996; Stice, 1994). Socio-cultural pressures are readily apparent in the gaunt images seen in television and magazines that portray the supposedly successful woman. During the past 30 years, fashion models and Miss America participants have gotten progressively taller and thinner and now weigh 13 to 19% under normal weight (Garner, Garfinkel, Schwartz, & Thompson, 1980; Wiseman, Gray, Mosimann, & Ahrens, 1992). The fashion and cosmetic industries make millions by instilling appearance anxiety and body dissatisfaction to sell their products, equating thinness with attractiveness, and success, and overweight bodies with unattractiveness and laziness (Rothblum, 1994). Given the impossibly stringent beauty standards portrayed in the media, nearly all women are at some risk of body dissatisfaction, an important etiological factor in the development of eating disorders.

Another message society promotes is the view that one's body can be "shaped and molded at will and that with only the right diet, exercise program, and personal effort, an individual can have the perfect weight and contours" (Brownell & Wadden, 1962, p. 507). The dieting industry makes billions selling weight loss plans that do not work to girls and women who often do not need them. Half of adolescent girls (Grigg, Bowman, & Redman, 1996), and 30% of adult women are dieting at any given time (Neumark-Sztainer, Jeffery, & French, 1997). In a large study of 14- to 16-year-old-girls, more than one-third reported using extreme

LINDA KRUG PORZELIUS • School of Professional Psychology, Pacific University, Forest Grove, Oregon 97116. BRITTA D. DINSMORE • Pacific University Student Counseling Center, Forest Grove, Oregon 97116. DARLENE STAFFELBACH • St. Vincent's Hospital Eating Disorder Program, Providence St. Vincent Hospital, Portland, Oregon 97225.

Advanced Abnormal Psychology, Second Edition, edited by Hersen and Van Hasselt. Kluwer Academic/Plenum Publishers, New York, 2001.

dieting measures in the past month, such as fasting, diet pills, diuretics, laxatives, and cigarette smoking (Grigg et al., 1996). Girls as young as six years old express weight concerns and report that they are dieting (Flannery-Schroeder & Chrisler, 1996). Women more than 60 years old continue to be concerned about weight issues and unhappy with their bodies (Hetherington & Burnett, 1994).

Substantial evidence indicates that body dissatisfaction and dieting are rampant and are important contributors to the development of eating disorders; yet not all women who are unhappy with their bodies develop serious eating disorders. Support can be found for a continuum of eating and weight symptoms, ranging from no body dissatisfaction to moderate dissatisfaction and dieting, to clinical eating disorders. The development of clinical eating disorders involves a complex interaction of biological, psychological, and social factors. In clinical eating disorders, body dissatisfaction and weight concerns are intense and pervasive and reflect a dread of being fat. Weight becomes the most important way in which the woman defines herself. Weight control practices are extreme and involve frequent fasting, abuse of laxatives, or self-induced vomiting. Health, social life, school, and work are often greatly impacted.

The major clinical eating disorders are Anorexia Nervosa (AN), Bulimia Nervosa (BN), and Binge Eating Disorder (BED) (*Diagnostic and Statistical Manual* [DSM-IV]; American Psychiatric Association [APA], 1994). AN is characterized by a refusal to maintain normal body weight due to fear of weight gain and to body image disturbance and can be either restricting or binge/purge type. BN involves recurrent binge eating and regular use of behaviors to compensate for calorie intake (APA). Individuals who have the purging type of BN use self-induced vomiting, laxatives, or diuretics to prevent weight gain. Individuals who have nonpurging BN use either extreme dieting or excessive exercise to prevent weight gain from binges. Individuals who have BED engage in frequent and regular binge eating but do not regularly use unhealthy methods to prevent weight gain.

EPIDEMIOLOGY

Anorexia Nervosa and Bulimia Nervosa

Many studies have assessed prevalence rates for eating disorders, most among groups of girls and women in Western countries where eating disorder rates are highest. Studies vary tremendously in methodology, definition of eating disorders, and samples and make interpretation difficult (Fairburn & Beglin, 1990; Hoek, 1993; Hsu, 1996). In a review of epidemiological studies of eating disorders, Hsu estimated the point prevalence of AN between 0.2% and 0.5%, and of BN between 2% to 3%. Lifetime prevalence rates are generally higher (Hoek, 1993). In a recent study using a general female sample, Gotestam and Agras (1995) found a lifetime prevalence of 8.7% across all eating disorder categories, 3% for EDNOS, and 2% for strictly defined AN and BN. Some evidence suggest that rates may be increasing among young women (Hoek, 1993). Eating disorder rates tend to be much higher among certain subgroups. Gymnasts, dancers, and models, who experience intense pressures to be thin, all have elevated rates of eating disorders (Hsu, 1996). Behaviors associated with eating disorders are much more common than full-blown eating disorders. Approximately 24% of women report having had eating binges, and 5% report self-induced vomiting (Sullivan, Bulik, & Kendler, 1998). Thus, many women have significant problems with binge eating and/or purging but do not meet criteria for BN or BED.

Men clearly experience fewer risk factors for eating disorders, including less media pressure to be thin (Andersen & DiDomenico, 1992), less body dissatisfaction (Feingold & Massella, 1998), and less dieting (Neumark-Sztainer, Jeffery, & French, 1997). Not surprisingly, men are also less likely to de diagnosed with an eating disorder (Hoek, 1993). In clinical samples, females account for about 93% of individuals diagnosed with AN and 96% of those with BN. In studies using community samples, the rates of males with eating disorders tend to be higher than in studies using clinical samples, suggesting that men are less likely to seek treatment (Carlat & Camargo, 1991). However, a recent study indicated that rates of men seeking treatment for an eating disorder may be increasing (Braun, Sunday, Huang, & Halmi, 1999). In general, boys and men who develop eating disorders show similar levels of body dissatisfaction, eating and weight symptoms, and associated pathology (Carlat, Camargo, & Herzog, 1997; Keel, Klump, Leon, & Fulkerson, 1998). Men tend to have a later onset of their eating disorders and are more likely to be involved in a sport, such as rowing, cross-country running, wrestling, and bodybuilding, where performance is influenced by weight (Braun et al., 1999; Carlat et al., 1997). Although disordered eating behaviors are common among male athletes, most do not have full blown eating disorders. In particular, men often do not have a morbid fear of fat typical of eating disorders (Hsu, 1996).

Eating disorders are relatively rare in nonindustrialized cultures (for reviews, see Fedoroff & McFarlane, 1998; Hoek, 1993; Hsu, 1996). Among immigrants from nonindustrialized countries, eating disorders rates increase in relation to the degree of acculturation to Western ideals. Rates are also lower among ethnic minority women within Western cultures, although research is needed to obtain accurate prevalence information (Fedoroff & McFarlane, 1998). However, eating disorders may be underdiagnosed if therapists assume that minority women do not experience body dissatisfaction and eating problems. To the extent that a minority woman "buys into" cultural pressures for thinness, she is likely to experience body dissatisfaction and weight concerns, which are risk factors for eating disorders. Additionally, society's marginalization of women of color may contribute to feelings of inadequacy and place these women at risk of developing eating disorders. Although eating disorders appear to occur less often among women of color, they do occur and should not be ignored. Women of color who develop eating disorders are similar to eating disordered white women in demographic characteristics, symptoms, and general psychopathology (le Grange, Telch, & Agras, 1997).

Both AN and BN tend to be thought of as affecting middle to upper class females, and some evidence supports this view (Hoek, 1993). However, not all studies find different rates of eating disorders across SES groups (Rogers, Resnick, Mitchell, & Blum, 1997). In their recent review on SES and eating disorders, Gard and Freeman (1996) found no relationship between AN and SES, and possibly an inverse relationship between BN an SES. It is clear that eating disorders can occur across all classes and exhibit similar patterns of symptomatology an psychopathology.

Binge Eating Disorder

As a relatively new diagnostic category, much less is know about rates of BED than of the traditional eating disorders. BED became a focus of attention when university-based weight control programs identified rates of 20 to 40% among participants (Castonguay, Eldredge, & Agras, 1995). Community studies find lifetime prevalence rates of approximately 1.5% among women (Gotestam & Agras, 1995), and 2% in women and men (Spitzer, Devlin, Walsh et al., 1992). Among overweight individuals, rates are 2.9%, almost double the rates among normal weight individuals (Smith, Marcus, Lewis, Fitzgibbon, & Schreiner, 1998).

Demographic correlates of BED are quite different from the traditional eating disorders. Rates of BED are only slightly higher for women than men (Spitzer et al., 1992; Spitzer, Yanovski, Wadden et al., 1993). Men and women who have BED are similar in demographic characteristics, eating symptoms, and associated psychopathology (Striegel-Moore, Wilson, Wilfley, Elder, & Brownell, 1998; Tanofsky, Wilfley, Spurrell, Welch, & Brownell, 1997). Rates of BED appear similar among Black, White, and Hispanic women (Bruace & Agras, 1992; Smith et al., 1998), although Hispanic women may experience more severe binge eating problems (Fitzgibbon, Spring, Avellone et al., 1998).

CLINICAL PICTURE

Case Descriptions

BULIMIA NERVOSA

Teresa was a 32-year-old married woman who had two small children and worked as a part-time waitress. Although of normal weight, she constantly dieted, hoping to get back down to her high school weight of 100 pounds. She remembers starting to worry about her weight at age 11, after her father teased her about getting fat. She went on her first diet at age 14 and dieted together with a friend. Although successful at keeping her weight below normal for several years, Teresa's hunger and cravings eventually weakened her control and she began binge eating. Extremely fearful of getting fat, she began making herself vomit after overeating. She was disgusted with herself for binge eating and vomiting, but also felt a strong sense of relief that she could overeat without gaining weight. Purging allowed her to binge on larger and larger amounts of food, without fear of weight gain.

On most mornings, Teresa vowed to quit binge eating and purging. She carefully counted calories, trying to follow a healthy diet plan. She usually failed. Hunger, stress, and loneliness combined, leading her to binge and purge. For years, Teresa kept her bulimia a secret from her parents, sisters, friends, and husband. She had two full-term pregnancies during which she did not vomit or use laxatives "for the baby's sake." However, she was extremely anxious about getting fat during the pregnancies and continued to restrict her eating. For a short time after the pregnancies, she quit binge eating or purging. However, her dieting continued and eventually the binges resumed. At age 32, she finally sought treatment for her eating disorder after multiple visits to the emergency room for dizziness and dehydration.

ANOREXIA NERVOSA

Katrina, a high school sophomore, was a straight "A" student, active in track and student government. At 5'6" and 100 pounds, she looked strikingly thin, have lost 30 pounds in the last four months. Coming from a health-conscience family, she had always tried to eat healthfully. However, she had become increasingly rigid about "healthy eating" since her track coach talked to her about getting her weight down four months ago. She was now eating only fruits and vegetables, eliminating all fats from her diet. She exercised regularly, running and lifting weights two to three hours per day. Recently, she had begun to participate less in school and social activities, preferring to use her time to exercise. She felt proud of the weight loss she had achieved, and fearful that, should she fail to maintain her behaviors, she would get fat. She weighed herself at least four time daily, feeling her pride when her weight was under 100 pounds, and intense fear when the scale indicated that her weight was higher. Katrina often felt cold and dressed in many layers of clothing to stay warm. The layers also offered protection from others' comments about how she looked. She had not had her period for four months. Although secretly relieved not to have them, she worried that something might be wrong. She was frequently dizzy but told no one.

Central Characteristics

BODY IMAGE DISTURBANCE

A large volume of research identifies body image disturbances as important in the etiology and maintenance and AN and BN (for a review, see Thompson, 1996). Although common in many non-eating-disordered girls and women, body image disturbances are much more severe among individuals who have eating disorders (Cash & Deagle, 1997). In AN, body image disturbance often involves a distorted perception of body shape or size, as evidenced in Katrina, who is emaciated yet continues to feel fat, and believes that her stomach is bulging. Another form of body image distortion is seen in young women who fail to recognize the seriousness of their weight loss. Dissatisfaction with weight or shape is a common type of body image disturbance found in all eating disorders but is more pronounced in BN than in AN (Cash & Deagle, 1997). Although not a criterion in the diagnosis of BED (APA, 1994), body dissatisfaction appears to be significant in this groups and is related to their obesity (Johnson & Torgrud, 1996). A final type of body image disturbance, typical of both AN and BN, involves overemphasis on weight and shape in defining self-worth (APA).

Given our society's obsession with thinness, it is not surprising that women who are genetically predisposed toward being heavier are more likely to be dissatisfied with their bodies. Longitudinal studies find that girls who have higher percentages of body fat are most at risk of developing eating disorders over time (for review see Hsu, 1997). Overweight girls are also more likely to have experienced teasing about their weight. Teasing about weight from peers and family members is a risk factor for both body dissatisfaction and eating disorders (Thompson, 1996). Overweight and teasing about weight appear to be particularly important risk factor for BED (Fariburn, Doll, Welch et al., 1998). Families who emphasize weight and appearance may also contribute to body dissatisfaction, dieting, and eating disorders, although research is mixed (Agras, Hammer, & McNicholas, 1999). Membership in groups that emphasize the importance of thinness and appearance, such as dancers, gymnasts, or models, also increases the risk of body dissatisfaction (Stice, 1994).

DIETING

Dieting has been clearly identified as a risk factor in the development of eating disorders (Hsu, 1996). In BN and AN, dieting almost always precedes the onset of binge eating, and usually continues between binges (Polivy & Herman, 1985). Furthermore, the prevalence of eating disorders in populations is increased in proportion to the prevalence of dieting behavior (Hsu, 1966). In one prospective study, adolescent girls who reported frequent dieting were three to eight times more likely to develop disordered eating behaviors than those who reported not dieting frequently (French, Perry, Leon, & Fulkerson, 1995). The role of dieting in the onset of BED appears to be less central. Many report an onset of dieting after the onset of binge eating (Howard & Porzelius, 1998; Santonasto, Ferrara, & Favaro, 1999).

The manner in which women who have eating disorders attempt to diet or restrict their eating varies considerably from highly selective and restrictive dieting, involving periods of fasting or severe calorie limits, to more moderate, healthful restriction in type or amount of food eaten. Dieting in AN is often obsessive. Food rituals may develop, such as cutting food into minute portions or taking an exact number of sips of water between each bite. Rituals for food preparation and consumption may be a result of starvation (Keys, Brozek, Henschel, Mickelson, & Taylor, 1950). In BN, skipping meals is common (Guertin, 1999). High-fat snacks and desserts are typically avoided, labeled as "unsafe" or "forbidden."

Although dieting is implicated in the development of eating disorders, not all who diet develop eating disorders. Dieting may be most problematic for women who lack a sense of competence and mastery in other areas of their lives. For these women, successful weight loss provides a source of self-worth and helps to combat feelings of inadequacy (Gayner, Vitousek, & Pike, 1997; Tiggeman & Raven, 1998). Unassertive and outwardly compliant in many areas, eating and weight offer an area where they are in control. As described in Katrina's case, a sense of accomplishment comes from achieving weight loss and controlling hunger, which serves as a strong positive reinforcer to maintain food restriction (Vitousek & Hollon, 1993). The attention and energy spent on weight loss may also help the individual to avoid dealing with many anxieties of adolescence, including sexuality and separation from parents (Strober, 1997; Vitousek & Hollon, 1993).

BINGE EATING

For many, chronic, rigid dieting cannot be sustained. Physiological, cognitive, or emotional events disrupt dietary restraint, resulting in a loss of control over eating or a binge (Grilo & Shiffman, 1994; Policy & Herman, 1995; Schlundt & Johnson, 1990). Typical triggers include stress, negative emotions, hunger, the presence of food cues, and eating a forbidden food. Triggers for BED are similar to those for BN and AN but are not often triggered by hunger (Agras & Talch, 1998; Johnson & Torgrud, 1996). Binges most typically occur in the afternoon or evening, during unstructured times, and when alone. In AN and BN, women are often very secretive, especially about purging. Binges in BED occur with and without others present (Johnson & Torgrud, 1996). Binges typically involve rapid consumption of avoided or "forbidden" foods (Guertin, 1999). The length of a binge episode is usually about 30 to 60 minutes, although longer bingers are not uncommon and may involve multiple purges during the episode. In BED, binges occur less often and involve smaller amounts of food than in BN (Hay & Fairburn, 1998).

Binge eating raises the mood in the short-term (Lingswiler, Crowther, & Stephens, 1989). However, shortly after the binge, the mood drops, and feelings of extreme guilt, depression, self-loathing, and intense anxiety about weight gain arise. Purging reduces anxiety about weight gain following a binge (Rosen & Leitenberg, 1988), and initial feelings of relief give way to feelings of shame and disgust, further contributing to poor self-esteem (Fairburn, Marcus, & Wilson, 1993). The individual then renews her commitment to dieting to overcome feelings of inadequacy. In BED, binge eating may be maintained by a "trade-off" (Kenardy, Arnow, & Agras, 1997). Negative moods before the binge are replaced by guilt and fear of weight gain, which are less aversive negative feelings than those that triggered the binge.

PURGING

Purging behaviors include self-induced vomiting, abuse of laxatives, diuretics, enemas, appetite suppressants, and other medications. Self-induced vomiting is the most commonly reported method of purging, followed by laxative use, although many women use multiple methods of purging (Schlundt & Johnson, 1990). Most methods do not effectively rid the body of calories eaten. Rather, they result in water loss, which temporarily makes the individual feel thinner.

Associated Characteristics

A substantial body of research has identified the characteristics of individuals who have eating disorders, though most of the research is correlational. Several etiological models have been developed and are beginning to be evaluated. Models generally include sociocultural factors, as previously described. Cultural pressures on women to achieve an overly thin weight clearly have an enormous impact on dieting and weight concerns for many women in our society. However, some women are particularly vulnerable to these pressures. Thus, etiological models must identify additional vulnerability factors. The following section briefly reviews psychological and environmental correlates of eating disorders, some of which are important in etiology. Because of the reciprocal relationship between eating symptoms and psychological features, it is difficult to distinguish between factors that are etiological and those that are merely correlates, possibly even themselves caused by abnormal eating practices. For example, starvation can cause many of the symptoms observed in AN, including food rituals, mood swings, cognitive functioning, fatigue, and decreased sleep (Keys, Brozek, Henschel, Mickelson, & Taylor, 1950).

The following section briefly reviews the characteristics commonly associated with eating disorders, including personality characteristics, problems with mood regulation, deficits in coping skills, and interpersonal difficulties. Environmental correlates of eating disorders are briefly summarized, focusing on family environment and sexual trauma.

PERSONALITY

A considerable amount of research has examined personality characteristics associated with eating disorders, which may play an important role in etiology. AN is typically associated with obsessive-compulsive features, harm avoidance, shyness, perfectionism, compliance, and dependency (for a review, see Vitousek & Manke, 1994). Obsessiveness commonly extends beyond the food and exercise domain and often includes fastidiousness with living space and personal hygiene. Although starvation symptoms may exacerbate these personality characteristics, traits are found before the onset of AN, and after treatment, when weight is restored. Unlike AN, BN is typically associated with emotional lability, novelty seeking, sociability, and impulsivity. Some traits are seen in both AN and BN, including perfectionism, negative affect, and harm avoidance. Binge/purge type of AN tends to be more similar to BN than to Restricting AN. Available research suggests that individuals who have BED have personality traits similar to individuals who have BN, but less extreme (Castonguay, Eldredge, & Agras, 1995).

MOOD REGULATION

Negative affect and mood instability are commonly associated with eating disorders, particularly when binge eating is present (Vitousek & Manke, 1994). Among early adolescents, self-reported negative emotionality and an inability to label emotional arousal act as risk factors in the development of an eating disorder (Leon, Fulkerson, Perry, & Cudek, 1993). Stress and negative affect are also common antecedents of binge eating (Davis, Freeman, & Garner, 1988; Elmore & deCastro, 1990; Rebert, Stanton, & Schwartz, 1991). In addition, binge eating is associated with reductions in negative mood states, including depression, anger, boredom, shame, and anxiety (Steinberg, Tobin, & Johnson, 1990; Teusch, 1988). Binge eating may soothe negative emotions or may be a means to avoid painful emotions by narrowing the individual's focus of attention and distracting from painful self-awareness (Heatherton & Baumeister, 1991; Polivy & Herman, 1993). Reduction in negative affect during and imme- diately after the binge reinforces eating as a way to cope with negative affect. Foods eaten during a binge may have particularly strong reward potential following restriction of food intake (Wardle, 1988).

Coping Skill Deficits

Deficits in coping skills among individuals who have eating disorders may contribute to frequent mood fluctuations and to the use of eating as a way to cope with emotions (for review, see Christiano & Mizes, 1997). Numerous studies have identified deficits in both appraisal and coping skills among individuals who have eating disorders (Cattanach & Rodin, 1988; Hansel & Wittrock, 1997; Soukup, Beiler, & Terrell, 1998). Women who have eating disorders report frequent use of avoidant coping and emotion-oriented strategies (Koff & Sangani, 1997; Paxton & Diggens, 1997; Troop, Holbrey, & Treasure, 1998), which tend to be ineffective in the long run (Wills, 1997). Individuals who have eating disorders are more likely to rate events as highly stressful and threatening than noneating disordered individuals, reflecting appraisal deficits. Another appraisal deficit involves difficulty in differentiating among emotional states or between emotional and physical states, such as hunger or fatigue (Cochrane, Brewerton, Wilson, & Hodges, 1993; De Groot, Rodin, & Olmsted, 1995). Alexithymia, which involves a disturbance in the ability to recognize and describe one's own feelings or to distinguish between internal emotional states, is associated with eating disorders (Smith, Amner, Johns- son, & Franck, 1997; Taylor, Parker, Bagby, & Rourke, 1996). The young woman who has difficulty identifying and distinguishing between internal emotional states is limited in her ability to respond with adaptive, goal-directed coping strategies.

Interpersonal Problems

Numerous studies have identified interpersonal problems among individuals who have AN and BN, including nonassertiveness, difficulties in expressing anger, elevated inter- personal conflict, and inadequate social support (Eldredge, Locke, & Horowitz, 1998; Grissett & Norvell, 1992; Herzog, Keller, Lavori, & Ott, 1987; Tiller et al., 1997). In addition to strong fears about negative evaluation of their bodies, individuals who have eating disorders also have general social evaluation concerns that may act as a risk factor (Striegel-Moore, Silber- stein, & Rodin, 1993). High levels of social anxiety are common among individuals who have AN and BN and usually appear years before the eating disorder (Schwalberg, Barlow, Alger, & Howard, 1992). Studies find a high need for acceptance and approval among individuals who have eating disorders (Bulik, Beidel, Duchmann, & Weltzin, 1991; Friedman & Whisman, 1998), which may cause apprehension about expressing their emotions or asserting their needs for fear of rejection. Preliminary evidence indicates that interpersonal factors also play a significant role in BED (Eldredge et al., 1998; Telch & Agras, 1994).

Sexual Trauma

The relationship between sexual abuse and eating disorders is a topic given much attention in clinical writing and research studies. Despite considerable research, no firm conclusions can be drawn because of methodological difficulties in conducting the research.

Recent reviews of the literature (Fallon & Wonderlich, 1997; Wonderlich, Brewerton, Jocic, Dansky, & Abbott, 1997) note preliminary evidence that childhood sexual abuse acts as a nonspecific risk factor for BN, but not for AN. Approximately one-third individuals who have BN report a history of childhood sexual abuse, much less than in AN (Welch & Fairburn, 1996). Individuals who have eating disorders and experienced sexual abuse have greater psychiatric comorbidity but do not have more severe eating disorder symptomatology. However, severity of the eating disorder is associated with the severity of the child abuse, the quality of the maternal relationship, and social competence. The mechanism by which sexual abuse may contribute to one's risk for an eating disorder is not yet understood.

COURSE AND PROGNOSIS

Eating disorders typically emerge during adolescence and early adulthood. The average age of onset is 17 years for AN (APA, 1994), 19 years for BN (Fairburn et al., 1997), and 25 years for BED (Spurrell, Wilfley, Tanofsky, & Brownell, 1997). AN can be seen in prepubertal children (Lask & Bryant-Waugh, 1997), whereas BN is rarely seen before age 14 (Stein, Chalhoub, & Hodes, 1998). Most cases of BN occur before age 25 (Woodside & Garfinkel, 1992). Most cases of AN occur between ages 14 and 20, although an older age of onset is not uncommon.

Eating disorders, particularly AN and BN, can be serious medical, social, and psychological consequences (Zerbe, 1996). Unfortunately, a good understanding of course and prognosis in eating disorders is limited by inconsistencies and shortcomings in available research (Herzog, Nussbaum, & Marmor, 1996; Pike, 1998). Left untreated, eating disorders may wax and wane for years (Franko & Erb, 1998). Disordered behaviors become more deeply ingrained. Over time, physiological changes related to starvation can increase the risk of poor outcome. Individuals who have eating disorders often avoid treatment, particularly in AN, denying the severity of the problem. Alarmingly, the annual mortality rate in AN is 5.9%, or 12 times the annual death rate due to all other causes in females ages 15–24 (Sullivan, 1995). Unfortunately, deaths are frequently sudden and unexpected (Isner, Roberts, Heymsfield, & Yager, 1985). The most common cause is starvation (Sullivan, 1995).

Medical consequences of AN are generally related to starvation and include low blood pressure, slow or irregular heart beat, slow digestion, muscle weakness, and lowered body temperature (Mitchell, Pomeroy, & Adson, 1997). Medical complications in BN usually result from vomiting or abuse of laxatives. The most serious complication is loss of potassium or other electrolytes, which can cause muscle weakness, fatigue, irregular heartbeat, and heart failure. Less is known about the death rate of BN, though some believe it may equal the rate of AN (Zerbe, 1996).

Accumulated data suggest that between 50 to 70% of patients who have AN attain good intermediate or long-term outcomes with treatment (Pike, 1998). However, complete recovery is rare because the majority continues to experience impairment in physical, psychological, and social functioning and is preoccupied with food and weight, even after weight has been restored (Herzog et al., 1996). Poorer prognosis is associated with the use of vomiting, lower body weight, longer duration of the problem before treatment, and later age of onset (Pike, 1998).

Individuals who have BN generally show good response to treatment. A review of outcome studies found recovery rates ranging from 13% to 71% (Herzog et al., 1996). The most consistent predictors of good outcomes are less severe eating symptoms and early age of onset (Herzog et al., 1996). Data from three studies of long-term outcome, more than 10 years after treatment, found that about approximately 46 to 70% were fully recovered, 30% to 40% were partially recovered, and 9% still met diagnostic criteria (Collings & King, 1994; Fichter & Quadflieg, 1997; Keel, Mitchell, Miller, Davis, & Crow, 1999). In general, those who have less severe symptoms at the onset of treatment tend to have a better prognosis than those who have more acute or disabling symptoms (APA, 1994). Poorer prognosis has also been associated with substance abuse and greater general psychopathology (Herzog et al., 1996).

Course and prognosis in BED are not well understood due to a dearth of research. A study of treatment outcome found poor outcome 1 to 3 years following treatment, but generally good outcome by 6-year follow-up (Fichter, Quadflieg, & Gnutzmann, 1998). A study of the natural history of BED in the community found a better short-term outcome for BED than BN (Hay & Fairburn, 1998). Predictors of short- and long-term prognosis are not yet known.

FAMILIAL AND GENETIC PATTERNS

Family Environment

Numerous studies that involve self-report and observational data have found problematic interactions in families of individuals who have eating disorders, compared to normal controls (for a review, see Connors, 1996). Dysfunctional family interactions appear to act as a risk factor for eating disorders but may not represent a specific risk factor (Friedmann, McDermut, Solomon et al., 1997). Compared to families of normal controls, family environments of individuals who have eating disorders have lower levels of cohesiveness that reflect less support, empathy, and understanding from parents. Poor communication or low expressiveness and high levels of conflict and hostility are also characteristic. In such families, the level of conflict is high, but conflicts are often not expressed constructively and worked through to resolution. A comparison of eating disorder subtypes indicated that BED is associated with the lowest level of cohesiveness and expressiveness (Hodges, Cochrane, & Brewerton, 1998). Families are also characterized as enmeshed and not supportive of their daughter's autonomy. According to this conceptualization, the developmentally appropriate need for increased autonomy in adolescence is viewed as a threat to the closeness of the family (Minuchin, Rosman, & Baker, 1978). Control of food thus represents a "safe" way for the adolescent to "be her own person" and to have control over something in his/her life.

Families may also influence the development and maintenance of eating disorders through their impact on body dissatisfaction and dieting. In a community study, families of women who had BN were more likely to diet and to be critical of weight and eating, compared to families of both normal and psychiatric controls (Fairburn, Welch, Doll, Davies, & O'Connor, 1997). Mothers of adolescent girls who have eating disorders tend to be chronic dieters and to be critical of their daughter's weight (Pike & Rodin, 1991). In a prospective study, modeling of abnormal eating behaviors predicted the onset of binge eating and purging among adolescent girls (Stice, 1998). Another study found support for a dual process model, in which family preoccupation with weight and appearance had a direct impact on body dissatisfaction and eating symptoms, whereas family dysfunction had indirect effects on eating symptoms (Leung, Schwartzman, & Steiger, 1996; Connors, 1996).

Genetic Factors

Genetic factors are important in the development of both anorexia and bulimia. Genetic studies on BED are lacking. The eating disorders AN and BN clearly run in families (Strober, 1991). In anorexia, first-degree relatives have an increased risk of both anorexia and bulimia. Similarly, first-degree relatives of individuals who have bulimia have an increased risk of both disorders. Twin studies of anorexia demonstrated concordance rates for monozygotic twins between 44% and 50% compared to 7% for dizygotic twin pairs (Hsu, Chesler, & Santhouse, 1990; Scott, 1986). In bulimia, concordance rates were 29% for monozygotic twins and only 9% for dizygotic twin pairs (Kendler et al., 1991). Environmental contributors seem to come from individual experiences, rather than experiences shared between the co-twins (Kendler et al., 1995). The genetic transmission of eating disorder risk is not known but could occur through transmission of behavioral, neurochemical, or metabolic risk factors.

DIAGNOSTIC CONSIDERATIONS

Anorexia Nervosa

The central characteristic of AN is starvation. The individual who has AN refuses to maintain normal body weight based on an intense, irrational fear of weight gain. DSM-IV provides a figure of 85% in determining low body weight, but calls for flexibility and use of clinical judgment (Walsh & Garner, 1997). Adolescent women in the process of developing may become underweight when they fail to gain weight as a normal part of development. Women who meet all but the weight criteria for AN are quite similar to women who have AN in measures of associated psychopathology (Geist, Davis, & Heinmaa, 1998). DSM-IV criteria also require body image disturbance, very broadly defined, but do not specify the extent of disturbance required (APA, 1994). Some measures of body image disturbance have successfully differentiated eating disorder groups from nonclinical groups (Rosen, Reiter, & Orosan, 1995).

The fourth criterion for AN requires amenorrhea, defined as the absence of three consecutive menstrual periods (APA, 1994). DSM-IV improved on previous editions by including only postmenarchal girls in this criterion, thereby allowing for greater diagnostic specificity (APA, 1994). DSM-IV also considers that women have amenorrhea if menstruation occurs as a result of oral contraceptive use (Walsh & Garner, 1997). Although DSM-IV improved on previous versions, the requirement of amenorrhea remains problematic. Amenorrhea may not be detected when young, premenarchal girls fail to begin menstruating due to insufficient weight gain. In addition, some women continue menstruating even at extremely low body weights (Cachelin & Maher, 1998a). Comparisons of amenorrheic AN and nonamenorrheic AN have found no differences in the severity of eating disorder symptoms or rates of comorbid psychopathology (Cachelin & Maher, 1998a; Garfinkel, Lin, Goering et al., 1996).

DSM-IV added subtypes of AN (APA, 1994). The Restricting type describes the "classical" presentation of AN, whereby the individual attempts to lose weight by dieting, fasting, or engaging in excessive exercise. The binge-eating/purging type regularly participates in binge eating and/or "purging" during an episode of AN. Although some studies find that the binge-eating/purging type is associated with greater psychological disturbance (e.g., Geist, Davis, & Heinmaa, 1998), other studies have found little or no differences between the subtypes (Nagata, McConaha, Rao, Sokol, & Kaye, 1997; Pryor, Wiederman, & McGilley, 1996). Some studies found that purging, but not binge eating, is related to more severe psychopathology in AN (Cachelin & Maher, 1998b; Garner, Garner, & Rosen, 1993).

Bulimia Nervosa

DSM-IV criteria for BN include the following: regular binge eating, undue importance placed upon body image and weight in self-evaluation, and regular use of inappropriate behaviors to compensate for calorie intake (APA, 1994). DSM-IV requires a binge-eating and purging frequency of at least two times per week for a 3 month duration. However, research does not strongly support this frequency cutoff. Individuals who meet BN criteria, but binge less than twice per week do not appear to differ in important ways from those with greater binge frequency (Walsh & Garner, 1997).

The central feature of BN, binge eating, is defined as eating a large quantity of food during a discrete period of time, while experiencing a lack of control. A large quantity of food is defined as "… more than most people would eat under similar circumstances" (APA, 1994, p. 549). Studies of calorie intake during binge episodes find that binges are generally large, more than 1000 calories, but also vary tremendously, ranging from 45 to 8,400 calories (for a review of empirical studies, see Guertin, 1999). DSM-IV excludes "subjective" binges in which food quantity is normal, but the individual feels out of control because she ate more than she intended or broke a dietary rule. Some argue that subjective binges should be included in the binge definition because research has not found a relationship between the quantity of food eaten during a binge and the associated psychopathology or treatment outcome (Niego, Pratt, & Agras, 1997; Smith, Marcus, & Eldredge, 1994).

DSM-IV introduced subtypes of BN according to type of compensatory behaviors used: purging and nonpurging types. Purging type individuals engage in self-induced vomiting or abuse of laxatives or diuretics. The nonpurging type uses compensatory behaviors of extreme dieting or excessive exercise. The utility of the subtypes is not yet clear. Some studies have found that purging BN is associated with lower body weight and higher levels of eating disorder and comorbid psychopathology (Garfinkel et al., 1996). Other research has failed to support the subtypes and found no difference in eating disorder symptoms or other psychopathology between purging and nonpurging BN (Hay & Fairburn, 1998; Tobin, Griffing, & Griffing, 1997).

Eating Disorder Not Otherwise Specified

Eating Disorder Not Otherwise Specified (EDNOS) is a frequently diagnosed category, and approximately 25% of eating disordered individuals are given this diagnosis (Hay & Fairburn, 1998; Mizes & Sloan, 1998). EDNOS includes individuals who have widely differing symptoms (APA, 1994). DSM-IV lists several examples of EDNOS. EDNOS is diagnosed when most AN criteria are met, but weight loss is insufficient or menstruation continues. An individual who meets criteria for BN but binges less than twice per week would receive a diagnosis of EDNOS. Another common pattern is the individual who binges on small or normal amounts of food, but experiences a lack of control, and engages in self-induced vomiting or other compensatory behaviors after the subjective binge. A greater understanding of this large and diverse group has been identified as a top research priority (Grilo, Devlin, Cachelin, & Yanovski, 1997).

Binge Eating Disorder

BED is a specific subtype of EDNOS, defined in the DSM-IV appendix to facilitate research and determine whether it should be included as an eating disorder category in future DSM versions. BED involves regular binge eating without regular use of compensatory behaviors. Binge eating is defined as it is for BN. As in BN, the individual must binge at least two times per week. However, studies have generally found no differences between BED and subclinical BED with lower frequency (Striegel-Moore, Wilson, Wilfley, Elder, & Brownell, 1998). A duration of 6 months is required for a BED diagnosis, rather than 3 months as with BN.

In addition to regular binge eating, the individual must be very distressed about the binge eating (APA, 1994). The individual must report three of the following: eating faster than normal; eating until uncomfortably full; eating a large amount of food when not hungry; eating alone due to embarrassment; and feeling disgust, depression, or guilt after overeating. These criteria help to distinguish BED from regular overeating, which is not of great concern to the individual. Studies suggest that BED is associated with less severe body dissatisfaction, fewer eating disorder symptoms, and less associated psychopathology than purging type BN (Hay & Fairburn, 1998; Molinari, Ragazzoni, & Morosin, 1997). Individuals with BED are older and of higher weight, on average, than individuals who have BN (Spitzer et al., 1993).

COMORBID PSYCHOPATHOLOGY

Anorexia and Bulimia

Eating disorders are associated with considerable comorbid psychopathology, leading to an impressive volume of research. Research indicates an association of AN and BN with affective disorders, anxiety disorders, personality disorders, and substance abuse. Two recent reviews summarize this literature (Herzog, Nussbaum, & Marmor, 1996; Wonderlich & Mitchell, 1997).

ANXIETY DISORDERS

Individuals who have eating disorders experience many symptoms of anxiety, including obsessions and compulsions about food and weight, morbid fear of fat, and social phobia. Lifetime prevalence rates of anxiety disorders are elevated in both AN and BN, but are somewhat higher in AN and range from 20% to 65% (Wonderlich & Mitchell, 1997). AN is most strongly related to obsessive-compulsive disorders, BN to social phobia. Some studies have found that anxiety disorders most often predate the eating disorder, leading to suggestions that eating disorders are related to obsessive-compulsive disorder or social phobia (Aragona & Vella, 1998; Bulik, Sullivan, Fear, & Joyce, 1997; Schwalberg et al., 1992). Among women who have both AN and OCD, OCD symptoms are similar in severity to symptoms in individuals who have OCD, but differ in type of OCD symptoms (Matsunaga, Kiriike, Iwasaki, Yamagami, & Kaye, 1999). The association of eating disorders with Posttraumatic Stress Disorder has received less attention, but recent studies find elevated rates of current and lifetime PTSD (Dansky, Brewerton, Kilpatrick, & O'Neil, 1997; Gleves, Eberenz, & May, 1998; Striegel-Moore, Garvin, Dohm, & Rosenheck, 1999).

DEPRESSION

The relationship between eating disorders and affective disorders has been a focus of considerable research because depressed mood is quite common in individuals who have eating disorders. Lifetime prevalence rates of major depression in eating disorders range from 25% to 80%, and rates are approximately equal across eating disorder classifications (for reviews, see Herzog, Nussbaum, & Marmor, 1996; Wonderlich & Mitchell, 1997). Depression symptoms in eating disorders may be less severe than in major depression and have fewer melancholic features (Wonderlich & Mitchell, 1997). Research has found that eating disorders usually predate depressive symptoms. Thus, depression is viewed as a reaction to the eating disorder rather than a vulnerability factor, although the relationship is likely to be complex.

PERSONALITY DISORDERS

Rates of personality disorders are also elevated in eating disorders and range from 20% to 80% in AN and from 22% to 77% in BN (for a review, see Dennis & Sansone, 1997). Purging in both AN and BN is most often associated with borderline and histrionic features. Restricting AN is associated with avoidant, obsessive-compulsive, and dependent personality disorders. However, Vitousek and Manke (1994) recommend caution in diagnosing personality disorders. Personality disorder symptoms may be a direct result of the eating disorder and will remit along with remission of the eating disorder.

SUBSTANCE ABUSE

Holderness, Brooks-Gunn, and Warren (1994) conducted a meta-analysis of 51 studies on substance abuse and eating disorders. Substance abuse appears to be more common in BN and in the binge-purge type of AN than in restricting AN. The rate of comorbid substance abuse among those who have BN is approximately 22.9% (Holderness et al., 1994), significantly higher than rates found among controls (Garfinkel et al., 1995). Men diagnosed with eating disorders have higher comorbid rates of substance abuse than women who have eating disorders (Striegel-Moore, Garvin, Dohm, & Rosenheck, 1999). Studies comparing BN with and without comorbid alcohol dependence have found that alcohol dependence is associated with higher attempted suicide rates, greater impulsiveness, and higher rates of borderline personality disorder (Bulik, Sullivan, Carter, & Joyce, 1997; Suzuki, Higuchi, Yamade, Komiya, & Takagi, 1994). A recent study found no relationship between bulimia and alcohol use when controlling for personality disorder (Kozyk, Touyz, & Beaumont, 1998). Some hypothesize that eating disorders and substance abuse may derive from similar underlying personality disturbances, representing features of an impulse-control problem. Preliminary evidence supports defining a subgroup of individuals who have BN, termed multi-impulsive BN, that involves excessive alcohol use, drug abuse, self-mutilation, and stealing (Fichter, Quadflieg, & Rief, 1994).

Binge Eating Disorder

Research on psychopathology associated with BED is sparse compared to that on anorexia and bulimia. Castonguay, Eldredge, and Agras (1995) provide a review of research on comorbidity in BED. The majority of available studies used clinical samples and compared obese individuals who had BED to obese individuals who did no binge eating. Results show higher rates of bulimia nervosa, major depression, panic disorder, substance abuse, borderline personality disorder, and avoidant personality among individuals who have BED. In a community study, individuals who had BED compared to non-eating-disordered overweight controls were significantly more likely to have received a lifetime diagnosis of major depression or of any Axis I or Axis II disorder (Telch & Stice, 1998). A few studies that compared BED to BN found that BED is associated with less psychopathology than BN, but more than among individuals who have no binge-eating pathology (Antony, Johnson, Carr-Nangle, & Abel, 1994; Dansky, Brewerton, Kilpatrick, & O'Neil, 1997; Hay & Fairburn, 1998).

SUMMARY

An expansion of research on eating disorders during the last 25 years has furthered our understanding of diagnosis, etiology, and treatment, yet many questions remain (Stunkard,

1997). Eating disorders are complex and chronic disorders. The complexity of the disorders is evidenced by high rates of comorbidity with anxiety disorders, depression, personality disorders, and substance abuse. Multiple etiological factors have been identified, including psychological, familial, biological, and sociocultural contributors, which combine in different ways for each individual. Sociocultural factors contribute to the development of eating disorders through their impact on dieting, body dissatisfaction, and fear of fat. However, etiological models must identify additional vulnerability factors because chronic dieting and body dissatisfaction do not always lead to eating disorders. Environmental factors implicated in the development of eating disorder include family relationships, the family's attitudes toward weight and appearance, and sexual trauma. Individual characteristics are also implicated, including personality characteristics, interpersonal and social difficulties, coping skills, and mood regulation. Increasingly complex and sophisticated etiological models are being developed and tested.

Left untreated, disordered behaviors often become more deeply ingrained. The physiological effects of starvation contribute to further deterioration and can result in death. Individuals whose symptoms improve often continue to experience distorted attitudes about food and eating. Fortunately, many patients do recover fully with treatment. The prevalence of eating disorders and disordered eating behaviors, combined with the potentially serious psychological and physical consequences, points to the crucial importance of research in this area.

REFERENCES

Agras, W. S., Hammer, L., & McNicholas, F. (1999). A prospective study of the influence of eating-disordered mothers on their children. *International Journal of Eating Disorders, 25,* 253–262.

Agras, W. S., & Telch, C. F. (1998). The effects of caloric deprivation and negative affect on binge eating in obese binge-eating disordered women. *Behavior Therapy, 29,* 491–503.

American Psychiatric Association. (1994). *Diagnostic and statistical manual of mental disorders,* 4th ed. Washington, DC: Author.

Andersen, A. E., & DiDomenico, L. (1992). Diet vs. shape content of popular male and female magazines: A dose–response relationship to the incidence of eating disorders? *International Journal of Eating Disorders, 11,* 283–287.

Antony, M. M., Johnson, W. G., Carr-Nangle, R. E., & Abel, J. (1994). Psychopathology correlates of binge eating and eating disorder. *Comprehensive Psychiatry, 35,* 386–392.

Aragona, M., & Vella, G. (1998). Psychopathological considerations on the relationship between bulimia and obsessive-compulsive disorder. *Psychopathology, 31,* 197–205.

Braun, D. L., Sunday, S. R., Huang, A., & Halmi, K. A. (1999). More males seek treatment for eating disorders. *International Journal of Eating Disorders, 25,* 415–424.

Brownell, K. D., & Wadden, T. A. (1992). Etiology and treatment of obesity: Understanding a serious, prevalent, and refractory disorder. *Journal of Consulting and Clinical Psychology, 60,* 505–517.

Bruce, B., & Agras, W. S. (1992). Binge eating in females: A population-based investigation. *International Journal of Eating Disorders, 12,* 365–373.

Bulik, C. M., Beidel, D. C., Duchmann, E., & Weltzin, T. E. (1991). An analysis of social anxiety in anorexic, bulimic, social phobic, and control women. *Journal of Psychopathology and Behavioral Assessment, 13*(3), 199–211.

Bulik, C. M., Sullivan, P. F., Carter, F. A., & Joyce, P. R. (1997). Lifetime comorbidity of alcohol dependence in women with bulimia nervosa. *Addictive Behaviors, 22,* 437–446.

Bulik, C. M., Sullivan, P. F., Fear, J. L., & Joyce, P. R. (1997). Eating disorders and antecedent anxiety disorders: A controlled study. *Acta Psychiatrica Scandinavica, 96*(2), 101–107.

Cachelin, F. M., & Maher, B. A. (1998a). Is amenorrhea a critical criterion for anorexia nervosa? *Journal of Psychosomatic Research, 44,* 435–440.

Cachelin, F. M., & Maher, B. A. (1998b). Restricters who purge: Implications of purging behavior for psychopathology and classification of anorexia nervosa. *Eating Disorders: The Journal of Treatment and Prevention, 6,* 51–63.

Carlat, D. J., & Camargo, C. A. (1991). Review of bulimia nervosa in males. *American Journal of Psychiatry, 148,* 831–843.

Carlat, D. J., Camargo, C. A., & Herzog, D. B. (1997). Eating disorders in males: A report on 135 patients. *American Journal of Psychiatry, 154*, 1127–1132.

Cash, T. F., & Deagle, E. A., III. (1997). The nature and extent of body-image disturbances in anorexia nervosa and bulimia nervosa: A meta-analysis. *International Journal of Eating Disorders, 22*, 107–125.

Cash, T. G., & Henry, P. (1995). Women's body images: The results of a national survey in the U.S.A. *Sex Roles, 33*, 19–28.

Castonguay, L. G., Eldredge, K. L., & Agras, W. S. (1995). Binge eating disorder: Current status and future directions. *Clinical Psychology Review, 15*, 865–890.

Cattanach, L., & Rodin, J. (1988). Psychosocial components of the stress process in bulimia. *International Journal of Eating Disorders, 7*(1), 75–88.

Christiano, B. A., & Mizes, J. S. (1997). Appraisal and coping deficits associated with eating disorders: Implications for treatment. *Cognitive and Behavioral Practice, 4*, 263–290.

Cochrane, C. E., Brewerton, T. D., Wilson, D. B., & Hodges, E. L. (1993). Alexithymia in the eating disorders. *International Journal of Eating Disorders, 14*, 219–222.

Collings, S., & King, M. (1994). Ten-year follow-up of 50 patients with bulimia nervosa. *British Journal of Psychiatry, 164*, 80–87.

Connors, M. E. (1996). Developmental vulnerabilities for eating disorders. In L. Smolak, M. P. Levine, & R. Striegel-Moore (Eds.), *The developmental psychopathology of eating disorders: Implications for research, prevention, and treatment* (pp. 285–310). Mahwah, NJ: Erlbaum.

Dansky, B. S., Brewerton, T. D., Kilpatrick, D. G., & O'Neil, P. M. (1997). The National Women's Study: Relationship of victimization and posttraumatic stress disorder to bulimia nervosa. *International Journal of Eating Disorders, 21*, 213–228.

Davis, R., Freeman, R. J., & Garner, D. M. (1988). A naturalistic investigation of eating behavior in bulimia nervosa. *Journal of Consulting and Clinical Psychology, 56*, 273–279.

De Groot, J. M., Rodin, G., & Olmsted, M. P. (1995). Alexithymia, depression, and treatment outcome in bulimia nervosa. *Comprehensive Psychiatry, 36*(1), 53–60.

Dennis, A. B., & Sansone, R. A. (1997). Treatment of patients with personality disorders. In D. M. Garner & P. E. Garfinkel (Eds.), *Handbook of treatment for eating disorders* (pp. 437–449). New York: Guilford.

Eldredge, K. L., Locke, K. D., & Horowitz, M. (1998). Patterns of interpersonal problems associated with binge eating disorder. *International Journal of Eating Disorders, 23*, 383–389.

Elmore, D. K., & deCastro, J. M. (1990). Self-related moods and hunger in relation to spontaneous eating behavior in bulimics, recovered bulimics, and normals. *International Journal of Eating Disorders, 9*, 179–190.

Fairburn, C. G., & Beglin, S. J. (1990). Studies of the epidemiology of bulimia nervosa. *American Journal of Psychiatry, 147*, 401–408.

Fairburn, C. G., Doll, H. A., Welch, S. L., Hay, P. J., Davies, B. A., & O'Connor, M. E. (1998). Risk factors for binge eating disorder: A community-based control study. *Archives of General Psychiatry, 55*, 425–432.

Fairburn, C. G., Marcus, M. D., & Wilson, G. T. (1993). Cognitive-behavioral therapy for binge eating and bulimia nervosa: A comprehensive treatment manual. In C. G. Fairburn & G. T. Wilson (Eds.), *Binge eating: Nature, assessment, and treatment* (pp. 361–404). New York: Guilford.

Fairburn, C. G., Welch, S. L., Doll, H. A., Davies, B. A., & O'Connor, M. E. (1997). Risk factors for bulimia nervosa: A community-based case-control study. *Archives for General Psychiatry, 54*, 509–517.

Fallon, P., & Wonderlich, S. A. (1997). Sexual abuse and other forms of trauma. In D. M. Garner & P. E. Garfinkel (Eds.), *Handbook of treatment of eating disorders*, 2nd ed. (pp. 394–414). New York: Guilford.

Federoff, I. C., & McFarlane, T. (1998). Cultural aspects of eating disorders. In S. S. Kazarian & D. R. Evans (Eds.), *Cultural clinical psychology: Theory, research and practice* (pp. 153–176). New York: Oxford University Press.

Feingold, A., & Mazzella, R. (1998). Gender differences in body image are increasing. *Psychological Science, 9*, 190–195.

Fichter, M. M., Quadflieg, N., & Gnutzmann, A. (1998). Binge eating disorder: Treatment outcome over a 6-year course. *Journal of Psychosomatic Research, 44*, 385–405.

Fichter, M. M., Quadflieg, N., & Rief, W. (1994). Course of multi-impulsive bulimia. *Psychological Medicine, 24*, 591–604.

Fitzgibbon, M. L., Spring, B., Avellone, M. E., Blackman, L. R., Pingitore, R., & Stolley, M. R. (1998). Correlates of binge eating in Hispanic, Black, and White women. *International Journal of Eating Disorders, 24*, 43–52.

Flannery-Schroeder, E. C., & Chrisler, J. C. (1996). Body esteem, eating attitudes, and gender-role orientation in three age groups of children. *Current Psychology: Developmental, Learning, Personality, Social, 15*, 235–248.

Franko, D. L., & Erb, J. (1998) Managed care or mangled care?: Treating eating disorders in the current healthcare climate. *Psychotherapy, 35*, 43–53.

French, S. A., Perry, C. L., Leon, G. R., & Fulkerson, J. A. (1995). Changes in psychological variables and health behaviors by dieting status over a three-year period in a cohort of adolescent females. *Journal of Adolescent Health, 16,* 438–447.

Friedmann, M. S., McDermut, W. H., Solomon, D. A., Ryan, C. E., Keitner, G. I., & Miller, I. W. (1997). Family functioning and mental illness: A comparison of psychiatric and nonclinical families. *Family Process, 36,* 357–367.

Friedman, M. A., & Whisman, M. A. (1998). Sociotropy, autonomy, and bulimic symptomatology. *International Journal of Eating Disorders, 23,* 439–442.

Gard, M. C. E., & Freeman, C. P. (1996). The dismantling of a myth: A review of eating disorders and socioeconomic status. *International Journal of Eating Disorders, 20,* 1–12.

Garfinkel, P., Lin, E., Goering, P., Spegg, C., Goldbloom, D. S., Kennedy, S., Kaplan, A. S., & Woodside, D. B. (1996). Purging and nonpurging forms of bulimia nervosa in a community sample. *International Journal of Eating Disorders, 20,* 231–238.

Garner, D. M., Garfinkel, P. E., Schwarz, D. M., & Thompson, M. M. (1980). Cultural expectations of thinness in women. *Psychological Bulletin, 47,* 483–491.

Garner, D. M., Garner, M. V., & Rosen, L. W. (1993). Anorexia nervosa "restricters" who purge: Implications for subtyping anorexia nervosa. *International Journal of Eating Disorders, 13,* 171–185.

Garner, D. M., Vitousek, K. M., & Pike, K. M. (1997). Cognitive-behavioral therapy for anorexia nervosa. In D. M. Garner & P. E. Garfinkel (Eds.), *Handbook of treatment for eating disorders* (pp. 94–144). New York: Guilford.

Geist, R., Davis, R., & Heinmaa, M. (1998). Binge/purge symptoms and comorbidity in adolescents with eating disorders. *Canadian Journal of Psychiatry, 43,* 507–512.

Gilbert, S., & Thompson, J. K. (1996). Feminist explanations of the development of eating disorders: Common themes, research findings, and methodological issues. *Clinical Psychology—Science and Practice, 3,* 183–202.

Gleaves, D. H., Eberenz, K. P., & May, M. C. (1998). Scope and significance of posttraumatic symptomatology among women hospitalized for an eating disorder. *International Journal of Eating Disorders, 24,* 147–156.

Gotestam, K. G., & Agras, W. S. (1995). General population-based epidemiological study of eating disorders in Norway. *International Journal of Eating Disorders, 18,* 119–126.

Grigg, M., Bowman, J., & Redman, S. (1996). Disordered eating and unhealthy weight reduction practices among adolescent females. *Preventive Medicine, 25,* 748–756.

Grilo, C. M., & Shiffman, S. (1994). Longitudinal investigation of the abstinence violation effect in binge eaters. *Journal of Consulting and Clinical Psychology, 62,* 611–619.

Grilo, C. M., Devlin, M. J., Cachelin, F. M., & Yanovski, S. (1997). Report of the National Institutes of Health (NIH) workshop on the development of research priorities in eating disorders. *Psychopharmacology Bulletin, 33,* 321–333.

Grissett, N. I., & Norvell, N. K. (1992). Perceived social support, social skills, and quality of relationships in bulimic women. *Journal of Consulting and Clinical Psychology, 60,* 293–299.

Guertin, T. L. (1999). Eating behavior of bulimics, self-identified binge eaters, and non-eating-disordered individuals: What differentiates these populations? *Clinical Psychology Review, 19,* 1–23.

Hansel, S. L., & Wittrock, D. A. (1997). Appraisal and coping strategies in stressful situations: A comparison of individuals who binge eat and controls. *International Journal of Eating Disorders, 21,* 89–93.

Hay, P., & Fairburn, C. (1998). The validity of the DSM-IV scheme for classifying bulimic eating disorders. *International Journal of Eating Disorders, 23,* 7–15.

Heatherton, T. F., & Baumeister, R. F. (1991). Binge eating as escape from self-awareness. *Psychological Bulletin, 110,* 86–108.

Herzog, D. B., Keller, M. B., Lavori, P. W., & Ott, I. L. (1987). Social impairment in bulimia. *International Journal of Eating Disorders, 6,* 741–747.

Herzog, D. B., Nussbaum, K. M., & Marmor, A. K. (1996). Comorbidity and outcome in eating disorders. *Psychiatric Clinics of North America, 19,* 843–859.

Hetherington, M. M., & Burnett, L. (1994). Ageing and the pursuit of slimness: Dietary restraint and weight satisfaction in elderly women. *British Journal of Clinical Psychology, 33,* 391–400.

Hodges, E. L., Cochrane, C. E., & Brewerton, T. D. (1998). Family characteristics of binge-eating disorder patients. *International Journal of Eating Disorders, 23,* 145–151.

Hoek, H. W. (1993). Review of the epidemiological studies of eating disorders. *International Review of Psychiatry, 5,* 61–74.

Holderness, C. C., Brooks-Gunn, J., & Warren, M. P. (1994). Co-morbidity of eating disorders and substance abuse review of the literature. *International Journal of Eating Disorders, 16,* 1–34.

Howard, C. E., & Porzelius, L. K. (1998). The role of dieting in binge eating disorder: Etiology and treatment implications. *Clinical Psychology Review, 19,* 25–44.

Hsu, L. K. G. (1996). Epidemiology of the eating disorder. *The Psychiatric Clinics of North America, 19*, 681–701.

Hsu, L. K. (1997). Can dieting cause an eating disorder? *Psychological Medicine, 27*, 509–513.

Hsu, L. G., Chesler, B. E., & Santhouse, R. (1990). Bulimia nervosa in eleven sets of twins: A clinical report. *International Journal of Eating Disorders, 9*, 275–282.

Isner, J. M., Roberts, W. C., Heymsfield, S. B., & Yager, J. (1985). Anorexia nervosa and sudden death. *Annals of Internal Medicine, 102*, 49–52.

Johnson, W. G., & Torgrud, L. J. (1996). Assessment and treatment of binge eating disorder. In J. K. Thompson (Ed.), *Body image, eating disorders, and obesity: An integrative guide for assessment and treatment* (pp. 321–343). Washington, DC: American Psychological Association.

Keel, P. K., Klump, K. L., Leon, G. R., & Fulkerson, J. A. (1998). Disordered eating in adolescent males from a school-based sample. *International Journal of Eating Disorders, 23*, 125–132.

Keel, P. K., Mitchell, J. E., Miller, K. B., Davis, T. L., & Crow, S. J. (1999). Long-term outcome of bulimia nervosa. *Archives of General Psychiatry, 56*, 63–69.

Kenardy, J., Arnow, B., & Agras, W. S. (1997). The aversiveness of specific emotional states associated with binge-eating in obese subjects. *Australian and New Zealand Journal of Psychiatry, 30*, 839–844.

Kendler, K. S., MacLean, C., Neale, M., Kessler, R., Heath, A., & Eaves, L. (1991). The genetic epidemiology of bulimia nervosa. *American Journal of Psychiatry, 148*, 1627–1637.

Kendler, K. S., Walters, E. E., Neale, M. C., Kessler, R. C., Heath, A. C., & Eaves, L. J. (1995). The structure of the genetic and environmental risk factors for six major psychiatric disorders in women. *Archives of General Psychiatry, 52*, 374–383.

Keys, A., Brozek, J., Henschel, A., Mickelson, O., & Taylor, H. I. (1950). *The biology of human starvation.* Minneapolis: University of Minnesota Press.

Koff, E., & Sangani, P. (1997). Effects of coping style and negative body image on eating disturbance. *International Journal of Eating Disorders, 22*, 51–56.

Kozyk, J. C., Touyz, S. W., & Beaumont, P. J. V. (1998). Is there a relationship between bulimia nervosa and hazardous alcohol use? *International Journal of Eating Disorders, 24*, 95–99.

Lask, B., & Bryant-Waugh, R. (1997). Prepubertal eating disorders. In D. M. Garner & P. E. Garfinkel (Eds.), *Handbook of treatment for eating disorders*, 2nd ed. (pp. 476–483). New York: Guilford.

le Grange, D., Telch, C. F., & Agras, W. S. (1997). Eating and general psychopathology in a sample of Caucasian and ethnic minority subjects. *International Journal of Eating Disorders, 21*, 285–293.

Leon, G., Fulkerson, J., Perry, C., & Cudeck, R. (1993). Personality and behavioral vulnerabilities associated with risk status for eating disorders in adolescent girls. *Journal of Abnormal Psychology, 102*, 438–444.

Leung, F., Schwartzman, A., & Steiger, H. (1996). Testing a dual-process family model in understanding the development of eating pathology: A structural equation modeling analysis. *International Journal of Eating Disorders, 20*, 367–375.

Lingswiler, V. M., Crowther, J. H., & Stephens, M. A. P. (1989). Emotional and somatic consequences of binge episodes. *Addictive Behaviors, 14*, 503–511.

Matsunaga, H., Kiriike, N., Iwasaki, Y., Miyata, A., Yamagamik, S., & Kaye, W. H. (1999). Clinical characteristics in patients with anorexia nervosa and obsessive-compulsive disorder. *Psychological Medicine, 29*, 407–414.

Minuchin, S., Rosman, B. L., & Baker, L. (1978). *Psychosomatic families: Anorexia in context.* Cambridge, MA: Harvard University Press.

Mitchell, J. E., Pomeroy, C., & Adson, D. E. (1997). Managing medical complications. In D. M. Garner & P. E. Garfinkel (Eds.), *Handbook of treatment for eating disorders*, 2nd ed. (pp. 383–393). New York: Guilford.

Mizes, J. S., & Sloan, D. M. (1998). An empirical analysis of eating disorder, not otherwise specified: Preliminary findings. *International Journal of Eating Disorders, 23*, 233–242.

Molinari, E., Ragazzoni, P., & Morosin, A. (1997). Psychopathology in obese subjects with and without binge-eating disorder and in bulimic subjects. *Psychological Reports, 80*, 1327–1335.

Nagata, T., McConaha, C., Rao, R., Sokol, M., & Kaye, W. (1997). A comparison of subgroups of inpatients with anorexia nervosa. *International Journal of Eating Disorders, 22*, 309–314.

Neumark-Sztainer, D., Jeffery, R. W., & French, S. A. (1997). Self-reported dieting: How should we ask? What does it mean? Association between dieting and reported energy intake. *International Journal of Eating Disorders, 22*, 437–449.

Niego, S. H., Pratt, E. M., & Agras, W. S. (1997). Subjective or objective binge: Is the distinction valid? *International Journal of Eating Disorders, 22*, 291–298.

Paxton, S. J., & Diggens, J. (1997). Avoidance coping, binge eating, and depression: An examination of the escape theory of binge eating. *International Journal of Eating Disorders, 22*, 83–87.

Pike, K. M. (1998). Long-term course of anorexia nervosa: Response, relapse, remission, and recovery. *Clinical Psychology Review, 18*, 447–475.

Pike, K. M., & Rodin, J. (1991). Mothers, daughters, and disordered eating. *Journal of Abnormal Psychology, 100*, 198–204.

Polivy, J., & Herman, C. P. (1995). Dieting and bingeing: A causal analysis. *American Psychologist, 40*, 193–201.

Pryor, T., Wiederman, M. W., & McGilley, B. (1996). Clinical correlates of anorexia subtypes. *International Journal of Eating Disorders, 19*, 371–379.

Rebert, W. M., Stanton, A. L., & Schwarz, R. M. (1991). Influence of personality attributes and daily moods on bulimic eating patterns. *Addictive Behaviors, 16*, 497–505.

Rogers, L., Resnick, M. D., Mitchell, J. E., & Blum, R. W. (1997). The relationship between socioeconomic status and eating-disordered behaviors in a community sample of adolescent girls. *International Journal of Eating Disorders, 22*, 15–23.

Rosen, J. C., & Leitenberg, H. (1988). The anxiety model of bulimia nervosa and treatment with exposure plus response prevention. In K. M. Pike, W. Vandereycken, & D. Ploog (Eds.), *The psychobiology of bulimia nervosa* (pp. 146–150). Heidelberg, Germany: Springer Verlag.

Rosen, J. C., Reiter, J., & Orosan, P. (1995). Assessment of body image in eating disorders with the Body Dysmorphic Disorder Examination. *Behaviour Research and Therapy, 33*, 77–84.

Rothblum, E. D. (1994). "I'll die for the revolution but don't ask me not to diet": Feminism and the continuing stigmatization of obesity. In P. Fallon & M. A. Katzman (Eds.), *Feminist perspectives on eating disorders* (pp. 53–76). New York: Guilford.

Santonasto, P., Ferrara, S., & Favaro, A. (1999). Differences between binge eating disorder and nonpurging bulimia nervosa. *International Journal of Eating Disorders, 25*, 215–218.

Schlundt, D. G., & Johnson, W. G. (1990). *Eating disorders: Assessment and treatment.* Boston: Allyn & Bacon.

Schwalberg, M. D., Barlow, D. H., Alger, S. A., & Howard, L. J. (1992). Comparison of bulimics, obese binge eaters, social phobics, and individuals with panic disorder on comorbidity across DSMIII-R anxiety disorders. *Journal of Abnormal Psychology, 101*, 675–681.

Scott, D. W. (1986). Anorexia nervosa: A review of possible genetic factors. *International Journal of Eating Disorders, 5*, 1–20.

Smith, G. J. W., Amner, G., Johnsson, P., & Franck, A. (1997). Alexithymia in patients with eating disorders: An investigation using a new projective technique. *Perceptual and Motor Skills, 85*, 247–257.

Smith, D. E., Marcus, M. D., & Eldredge, K. L. (1994). Binge eating syndromes: A review of assessment and treatment with an emphasis on clinical application. *Behavior Therapy, 25*, 635–658.

Smith, D. E., Marcus, M. D., Lewis, C. E., Fitzgibbon, M., & Schreiner, P. (1998). Prevalence of binge eating disorder, obesity, and depression in a biracial cohort of young adults. *Annals of Behavioral Medicine, 20*, 227–232.

Soukup, V. M., Beiler, M. E., & Terrell, F. (1998). Stress, coping style, and problem solving ability among eating-disordered inpatients. *Journal of Clinical Psychology, 46*, 592–599.

Spitzer, R. L., Devlin, M., Walsh, B. T., Hasin, D., Wing, R., Marcus, M., Stunkard, A., Wadden, T., Yanovski, S., Agras, S., Mitchell, J., & Nonas, C. (1992). Binge eating disorder: A multisite field trial of the diagnostic criteria. *International Journal of Eating Disorders, 11*, 191–203.

Spitzer, R. L., Yanovski, S., Wadden, T., Wing, R., Marcus, M. D., Stunkard, A., Devlin, M., Mitchell, J., Hasin, D., & Horne, R. L. (1993). Binge eating disorder. Its further validation in a multisite study. *International Journal of Eating Disorders, 13*, 137–153.

Spurrell, E. B., Wilfley, D. E., Tanofsky, M. B., & Brownell, K. D. (1997). Age of onset for binge eating: Are there different pathways to binge eating? *International Journal of Eating Disorders, 21*, 55–65.

Stein, S., Chalhoub, N., & Hodes, M. (1998). Very early-onset bulimia nervosa: Report of two cases. *International Journal of Eating Disorders, 24*, 323–327.

Steinberg, S., Tobin, D. L., & Johnson, C. (1990). The role of bulimic behaviors in affect regulation: Different functions for different patient subgroups? *International Journal of Eating Disorders, 9*, 51–55.

Stice, E. (1994). Review of the evidence for a sociocultural model of bulimia nervosa and an exploration of the mechanisms of action. *Clinical Psychology Review, 14*, 633–661.

Stice, E. (1998). Modeling of eating pathology and social reinforcement of the thin-ideal predict onset of bulimic symptoms. *Behaviour Research and Therapy, 36*, 931–944.

Striegel-Moore, R. H., Garvin, V., Dohm, F. A., & Rosenheck, R. A. (1999). Eating disorders in a national sample of hospitalized female and male veterans: Detection rates and psychiatric comorbidity. *International Journal of Eating Disorders, 25*, 405–414.

Striegel-Moore, R. H., Silberstein, L. R., & Rodin, J. (1986). Toward an understanding of risk factors for bulimia. *American Psychologist, 41,* 246–263.

Striegel-Moore, R. H., Silberstein, L. R., & Rodin, J. (1993). The social self in bulimia nervosa: Public self-consciousness, social anxiety, and perceived fraudulence. *Journal of Abnormal Psychology, 102,* 297–303.

Striegel-Moore, R. H., Wilson, G. T., Wilfley, D. E., Elder, K. A., & Brownell, K. A. (1998). Binge eating in a community sample. *International Journal of Eating Disorders, 23,* 27–37.

Strober, M. (1991). Family-genetic studies of eating disorders. *Journal of Clinical Psychiatry, 52,* 9–12.

Strober, M. (1997). Consultation and therapeutic engagement in severe anorexia nervosa. In D. M. Garner & P. E. Garfinkel (Eds.), *Handbook of treatment for eating disorders* (pp. 229–247). New York: Guilford.

Stunkard, A. (1997). Eating disorders: The last 25 years. *Appetite, 29,* 181–190.

Sullivan, P. F. (1995). Mortality in anorexia nervosa. *American Journal of Psychiatry, 152,* 1073–1074.

Sullivan, P. F., Bulik, C. M., & Kendler, K. S. (1998). The epidemiology and classification of bulimia nervosa. *Psychological Medicine, 28,* 599–610.

Suzuki, K., Higuchi, S., Yamada, K., Komiya, H., & Takagi, S. (1994). Bulimia nervosa with and without alcoholism: A comparative study in Japan. *International Journal of Eating Disorders, 16,* 137–146.

Tanofsky, M. B., Wilfley, D. E., Spurell, E. B., Welch, R., & Brownell, K. D. (1997). Comparison of men and women with binge eating disorder. *International Journal of Eating Disorders, 21,* 49–54.

Taylor, G. J., Parker, J. D., Bagby, R. M., & Rourke, M. P. (1996). relationships between alexithymia and psychological characteristics associated with eating disorders. *Journal of Psychosomatic Research, 41,* 561–568.

Telch, C. F., & Agras, W. S. (1994). Obesity binge eating and psychopathology: Are they related? *International Journal of Eating Disorders, 15,* 53–61.

Telch, C. G., & Stice, E. (1998). Psychiatric comorbidity in women with binge eating disorder: Prevalence rates from a non-treatment-seeking sample. *Journal of Consulting and Clinical Psychology, 66,* 768–776.

Teusch, R. (1988). Level of ego development and bulimics' conceptualizations of their disorder. *International Journal of Eating Disorders, 7,* 607–615.

Thompson, J. K. (1996). Introduction: Body image, eating disorders, and obesity—an emerging synthesis. In J. K. Thompson (Ed.), *Body image, eating disorders, and obesity: An integrative guide for assessment and treatment* (pp. 1–22). Washington, DC: American Psychological Association.

Tiggemann, M., & Raven, M. (1998). Dimensions of control in bulimia and anorexia nervosa: Internal control, desire for control, or fear of losing self-control? *Eating Disorders: The Journal of Treatment and Prevention, 6,* 65–71.

Tiller, J. M., Sloane, G., Schmidt, U., Troop, N., Power, M., & Treasure, J. L. (1997). Social support in patients with anorexia nervosa and bulimia nervosa. *International Journal of Eating Disorders, 21,* 31–38.

Tobin, D. L., Griffing, A., & Griffing, S. (1997). An examination of subtype criteria for bulimia nervosa. *International Journal of Eating Disorders, 22,* 179–186.

Troop, N. A., Holbrey, A., & Treasure, J. L. (1998). Stress, coping, and crisis support in eating disorders. *International Journal of Eating Disorders, 24,* 157–166.

Tylka, T. L., Subich, M., & Mezydlo, L. (1999). Exploring the construct validity of the eating disorder continuum. *Journal of Counseling Psychology, 46,* 268–276.

Vitousek, K. B., & Hollon, S. D. (1990). The investigation of schematic content and processing in eating disorders. *Cognitive Therapy and Research, 14,* 191–214.

Vitousek, K., & Manke, F. (1994). Personality variables and disorders in anorexia nervosa and bulimia nervosa. *Journal of Abnormal Psychology, 103,* 137–147.

Walsh, B. T., & Garner, D. M. (1997). Diagnostic issues. In D. M. Garner & P. E. Garfinkel (Eds.), *Handbook of treatment for eating disorders,* 2nd ed. (pp. 25–33). New York: Guilford.

Wardle, J. (1988). Cognitive control of eating. *Journal of Psychosomatic Research, 32,* 607–612.

Welch, S. L., & Fairburn, C. G. (1996). Childhood sexual and physical abuse as risk factors for the development of bulimia nervosa: A community-based case control study. *Child Abuse and Neglect, 20,* 633–642.

Wills, T. A. (1997). Modes and families of coping: An analysis of downward comparison in the structure of other cognitive and behavioral mechanisms. In B. P. Buunk & F. X. Gibbons (Eds.), *Health, coping, and well-being: Perspectives from social comparison theory.* Mahwah, NJ: Erlbaum.

Wiseman, C. V., Gray, J. J., Mosimann, J. E., & Ahrens, A. H. (1992). Cultural expectations of thinness in women: An update. *International Journal of Eating Disorders, 11,* 85–89.

Wonderlich, S. A., Brewerton, T. D., Jocic, Z., Dansky, B. S., & Abbott, D. W. (1997). Relationship of childhood sexual abuse and eating disorders. *Journal of the American Academy of Child and Adolescent Psychiatry, 36,* 1107–1115.

Wonderlich, S. A., & Mitchell, M. D. (1997). Eating disorders and comorbidity: Empirical, conceptual, and clinical implications. *Psychopharmacology Bulletin, 33*(3), 381–390.

Woodside, D. B., & Garfinkel, P. E. (1992). Age of onset in eating disorders. *International Journal of Eating Disorders, 12,* 31–36.

Yanovski, S. Z., Nelson, J. E., Dubbert, B. K., & Spitzer, R. L. (1993). Association of binge eating disorder and psychiatric comorbidity in obese subjects. *American Journal of Psychiatry, 150,* 1472–1479.

Zerbe, K. J. (1996). Anorexia nervosa and bulimia nervosa: When the pursuit of bodily "perfection" becomes a killer. *Postgraduate Medicine, 99,* 161–169.

III

Adult and Older Adult Disorders: Introductory Comments

The past several years have witnessed a dramatic upsurge of clinical and investigative interest in the epidemiology, prevention, assessment, and treatment of adult disorders. The increased activity in this area is partly attributable to improvements in the primary classification system used to diagnose these problems: the *Diagnostic and Statistical Manual of Mental Disorders* (DSM). Since the inception of nosological precision and prediction, adult research efforts have burgeoned. In addition to this, the growing awareness of the need to consider psychological, biological, and environmental factors in psychopathology has (1) greatly expanded the range of specialty areas (e.g., neurology, biochemistry, and endocrinology) involved in the study of the various disorders and (2) underscored the need for interdisciplinary approaches that consider the multiple and complex factors responsible for their occurrence.

The chapters in this part of the book cover the major adult and older adult disorders. In Chapter 14, Paul M. G. Emmelkamp and Patricia Van Oppen review the major anxiety disorders, including specific phobia, panic disorder with and without agoraphobia, social phobia, generalized anxiety disorder, obsessive–compulsive disorder, and acute and posttraumatic stress disorder. Case illustrations of assessment and intervention approaches for each of these difficulties are provided. Lynn P. Rehm, Paras Mehta, and Carrie L. Dodrill discuss current strategies and issues in the assessment and treatment of depression (Chapter 15). Further, they underscore the importance of a biopsychosocial perspective in studying the problem. Schizophrenia, one of the most disabling psychiatric disturbances, is covered by Michelle P. Salyers and Kim T. Mueser (Chapter 16). These authors provide an overview of psychosocial and pharmacological treatments, in addition to a discussion of major etiological theories.

Substance use disorders are the most common group of psychiatric disorders in the United States. In Chapter 17, Timothy J. O'Farrell outlines heuristic evaluation and remediation strategies for alcohol and drug problems. William O'Donohue, Tamara Penix, and Lisa Regev discuss the two categories of sexual problems: sexual dysfunctions and sexual deviations. The authors document research confirming the efficacy of various treatment techniques with these disorders. In Chapter 19, Brian P. O'Connor and Jamie A. Dyce describe the extreme and inflexible manifestations of personality characteristics known as personality disorders. They present symptom pictures for each disorder and highlight the evidence for both genetic and specific environmental influences. In Chapter 20, Kristine L. Brady and Patricia L. Fiero define psychophysiological disorders as physical or medical problems that are significantly influenced by psychological, behavioral, and/or environmental factors. They review clinical and research findings pertaining to the most prevalent difficulties under this rubric: headache, insomnia, and essential hypertension. Finally, Gerald Goldstein covers organic mental disorders (Chapter 21). This category includes the constellation of severely disabling conditions caused by impaired brain functions. Delirium, dementia, amnesia, and other syndromes that alter personality, mood, or anxiety level are also reviewed.

14

Anxiety Disorders

Paul M. G. Emmelkamp and Patricia Van Oppen

Introduction

This chapter discusses the description, epidemiology, clinical features, course and prognosis, familial and genetic patterns, and differential diagnosis of anxiety disorders. The various anxiety disorders (i.e., specific phobia, panic disorder with and without agoraphobia, social phobia, generalized anxiety disorder, obsessive–compulsive disorder, and acute and post-traumatic stress disorder) are dealt with separately.

Specific Phobia

Description of the Disorder

One of the most widespread anxiety disorders is the specific or simple phobia. The term specific phobia refers to a broad scale of phobias associated with different stimuli. Specific phobias are restricted to specific situations. According to the diagnostic criteria of DSM-IV (American Psychiatric Association, 1993), specific phobia should be diagnosed in the case of a persistent excessive or irrational fear of a circumscribed stimulus (object or situation), which is avoided or endured with intense anxiety. The fear or the avoidance behavior has to interfere significantly with the person's normal life. The fear-related stimulus of specific phobia has to be different from panic disorder/agoraphobia or social phobia stimuli and unrelated to the content of the obsessions of obsessive–compulsive disorder or the trauma of posttraumatic stress. The DSM-IV distinguishes four types of specific phobias: animal type (e.g., spiders, dogs, cats, snakes, and birds), natural environment type (e.g., storms, heights, or water), blood-injection-injury type (e.g., dental phobia), and situational type (e.g., tunnels, bridges, elevators, flying, driving, or enclosed places).

Paul M. G. Emmelkamp • Department of Clinical Psychology, University of Amsterdam, 1018 WB Amsterdam, The Netherlands.   **Patricia Van Oppen** • Department of Psychiatry, Valeriuskliniek, 1075 BG Amsterdam, The Netherlands.

Advanced Abnormal Psychology, Second Edition, edited by Hersen and Van Hasselt. Kluwer Academic/Plenum Publishers, New York, 2001.

Epidemiology

In the last decade, several epidemiological studies investigated the prevalence rate of simple phobia according to the DSM-III (Bijl, van Zessen, & Ravelli, 1997; Bland, Orn, & Newman, 1988; Burnam et al., 1987; Karno et al., 1987; Kessler et al., 1994; Myers et al., 1984; Robins et al., 1984; Wittchen, 1988). These data are presented in Table 1. Specific phobia is the most common anxiety disorder. The mean lifetime prevalence of specific phobias is just over 10%.

The situational and the natural environment type had the highest point-prevalence rate (13%), followed by animal phobias (8%). Finally, the point-prevalence rate of blood-injection-injury phobias was 3%. The prevalence of specific phobias is higher among females than among males, especially for animal, situational, and natural environment phobias (Frederik-son et al., 1996).

Clinical Picture

Angela is a 29-year-old unmarried woman. She is employed in a large business firm. For several years she has had a flight phobia. She particularly fears a crash. Angela avoids going by plane. Besides this phobia, she has cat and insect phobias, but the latter phobias do not restrict her life. Angela does not know how these phobias developed. The anxiety increased over the years. Recently, she received a promotion, and her new job requires several distant trips; therefore, she is now seeking treatment for her flight phobia.

A specific phobia can lead to intense panic and extreme avoidance of the specific situations. In some cases, this might have severe consequences, for example, when a blood phobic avoids medical treatment or a claustrophobic refuses to have a scan taken. Rarely are the fears strong enough to motivate individuals to refer themselves for treatment. When specific phobics do seek treatment, it is often because they anticipate that circumstances will force confrontation with a dreaded cue stimulus.

Originally, behavior theorists held that specific phobias were acquired through a process

TABLE 1. Prevalence Rate of Anxiety Disorders

Authors/study	Any anxiety disorder[a] (%)	Agoraphobia (%)	Panic disorder (%)	Social phobia (%)	Specific phobia (%)	Obsessive–compulsive disorder (%)	GAD (%)
Robins et al. (1984)							
Myers et al. (1984)							
New Haven	7.8	3.5	1.4	—	6.3	2.6	—
Baltimore	23.3	9.0	1.4	—	20.4	3.0	—
St. Louis	9.4	4.0	1.5	—	6.8	1.9	—
Karno et al. (1987) Burnam et al. (1987)	11.7	—	1.5	—	—	2.1	—
Wittchen (1988)	13.9	5.7	2.4	8.0		2.0	—
Bland et al. (1988)	8.9	2.9	1.2	1.7	7.2	3.0	—
Kessler et al. (1994)	24.9	5.3	3.5	13.3	11.3	—	5.1
Bijl et al. (1997)	19.3	3.4	3.8	7.8	10.1	0.9	2.3

[a]Apart from posttraumatic and acute stress disorders.

of conditioning, in which CS and UCS are paired, but the conditioning model of fear acquisition does not seem to be tenable (e.g., Emmelkamp, 1982). More recently it is accepted that many factors other than the experienced pairings of CS and UCS can affect the strength of the association between these events, including beliefs and expectancies about possible danger associated with a particular CS, and culturally transmitted information about the CS-UCS contingency (Davey, 1997).

It is remarkable that a selection of objects or situations exists that specific phobics fear. Surprisingly, some phobias such as gun phobias, mixer phobias, car phobias, mower phobia, and hammer phobia, never occur. The preparedness theory attempts to explain this phenomenon. According to this perspective, most phobias are based on a genetic disposition or preparedness to develop fear of those objects and situations (e.g., snakes, spiders, and enclosed places) that were threatening to our prehistoric ancestors. Although several experimental laboratory studies have been conducted to test this theory, the results are inconclusive (Merkelbach & de Jong, 1997).

When specific phobics are confronted with the phobic object or situation, this immediately induces extreme distress and panic. When the phobic stimulus is taken away, the anxiety decreases. Confrontation with the phobic stimuli leads to a sympathetically mediated increase in blood pressure and heart rate. However, blood-injury phobics show a very short sympathetic activation followed by a parasympathetic activation (a drop in heart rate and/or blood pressure) (Öst & Hellström, 1997).

There is a considerable overlap between anxiety and affective syndromes. This overlap is not seen for specific phobics. Only 9% of patients who had specific phobia reported past depressive episodes (Monroe, 1990).

Course and Prognosis

In young children (2–6 years), simple phobias (mostly fears of animals) often improve "spontaneously" without any treatment. Those who have phobias that continue into adulthood seldom recover spontaneously. The mean onset age for animal phobia and blood-injury phobia is about 8 years (Öst & Hellström, 1997), 12 years for dental phobia, and 20 years for claustrophobia (Öst, 1987). Specific phobias are especially responsive to behavioral treatment (Emmelkamp, 1994). However, there may be problems in arranging exposure for less approachable stimuli (e.g., storms).

Familial and Genetic Patterns

Clearly there are familial influences on fears during childhood and adulthood. Positive correlations have been found routinely between the fears of children and their mothers (Emmelkamp & Scholing, 1997a). The influence of mothers' and siblings' fears on the fears of children is probably greater among younger than among older children. Familial influences also might be relatively stronger among children from lower socioeconomic strata. These data suggest that social learning factors are important in the development of specific phobias (Chapman, 1997).

The concordances of blood-injury phobias and animal phobias were higher among monozygotic than among dizygotic twins (Torgersen, 1979). In family studies, Fyer and his colleagues present evidence for a specific genetic contribution to specific phobias (Fyer et al., 1990, 1995). Relatives of probands who have specific phobias were at increased risk for specific phobias, but not for other phobias. In contrast, results of the studies of Skre et al.

(1993) and Kendler et al. (1992a) suggest that there is a common genetic variance for anxiety disorders in general, rather than that there is a specific genetic vulnerability.

Finally, blood-injury phobics have more relatives who have similar problems than other phobics do. Among blood phobics, about 60% had first-degree relatives who were also blood phobic; this is three to six times more frequently than panic disorder, obsessive–compulsive disorder, and agora-, social, dental, or animal phobics (Marks, 1987; Öst, 1992).

Diagnostic Considerations

In general, the diagnosis of a specific phobia provides little difficulty. For the differential diagnosis, it is important that the fear is unrelated to agoraphobia, social phobia, posttraumatic stress disorder, and obsessive–compulsive disorder. A specific phobia can be a part of another anxiety disorder. For example, a patient who had obsessive–compulsive problems also had an AIDS phobia. She had many cleaning rituals and obsessional concerns with germs and contamination. One of her obsessional concerns pertained to the fear of developing AIDS. In this case, the diagnosis of a specific phobia should not be made. Further, anxiety related to a severe trauma is not diagnosed as a specific phobia but may be associated with posttraumatic stress disorder. Finally, the fear of being scrutinized by other persons or feeling embarrassed is not referred to as specific phobia but as social phobia.

PANIC DISORDER

Description of the Disorder

Panic disorder is characterized by recurrent unexpected panic attacks and at least one month of persistent apprehension about the recurrence of panic. A panic attack is a discrete period of intense fear or discomfort. According to DSM-IV, attacks (1) do not occur immediately before or after exposure to a situation that nearly always causes anxiety and (2) are not the result of situations in which the person is the focus of others' attention (as in social phobia). During a panic attack, four of the following symptoms occur: shortness of breath (dyspnea); dizziness or unsteady feelings; palpitations (tachycardia); trembling or shaking; sweating; feelings of choking; nausea or abdominal distress; depersonalization or derealization; paresthesias; (hot) flushes or chills; chest pain or discomfort; fear of dying; and fear of losing control. These symptoms should not be due to any organic factor, such as amphetamine, caffeine intoxication, or hyperthyroidism. Many panic patients tend to avoid situations or activities that trigger panic attacks. Although avoidance behavior may prevent a person from having a panic attack, it usually leads to a very restricted lifestyle. A diagnosis of panic disorder with agoraphobia is made when the complaints meet the criteria of panic disorder and those of agoraphobia as well. DSM-IV distinguishes between agoraphobia in connection with panic disorder and agoraphobia without a history of panic attacks. Agoraphobia connected with panic disorder is described as a fear to be in places or situations from which it is difficult to escape or in which there is no help at hand in case of a panic attack. In agoraphobia without panic disorder, there is a fear of suddenly emerging symptoms that may embarrass the persons or make them need help, such as losing control over bladder or bowel, vomiting, depersonalization or derealization, and dizziness. This fear leads to avoidance of a number of situations, such as walking, standing in a queue, being in a large shop, mall, or crowded and busy streets, traveling in public transport, and driving a car.

Epidemiology

Panics are occasionally experienced by nearly 30% of the adult population, but most of these attacks are only mildly distressing (Norton, Cox, & Malan, 1992). An important difference between nonclinical panickers and panic patients is that the latter group responds with anxiety and catastrophic cognitions to the physical sensation whereas the former group does not (Telch, Lucas, & Nelson, 1989). The mean lifetime prevalence rate of panic disorder is 2.1%, and of agoraphobia about 4% in the community surveys summarized in Table 1. Note that the prevalence figure of agoraphobia and panic disorder is somewhat unreliable due to the definitions used in the particular interview (the DIS) employed in the Epidemiology Catchment Area Studies. Studies using the CIDI (e.g., Bijl et al., 1997; Kessler et al., 1994) found a higher prevalence of panic disorder than studies that used the DIS. Agoraphobia was more prevalent than panic disorder. Agoraphobia and panic disorder constitute about 50 to 80% of patients with anxiety disorders seen in clinical practice. Both disorders are much more common among females than among males. There may be important differences between clinic samples and community samples. For example, although agoraphobia without a history of panic attacks is apparently quite common in community surveys (5.3% lifetime prevalence in the study of Kessler et al., 1994), such patients are hardly seen in clinical settings (Craske, 1999).

Clinical Picture

> Jeanette (28 years of age) is referred for anxiety complaints, which have prevented her from doing her job in the past year. For 5 years, she has been suffering from panic attacks and symptoms of breathlessness, palpitations, and dizziness. She is afraid of having a heart attack. During the past six months, she has had attacks on the average of 12 a month, characterized by a sudden increase of panic, which subsides after about 15 minutes. The attacks predominantly occur in crowded situations: crowded streets, shopping malls, and supermarkets. Recently, the patient has not been going out of the house on her own; she needs to be accompanied by a friend. Sometimes, at home, she becomes panicky without any apparent reason.

Although the somatic symptoms of panic attacks are well defined, the cognitive concomitants of patients may vary from patient to patient. A number of panic patients' fears are focused on the somatic consequences: They fear a heart attack, a stroke, or fainting. When patients fear loss of psychic control, the anxiety centers around patients' belief that they are possibly going mad; often as a result of the depersonalization and derealization that a patient may experience during a panic attack. Finally, a number of panic patients are afraid of criticism from other people who react to their panic attack. A number of investigators suggest that biological mechanisms may predispose subjects to experience panic attacks.

Although it has been found that heightened levels of activation in autonomic measures (e.g., heart rate and skin conductance) characterize panic patients (Craske, 1999), the significance of this for the development of panic disorder remains unclear. Such heightened physiological arousal may be the result of anxiety elicited by the laboratory situation, rather than evidence of a biological vulnerability. Further, rather than being a causative agent, physiological activation can be secondary to the development of panic attacks.

There are two related vulnerability factors that may be associated with the development of panic disorder: (1) anxiety sensitivity and (2) heightened awareness of bodily sensations. The Anxiety Sensitivity Index was able to predict the occurrence of panic attacks one year

(Ehlers, 1995) to three years (Maller & Reiss, 1992) later, thus supporting the notion that anxiety sensitivity may be important in predisposing individuals to the development of panic attacks. Further, there is now some evidence that panic patients are more hypervigilant to bodily sensations (e.g., Ehlers & Breuer, 1996; Ehlers, Breuer, Dohn, & Fiegenbaum, 1995), but it is questionable whether they are more accurate in detecting them (Craske, 1999). Why some individuals who have recurrent panic attacks develop agoraphobia and others do not is not yet really understood. The acute and intense experience of anxiety is held responsible for the tendency to escape, which is characteristic of the panic attack. It has been suggested that the severity of panic attacks and catastrophic cognitions associated with them determine whether patients maintain a panic disorder without avoidance behavior or develop agoraphobia. Comparisons between patients having panic disorder with agoraphobia and those having panic disorder without agoraphobia have found few consistent disparities between groups (Craske, 1999; de Jong & Bouman, 1995). The most robust predictor of agoraphobia is gender; most agoraphobic patients are female. The preponderance of agoraphobia in women may be due to psychosocial factors such as sex-role stereotyping or biological factors (e.g., sex hormones). There is not yet convincing evidence for either a social learning or a biological interpretation of the sex difference in the prevalence of agoraphobia.

More than half of the panic patients with or without agoraphobia also qualify for the diagnosis of another anxiety disorder or depression (Craske, 1999; Goisman et al., 1994; de Ruiter et al., 1989). There is considerable symptom overlap between panic disorder and generalized anxiety, which suggests that the differences between generalized anxiety and panic are more quantitative than qualitative. Agoraphobia and panic are associated with depression and hypochondriasis. The rate of primary major depression is about 30%, and the range for secondary depression is 30 to 53% (Lesser, 1988). It is questionable whether depressive symptoms should be viewed as an independent disorder or as merely the result of the severe restrictions imposed on one's life by panic disorder.

The somatic complaints and preoccupations may be related to hyperventilation in some patients, which can result in heart palpitations, chest pains, sweating, and lightheadedness; these may play a causal role in provoking a panic attack. A hyperventilation attack and the concomitant bodily sensations often are accompanied by severe anxiety, which by itself may provoke hyperventilation in the future. This fear of panic may lead to avoidance of a number of situations, which ultimately may result in agoraphobia. In a number of patients, abnormalities in the vestibular system are involved, but to how many of the panic patients this applies is unclear (Jacob et al., 1989).

Alcohol abuse is common among panic patients. In a sample of panic patients with agoraphobia gathered from the Epidemiologic Catchment Area Study, nearly 30% qualified for the diagnosis of alcohol abuse or dependence (Himle & Hill, 1991). Patients who have agoraphobia without panic attacks are also less likely to have an alcohol problem. In general, substance abuse follows rather than precedes the panic disorder, suggesting that in these cases substance abuse might be considered avoidance behavior.

Most panic patients report catastrophic cognitions related to physical sensations during panic attacks. Patients who have chest pain, breathlessness, numbness and tingling, blurred vision, and choking typically have thoughts about having a brain tumor, heart attack, or a stroke. Other patients have thoughts about the psychosocial consequences of their anxiety. For example, depersonalization is often related to thoughts about losing control, acting foolishly, and going crazy.

It has been suggested that the intimate relationship of agoraphobic patients with their partner may be of critical importance in the development and maintenance of agoraphobic symptoms (Hafner, 1982). Controlled studies, however, found that agoraphobics and their partners tend to be comparably happily married (Emmelkamp & Gerlsma, 1994). Although agoraphobics have been found to be more socially anxious, more externally controlled, and more introverted than controls, it is unclear whether these are premorbid personality features or whether these personality characteristics are merely the result of the panic and agoraphobic complaints. The same applies to the finding that nearly 20% of agoraphobics qualify for the diagnosis of avoidant personality disorder (Van Velzen & Emmelkamp, 2000).

Course and Prognosis

The mean age of onset of agoraphobia is approximately 28 (Mannuzza, Fyer, Liebowitz, & Klein, 1990). In a large series of clinical patients, agoraphobia started mainly between ages 17 and 29, but with a few (16%) it started only after age 40 (Lelliott, McNamee, Marks, 1991). It has been suggested that agoraphobia has its precursor in separation anxiety in childhood; however, there is little evidence to substantiate such clinicians' claims (Shear, 1996). Moreover, separation anxiety is not specifically related to panic disorder but is also associated with other anxiety disorders and with depression (Moreau & Follett, 1993). Although agoraphobics may have their good days and their bad days, in only a few persons will agoraphobia remit spontaneously after a year. Treatment consisting of *in vivo* exposure is effective in nearly 75% of agoraphobics (Emmelkamp, 1994). Panic can be effectively treated by cognitive-behavior therapy, high-potency benzodiazepines, tricyclic antidepressants, and selective serotonin reuptake inhibitors (Craske, 1999). If patients discontinue medication, relapse is the rule rather than the exception.

Familial and Genetic Patterns

Reich and Yates (1988) found that the rate of panic disorder was higher among the relatives of panic patients (9.3%) than among the relatives of social phobics (1.3%) and of controls (0%). A family history of agoraphobia is reportedly more common in panic patients who have agoraphobia than in patients who have uncomplicated panic disorder (Harris et al., 1983; Noyes et al., 1986). Skre, Onstad, Torgersen, Lygren, and Kringlen (1993) and Torgersen (1983) found a significantly higher concordance rate for agoraphobia and panic disorder in monozygotic twins than in dizygotic twins. Taken together, these results suggest that genetic factors play some role in panic disorder.

Diagnostic Considerations

Clinicians need to be attuned to the possibility of comorbid alcohol dependence among panic patients. Because a number of panic patients do not report alcohol problems spontaneously, sensitive questioning is needed.

Although a number of agoraphobics also have specific phobias, closer scrutiny may reveal that these phobias are actually part of the agoraphobic symptomatology and the result of a panic attack in particular situations. A close temporal relationship between a panic attack and fear in a particular situation may alert clinicians to the possibility that the phobia developed in the context of a panic attack. It is also important to realize that most specific phobias develop at a relatively young age. In a number of patients, however, specific phobias, such as fear of heights and fear of enclosed spaces, may exist long before the onset of their first panic attack, in which case an additional diagnosis of specific phobia is justified. Panic should be distinguished from hypochondriasis, which is characterized by a persistent conviction and fear of a serious disease. Panic patients are usually less concerned about having a serious disease between panic attacks.

Some social phobics avoid the same situations as agoraphobics. Agoraphobia can be differentiated from social phobia by detailed inquiry into the reasons that people avoid certain situations. Anxiety is triggered in social phobics by the fear of criticism and (negative) evaluation. The fear is not for the symptoms as such but for possible scrutiny by other people. In agoraphobia (with panic), the fear involves having a panic attack or losing control. There is also some difference in the physical symptoms experienced. Blushing is common in social phobics, whereas difficulty in breathing, dizziness, and weakness in limbs are more characteristic somatic symptoms of agoraphobics.

SOCIAL PHOBIA

Description of the Disorder

In DSM-IV, "social phobia" is described as a persistent fear of one or more social or performance situations in which the person is exposed to possible scrutiny by others and fears to behave in a way that will be humiliating and embarrassing. Social phobics are anxious when confronted with the feared situation, and those situations will generally be avoided or endured only with intense anxiety, if avoidance is impossible. The avoidance behavior interferes with occupational or social functioning. The fear must be unrelated to panic disorder or to somatic disorders. As an example, fear of trembling that results from Parkinson's disease does not justify a diagnosis of social phobia. In DSM-III, social phobia was described as a persistent irrational fear of one specific social situation: Fears of more than one social situation were classified as "avoidant personality disorder" rather than as social phobia. In DSM-IV, fear of several social situations is classified as "social phobia" with the addition of "generalized type."

Epidemiology

The results of epidemiological studies with respect to lifetime diagnosis are summarized in Table 1. The lifetime prevalence of social phobia in the Bijl et al. (1997) and the Kessler et al. (1994) studies is much higher than in previous studies, presumably due to the requirement of DSM-III that there should be actual avoidance before the diagnosis social phobia could be established. There is an equal sex ratio in both community surveys (Bourdon et al., 1988) and in clinical samples.

Clinical Picture

John is a 20-year-old male who is extremely bothered by social phobia. At first sight, the complaints look like agoraphobia. He does not leave the house and is afraid of going to shops because it makes him anxious. On inquiry, it appears that it is not so much a matter of fear of a panic attack, but rather a fear of what other people might think of him. He is very discontent about his appearance although there is nothing wrong with it. And he is preoccupied with the idea that everybody finds him stupid. Recently, he would not dare to open the door or to answer the phone. He is still living with his mother, who takes care of shopping and such chores. When his mother has visitors, which happens rarely, he remains in his room. As a child, John was very withdrawn and always had a feeling of not belonging. For a brief period, he worked at a warehouse; however, when his boss made a very critical remark once, he did not return to work. Since that time his complaints have worsened.

The essential feature of social phobia is "a marked or persistent fear of one or more social or performance situations in which the person is exposed to possible scrutiny by others and fears that he or she may do something or act in a way that will be humiliating or embarrassing." A number of social phobics experience fear in any situation; however, fears in other patients are limited to specific situations. For example, some patients fear that their hands may tremble when writing or holding a cup in front of others. Others may be afraid of blushing or of eating in public places. Most social phobics have difficulty in at least two different situations, and nearly half feel anxious in three or more situations. Holt, Heimberg, Hope, and Liebowitz (1992) distinguished four different situational domains of social phobia: (1) formal speaking and interaction, (2) informal speaking and interaction, (3) observation by others, and (4) assertion. Seventy-five percent of social phobics experienced anxiety in more than one domain. Nearly all social phobics had significant problems in the formal speaking/ interaction domain, which corroborates the clinical impression that public speaking anxiety is prevalent among social phobics. Although earlier research suggested that social phobics lacked adequate social skills, other studies do not support this for specific interpersonal behaviors such as eye contact and length of speaking time (Monti et al., 1984). Cognitive factors, such as negative self-statements and irrational beliefs, are more important (Sanderman et al., 1987). Social phobics display considerably more negative self-statements in social contacts than nonanxious persons (Stopa & Clark, 1993). Socially anxious people misallocate limited attentional resources to social threat cues (Elting & Hope, 1995). Further, they tend to evaluate their own (social) behavior excessively negatively and selectively attend to negative experiences in social situations. Finally, social phobics interpret ambiguous social situations as more negative and more catastrophic than other anxious patients (Wells & Clark, 1997).

Based on the research findings discussed here, Clark and Wells (1995) formulated a cognitive model of social phobia. According to this model, social phobics are eager to present favorable impressions of themselves, but they are insecure in their performance in social situations. This social insecurity is fed by negative self-focused processing and leads to "safety behaviors" intended to avoid negative evaluations of others and to protect self-esteem. Being self-conscious leads to clumsy behavior in social situations, thus reinforcing negative impressions of the self.

Generally, there is a high comorbidity with other anxiety disorders (Craske, 1999; Lepine & Lelouche, 1995), with depression, and with avoidant personality disorder (van Velzen & Emmelkamp, 1999). Alcohol abuse and dependence is often a problem in social phobics, and the prevalence might be even higher among social phobics than among panic patients (Norton et al., 1996). Social phobics who concurrently abuse alcohol are more anxious than social phobics without alcohol problems (Schneier et al., 1989). Retrospective studies that focused on the antecedent factors of social phobia have found problematic relationships with parents: relationships lacking in emotional warmth and marred by rejection and overprotection (Arrindell et al., 1983).

Course and Prognosis

The onset of social phobia is usually in adolescence (around the age of 18), which is much earlier than the mean age of onset in agoraphobia. When patients report both alcohol abuse and social phobia, the social phobia precedes the onset of the alcohol problem in nearly all cases (Schneier et al., 1989). The prognosis for patients treated with cognitive and behavior therapy is relatively good (Emmelkamp & Scholing, 1997b).

Familial and Genetic Patterns

Few systematic studies exist. Fyer et al. (1995) and Reich and Yates (1988) found a higher prevalence of social phobia among the relatives of social phobics than among the relatives of patients who have other anxiety disorders. However, these studies provide only meager evidence of a genetic disposition because environmental factors can account equally well for the differences obtained. Torgersen (1988) garnered some support in twin studies for a genetic contribution to social fears in normals.

Diagnostic Considerations

Social phobia is distinguished from the shyness and social anxiety that many individuals experience by the intensity of the fears and the abnormal avoidance of the social situations involved. There is considerable overlap among social phobia, panic disorder, and generalized anxiety. Rather than being considered as distinct diagnostic categories, phobic symptoms are better viewed as lying in a number of different continua. The actual primary diagnosis depends on the predominant features in a particular patient. Many social phobics meet criteria for avoidant personality disorder, and it is questionable whether social phobia and avoidant personality disorder are two separate categories (van Velzen & Emmelkamp, 1996). However, there is some evidence that individuals who have avoidant personality disorders are less socially skilled and more socially anxious than social phobics. It has been suggested that individuals who have avoidant personality disorders are more accepting of their limitations in social situations than social phobics without this personality disorder. Social phobia may, in a number of cases, be related to body dysmorphic disorder and be difficult to distinguish from this disorder. In other cases, the diagnosis of body dysmorphic disorder rather than social phobia is more appropriate. In DSM IV, body dysmorphic disorder is not classified among the anxiety disorders but among the somatoform disorders. Patients qualify for the diagnosis of body dysmorphic disorder when they are preoccupied by a presumed physical anomaly of their bodies, with no objective basis. Most patients who have a body dysmorphic disorder experience anxiety in social contacts and tend to avoid these situations.

GENERALIZED ANXIETY DISORDER

Description of the Disorder

Generalized anxiety disorder (GAD) is defined in DSM-IV as excessive or unrealistic anxiety and worry for a period of 6 months or more about a number of events or activities. Although a patient may have "good days" without much worrying, there should be more "worry days" than days on which the individual is not bothered by these concerns. Most worries of generalized anxiety patients involve anxious apprehension with respect to finances, work, interpersonal problems, accidents, or illnesses and health issues.

GAD, which before its introduction in DSM-III was known as free-floating anxiety, has poor diagnostic reliability and is not easily distinguished from other anxiety disorders. Many patients who have GAD also meet criteria for another anxiety disorder, usually social or simple phobia (Brown & Barlow, 1992). Most panic patients, agoraphobics, obsessive–compulsives, and social phobics present symptoms that belong to the generalized anxiety cluster. There is considerable symptom overlap with depression (Wittchen et al., 1994). Many depressed persons have concomitant symptoms of GAD.

Epidemiology

Generalized anxiety is very common in the general population. In the National Co-morbidity Survey, the lifetime prevalence was 5.1% and the 12-month prevalence was 3.1% (Kessler et al., 1994). Estimates may be even higher in the elderly (Brawman-Mintzer & Lydiard, 1996). As in panic disorder and specific phobia, there is a clear preponderance of GAD among females. Although it is one of the most frequent anxiety disorders in the community, most patients do not seek treatment other than that provided by their general practitioners (Edelmann, 1992; Wittchen et al., 1994).

Clinical Picture

Judith is a 34-year-old woman with two children, who has sought treatment because of anxiety complaints. In fact, she has felt anxious as long as she can remember. She describes herself as the worrying type. In elementary school, she was afraid of being teased, and during her adolescence she hardly went out because she thought other people would not like her anyway. As a child, she was afraid of accidents, thunder, and being home alone. These fears have persisted over the years. Since she got married, she has been constantly worried about financial matters although her husband has a well-paying job. Since the children arrived, she has been constantly afraid that they might meet with an accident or be taken away by strangers. Further, Judith cannot stand loud noises, and she is very frightful. She makes a very tense impression and startles at the sound of a telephone. The immediate reason for referral is that her eldest son (12 years old) has to go to school by bike, but she would not allow this until now because she is afraid that he might have an accident. This has led to a severe row with her husband, who thinks she is overprotective.

Worry is the central characteristic of GAD. However, before meeting full criteria, persons also need to have a number of anxiety symptoms. Three out of the following symptoms are required: (1) restlessness or feeling keyed up or on edge, (2) being easily fatigued, (3) difficulty concentrating, (4) irritability, (5) muscle tension, and (6) sleep disturbance.

Most generalized anxiety patients are seen by general practitioners, who usually prescribe tranquilizing drugs. Few patients are referred to clinical psychologists or psychiatrists.

Some have argued that generalized anxiety should not be considered a separate anxiety disorder. According to these investigators, the difference between GAD and other anxiety disorders, particularly panic disorder, is more quantitative than qualitative. There is some evidence, however, that generalized anxiety can be differentiated from panic by physiological measures. Hoehn-Saric and McLeod (1988) suggested that generalized anxiety is associated with an inhibition in some sympathetic systems. Panic patients had higher EMGs and higher heart rates than generalized anxiety patients when tested in the laboratory (Barlow et al., 1984). Other differences between panic disorder and GAD are the sudden onset in panic patients in contrast with the more gradual onset in generalized anxiety and a presumably genetic component in panic disorder, which has not been found in GAD.

Barlow (1988) contended that GAD is the end result of a process in which multiple etiological factors are involved. According to Barlow, generalized anxiety patients have a biological vulnerability and experience external stressors (life events and daily hassles) as uncontrollable and unpredictable, eventually culminating in a spiral of worrying. Although this model has some appeal, it is yet far from proven.

Finally, there is some evidence that generalized anxiety patients are characterized by selective processing of emotional stimuli. There is considerable evidence that selective attentional attraction to threat cues is characteristic of patients who have generalized anxiety (Eysenck, 1997).

Course and Prognosis

The onset of generalized anxiety is usually earlier than in panic disorder and, as a rule, is slow and gradual. However, this picture is based on GAD patients seen by clinicians. Whether the same applies to generalized anxiety patients who are not referred to clinicians is unclear. Generally, results of cognitive-behavioral treatments (CBT) are positive (Borkovec & Newman, 1998), but whether the effects of CBT are due to specific cognitive and behavioral components or could be accounted for by nonspecific factors has not yet been satisfactorily settled. No reliable data exist on the long-term outcome of treated patients who have GAD.

Familial and Genetic Patterns

Until recently, there was no evidence of a genetic component in GAD (Torgersen, 1983, 1986). Family studies did not reveal a higher prevalence of generalized anxiety among family members of generalized anxiety patients than among family members of controls (Anderson, Noyes, & Crowe, 1984). More recently, two studies found some evidence for a genetic contribution to GAD. Kendler, Neale, Kessler, Heath, and Eaves (1992b) and Skre et al. (1993) found that the concordance for GAD was higher in monozygotic twins than in dizygotic twins.

Diagnostic Considerations

Given the symptom overlap with mood disorders, such as major depression and dysthymia, and with anxiety disorders (e.g., agoraphobia, panic disorder, obsessive–compulsive disorder, and social phobia), the diagnosis of GAD often presents problems, even for the experienced clinician. An important diagnostic difference is the focus of the worries. Panic patients are primarily concerned with having a panic attack. They report catastrophic cognitions associated with disastrous consequences primarily related to malfunctioning of their own body. Social phobics are primarily concerned about social evaluation and criticism from others, and obsessive–compulsives are concerned about contamination, harming, etc. In contrast, generalized anxiety patients worry excessively about minor and often futile things and are not primarily concerned about bodily symptoms. However, a number of generalized anxiety patients are concerned about social evaluation and criticism, thus blurring a clear-cut difference with social phobics. In such cases, the degree of avoidance of social situations may help in differentiating between social phobia and GAD. Although patients who have generalized anxiety tend to avoid a number of situations, the avoidance is less focused than in social phobia, agoraphobia, and simple phobia.

OBSESSIVE–COMPULSIVE DISORDER

Description of the Disorder

Either recurrent obsessions or compulsions have to occur for a diagnosis of obsessive–compulsive disorder (OCD). Essential for the diagnosis of OCD is that the complaints cause marked distress, are time-consuming (take more than an hour), or interfere with the social or work functioning. The content of the obsession or compulsion must be unrelated to any other Axis I disorder. Obsessions are repetitive, recurring thoughts, ideas, images, or impulses that are experienced as intrusive. The person recognizes that the obsessions are the product of his or her own mind. Obsessions are experienced as senseless or repugnant, which the patient attempts to ignore or suppress. Compulsions, on the other hand, are repetitive, apparent, purposeful behaviors that are performed according to certain rules, or in a stereotyped fashion. Compulsions have the function of neutralizing or preventing discomfort and/or anxiety.

Epidemiology

Community surveys have shown a relatively high prevalence rate of OCD. The lifetime prevalence rate of different surveys is presented in Table 1. The mean lifetime prevalence was 2.2. In these community surveys, the prevalence of OCD was slightly higher among females than among males. Checking, however, is more prevalent among males, and washing and cleaning are more common among females (Hoekstra, Visser, & Emmelkamp, 1989). These investigators provide some evidence that the type of obsessive–compulsive behavior is related to the tasks for which the individual is responsible.

Clinical Picture

> Sophia, a 30-year-old unmarried woman, has been suffering from compulsive checking and obsessions. Over the past month, she also felt very depressed. She had an apartment of her own but lived with her parents as a result of her fear of losing control over her behaviors. When leaving home, she had to return several times to check the gas, taps, doors, and windows repeatedly. In addition, her father had to check everything to make sure that she did not do anything wrong. Apart from such checking, she suffered from obsessions. She had the idea that she would do some horrible things on purpose and that other people would be harmed. For example, she had to check letters over and over again because she was afraid that she would write down Stupid Mrs. X instead of Dear Mrs. X. She developed her obsessive–compulsive problems at age 26, shortly after her boyfriend broke up their relationship. Soon after her complaints started, she was unable to perform her job. She worked in a day-care center and her obsessions concerned doing irresponsible things in her job. She had never had any checking compulsions or obsessions before, but she used to be very perfectionistic. She hardly had any relationships apart from her parents.

Rituals or compulsions mostly accompany obsessions. A majority (nearly 80%) of the obsessive–compulsive patients has obsessions as well as compulsions. A minority of such patients suffers from obsessions only, most often harming obsessions. Patients who have harming obsessions are afraid of harming others (e.g., by strangling) and avoid ropes and sharp objects—such as knives, scissors, pieces of glass—or being alone with young children or helpless elderly people. A few are concerned only about harming themselves (e.g., by committing suicide). Patients who have only rituals are seen very rarely. Generally, the obsessions induce anxiety, and the performance of compulsions leads to anxiety reduction. The most common compulsions involve "cleaning" and "checking." Less common complaints are compulsive slowness, orderliness, hoarding, buying, and counting. A person who suffers from compulsive hoarding collects all kinds of things and may have cupboards filled with old bills, notes, hundreds of pairs of shoes, and underwear. These objects are not used, but the patient is afraid of throwing them away because they may come in handy one day. Compulsive buying implies that the person has a strong inclination to buy a wide variety of items. Compulsive counting often accompanies checking and washing. In some patients, counting is the main problem. In a number of patients, neutralizing thoughts have the same function as rituals, that is, the undoing of the harmful effects of the obsession. Two types of avoidance behavior are distinguished: active and passive avoidance. The obsessive–compulsive person avoids stimuli that might provoke anxiety and discomfort (passive avoidance). Active avoidance is the motor component of obsessive–compulsive behavior (e.g., cleaning and washing) in case the passive avoidance failed (Emmelkamp, 1982). Examples of passive avoidance are people with checking compulsions who avoid situations that provoke their rituals, such as being alone, driving a car, using matches, or being the last one to bed. Individuals who have a cleaning or washing obsession take many precautions to avoid contamination. When obsessions are related to death, people avoid all kinds of situations that suggest the notion of death, such as reading papers (obituaries), watching TV, and going to a funeral.

Considerable comorbidity exists between OCD and other disorders. For example, depression and OCD overlap one another. Studies of comorbidity suggest that 23–38% of obsessive–compulsive patients report major depression (Steketee, 1993). An additional number of patients also qualify for the diagnosis of dysthymia (Antony, Downie, & Swinson, 1998). The obsessive–compulsive symptoms often worsen during a depressed mood, and severe depression may influence the prognosis badly (Marks, 1987). Transition from obsession to depression occurs three times more often than the opposite (Marks, 1987).

There is also a considerable overlap between OCD and other anxiety disorders. Rasmussen and Tsuang (1986) found that 58% of 100 obsessive–compulsive patients had a lifetime prevalence of simple phobia, social phobia, or panic disorder. Further, GAD is a comorbid disorder in 20% of the OCD patients (Abramowitz & Foa, 1998).

The frequency of personality disorders among obsessive–compulsives is high (van Velzen & Emmelkamp, 1999). The diagnosis of obsessive–compulsive personality disorder is given in 25% of patients, which is not more than in other anxiety disorders. There is also a marked history of anorexia nervosa (Kasvikis et al., 1986) and bulimia (Steketee, 1993) in women who have OCD. Although it has been suggested that OCD is often associated with the Gilles de la Tourette syndrome, Rasmussen and Tsuang (1986) reported only a 5% incidence of Tourette's syndrome in patients who have OCD; this is consistent with our own clinical observation. Previously, many investigators suggested that OCD and schizophrenia were related; however, longitudinal studies have not found an increased incidence of schizophrenia either in obsessive–compulsive patients or in their relatives (Black & Noyes, 1990).

In the last decade an increasing number of studies have focused on beliefs and cognitive processes characteristic of obsessive–compulsive patients, including Inflated Responsibility, Thought Action Fusion, Indecisiveness, Magical Thinking, Aversion to Risk Taking, Pollution of the Mind, and Guilt. There is some evidence that specific beliefs are associated with specific obsessive–compulsive behaviors. For example, beliefs related to contamination (e.g., Pollution of the Mind) play an important part in washing but not in other obsessive–compulsive behaviors. Thought Action Fusion appeared to be important in washing and checking, but not in impulses, precision and rumination. Guilt is related to rumination and checking, but not to other obsessive–compulsive behaviors (Emmelkamp & Aardema, 1999).

Course and Prognosis

Mean age of onset is 20 to 25 years, 10% starts before age 10, and 9% starts after age 40 (Emmelkamp, 1990). The age at onset among males (20 years) is earlier than among females (25 years) (Minichiello, Baer, Jenike, & Holland, 1990). Data from this study revealed that cleaners had a later age of onset than checkers. Sometimes the onset of OCD is immediate; typically, however, problems arise insidiously during several years.

If the obsessive–compulsive patients do not get adequate treatment, the disorder tends to have a chronic, fluctuating course. Treatment of choice consists of behavior therapy, namely, *in vivo* exposure plus response prevention. When this treatment was given, approximately 75% of the patients improved and about 25% of the patients remained unchanged on self-ratings of obsessive–compulsive symptoms, anxiety, and depression (Emmelkamp & Scholing, 1997a). Recent studies suggest that cognitive therapy (van Oppen et al., 1995) and pharmacotherapy (tricyclic antidepressants and selective serotonin reuptake inhibitors; Pigott & Seay, 1998) are also promising, but long-term studies are needed before more definite conclusions are warranted.

Familial and Genetic Patterns

Studies showed that relatives of obsessive–compulsives have an increased risk of developing an anxiety disorder (Black, Noyes, Goldstein & Blum, 1992; McKeon & Murray, 1987), but did not show that relatives of OCD patients have an increased risk of getting OCD. More recently, Pauls, Alsobrook, Goodman, Rasmussen, and Leckman (1995) found evidence for elevated risk of obsessive compulsive disorder in probands of OCD patients. Thus, the results with respect to a genetic contribution in OCD are inconclusive.

Diagnostic Considerations

Certain obsessive thoughts should not be diagnosed as OCD (e.g., worrying in GAD and obsessive concern with one's own health in hypochondriasis). It is not always simple to distinguish agoraphobia from OCD, especially when the OCD patient avoids situations that are characteristic of avoidance in agoraphobics, such as going outdoors. However, the evoking stimuli of obsessive–compulsives differ from those of agoraphobics. And when passive avoidance fails, exposure will lead to compulsions in OCD. Although an obsessive–compulsive patient may avoid going outdoors, the reason for such avoidance is totally different from that of an agoraphobic. Agoraphobic patients are often afraid of having a panic attack; obsessive–compulsive patients may avoid going outdoors out of fear of contamination or to prevent checking rituals when they have to leave the house. Depression is very common in people who have obsessions and compulsions. In most cases, depression is secondary to the obsessive–compulsive disorder, which is not surprising considering the severity of the complaints. When obsessive thoughts are part of a depressive episode and disappear when the depression subsides, the diagnosis of depression is more appropriate than the diagnosis of OCD. Similarly, obsessions as part of a psychotic episode are not classified as OCD. Hallucinations and delusions need to be differentiated from obsessions. The main diagnostic question here is whether people recognize that their thoughts or ideas are unreasonable. Obsessive–compulsive personality traits are differentiated from OCD in that they are ego-syntonic, rarely provoke resistance, and are seldom accompanied by compulsions. In OCD patients, symptoms are ego-dystonic and usually provoke resistance; compulsions are very common. When patients have tics, these are diagnosed as tic disorder. Tics are seen as involuntary behaviors, whereas compulsions are intentional behaviors (Emmelkamp, 1990).

POSTTRAUMATIC AND ACUTE STRESS DISORDER

Description of the Disorder

Posttraumatic stress disorder (PTSD) is characterized by a number of stress symptoms that result from exposure to a recognizable stressor of sufficient magnitude to evoke stress in almost anyone. Characteristic symptoms include (1) reexperiencing of the trauma (e.g., flash-backs), and intrusive thoughts related to the traumatic event (e.g., nightmares), (2) avoidance of stimuli related to the trauma (e.g., psychogenic amnesia) and numbing symptoms (e.g., constricted affect and feelings of detachment), and (3) indexes of increased tension (e.g., sleep disturbance, irritability and anger, difficulty in concentrating, exaggerated startle response, and hypervigilance). The duration of the disturbance is more than 1 month. The symptoms result from extreme stress following a trauma, such as rape, assault, severe accident, airplane crash, natural disasters, and war atrocities. Although this disorder previously has been de-scribed as "war neurosis," KZ-syndrome, " shell shock," or traumatic neurosis, it was not until 1980 that it was recognized as a specific diagnostic category in DSM-III.

In DSM-IV, Acute Stress Disorder was introduced as a separate diagnosis. The essential feature of Acute Stress Disorder is the development of anxiety and dissociation that occurs within 1 month after exposure to an extreme traumatic stressor. This diagnosis is applied when the disorder lasts no longer than 4 weeks immediately after the traumatic stressor. For individuals who have the diagnosis Acute Stress Disorder and whose symptoms persist for longer than 1 month, the diagnosis of PTSD should be considered. Because the diagnosis Acute Stress Disorder is rather new, so far hardly any study has been conducted into its etiology and treatment. Therefore, the following discussion is restricted to PTSD.

Epidemiology

The prevalence of PTSD in the community is estimated at about 1% (Helzer, Robins, & McEnroy, 1987; Davidson, Hughes, Blazer, & George, 1991), although this figure is probably an underestimate. In a large representative sample of Vietnam veterans, the incidence of PTSD was 15% and 8.5%, and the lifetime prevalences were 30.9% and 26.9% for males and females, respectively (Jordan et al., 1991). Similar figures were reported for crime victims: 27.8% lifetime prevalence and 7.5% incidence (Kilpatrick et al., 1987). The lifetime prevalence of PTSD in women after rape has been estimated at 35% (Kilpatrick & Resnick, 1993). Thus, PTSD is a common disorder among persons who have undergone severe traumas. Neverthe-less, nearly two-thirds of individuals who have undergone extreme traumatic stressors do not develop severe psychological disturbances (Kamphuis & Emmelkamp, 1998).

Clinical Picture

Diana (22-years old) works behind the desk at a bank. One day, a disguised man appeared at her desk with a gun and threatened to kill her if she would not immediately hand over all the money to him. It was ruled, according to the bank's regulations, that Diana provided the attacker with the money. After this event, she stayed at home for a couple of days. The manager had to coerce her to resume her activities after a few days. In the course of a month, she reported being sick because of an increase in complaints. She had inexplicable attacks of anger at home as well as at work. Several times at night she suffered from nightmares, wherein she was being threatened or being followed by a man with a balaclava. She would awaken totally perspiring. Her relationship with her boyfriend was negatively influenced by this course of events. He became much like a stranger to her. Upon seeing violent scenes on television, she became extremely anxious, which was also the case upon seeing men on mopeds (the bank robber disappeared on a moped). Diana does not go to work, out of fear of being attacked again. During the past year, the office had been robbed three times. Apart from this, she no longer watches television, out of fear of being confronted with violence; she reads only the sports pages of the newspaper for the same reason.

Immediate stress reactions are common and normal after a traumatic event. These symptoms include nightmares, heightened startle responses, or dissociative reactions; they frequently disappear without any treatment. A number of studies suggest that PTSD is associated with drug and alcohol abuse; these findings, however, are primarily based on Vietnam veterans. Although alcohol and drug abuse may occur in other PTSD sufferers (e.g., rape victims), this is more often the exception than the rule.

Many factors are involved in the etiology of PTSD, including the degree of exposure to the stressor, biological and psychological vulnerability, social support, and coping style. Generally, the degree of exposure to the stressor, the duration of the traumatic event, and the degree of the life threat are all directly related to the severity of the disturbance. Although it is generally agreed that stressor severity is related to posttraumatic stress reactions, there is considerable evidence that individual vulnerability and buffer factors can facilitate, or respectively, protect against the development of posttraumatic morbidity. More specifically, coping behavior was an important mediator between disaster impact and psychological distress (Joseph, Williams, & Yule, 1995; Kamphuis & Emmelkamp, 1998; Valentiner et al., 1996). Further, there is some evidence that persons who experience other negative life events are especially vulnerable to develop PTSD (e.g., Creamer et al., 1993; Bryant & Harvey, 1996; Kamphuis & Emmelkamp, 1998). Finally, degree of controllability and social support seem to buffer against the development of PTSD (Craske, 1999).

Course and Prognosis

In many individuals who originally received a diagnosis of PTSD, symptoms decrease over time without any treatment. This has been found in victims of bank robbery (Kamphuis & Emmelkamp, 1998), victims of motor vehicle accidents (Blanchard et al., 1995), and victims of assault and rape (e.g., Valentiner et al., 1996). Further, recent developments in cognitive-behavior therapy look promising, especially for combat- and crime-related PTSD (Emmelkamp, 1994; Etten & Taylor, 1999). However, long-term follow-up investigations are needed before firm statements can be made regarding the prognosis.

Familial and Genetic Patterns

Few studies have addressed this issue. Davidson et al. (1985) found a lower prevalence of family disorder in PTSD among Vietnam veterans than in major depression and GAD. The most common disorders of PTSD family members were alcohol/drug abuse (60%) and other anxiety disorders (22%). Although Foy, Resnick, Sipprelle, and Carroll (1987) reported a higher prevalence of family psychopathology among Vietnam veterans who had PTSD than among Vietnam veterans without PTSD, they found that under conditions of high combat exposure, the influence of familial disposition was negligible. However, more recently, two studies suggest a much stronger genetic contribution in PTSD (Skre et al., 1993; True et al., 1993).

Diagnostic Considerations

Although PTSD and Acute Stress Disorder (ASD) are disorders in which an etiological agent (traumatic event) is part of the diagnostic criteria, a traumatic event by itself is an insufficient basis to warrant the diagnosis of ASD or PTSD. For every sufferer of a traumatic event who has ASD or PTSD, there are many more persons who have undergone the same trauma but do not qualify for the diagnosis of ASD or PTSD. Generally, the diagnosis of ASD or PTSD does not offer special difficulties. In some cases, depression may be more in the forefront of the clinical picture, and the posttraumatic stress symptomatology may be overlooked. In other instances, the distinction from GAD can be difficult. In contrast with GAD, PTSD patients do not worry about the future; rather, they worry about the past, and the (cognitive) avoidance and numbness of feelings are not characteristic of GAD. Further, PTSD can be distinguished from adjustment disorder by the reexperiencing of the traumatic event and by the severity of the stressor.

SUMMARY

Since the introduction of DSM-III in 1980, considerable research has been conducted on the characteristics and clinical features of anxiety disorders. As a result of these efforts, reliable data are now available on such issues as onset age, comorbidity, and the prevalence of the various anxiety disorders. The onset age varies across the different anxiety disorders.

Comorbidity is a frequent phenomenon in the general population and even more common in clinical samples. Many patients who have one anxiety disorder qualify for a diagnosis of another anxiety disorder as well. Depression and alcohol abuse are often comorbid disorders, especially in panic patients and social phobics. Epidemiological studies have revealed that anxiety disorders are much more frequent among the general population than once thought. Actually, anxiety disorder is the most prevalent disorder among females and the second most prevalent disorder among males.

Few long-term follow-up studies have been conducted on course and prognosis of anxiety disorders. Consequently, our knowledge regarding the natural course of untreated anxiety disorders is limited (Wittchen & Essau, 1989). Generally, spontaneous remission from the various anxiety disorders is infrequent (Wittchen, 1991). A number of long-term follow-up studies with obsessive–compulsives and agoraphobics reveal that the positive results of behavioral treatment are maintained up to 6 and 9 years (Emmelkamp & Scholing, 1997b). Long-term follow-up studies with respect to the other anxiety disorders and to other treatment approaches are lacking.

Although there is some evidence for a genetic contribution, further investigations are needed before more definitive conclusions can be reached. It is now a well-established finding that there is a higher family prevalence of anxiety disorders than would be expected by chance. However, the results of such family studies have to be qualified. First, there is a serious risk of overdiagnosis when carrying out family studies in an unblind fashion. Second, such studies provide meager evidence of a genetic disposition because, in a number of instances, environmental factors can account equally well for the differences found.

REFERENCES

Abramovitz, J. S., & Foa, E. B. (1998). Worries and obsessions in individuals with obsessive–compulsive disorder with and without comorbid generalized anxiety disorder. *Behaviour Research and Therapy, 36,* 695–700.

American Psychiatric Association. (1994). *Diagnostic and statistical manual of mental disorders,* 4th ed. Washington, DC: Author.

Anderson, D., Noyes, R. J., & Crowe, R. R. (1984). A comparison of panic disorder and generalized anxiety disorders. *American Journal of Psychiatry, 141,* 572–575.

Antony, M. M., Downie, F., & Swinson, R. P. (1998). Diagnostic issues and epidemiology in obsessive–compulsive disorder. In R. P. Swinson, M. M. Antony, S. Rachman, & M. A. Richter (Eds.), *Obsessive–compulsive disorder: Theory, research, and treatment* (pp. 3–32). New York: Guilford.

Arrindell, W. A., Emmelkamp, P. M. G., Monsma, A., & Brilman, E. (1983). The role of perceived parental rearing practices in the aetiology of phobic disorders: A controlled study. *British Journal of Psychiatry, 143*, 183–187.

Barlow, D. H. (1988). *Anxiety and its disorders*. New York: Guilford.

Barlow, D. H., Cohen, A. S., Waddell, M. T., Vermilyea, B. B., Klosko, J. S., Blanchard, E. B., & DiNardo, R. A. (1984). Panic and generalized anxiety disorders: Nature and treatment. *Behavior Therapy, 15*, 431–449.

Bijl, R. V., Zessen G. van, & Ravelli, A. (1997). Psychiatrische morbiditeit onder volwassenen in Nederland: Het NEMESIS-onderzoek. II. Prevalentie van psychiatrische stoornissen. *Nederlands Tijdschrift voor Geneeskunde, 141*, 2453–2460.

Black, D. W., & Noyes, R. (1990). Co-morbidity of the obsessive compulsive disorder. In J. D. Maser & C. R. Cloninger (Eds.), *Comorbidity of mood and anxiety disorders* (pp. 463–543). Washington, DC: American Psychiatric Press.

Black, D. W., Noyes, R., Goldstein, R. B., & Blum, N. (1992). A family study of obsessive–compulsive disorder. *Archives of General Psychiatry, 49*, 362–368.

Blanchard, E. B., Hickling, E. J., Vollmer, A. J., Loos, W. R., Buckley, T. C., & Jaccard, J. (1995). Short-term follow-up of post-traumatic stress symptoms in motor vehicle accident victims. *Behaviour Research and Therapy, 33*, 369–377.

Bland, R. C., Orn, H., & Newman, S. C. (1988). Lifetime prevalence of psychiatric disorders in Edmonton. *Acta Psychiatrica Scandinavica, 77*, 24–32.

Borkovec, T. D., & Newman, M. G. (1998) Worry and generalized anxiety disorder. In A. S. Bellack & M. Hersen (Eds.), *Comprehensive clinical psychology*, Vol. 6 (pp. 439–459). Oxford, England: Elsevier.

Bourdon, K. H., Boyd, J. H., Rae, D. S., Burns, B. J., Thompson, I. W., & Locke, B. Z. (1988). Gender differences in phobias: Results of the ECA Community Survey. *Journal of Anxiety Disorders, 2*, 227–241.

Brawman-Mintzer, O., & Lydiard, B. (1996). Generalized anxiety disorder: Issues in epidemiology. *Journal of Clinical Psychiatry, 57*, 3–8.

Brown, T. A., & Barlow, D. H. (1992). Comorbidity among anxiety disorders: Implications for treatment and DSM-IV. *Journal of Consulting and Clinical Psychology, 60*, 835–844.

Bryant, R. A., & Harvey, A. G. (1996). Posttraumatic stress reactions in volunteer firefighters. *Journal of Traumatic Stress, 9*, 51–62.

Burnam, M. A., Hough, R. L., Escobar, J. I., Karno, M., Timbers, D. M., Telles, C. A., & Locke, B. Z. (1987). Six-month prevalence of specific psychiatric disorders among Mexican Americans and non-Hispanic whites in Los Angeles. *Archives of General Psychiatry, 44*, 687–694.

Chapman, T. F. (1997). The epidemiology of fears and phobias. In G. C. L. Davey (Ed.), *Phobias: A handbook of theory, research and treatment* (pp. 416–434). New York: Wiley.

Clark, D. M., & Wells, A. (1995). A cognitive model of social phobia. In R. G. Heimberg, M. Liebowitz, D. Hope, & F. Schneier (Eds.), *Social phobia: Diagnosis, assessment, and treatment*. New York: Guilford.

Craske, M. G. (1999). *Anxiety disorders: Psychological approaches to theory and treatment*. Boulder, CO: Westview Press.

Creamer, M., Burgess, P., Buckingham, W., & Pattison, P. (1993). Posttrauma reactions following a multiple shooting. In J. P. Wilson & B. Raphael (Eds.), *International handbook of traumatic stress syndromes* (pp. 201–212). New York: Plenum.

Davidson, J. R. T., Hughes, D. L., Blazer, D. G., & George, L. K. (1991). Post-traumatic stress disorder in the community: An epidemiological study. *Psychological Medicine, 21*, 713–721.

Davidson, J., Swartz, M., Stork, M., Krishman, R. R., & Hammett, E. (1985). A diagnostic and family study of posttraumatic stress disorder. *American Journal of Psychiatry, 142*, 90–93.

Davey, G. C. L. (1997). A conditioning model of phobias. In G. C. L. Davey (Ed.), *Phobias: A handbook of theory, research and treatment* (pp. 301–318). New York: Wiley.

Edelmann, R. J. (1992). *Anxiety: Theory, research and intervention in clinical and health psychology*. Chichester, England: Wiley.

Ehlers, A. (1995). A 1-year prospective study of panic attacks: Clinical course and factors associated with maintenance. *Journal of Abnormal Psychology, 104*, 164–172.

Ehlers, A., & Breuer, P. (1996). How good are patients with panic disorder at perceiving their heartbeats? *Biological Psychology, 42*, 165–182.

Ehlers, A., Breuer, P., Dohn, D., & Fiegenbaum, W. (1995). Heartbeat perception and panic disorder. Possible explanations for discrepant findings. *Behaviour Research and Therapy, 33*, 69–76.

Elting, D. T., & Hope, D. A. (1995). Cognitive assessment. In R. G. Heimberg, M. Liebowitz, D. Hope, & F. Schneier (Eds.), *Social phobia: Diagnosis, assessment, and treatment* (pp. 232–258). New York: Guilford.

Emmelkamp, P. M. G. (1982). *Phobic and obsessive–compulsive disorders*. New York: Plenum.

Emmelkamp, P. M. G. (1990). Obsessive compulsive disorder in adulthood. In M. Hersen & C. G. Last (Eds.), *Handbook of child and adult psychopathology* (pp. 221–234). New York: Pergamon.

Emmelkamp, P. M. G. (1994). Behavior therapy with adults. In S. Garfield & A. Bergin (Eds.), *Handbook of psychotherapy and behavior change*, 4th ed. New York: Wiley.

Emmelkamp, P. M. G. & Aardema, A. (1999). Metacognition, specific obsessive–compulsive beliefs and obsessive–compulsive behaviour. *Clinical Psychology and Psychotherapy, 6*, 139–145.

Emmelkamp, P. M. G., & Gerlsma, C. (1994). Marital functioning and the anxiety disorders. *Behavior Therapy, 25*, 407–429.

Emmelkamp, P. M. G., & Scholing, A. (1997a). Anxiety disorders. In C. Essau & F. Petermann (Eds.), *Developmental psychopathology*. Amsterdam: Harwood.

Emmelkamp, P. M. G., & Scholing, A. (1997b). Behavioral treatment strategies for panic disorder, social phobia, and obsessive compulsive disorder. In J. A. den Boer (Ed.), *Clinical management of anxiety*. New York: Dekker.

Etten, van, M. L., & Taylor, S. (1998). Comparative efficacy of treatments for post-traumatic stress disorder: A meta-analysis. *Clinical Psychology and Psychotherapy, 5*, 126–144.

Eysenck, M. W. (1997). *Anxiety and cognition*. Hove: Psychology Press.

Foy, D. W., Resnick, H. S., Sipprelle, R. C., & Carroll, E. M. (1987). Premilitary, military, and postmilitary factors in the development of combat-related stress disorders. *The Behavior Therapist, 10*, 3–9.

Frederikson, M., Annas, P., Fischer, H., & Wik, G. (1996). Gender and age differences in the prevalence of specific fears and phobias. *Behaviour Research and Therapy, 34*, 33–39.

Fyer, A. J., Mannuzza, S., Chapman, T. F., Martin, L. Y., & Klein, D. F. (1995). Specificity in familial aggregation of phobic disorders. *Archives of General Psychiatry, 52*, 564–573.

Fyer, A. J., Mannuzza, S., Martin, L. Y., Gallops, M. S., Endicot, J., Schleyer, B., Gorman, J. M., Liebowitz, M. R., & Klein, D. F. (1990). Familial transmission of simple phobias and fears. *Archives of General Psychiatry, 47*, 252–256.

Goisman, R. M., Warshaw, M. G., Peterson, L. G., Rogers, M. P., Cuneo, P., Hunt, M. F., Tolin-Albanese, J. M., Kazim, A., Gollan, J. K., Epstein-Kaye, T., Reich, J. H., & Keller, M. B. (1994). Panic, agoraphobia, and panic disorder with agoraphobia: Data from a multicenter anxiety disorders study. *Journal of Nervous and Mental Disease, 182*, 72–79.

Hafner, J. (1982). The marital context of the agoraphobic syndrome. In D. L. Chambless & A. J. Goldstein (Eds.), *Agoraphobia: Multiple perspectives on theory and treatment* (pp. 77–118). New York: Wiley.

Harris, E. L., Noyes, R., Crowe, R. R., & Chaudry, D. R. (1983). A family study of agoraphobia: Report of a pilot study. *Archives of General Psychiatry, 40*, 1061–1064.

Helzer, J. E., Robins, L. N., & McEnroy, M. A. (1987). Post-traumatic stress disorder in the general population. *The New England Journal of Medicine, 317*, 1630–1634.

Himle, J. A., & Hill, E. M. (1991). Alcohol abuse and the anxiety disorders: Evidence from the Epidemiologic Catchment Area Survey. *Journal of Anxiety Disorders, 5*, 237–245.

Hoehn-Saric, R., & McLeod, D. R. (1988). The peripheral sympathetic nervous system: Its role in normal and pathologic anxiety. *Psychiatric Clinics of North America, 11*, 375–386.

Hoekstra, R. J., Visser, S., & Emmelkamp, P. M. G. (1989). A social learning formulation of the etiology of obsessive–compulsive disorders. In P. M. G. Emmelkamp, W. T. A. M. Everaerd, R. W. Kraaimaat, & M. J. M. van Son (Eds.), *Fresh perspectives on anxiety disorders*. Lisse, The Netherlands: Swets and Zeitlinger.

Holt, C. S., Heimberg, R. G., Hope, D. A., & Liebowitz, M. R. (1992). Situational domains of social phobia. *Journal of Anxiety Disorders, 6*, 63–77.

Jacob, R. G., Lilienfeld, S. O., Furman, J. M. R., Durrant, J. D., & Turner, S. M. (1989). Panic disorder with vestibular dysfunction: Further clinical observations and description of space and motion phobic stimuli. *Journal of Anxiety Disorders, 3*, 117–130.

de Jong, G. M., & Bouman, T. K. (1995). Panic disorder: Predictability of agoraphobic avoidance behavior. *Journal of Anxiety Disorders, 9*, 185–199.

Jordan, B. K., Schlenger, W. E., Hough, R., Kulka, R. A., Weiss, D., Fairbank, J. A., & Marmar, C. E. (1991). Lifetime and current prevalence of specific psychiatric disorders among Vietnam veterans and controls. *Archives of General Psychiatry, 48*, 207–215.

Joseph, S. A., Williams, R., & Yule, W. (1995). Psychosocial perspectives on post-traumatic stress. *Clinical Psychology Review, 15*, 515–544.

Kamphuis, J. H., & Emmelkamp, P. M. G. (1998). Crime-related trauma: Psychological distress in victims of bank robbery. *Journal of Anxiety Disorders, 12*, 199–208.

Karno, M., Hough, R. L., Burnam, A., Escobar, J. I., Timbers, D. M., Santana, F., & Boyd, J. H. (1987). Lifetime prevalence of specific psychiatric disorders among Mexican Americans and non-Hispanic whites in Los Angeles. *Archives of General Psychiatry, 44*, 695–701.

Kasvikis, G. Y., Tsakiris, F., Marks, I. M., Basoglu, M., & Noshirvani, H. F. (1986). Past history of anorexia nervosa in women with obsessive–compulsive disorder. *International Journal of Eating Disorders, 5*, 1069–1075.

Kendler, K. S., Neale, M. C., Kessler, R. C., Heath, A. C., & Eaves, L. J. (1992a). The genetic epidemiology of phobias in women: The interrelationship of agoraphobia, social phobia, situational phobia, and simple phobia. *Archives of General Psychiatry, 49*, 273–281.

Kendler, K. S., Neale, M. C., Kessler, R. C., Heath, A. C., & Eaves, L. J. (1992b). Generalized anxiety disorder in women: A population-based twin study. *Archives of General Psychiatry, 49*, 267–272.

Kessler, R. C., McConagle, K. A., Zhao, S., Nelson, C. B., Hughes, M., Eshleman, S., Wittchen, H. U., & Kendler, K. S. (1994). Lifetime and 12-month prevalence of DSM-III-R psychiatric disorders in the United States. *Archives of General Psychiatry, 51*, 8–19.

Kilpatrick, D. G., & Resnick, H. S. (1993). Posttraumatic stress disorders associated with exposure to criminal victimization in clinical and comunity populations. In J. R. T. Davidson & E. B. Foa (Eds.), *Posttraumatic stress disorders: DSM IV and beyond* (pp. 113–143). Washington, DC: American Psychiatric Press.

Kilpatrick, D. G., Saunders, B. E., Veronen, L., Best, C. L., & Von, J. M. (1987). Criminal victimization: Lifetime prevalence, reporting to police, and psychological impact. *Crime and Delinquency, 33*, 479–489.

Lelliott, P., McNamee, G., & Marks, I. (1991). Features of agora-, social, and related phobias and validation of the diagnoses. *Journal of Anxiety Disorders, 5*, 313–322.

Lepine, J. P., & Lelouch, J. (1995). Classification and epidemiology of social phobia. *European Archives of Psychiatry and Clinical Neuroscience, 24*, 290–296.

Lesser, I. M. (1988). The relationship between panic disorder and depression. *Journal of Anxiety Disorders, 2*, 3–15.

Maller, R. G., & Reiss, S. (1992). Anxiety sensitivity in 1984 and panick attacks in 1987. *Journal of Anxiety Disorders, 6*, 241–247.

Mannuzza, S., Fyer, A. J., Liebowitz, M. R., & Klein, D. F. (1990). Delineating the boundaries of social phobia: Its relationship to panic disorder and agoraphobia. *Journal of Anxiety Disorders, 4*, 41–59.

Marks, I. M. (1987). *Fears, phobias, and rituals. Panic, anxiety and their disorders.* New York: Oxford University Press.

McKeon, P., & Murray, R. (1987). Familial aspects of obsessive–compulsive neurosis. *British Journal of Psychiatry, 151*, 528–534.

Merkelbach, H., & de Jong. P. J. (1997). Evolutionary models of phobias. In G. C. L. Davey (Ed.), *Phobias: A handbook of theory, research and treatment* (pp. 323–348). New York: Wiley.

Minichiello, W. E., Baer, L., Jenike, M. A., & Holland, A. (1990). Age of onset of major subtypes of obsessive–compulsive disorder. *Journal of Anxiety Disorders, 4*, 147–150.

Monroe, S. M. (1990). Psychosocial factors in anxiety and depression. In J. D. Maser & C. R. Cloninger (Eds.), *Comorbidity of mood and anxiety disorders* (pp. 463–543). Washington, DC: American Psychiatric Press.

Monti, P. M., Boice, R., Fingeret, A. L., Zwiek, W. R., Kolko, D., Munroe, S., & Grunberger, A. (1984). Mid-level measurement of social anxiety in psychiatric and nonpsychiatric samples. *Behaviour Research and Therapy, 22*, 651–660.

Moreau, D., & Follett, C. (1993). Panic disorder in children and adolescents. *Child and Adolescent Psychiatry Clinics of North America, 2*, 581–602.

Myers, K. M., Weissman, M. M., Tischler, G. L., Holzer, C. E., Leaf, P. J., Orvaschel, H., Anthony, I. C., Boyd, J. H., Burke, I. D., Kramer, M., & Stoltzman, R. (1984). Six-month prevalence of psychiatric disorders in three communities. *Archives of General Psychiatry, 41*, 959–967.

Norton, G. R., Cox, B., & Malan, J. (1992). Non-clinical panickers. A critical review. *Clinical Psychology Review, 12*, 121–139.

Norton, G. R., McLeod, L., Guertin, J., Hewitt, P. L., Walker, J. R., & Stein, M. B. (1996). Panic disorder or social phobia: Which is worse? *Behaviour Research and Therapy, 34*, 273–276.

Noyes, R., Crowe, R. R., Harris, E. L., Hamra, B. J., McChesney, C. M., & Chaudry, D. R. (1986). Relationship between panic disorder and agoraphobia: A family study. *Archives of General Psychiatry, 43*, 227–232.

van Oppen, P., de Haan, E., van Balkom, A. J. M. L., Spinhoven, P., Hoogduin, C. A. L., & van Dyck, R. (1995). Cognitive therapy and exposure in vivo in the treatment of obsessive–compulsive disorder. *Behaviour Research and Therapy, 33*, 379–390.

Öst, L.-G. (1987). Age of onset in different phobias. *Journal of Abnormal Psychology, 96*, 223–229.

Öst, L.-G. (1992). Blood and injection phobia: Background and cognitive, physiological, and behavioral variables. *Journal of Abnormal Psychology, 101*, 68–74.

Öst, L.-G., & Hellström, K. (1997). Blood-injury-injection phobia. In G. C. L. Davey (Ed.), *Phobias: A handbook of theory, research and treatment* (pp. 63–80). New York: Wiley.

Pauls, D. L., Alsobrook, J. P., Goodman, W., Rasmussen, S., & Leckman, J. F. (1995). A family study of obsessive compulsive disorder. *American Journal of Psychiatry, 71*, 124–135.

Pigott, T. A., & Seay, S. (1998). Biological treatments for obsessive–compulsive disorder: Literature review. In R. P. Swinson, M. M. Antony, S. Rachman, & M. A. Richter (Eds.), *Obsessive–compulsive disorder: Theory, research, and treatment* (pp. 298–326). New York: Guilford.

Rasmussen, S. A., & Tsuang, M. T. (1986). Clinical characteristics and family history in DSM-III obsessive–compulsive disorder. *American Journal of Psychiatry, 143*, 317–322.

Reich, J., & Yates, W. (1988). Family history of psychiatric disorders in social phobia. *Comprehensive Psychiatry, 29*, 72–75.

Robins, L. N., Helzer, J. E., Weissman, M. M., Orvaschel, H., Gruenberg, E., Burke, J. D., & Regier, D. A. (1984). Lifetime prevalence of specific psychiatric disorders in three sites. *Archives of General Psychiatry, 41*, 949–958.

de Ruiter, C., Rijken, H., Garssen, B., van Schaik, A., & Kraaimaat, E (1989). Comorbidity among the anxiety disorders. *Journal of Anxiety Disorders, 3*, 57–68.

Sanderman, R., Mersch, P. P., van der Sleen, J., Emmelkamp, P. M. G., & Ormel, J. (1987). The rational behavior inventory (RBI): A psychometric evaluation. *Personality and Individual Differences, 8*, 561–569.

Schneier, R., Martin, L. Y., Liebowitz, M. R., Gorman, J. M., & Fyer, A. J. (1989). Alcohol abuse in social phobia. *Journal of Anxiety Disorders, 3*, 15–23.

Shear, M. K. (1996). Factors in the etiology and pathogenesis of panic disorder: Revisiting the attachment-separation paradigm. *American Journal of Psychiatry, 153*, 125–136.

Skre, L., Onstad, S., Torgersen, J., Lygren, S., & Kringlen, E. (1993). A twin study of DSM-III-R anxiety disorders. *Acta Psychiatrica Scandinavica, 88*, 85–92.

Steketee, G. S. (1993). *Treatment of obsessive–compulsive disorder*. New York: Guilford.

Stopa, L., & Clark, D. M. (1993). Cognitive processes in social phobia. *Behaviour Research and Therapy, 31*, 255–267.

Telch, M. J., Lucas, J. A., & Nelson, P. (1989). Nonclinical panic in college students: An investigation of prevalence and symptomatology. *Journal of Abnormal Psychology, 98*, 300–306.

Torgersen, S. (1979). The nature and origin of common phobic fears. *British Journal of Psychiatry, 134*, 343–351.

Torgersen, S. (1983). Genetic factors in anxiety disorders. *Archives of General Psychiatry, 40*, 1085–1089.

Torgersen, S. (1986). Childhood and family characteristics in panic and generalized anxiety disorders. *American Journal of Psychiatry, 143*, 630–632.

Torgersen, S. (1988). Genetics. In C. G. Last & M. Hersen (Eds.), *Handbook of anxiety disorders* (pp. 159–170). New York: Pergamon Press.

True, W. R., Rice, J., Eisen, S. A., Heath, A. C., Goldberg, J., Lyons, M. J., & Nowak, J. (1993). A twin study of genetic and environmental contributions to liability for posttraumatic stress symptoms. *Archives of General Psychiatry, 50*, 257–264.

Valentiner, D. P., Foa, E. B., Riggs, D. S., & Gershunny, B. S. (1996). Coping strategies and posttraumatic stress disorder in female victims of sexual and nonsexual assault. *Journal of Abnormal Psychology, 105*, 455–458.

van Velzen, C., & Emmelkamp, P. M. G. (1996). The assessment of personality disorders: Implications for cognitive and behaviour therapy. *Behaviour Research and Therapy, 34*, 655–668.

van Velzen, C., & Emmelkamp, P. M. G. (1999). The relationship between anxiety disorders and personality disorders: Prevalence rates and co-morbidity models. In J. Derksen et al. (Eds.), *Treatment of personality disorders*. New York: Plenum.

Wells, A., & Clark, D. M. (1997). Social phobia: A cognitive approach. In G. C. L. Davey (Ed.), *Phobias: A handbook of theory, research and treatment* (pp. 3–26). New York: Wiley.

Wittchen, H. U. (1988). Natural course and spontaneous remissions of untreated anxiety disorders. In I. Hand & H. U. Wittchen (Eds.), *Panic and phobias*, Vol. 2. New York: Springer.

Wittchen, H. U. (1991). Der langzeitverlauf unbehandelter Angststorungen (Follow-up of untreated anxiety disorders). *Verhaltenstherapie, 1*, 273–282.

Wittchen, H. U., & Essau, C. A. (1989). Comorbidity of anxiety disorders and depression: Does it affect course and outcome? *Psychiatry and Psychobiology, 4*, 315–323.

Wittchen, H. U., Zhao, S., & Kessler, R. C. (1994). DSM-III-R generalized anxiety disorder in the National Comorbidity Survey. *Archives of General Psychiatry, 51*, 355–364.

15

Depression

Lynn P. Rehm, Paras Mehta, and Carrie L. Dodrill

Introduction

Disorders of mood include various syndromes of depression and of mania, separately and in combination. These are ordinarily distinguished from anxiety syndromes, although the boundaries between depression and anxiety are indistinct and much overlap in symptoms exists. The term affective disorders is sometimes applied to depression, mania, and anxiety disorders. Although mood disorders are characterized as disturbances of mood, which range from profound sadness to grandiose elation, the syndromes also include symptoms in cognitive, behavioral, and somatic domains.

Among the mood disorders, there is a great deal of heterogeneity in symptomatology. The distinction between normal, sad and elated states and pathological states of depression and mania is itself complex. Symptoms overlap other disorders, and comorbid diagnoses are common. Differential diagnosis from anxiety disorders, certain personality disorders, and schizophrenia is often difficult. To make sense of the complex phenomena involved, many different syndromes have been defined and many distinctions made among subtypes of mood disorders. Distinctions have often been made based on theoretical models of etiology.

Our discussion of mood disorders follows the classification scheme of the American Psychiatric Association's (1993) DSM-IV. We also describe some additional categorizations. A diagnostic system evolves over time, and definitions of disorders and boundaries between them change. We comment on some of these changes. The DSM system attempts to distinguish among disorders based on observed co-occurrence of symptoms without invoking putative cause. Nevertheless, a number of causal assumptions underlie the DSM system, and we attempt to make these explicit. We will also critique the DSM and point out the ways in which it is at times arbitrary and inexact.

Our conceptualization of this chapter approaches the issues of etiology from a biopsychosocial perspective. We assume that biological variables, psychological variables, and environ-

Lynn P. Rehm, Paras Mehta, and Carrie L. Dodrill • Department of Psychology, University of Houston, Houston, Texas 77204-5341.

Advanced Abnormal Psychology, Second Edition, edited by Hersen and Van Hasselt. Kluwer Academic/Plenum Publishers, New York, 2001.

mental variables interact in various ways to produce mood disorders. The importance of each set of variables may vary from one syndrome to another, but all three sets contribute to each disorder. Within a disorder, the contributions of biology, psychology, and environment may vary tremendously from case to case. Many theories of etiology are posed within single dimensions of causality (biological theories, psychological theories, or environmental theories) and are often pitted against one another (e.g., the biological versus the psychological explanation). Two dimensional diathesis-stress models posit interactions between either biological or psychological predispositions and life stress. We try to maintain a three-dimensional view that acknowledges interactions between biology and psychology as well as the interactions of both with the environment.

Although we want to stress interaction among etiological factors from the biopsychosocial perspective, sections of the chapter highlight different contributing causes. In "Familial and Genetic Pattern," we review evidence for biological contributions. The "Diagnostic Considerations" section holds most of our discussion of psychological models and the "Epidemiology" and "Course of the Disorder" sections of the chapter highlight social, environmental, or life stress factors. Each section shows how various components fit with the biopsychosocial perspective.

DESCRIPTION OF THE DISORDERS

The description of mood disorders depends on the many diagnostic distinctions made in DSM-IV and other nosological systems. To begin with, it is useful to distinguish among mood *per se*, mood syndromes, and mood disorders. Mood is the normal affective states experienced by all people on a day-to-day, hour-to-hour, or even moment-to-moment basis. It is important to note that mood is a normal part of human existence and a contrast, in either degree or quality, to syndrome or disorder. As a syndrome, extreme mood states are part of a constellation of symptoms that remain relatively stable during a longer period of time. An episode of depression or mania is diagnosed when a set of symptoms that includes altered mood exists for a relatively enduring period. A specific mood disorder is diagnosed on the basis of the pattern of mood syndromes in the person's past history. Many different mood disorders have been defined historically. Among the most important is the distinction between unipolar and bipolar mood disorders.

Unipolar and Bipolar Mood Disorders

Emil Kraepelin (1921) first made the distinction between manic-depressive illness and dementia praecox (schizophrenia) on the basis of syndrome, course, and prognosis. Manic-depressive disorder was seen as encompassing recurrent syndromes of depression, mania or both, and as episodic with relatively complete recovery between episodes. In contrast, schizophrenia was viewed as having a chronic, deteriorating course. DSM-II adapted Kraepelin's distinction but also included neurotic depression, which was defined as a less severe though often more chronic depressive syndrome than manic depression.

In the late 1950s, Leonhard (1957) and others began arguing that recurrent episodes of only depression should be distinguished from disorders that included episodes of both mania and depression. The distinction was based on differences in age of onset, genetics, and depressive symptomatology, as well as course. Unipolar disorder (deviation toward only one pole of the mood spectrum) was broadened to include some of what earlier was considered neurotic depression. Bipolar disorder (deviation toward both manic and depressive poles) was a narrower category than Kraepelin's manic-depressive category. DSM-III incorporated the unipolar–bipolar distinction, basing the diagnoses solely on a history of at least one manic episode with depressive episodes.

Syndromes of Depression and Mania

The DSM-IV criteria for depression and mania have several changes from previous DSMs. Pervasively sad mood was a required criterion symptom in DSM-III. DSM-III-R and DSM-IV recognized an alternate form of mood disturbance, anhedonia. Anhedonia is the inability to experience emotion, particularly pleasure. Apathy predominates, and expression of affect is blunted and "flat." Other affective states, including anxiety and anger, can coexist with sadness. Anxiety is so common in depressive disorders that it makes differentiation from anxiety disorders (particularly Generalized Anxiety Disorder) difficult. DSM-IV allows diagnosing combined depression-anxiety disorder. Especially among children and adolescents, sadness is often accompanied by irritability or an angry mood.

DSM-IV requires five out of nine symptoms, including either (1) sad mood or (2) anhedonia. Somatic symptoms include (3) appetite and (4)sleep disturbances, (5) psychomotor agitation/retardation, and (6) fatigue or loss of energy. Cognitive symptoms include (7) feelings of worthlessness or excessive guilt, (8) complaints of difficulty concentrating or thinking, and (9) recurrent thoughts of death or suicide.

Several among these symptoms may vary from the norm in either direction. Insomnia is the more common symptom, but hypersomnia is also seen in depression. Loss of appetite is more common than increased appetite, and each may be assessed by corresponding changes in weight. Middle or terminal insomnia (waking up in the middle of the night or early morning and inability to return to sleep) is distinguished from the more common initial insomnia, or difficulty falling asleep. Feeling slowed down and energyless is common. Agitation involves anxious, unproductive hyperactivity and, if present, is often noticeable in an interview where patients fidget or pace while reporting their complaints. Loss of libido, like many of the other symptoms mentioned, may have cognitive and behavioral, as well as somatic components (see disorders of sexual dysfunction). Increased libido does not occur as a symptom of depression.

Depressive episodes associated with bipolar disorder are often marked by anhedonia, middle or terminal insomnia, and motor retardation. In contrast, unipolar depressions are often marked by anxiety, agitation, and initial insomnia. Syndromes with hypersomnia and weight gain are sometimes called Atypical Depression and may be treated with different medications.

Other symptoms include impaired cognitive functioning, depressive ruminations, and in extreme cases, psychotic features. Impaired cognitive function includes inability to concentrate and indecisiveness. Depressive thinking is unrealistically negative and biased and has been described as the cognitive triad (Beck, 1972) of negative views of self, world, and future. Depressed people are overly self-critical and perceive themselves as guilty, worthless, and helpless. The world is perceived as full of loss and lacking in obtainable gratification. The future looks hopeless. Preoccupation with death and suicidal ideation may be the result of perceptions of hopelessness. Psychotic symptoms, hallucinations, or delusions may be present in very severe episodes. The content of the delusions or hallucinations in a depressive episode is typically mood congruent (i.e, the content reflects themes of guilt, persecution, punishment, ruin, and disaster).

The apathy and lack of motivation felt in depression are reflected in psychomotor retardation and lowered activity level. Other behavioral symptoms of depression include social withdrawal and lack of communication with others. Interpersonal relationships may be disrupted in various ways from increased dependency to irritable hostility.

The typical mood in mania is described as elevated, expansive, or euphoric. Irritability is common here as well, and mood may be very labile or, paradoxically, even depressed. The DSM requires three of a list of seven symptoms for a diagnosis of a manic episode. In contrast to depression, the content of manic thinking is often (1) grandiose, ranging from unrealistic self-confidence to delusions of grandeur. Other forms of delusion occur but are usually congruent with elevated mood, for example, delusions of persecution based on beliefs in other's jealousy. Hallucinations are infrequent and are predominantly auditory. Patients in a manic episode experience (2) a decreased need for sleep or feeling rested after only two or three hours in a night. Cognitive functioning is also impaired. The person in a manic episode may be (3) very talkative and feel a pressure to express all of their ideas. Patients report (4) that their thoughts are racing and jumping from one topic to another, described as a "flight of ideas." In mild cases, thinking is experienced as more fluid and creative. In more severe cases, thinking may become confused and the person may have (5) difficulty in concentrating and may be highly distractable. Behaviorally, people in manic episodes display (6) increases in goal-directed activity or agitation, and (7) may become excessively involved in pleasurable activities.

The grandiose outlook of a manic episode may result in poor judgment that has negative social consequences, such as precipitous business decisions, gambling, spending sprees, or hypersexuality. The distinction between a full manic episode and a lesser hypomanic episode is based on negative social consequences in mania. Hypomania may actually be associated with high levels of productivity and gregarious sociality. Activity level increases in either form of episode, and the need for sleep decreases, often to only 2 or 3 hours per night.

A formal diagnosis in DSM-IV assumes that episodes of mood disorder are distinct periods of changed mood. For depression, a minimum duration of 2 weeks is specified. DSM-III-R included a criterion that instructed clinicians to rule out "organic causes" of depressive symptoms. However, DSM-IV changed this criterion. Now, clinicians are instructed to rule out substance-induced depression or depression due to a general medical condition. This criterion was made more specific because of concern that the "organic" rule-out implied a greater distinction between mental and biological conditions than actually exists. The new criterion also has the advantage of allowing a mood disorder to be diagnosed and considered clinically significant in its own right, even if the symptoms are thought to be caused by a substance or medical condition. Diagnosis of a mood disorder also requires that psychotic symptoms must occur only during the mood episode to rule out other psychotic diagnoses. DSM-IV also includes a criterion specifying that the mood disturbance must also cause marked distress or significant impairment in social or occupational functioning. The reason for the addition was a concern that the diagnosis was overinclusive in the general population by diagnosing individuals who met minimal criteria but were not concerned or impaired by the symptoms.

DSM-IV distinguishes between bipolar disorder and depressive disorder (unipolar depression). The essential feature of bipolar disorder is the presence of at least one episode each of mania and depression. Episodes of depression alone, without a history of mania, are classified as major depressive disorder—either single or recurrent. Exclusion of a manic or hypomanic episode is necessary for diagnosis of a depressive disorder. Specific bipolar episodes are classified as depressed, manic, or mixed depending upon the nature of symptoms. Bipolar I disorder denotes a disorder that involves full manic and depressive episodes, whereas bipolar II disorder involves hypomanic and depressive episodes. Some authorities classify individuals who have only depressive episodes, but with bipolar relatives, as Bipolar III's. The assumption is that their underlying biochemical and medication responses would be similar to those of bipolar patients.

The DSM-IV also includes a milder, but more persistent form of unipolar disorder, called dysthymia. Dysthymia is defined as a disorder that has a minimum duration of two years during which depression never remits for more that two months. Depression is lesser in severity than in major depression, but at least two of the criteria for major depressive episode should be present during the course of the disorder. Similarly in parallel with bipolar disorder, cyclothymia is conceptualized as frequent hypomanic symptoms, as well as mild depressive symptoms. Individuals who have this diagnosis are often characterized as very moody with ups and downs from day to day. Dysthymia and cyclothymia were formerly classified as personality disorders because of their long duration and typical early onset.

DSM-IV focuses on issues of severity and course of episodes in several ways. Major depressive disorder is now separated into single episode and recurrent subtypes, and bipolar I is separated into subtypes based on the nature of the most recent episode: single manic episode and most recent episode either hypomanic, manic depressed, or unspecified. New sections on course specifiers identify rapid cycling (4 episodes of any kind in 12 months), seasonal pattern (regular seasonal onsets and remissions outnumbering other episodes), and postpartum onset (applicable to major depressive disorder, bipolar I, bipolar II, or acute psychotic disorder). Longitudinal course specifiers differentiate (1) single and recurrent episodes, (2) with or without antecedent dysthymia, and (3) with or without full interepisodic recovery. Minor depressive disorder (less than four symptoms) and recurrent brief depressive disorder (less than 2 weeks) has been added to the DSM-IV appendix for further study.

Other Diagnostic Distinctions

Former versions of the DSM included diagnostic distinctions based on putative cause. One such distinction is between endogenous and exogenous or reactive depressions. Endogenous depressions are presumed to be caused by internal biological mechanisms in contrast to reactive depressions which are seen as reactions to external events. Endogenous depressions, it is believed, are more severe, characterized by predominant somatic symptoms, and more medication-responsive. Reactive depressions are seen as milder and often self-limiting, characterized by more psychological symptoms, and responsive to psychotherapy. Endogenous depression is essentially a negative diagnosis because it is based on the absence of an identifiable external cause. This determination is unreliable and is an unsatisfactory basis for a diagnosis. Therefore, the distinction was not included in DSM-III.

DSM-III-R and DSM-IV do, however, include a subtype of major depressive disorder, melancholic subtype, that parallels endogenous depression. In DSM-IV, melancholic type is defined by symptoms of either anhedonia or lack of reactivity to normally pleasurable stimuli and three or more of the following: quality of depressed mood that is experienced as distinctly different from bereavement, diurnal variation with depression worse in the morning, early morning insomnia, loss of appetite or weight, psychomotor retardation or agitation, and excessive or inappropriate guilt. The melancholic type distinction has been difficult to support empirically, first, because it is confounded with severity. To diagnose melancholic subtype, DSM-III-R also required that previous good response to antidepressant medication was evident (seen as evidence for a biological basis).

The result of using the old criterion was to create a definition that was partly circular (i.e., a pharmacologically responsive subtype is defined in terms of previous pharmacological response). The biological component of depression is complex, polygenic, and variable in the risk it imparts. The expression of biologic vulnerability depends on environmental and psychological factors. As such, any distinction between internally versus externally caused biological versus psychological types of depression is overly simplistic.

In DSM-IV, two additional subtypes of depression besides melancholia are included under the heading of cross-sectional symptom features. Atypical features are characterized by mood reactivity and two symptoms out of a list, including significant weight gain or increase in appetite, hypersomnia, leaden paralysis, and a long-standing pattern of interpersonal rejection sensitivity. "With catatonia" is a symptomatic feature characterized by motoric immobility, purposeless excessive activity, extreme negativism or mutism, movement peculiarities, echo-lalia, or echopraxia.

Postpartum depression or mania is another diagnosis based on putative causation. Although some controversy remains, the idea that biological events associated with childbirth cause postpartum mood disorders is poorly supported. Childbirth is associated with a variety of physical and psychosocial stresses and changes in life patterns. Depression or mania in the postpartum period may be at least partly stress-induced. Therefore, the DSM-III-R took the position that a separate category for postpartum mood disorders is not necessary. DSM-IV has reinstated Postpartum Onset, however, as a course specifier.

Death of a loved one may be followed by a condition that is similar to a depressive episode; however, it was excluded from the mood disorders in DSM-III-R. Labeled "uncomplicated bereavement," it is assumed that grief is a natural and normal depressive reaction. From a biopsychosocial perspective, death of a loved one can be viewed as a form of psychosocial stressor or loss. It is not clear why this form of stress or loss should differ from others in producing normal versus abnormal depression. In some cases, duration, severity, and symptomatology are sufficient to warrant intervention, so that the distinction may be quite arbitrary.

Major Depressive Disorder may be diagnosed after the death of a loved one if the depressive episode lasts beyond two months after the loss or if there are symptoms that are uncharacteristic of a typical grief reaction (i.e., guilt about things unrelated to actions taken or not taken by the client at the time of the death of the loved one, prolonged and marked functional impairment, hallucinatory experiences unrelated to the death of the loved one, etc.).

DSM-IV includes two additional diagnostic categories based on presumed etiology. Secondary mood disorder due to a medical condition assumes that some medical conditions cause mood disorders directly, that is, the depression is not merely a reaction to the stress of being ill. Substance-induced mood disorder is associated with intoxication, withdrawal, or cessation of use. Again, the assumption is that the depression is not merely a response to the stressors and life events involved in substance abuse.

EPIDEMIOLOGY

The Epidemiologic Catchment Area (ECA) program of NIMH is the major source of epidemiological data in the United States (Regier et al., 1988). Data from all five sites were used to calculate one-month and lifetime prevalences of mood disorders. One-month prevalence is the number of new and continuing cases identifiable in a one-month period. Lifetime prevalence is the number of people who will develop the disorder during their lifetimes. Estimates were 5.1 and 8.3% for all affective disorders, 2.2 and 5.8% for major depressive episode, 0.4 and 0.8% for manic episode, and 3.3 and 3.3% for dysthymia. Mood disorders are the most prevalent psychiatric disorders after anxiety disorders.

The risk of affective disorders in general is about twice as high in females as in males. This conclusion has been supported for unipolar depression in a number of studies, but the data for bipolar depression are less conclusive. In bipolar disorder, estimates of prevalence vary from equal for the sexes to slightly higher rates for women. Many explanations have been offered for the sex differences in the prevalence of affective disorders. These range from suggestions that criteria may be biased or that reporting biases may make depression more likely to be reported by women, to sex linked genetic explanations, and to differences in sex role socialization that make women more psychologically vulnerable to depression.

Findings from the ECA program suggest that the risk of depression is greater for people born in more recent decades. The incidence of depression is highest for young people, especially for ages 25 to 34. A recent study of depression in adolescence (Lewinsohn, 1991) indicates that their disorder is about twice as prevalent in girls as in boys between ages 14 and 18, and prevalence rates are much higher than in the general adult population.

Unipolar depression is considered more prevalent among lower socioeconomic classes, and bipolar disorder in the higher socioeconomic class. Increased prevalence of unipolar depression in lower SES can be attributed to environmental stressors, but the increased prevalence of bipolar disorder in the upper SES is often attributed to reporting bias and unreliable diagnosis. Among higher socioeconomic classes, bipolar disorder may be diagnosed more than schizophrenia, whereas lower SES individuals may be more likely to receive a diagnosis of schizophrenia. Higher rates of depression in urban versus rural areas are often found, but these differences are probably attributable to socioeconomic and stress factors.

The relationship between depression and marital status is complex. Rates of depression for men are higher for single and divorced individuals, but among women rates are higher for married persons. The differences seem to relate to different stress and support factors for men and women. For example, among married women depression is far less frequent in women whose jobs are outside the home, presumably because the jobs offer additional sources of gratification. Job status, housekeeping duties, and marital satisfaction also contribute to the differences (Radloff, 1975).

Findings of the ECA program suggest that prevalence rates for mood disorders are fairly equal across racial and ethnic groups in the United States. There are relatively few cross-cultural studies, and those that exist are hard to interpret because of differences in methodology. The picture is further complicated by differences in the cultural expression of symptoms and syndromes (Castillo, 1997). The data available suggest that depression is common and that rates are comparable around the world. Sex differences are the same in industrialized countries but perhaps less discrepant in less developed countries (Nolen-Hoeksema, 1987).

CLINICAL PICTURE

Case Description

Six months ago Dan, 32, was hospitalized for depression after he told his half-brother that he was considering suicide. For several months before, following a break up with a girlfriend, he had been feeling increasingly depressed and unable to handle the demands of his daily life. Before his hospitalization, Dan complained that he did not derive pleasure from anything he did. He was constantly fatigued and felt slowed down in his activities. Dan was quite worried about his health, citing difficulty getting to sleep at night and loss of appetite resulting in unplanned weight loss. He told his half-brother that he felt worthless, guilty about things that he had done or not done for the family and that he saw no hope for improving his life in the future.

As a child Dan was close to his mother, who also suffered from bouts of depression. He was the only child of his father's second marriage, but he had a much older half-brother. His mother was hospitalized several times for depression during Dan's childhood, and she died when he was 12 of what may or may not have been an intentional overdose of sleeping medication. His father was never close, but became more distant and critical of Dan after his mother's death. Although Dan did well in school, his grades always fell short of his father's expectations.

Dan went off to college and felt a new experience of independence, acceptance for his accomplishments, and self-confidence. However, he had to drop out of school to care for his father who was disabled following a stroke. For the last several years, he has been living with his elderly father who recently has undergone bypass surgery and needs constant attention. His brother provides minimal financial support but does not participate in taking care of the father.

Before his hospitalization, a typical day for Dan started at 5 in the morning when he woke up to give his father his medications and ended at midnight making sure that the kitchen was clean. During the day, he attended to his father's complaints and constant demands for attention. Even though he handled his father's demands, Dan described himself as incompetent and unable to reach his own standards for performing even the simplest tasks. Although he would occasionally admit resentment for having to take care of his father, he also said at times that he was grateful to do it because otherwise his life would be meaningless.

During his hospitalization, Dan was diagnosed as experiencing major depressive disorder as an exacerbation of a long-time dysthymia. He was started on one of the new selective serotonin re-uptake inhibitor antidepressants which improved his energy, mood, and sleep. With the help of a therapist, he negotiated with his brother for more help in caring for the father, giving him more time for himself and the possibility of looking for a job outside the home.

Therapy after hospitalization began with efforts to increase Dan's activities and social interactions outside the family. As he made more contacts with people, therapy focused on his skills in certain social situations and proceeded to examine the ways in which he interpreted the behavior of others as rejecting and critical. His relationship with his father has been discussed as a source of this feelings about himself and his assumptions about his tendency to put the needs of others over any needs of his own. He has begun to question these assumptions and test them in his new relationships. Dan has found a job and is making progress in forming friendships while sharing responsibilities for his father's care with his half-brother.

COURSE AND PROGNOSIS

Part of the definition of mood disorders is that they are considered relatively constant over fairly long periods. DSM-IV requires that an episode of depression last a minimum of two weeks. An episode of mania must last for at least one week. Time course, including age of onset, duration, and spacing of episodes, varies among disorders and differences in time course may be part of the validation of the distinction between two disorders, that is, if they have different time courses, they are seen as different disorders.

In a prospective study of 400 patients who had mood disorder, Angst et al. (1973) demonstrated differences in the time course of unipolar disorder, bipolar I, and bipolar II (hypomania only). There were significant differences in the age of onset among the three groups. The average age of onset for unipolar disorder was 45, whereas for bipolar disorder it was 28 for bipolar I's and 32 for bipolar II's. About half of bipolar disorders occur before age 30, but only about a fourth of unipolar depression occurs by age 30. About 64% of bipolar I and 80% of bipolar II disorders began with a depressive episode. The first manic episode occurs later for bipolar II's. The average durations of unipolar and bipolar I episodes were 5.3 and 4.4 months, respectively. Bipolar I has the shortest interval between the onset of two consecutive episodes, 2.5 years, compared to 4.7 years average for unipolar disorder.

Stress and Depression

Many psychological and biological theories of depression posit vulnerability factors that interact with life stress to produce an episode of the disorder. Stress is often defined in terms of major life events that are occurrences that require major readjustment in the person's life. Therefore, stress can result from adverse events such as loss of a job or the exit of an important other person in the individual's life, but stress can also result from positive events that require major readjustment, such as moving one's residence or changing jobs. Stress can accumulate over a period of time to increase vulnerability to depression and other psychological and physical disorders. It can also be the precipitating factor for the origination of an episode. Stressful life events have been associated with increased risk of relapse after treatment and with increased risk of suicide attempts (Nezu & Roman, 1985). The role of negative life events has been frequently demonstrated in the etiology of unipolar depression, and Ellicot, Hammen, Gitlin, Brown, and Jamison (1990) demonstrated the relationship between stressful life events and bipolar depressive and manic episodes.

In addition to major life events, minor events that occur daily may also be important in depression. Daily mood is affected negatively by adverse events and positively by pleasant events. This is true for normal and clinical populations. Changing daily minor life events is the basis for therapy interventions as described later under diagnostic considerations.

Past Depressive Episodes as a Vulnerability Factor

Depression is often a recurring disorder. A past episode of depression represents a risk factor for developing subsequent episodes of depression. This suggests that factors responsible for the first episode may be different from those for the subsequent episodes. Life events may be less important, or lesser events may precipitate later episodes. Depression itself creates problems by interfering with adequate performance in many areas of life. Depression can produce events that are stressful and, thus, negative life events and depression may be reciprocally related.

FAMILIAL AND GENETIC PATTERNS

Family Studies

Depression is known to run in families. The problem is to separate the biological effects of genetics from the psychological effects of family environment. In general, there is a higher risk of having an affective disorder among relatives of a unipolar/bipolar patient compared to the relatives of a normal control person. Data from the NIMH Collaborative Study of the Psychobiology of Depression (Andreasen et al., 1987) indicate that unipolar depression is common among first-degree relatives of both unipolar and bipolar patients, but relatives of unipolar patients have higher rates of unipolar disorder than bipolar disorder. These data have been taken as an indication that the two disorders run relatively true in families, or that the rarer bipolar disorder may be a more severe form of the same genetic vulnerability. Bipolar patients have severe and less severe relatives, whereas unipolar patients have mostly less severe relatives.

The NIMH Epidemiological Catchment Area study (Regier et al., 1988) showed that individuals in more recent age cohorts generally have earlier ages of onset and increased rates of affective illness. These facts are inconsistent with a purely genetic explanation. This cohort effect may be attributable to methodological artifact or to increasing social, financial, and environmental stressors in a rapidly changing world, along with increasing psychological emphasis on individual responsibility (Seligman, 1989).

Twin Studies

Monozygotic twins (MZ) are genetically identical whereas dizygotic twins (DZ) share, on average, 50% of the genetic material. Because pairs of twins usually have similar environments, comparing MZ and DZ twins allows measuring the effect of genetics, and environment is held constant. If affective disorders have a genetic component, a MZ twin of a unipolar/ bipolar patient is more likely than a DZ twin to have the disorder. Data from the Danish twin study (Bertelsen, Harvald, & Hauge, 1977) indicate that the rates of concordance (co-occurrence) for MZ and DZ twins for bipolar probands were 79% and 24%, respectively. Corresponding rates for unipolar patients were 54% and 19%, respectively. This is indicative of a strong genetic component for affective illness, especially for bipolar disorders. However, it also demonstrates that genetics does not provide the entire answer for a cause of mood disorder because a large percentage of risk is not accounted for by common genes.

Adoption Studies

Even though twin studies provide strong evidence for genetic bases of affective disorders, they do not rule out the contribution of environmental factors. MZ twins may be reared similarly and DZ twins differently. Adoption studies attempt to tease apart the genetic from the environmental influences by comparing the biological with the adoptive parents of patients. If environment is more important, then adoptive parents would be more likely to have mood disorders. If genetics is more important, then biological parents would have higher rates of mood disorder. Mendlewicz and Rainer (1977) studied 29 bipolar adoptees. Thirty-one percent of biological parents of these patients had bipolar disorders, compared to 12% in the adoptive parents. The higher risk of affective illness in biological parents of bipolar adoptees is comparable to the risk for parents of nonadopted bipolars (26%). This suggests a strong genetic component in bipolar illness.

Mode of Genetic Transmission

If affective disorders have a genetic basis, the ultimate goal would be to identify the particular genes and the specific mode of transmission. Hints of specific modes of transmission have been stronger in bipolar than unipolar disorder. Winokur, Clayton, and Reich (1969) suggested a sex-linked connection to the X chromosome for bipolar illness. The higher risk for female first-degree relatives of bipolar patients and the low rate of father to son transmissions suggested a dominant X-linked illness. This effect has proven to be weak and suggests that only some component of the transmission may be sex-linked.

Egeland et al. (1987) studied genetic patterns in a large sample from the Old Order Amish, an ideal population to study because of the ability to identify and locate relatives of patients in a stable society. They appeared to show the contribution of a single-gene, dominant transmission of a specific gene for bipolar disorder. As more data were collected, however, it became clear that this effect was doubtful.

Presently, the mode of transmission for both bipolar and unipolar disorder is best seen as the sum of many genetic factors that accumulate to create differences in the risk of disorder. Expression of genetic risk may depend on other factors, including psychosocial vulnerability and environmental stressors.

DIAGNOSTIC CONSIDERATIONS

Comorbidity

When making treatment decisions, several diagnostic issues need to be taken into account. Depression is often comorbid with other disorders. For example, it is frequently encountered along with alcoholism or other substance abuse. Clinical lore suggests that the primary disorder (i.e., the one that occurred first) needs to be the primary target of treatment. It is assumed that treating the primary disorder will also treat the secondary disorder. This is based on the idea that primary depressed persons may be self-medicating their depressions with alcohol, and the primary alcoholics may be depressed over the consequences of their alcoholism. In practice, it may be difficult to determine a sequence of occurrence, and practical issues such as need for detoxification may take precedence in treatment.

Anxiety is also frequently seen in conjunction with depression. The DSM system may in fact be making artificial distinctions among problems of dysphoric affect that blend along a continuum. Problematic anxiety may precede depression in the history of many depressed persons. Medication choice may be predicated on the predominance of depressive or anxious symptoms. Psychological approaches may deal with combined themes or techniques, for example, identifying cognitive distortions concerning loss and danger or combining social skills training and relaxation training.

Depression in conjunction with medical disorders is common, and though it may be secondary to the medical condition, it should not be ignored. Depression is a negative prognostic sign for recovery and rehabilitation, so that treatment for depression can usefully be an adjunct to medical treatment. Few controlled studies exist, but psychotherapy for depression in conjunction with cancer treatment or cardiac rehabilitation can be very helpful.

Personality disorders are typically seen as a complicating factor in treating depression or any other Axis I disorder. Developing a working collaboration may take more effort, relationship issues may be more prominent in therapy, and therapy may take longer in dealing with maladaptive interpersonal styles and chaotic interpersonal relationships. Empirical evidence for the efficacy of treatments for depression in the presence of personality disorders is sparse, and more attention to this form of comorbidity would advance the field. The so-called personality disorders should be looked at in terms of extremes on basic dimensions of personality. They may represent personality styles or dimensions relevant to depression or to general psychopathology proneness. They may also be conceptualized at more basic levels of behavioral analysis as patterns of skill deficits and excesses.

Severity

Severity is another issue of diagnostic and treatment planning significance. Hospitalization may be required for severe depression or mania. In mania, hospitalization may be necessary to protect individuals and others around them from the adverse social consequences of poor decision making and impulsive behavior. In depression, the reasons for hospitalization are more likely to be deterioration in self-care or protection from suicide. Suicide is a risk in both unipolar and bipolar forms of depression, and it is important to note that risk increases during the period when the person appears to be recovering from an episode of depression. Medication management is also a reason for hospitalization. Research on psychotherapies with inpatients is beginning to appear (e.g., Miller, Norman, Keitner, Bishop, & Dow, 1989) and suggests that it can be a useful adjunct in the hospital, especially if maintained on an outpatient basis after discharge.

There is some evidence that more severe depressions respond better to pharmacotherapy and moderate depressions respond equally or better to psychotherapies (Elkin et al., 1989). People who have more severe depressions may comply better with medication regiments, whereas moderately depressed subjects are less likely to drop out of psychotherapy interventions. Combinations of pharmacotherapy and psychotherapy have been found superior to either intervention alone in a few studies but not so in others. Medication may be necessary or useful in severe depression to energize the patient sufficiently to take advantage of psychotherapeutic intervention, and sequencing may be a useful strategy. Psychotherapy has an advantage over pharmacotherapy in preventing relapse or recurrence, though recurrence is frequent in either form of treatment.

Diagnostic Subtypes

Diagnostic subtypes, such as the distinctions made by the DSM system, have significance for the choice of treatment among medications, but less so for the choice of psychotherapies. Bipolar disorders are generally considered of largely biological origin, and lithium salts (e.g., lithium carbonate) are the usual treatment of choice, sometimes enhanced by other medications. Lithium has a prophylactic effect in preventing future episodes of depression and mania and is prescribed as a maintenance treatment over long periods of time. Little attention has been given to bipolar disorder in the psychotherapeutic literature; most studies that assess the efficacy of psychotherapy exclude bipolars. Psychological treatments that are offered in practice are typically aimed at social support for patients and/or family members and involve the consequences of the disorder and medication education and management.

The possibility of more specific treatment of bipolar disorders via psychotherapy is beginning to be examined by researchers. Psychotherapies effective in treating unipolar depressive episodes may also be effective in treating bipolar depressive episodes. Psychotherapeutic strategies that target manic episodes have not been developed to date. Recent evidence indicates that bipolar episodes, like unipolar episodes, are often preceded by stress (Ellicott et al., 1990). Psychotherapies aimed at coping skills and stress reduction could be useful in reducing episodes. Evidence for such prophylactic effects in unipolar depression should be cause for exploring similar effects in bipolar disorder.

Unipolar depression is treated with a wide variety of medications, including tricyclic antidepressants, newer heterocyclic antidepressants, and monoamine oxidase inhibitors (MAOIs). The efficacy of tricyclics, such as amitriptyline (Elavil) or imipramine (Tofranil) for treating many forms of unipolar depression is well established in the research literature. Tricyclics have a special advantage for the more severe depressions. They have the disadvantage of some unpleasant side effects and the danger of precipitating manic episodes in bipolar I and II patients. The newer classes of antidepressants, such as the SSRIs (selective serotonin reuptake inhibitors), for example, fluoxetine (Prozac), have fewer side effects and less danger of inducing a manic episode. The MAOIs, such as isocarboxazid (Marplan) or tranylcypromine sulfate (Parnate), are usually reserved for tricyclic nonresponders because of severe dietary restrictions which must be followed by patients who take these medications. MAOIs may have special advantage for treating atypical depressions, those that involve increased appetite and sleep.

Dysthymia is a particular diagnostic problem in terms of recommended treatment. Dysthymia is seen by some as a biological disorder difficult to treat with antidepressant medications. On the other hand, it may be viewed as a problem of chronic pessimism, low self-esteem, and poor coping skills, akin to the personality disorders. Skill-oriented psychotherapies may be useful if they take into account the same concerns that are relevant to personality disorder comorbidity. Unfortunately, the dysthymia distinction has generally not been studied as a distinct population in the psychotherapy literature.

Psychotherapeutic Strategies

Psychotherapy is often the treatment preferred by patients and may be recommended for individuals who do not tolerate the side effects of antidepressant medications. Psychotherapy may be indicated instead of, or in addition to, medication for individuals who are dealing with significant life events or interpersonal problems or who have a history of poor coping skills.

Several psychotherapeutic strategies have been assessed and have proven effective in treating nonpsychotic, nonbipolar depression. Five general psychotherapeutic strategies can be identified in the psychotherapy research literature: (1) Reinforcement, (2) Social Skill, (3) Learned Helplessness, (4) Self-Management, and (5) Cognitive Therapies. Logically, the rationales and targeted symptoms could be considered a basis for making recommendations for specific individuals, that is, it would make sense to match the individual patient to the psychotherapy that best targets the person's deficits. Empirical evidence for matching strategies is weak at best (e.g., Zeiss, Lewinsohn, & Munoz, 1979; Rehm, Kaslow, & Rabin, 1987; Jacobson et al., 1996). Most therapies are actually complex programs that target multiple symptoms, and the programs may have more commonalities than differences. Matching psychotherapies to patient strengths may actually be a better matching strategy because available evidence suggests that individuals whose skills and attitudes are consistent with therapy approaches do better in those therapies (Rude & Rehm, 1991).

REINFORCEMENT

Reinforcement strategies are based on the behavioral rationale that depression is a deficiency in reinforcement for important response chains in the person's life. This approach is most closely associated with the work of Peter Lewinsohn (1974), who defines depression as a response to a loss or lack of response-contingent reinforcement. When behavior decreases due to nonreinforcement, the other symptoms of depression, such as low self-esteem or feelings of fatigue, follow as secondary sequelae. Lewinsohn argues that there are three primary reasons for such a condition of nonreinforcement: (1) reinforcement is not available from the person's environment, as in lack of employment opportunities or loss of a significant figure in the person's life; (2) the person lacks essential skills to obtain reinforcement, such as job skills or interpersonal skills required to satisfy interpersonal relationships; and (3) reinforcement is available, but the person is not able to experience it, for example, when social anxiety interferes with otherwise rewarding interpersonal relationships.

Each of these three conditions leads to a different therapeutic strategy. Deficient reinforcement in the environment leads to a strategy that encourages the person to engage in new or old behaviors that lead to reinforcement. Behaviors are identified that are potentially reinforcing, and the person develops a schedule for increasing these behaviors. For example, the person who has lost a significant friend might be encouraged to increase activities that previously were reinforcing before meeting the friend or to increase similar activities with other friends. The purpose would be to reengage the person with reinforcing social activities.

The therapeutic strategy to treat lack of important social skills is some form of skill training. For example, job skill programs, assertiveness training, or communication skill training might be recommended. This form of therapeutic strategy overlaps the next section where additional alternatives are described. If the identified deficit is interfering social anxiety, it follows logically that an anxiety reduction program, such as relaxation training or systematic desensitization, would be recommended.

Lewinsohn and his colleagues developed a Pleasant Event Schedule (PES; MacPhillamy & Lewinsohn, 1974, 1982) to assess the therapeutic strategy that best fits the individual's pattern of depression. The PES consists of a lengthy list of events that many people find reinforcing. Subjects indicate the degree to which the event would be potentially reinforcing to them and the frequency with which the event has occurred in the last month. Scores of reinforcement potential, activity level, and reinforcement obtained are useful in choosing the appropriate therapeutic strategy.

Note, however, that a study of matching by this strategy (Zeiss, Lewinsohn, & Munoz, 1979) did not find it useful. Subjects who were theoretically mismatched did just as well as subjects who were theoretically matched. In more recent years, therapeutic strategies have been combined into a larger therapy program that targets a series of behavioral deficits. The program has been effective in group, individual, and self-help formats (Brown & Lewinsohn, 1984).

SOCIAL SKILLS

Social skill approaches share the general assumption that depressed individuals suffer from deficiencies in social skills. A variety of deficiencies and conceptions of depression are involved. Gotlib and Colby (1987) make a general case that depression is an interpersonal phenomenon. Several researchers have taken the approach that depression occurs in the context of a marital relationship and have employed marital communication skill training as a therapeutic approach (e.g., Beach & O'Leary, 1986; McLean & Hakstian, 1979). Deficits in problem-solving skills are posited by Nezu, Nezu, and Perri (1989) as central to depression. Klerman, Weissman, Rounsaville, and Chevron (1984) developed a dynamically oriented, interpersonal psychotherapy based on the idea that depression results from disturbances in interpersonal relationships.

Each of these interpersonal approaches has implications for assessment and treatment matching. Marital dissatisfaction, interpersonal loss or conflict, and problem-solving deficits are constructs that are associated with their own assessment domains. It is entirely consistent with the biopsychosocial model to assess the interpersonal environment and the persons skills in interacting with that environment.

Learned Helplessness

The learned helplessness theory of depression has gone through several revisions (Seligman, 1975; Abramson, Seligman, & Teasdale, 1978; Alloy, Clements, & Kolden, 1985). The basic concept of learned helplessness is that depressed people have acquired a belief that they cannot affect important outcomes in their lives, that is, outcomes are independent of their actions. Drawing such a helpless conclusion typically follows a major aversive event. The likelihood of drawing a helpless conclusion is heightened if the person has a depressogenic attributional style. Such psychological diathesis consists of a predisposition to conclude that negative events are due to internal, stable, and global causes, that is, the adverse event is due to something about oneself, is due to something that is true about oneself now and continuing into the future, and is due to something about oneself that is true in all or many circumstances. If adverse events occur because of internal, stable, global causes, the person feels helpless to control future outcomes. In its most recent form (Alloy, Clements, & Kolden, 1985), the theory states that helplessness leads to hopelessness about the future which, in turn, produces depression.

Although the learned helplessness theory has not led to a specific form of therapy, Seligman (1981) argues that four therapeutic strategies are consistent with the theory. First, environmental enrichment could be used to put the person in an environment that is more controllable, allowing the person to regain a sense of control over outcomes. Second, skill training might be used to realistically increase the person's control in specific areas, such as job or interpersonal skills. Third, resignation training might be appropriate in situations where the helplessness is based on an unrealistically hopeless goal. The tactic is to help the persons resign themselves to more appropriate and attainable goals. Finally, the fourth strategy is attribution retraining, whereby the person is made aware of their depressogenic attributional style and is taught to make more optimistic causal attributions for failures and successes.

Self-Management

The self-control model of depression (Rehm, 1977) was intended to be an integrative model that brings together cognitive and behavioral elements under the framework of Kanfer's (1970) model of self-control. The model suggests that depression or depression proneness can be thought of in terms of one or more deficits in self-control behavior. Specifically, depression involves (1) selective attention to negative events to the relative exclusion of positive events; (2) selective attention to the immediate as opposed to the long-term outcomes of behavior; (3) setting stringent, perfectionistic self-evaluative standards; (4) depressive attributions for successes and failures; (5) insufficient contingent self-reward; and (6) excessive self-administered punishment. The model integrates concepts about depression from other models but adds an emphasis on looking at depression as a disconnection from goals that organize and give coherence and meaning to life.

Several scales have been developed that assess the deficits identified by the model to determine whether the program is appropriate. The Self-Control Questionnaire was developed by Rehm and his colleagues (Fuchs & Rehm, 1977) to assess all of the depressive deficits hypothesized by the model. The scale has been used primarily as an outcome measure in therapeutic studies generally.

Specific components of the model may be assessed by other scales. Self-evaluation and attributions can be assessed by self-esteem and attributional style measures. Heiby (1982) published a Self-Reinforcement Questionnaire and Lewinsohn, Larson, and Munoz (1982) developed the Cognitive Events Scale to assess self-reinforcing thoughts.

Cognitive Therapy

Aaron Beck's (1972) cognitive therapy is based on a cognitive model of depression and psychopathology generally. It assumes that depression is the product of negative distortions of events in daily life. For Beck, depression's primary components are the *cognitive triad*: (1) a negative view of self, (2) a negative view of world, and (3) a negative view of the future. Distortions occur when people view their world through the filter of depressive schemata, which are organized sets of assumptions and rules about the world stored in memory and accessed during depressive episodes. Interpretive *automatic thoughts* occur at the edge of awareness and lead to negative affect.

Several typical forms of negative distortion are identified. *Arbitrary inference* involves the automatic assumption that one is to blame for any negative life event. *Selective abstraction* occurs when the person focuses on minor negative information in an otherwise positive situation. A third example is *inexact labeling* where the person attaches a negative label to an experience and then reacts emotionally to the label.

Therapy is aimed at helping the patient to identify negative automatic thoughts and challenge them rationally and empirically. Gradually, as automatic thoughts are identified, the negative underlying assumptions and rules of the depressive schemata become apparent and can be challenged and modified by similar means.

Several instruments have been developed to assess negative automatic thoughts and underlying assumptions. The Automatic Thoughts Questionnaire (Hollon & Kendall, 1980) was developed to assess the symptomatic thoughts experienced daily by depressed persons. The Dysfunctional Attitudes Scale (Weissman & Beck, 1978) was developed to assess more basic assumptions presumed to reflect depression vulnerability. Both reflect depressive symptoms, but Miranda and Persons (1986) found that formerly depressed people score much higher on the Dysfunctional Attitudes Scale when a mild negative mood has been induced. Their interpretation of this finding is that depression prone people access alternative depressive schemata when they are in a depressed mood. "Affect priming," as this procedure has come to be called, is a promising assessment technique for assessing cognitive vulnerability to depression and perhaps the suitability of cognitive therapy.

Summary

A biopsychosocial approach to depression takes into account biological, psychological, and environmental factors in etiology, maintenance, symptomatology, underlying mechanisms, and intervention. Different subtypes of depression may represent different loadings of these factors, but all three factors may contribute to each individual's depression in a unique combination and interaction. We need more comprehensive theoretical approaches to understanding depression that take into account both biological and psychological diatheses as they interact with stress. We need a better understanding of the processes whereby these factors interact reciprocally over the development, course, and treatment of the depression.

References

Abramson, L. Y., Seligman, M. E. P., & Teasdale, J. D. (1978). Learned helplessness in humans: Critique and reformulation. *Journal of Abnormal Psychology, 87,* 32–48.

Alloy, L. B., Clements, C., & Kolden, G. (1985). The cognitive diathesis-stress theories of depression: Therapeutic implications. In S. Reiss & R. R. Bootzin (Eds.), *Theoretical issues in behavior therapy* (pp. 379–410). Orlando, FL: Academic Press.

American Psychiatric Association. (1980). *Diagnostic and statistical manual of mental disorders*, 3rd ed. Washington, DC: Author.

American Psychiatric Association. (1987). *Diagnostic and statistical manual of mental disorders*, 3rd ed., rev. Washington, DC: Author.

American Psychiatric Association. (1994). *Diagnostic and statistical manual of mental disorders*, 4th ed. Washington, DC: Author.

Andreasen, N. C., Rice, J., Endicott, J., Coryell, W., Grove, W. M., & Reich, T. (1987). Familial rates of affective disorder. A report from the National Institute of Mental Health Collaborative Study. *Archives of General Psychiatry, 44*, 461–469.

Angst, J., Bastrup, P., Grof, P., Hippius, H., Poldinger, W., & Weiss, P. (1973). The course of monopolar and bipolar psychoses. *Psychiatrica, Neurologica, and Neurochirurgia, 76*, 489–500.

Baron, M. (1977). Linkage between X-chromosome marker (deutan colorblindness) and bipolar affective illness. *Archives of General Psychiatry, 24*, 721–727.

Beach, S. R. H., & O'Leary, K. D. (1986). The treatment of depression occurring in the context of marital discord. *Behavior Therapy, 17*, 43–49.

Beck, A. T. (1972). *Depression: Causes and treatment*. Philadelphia: University of Pennsylvania Press.

Bertelsen, A., Harvald, B., & Hauge, M. (1977). A Danish twin study of manic depressive disorders. *British Journal of Psychiatry, 130*, 330–351.

Brown, R. A., & Lewinsohn, P. M. (1984). A psychoeducational approach to the treatment of depression: Comparison of group, individual, and minimal contact procedures. *Journal of Consulting and Clinical Psychology, 52*, 774–783.

Castillo, R. J. (1997) Culture & mental illness: A client centered approach. Pacific Grove, CA: Brooks/Cole.

Egeland, J. A., Gerhard, D. S., Pauls, D. S., Sussex, J. N., Kidd, K. K., Allen, C. R., Hostetter, A. M., & Housman, D. (1987). Bipolar affective disorders linked to DNA markers on chromosome II. *Nature, 325*, 783–787.

Elkin, I., Shea, M. T., Watkins, J. T., Imber, S. D., Sotsky, S. M., Collins, J. F., Glass, D. R., Pilkonis, P. A., Leber, W. R., Docherty, J. P., Fiester, S. J., & Parloff, M. B. (1989). National Institute of Mental Health treatment of depression collaborative research program: General effectiveness of treatments. *Archives of General Psychiatry, 46*, 971–982.

Ellicot, A., Hammen, C., Gitlin, M., Brown, G., & Jamison, K. (1990). Life events and course of bipolar disorder. *American Journal of Psychiatry, 147*, 1194–1198.

Fuchs, C. Z., & Rehm, L. P. (1977). A self-control behavior therapy program for depression. *Journal of Consulting and Clinical Psychology, 45*, 206–215.

Gotlib, I. H., & Colby, C. A. (1987). *Treatment of depression: An interpersonal systems approach*. New York: Pergamon.

Heiby, E. M. (1982). A self-reinforcement questionnaire. *Behaviour Research and Therapy, 20*, 397–401.

Hollon, S. D., & Kendall, P. C. (1980). Cognitive self-statements in depression: Development of an automatic thoughts questionnaire. *Cognitive Therapy and Research, 4*, 383–397.

Jacobson, N. S., Dobson, K. S., Truax, P. A., Addis, M. E., Koerner, K., Gollan, J. K., Gortner, E., & Prince, S. E. (1996). A component analysis of cognitive-behavioral treatment for depression. *Journal of Consulting and Clinical Psychology, 64*, 295–304.

Kanfer, F. H. (1970). Self-regulation: Research, issues and speculations. In C. Neuringer & J. L. Michael (Eds.), *Behavior modification in clinical psychology* (pp. 178–220). New York: Appleton-Century-Crofts.

Klerman, G. L., Weissman, M. M., Rounsaville, B. J., & Chevron, E. S. (1984). *Interpersonal psychotherapy of depression*. New York: Basic Books.

Kraeplin, E. (1921). *Manic-depressive insanity and paranoia*. Edinburgh, Scotland: Livingstone.

Leonhard, K. (1957). *Aufteilung der Endogenen Psychosen*, 4th ed. Berlin: Akademieverlag.

Lewinsohn, P. M. (1974). A behavioral approach to depression. In R. M. Friedman & M. M. Katz (Eds.), *The psychology of depression: Contemporary theory and research* (pp. 157–185). New York: Wiley.

Lewinsohn, P. M. (1991). Depression in adolescents. Paper presented at the *Meeting of the American Psychological Association*, August 1991, San Francisco.

Lewinsohn, P. M., Larson, D. W., & Munoz, R. F. (1982). The measurement of expectancies and other cognitions in depressed individuals. *Cognitive Therapy and Research, 6*, 437–446.

MacPhillamy, D. J., & Lewinsohn, P. M. (1974). Depression as a function of levels of desired and obtained pleasure. *Journal of Abnormal Psychology, 83*, 651–657.

MacPhillamy, D. J., & Lewinsohn, P. M. (1982). The pleasant events schedule: Studies on reliability, validity, and scale intercorrelation. *Journal of Consulting and Clinical Psychology*, *50*, 363–380.

McLean, P. D., & Hakstian, A. R. (1979). Clinical depression: Comparative efficacy of outpatient treatments. *Journal of Consulting and Clinical Psychology*, *47*, 818–836.

Mendlewicz, J., & Ranier, J. D. (1977). Adoption studies in manic-depressive illness. *Nature*, *268*, 327–329.

Miller, I. W., Norman, W. H., Keitner, G. I., Bishop, S. B., & Dow, M. G. (1989). Cognitive-behavioral treatment of depressed inpatients. *Behavior Therapy*, *20*, 25–47.

Miranda, J., & Persons, J. B. (1986). Relationship of dysfunctional attitudes to current mood and history of depression. Paper presented at the *Meeting of the Association for the Advancement of Behavior Therapy*, November 1986, Chicago.

Nezu, A. M., Nezu, C. M., & Perri, M. G. (1989). *Problem-solving therapy for depression: Theory research and clinical guidelines*. New York: Wiley.

Nezu, A. M., & Ronan, G. F. (1985). Life stress, current problems, problem solving and depressive symptoms: An integrative model. *Journal of Consulting and Clinical Psychology*, *53*, 693–697.

Nolen-Hoeksema, S. (1987). Sex differences in unipolar depression: Evidence and theory. *Psychological Bulletin*, *101*, 259–282.

Radloff, L. (1975). Sex differences in depression: The effects of occupation and marital status. *Sex Roles*, *1*, 249–265.

Regier, D. A., Boyd, J. H., Burke, J. D., Jr., Rae, D. S., Myers, J. K., Kramer, M., Robins, L. N., George, L. K., Karno, M., & Locke, B. Z. (1988). One-month prevalence of mental disorders in the United States: Based on five Epidemiological Catchment Area sites. *Archives of General Psychiatry*, *45*, 977–986.

Rehm, L. P., Kaslow, N. J., & Rabin, A. S. (1987). Cognitive and behavioral targets in a self-control therapy program for depression. *Journal of Consulting and Clinical Psychology*, *55*, 60–67.

Rehm, L. P. (1977). A self-control model of depression. *Behavior Therapy*, *8*, 787–804.

Rude, S., & Rehm, L. P. (1991). Cognitive and behavioral predictors of response to treatments of depression. *Clinical Psychology Review*, *11*, 493–514.

Seligman, M. E. P. (1975). *Helplessness: On depression, development and death*. San Francisco: Freeman.

Seligman, M. E. P. (1981). A learned helplessness point of view. In L. P. Rehm (Ed.), *Behavior therapy for depression: Present status and future directions*. New York: Academic Press.

Seligman, M. E. P. (1989). Research in clinical psychology: Why is there so much depression today? In I. S. Cohen (Ed.), *The G. Stanley Hall Lecture Series*, Vol. 9. Washington, DC: American Psychological Association.

Weissman, A. N., & Beck, A. T. (1978). Development and validation of the Dysfunctional Attitude Scale. Paper presented at the *Annual Convention of the Association for the Advancement of Behavior Therapy*, November 1978, Chicago.

Winokur, G., Clayton, P. J., & Reich, T. (1969). *Manic-depressive disease*. St. Louis, MO: Mosby.

Zeiss, A. M., Lewinsohn, P. M., & Munoz, R. F. (1979). Nonspecific improvement effects in depression using interpersonal skills training, pleasant activity schedules, or cognitive training. *Journal of Consulting and Clinical Psychology*, *47*, 427–439.

16

Schizophrenia

Michelle P. Salyers and Kim T. Mueser

Schizophrenia is the most severely debilitating of all adult psychiatric illnesses. Despite the recent trend toward community-oriented treatment, more psychiatric hospital beds are occupied by patients with schizophrenia than any other disorder. Even when patients receive optimal treatments, they usually continue to experience substantial impairments throughout most of their lives.

Since schizophrenia was first described more than 100 years ago, the nature of the disorder has been hotly debated, and public misconceptions about it have been commonplace. In recent years, there has been a growing consensus among clinicians and researchers to redefine the psychopathology and diagnostic features of this disorder. Once referred to as a "wastebasket diagnosis," the term *schizophrenia* is now used to describe a specific clinical syndrome. An understanding of the core clinical features of schizophrenia is necessary for differential diagnosis and treatment planning. After many years of struggling to improve the long-term course of schizophrenia, there is now abundant evidence that combined pharmacological and psychosocial interventions can have a major impact on improving functioning. This chapter provides an up-to-date review of schizophrenia and a particular focus on the psychopathology of the illness and its impact on other domains of functioning.

Description of the Disorder

Schizophrenia is characterized by impairments in social functioning, including difficulty establishing and maintaining interpersonal relationships, problems working or fulfilling other instrumental roles (e.g., student and homemaker), and the inability to care for oneself (e.g., poor grooming and hygiene). These problems in daily living, in the absence of significant impairment in intellectual functioning, are the most distinguishing characteristics of schizophrenia and are a necessary criterion for diagnosing it according to most diagnostic systems (e.g., *Diagnostic and Statistical Manual of Mental Disorders*, 4th ed. [DSM-IV], American

Michelle P. Salyers • Department of Psychology, Indiana University-Purdue University, Indianapolis, Indianapolis, Indiana 46202-3275.   **Kim T. Mueser** • Department of Psychiatry and Community and Family Medicine, Dartmouth Medical School, Dartmouth College, Concord, New Hampshire 03301-3852.

Advanced Abnormal Psychology, Second Edition, edited by Hersen and Van Hasselt. Kluwer Academic/Plenum Publishers, New York, 2001.

Psychiatric Association, 1994). Consequently, many patients who have the illness depend on others to meet their daily living needs. For example, estimates suggest that between 40 and 60% of patients with schizophrenia live with relatives, and an even higher percentage rely on relatives for caregiving (Goldman, 1982; Torrey, 1995). Patients without family contact typically rely on mental health, residential, and case management services. In the worst case scenario, patients who have insufficient contact with relatives and who fall between the cracks of the social service delivery system end up in jail (Torrey et al., 1992) or become homeless, and between 10 and 20% of homeless persons have schizophrenia (Susser, Stuening, & Conover, 1989).

In addition to the problems in daily living that characterize schizophrenia, patients who have the illness experience a range of different symptoms. The most common symptoms include positive symptoms (e.g., hallucinations and delusions), negative symptoms (e.g., social withdrawal, apathy, and anhedonia), cognitive impairments (e.g., memory difficulties and planning ability), and problems with mood (e.g., depression, anxiety, and anger). The specific nature of these symptoms is described in greater detail in the section titled *Clinical Picture*. The symptoms of schizophrenia account for some, but not all of the problems in social functioning (Glynn, 1998).

The various impairments associated with schizophrenia tend to be long-term, punctuated by fluctuations in severity over time. For this reason, schizophrenia has a broad impact on the family, and patients are often impeded from pursuing personal life goals. Despite severity of the disorder, advances in the treatment of schizophrenia provide solid hope for improving the outcome.

EPIDEMIOLOGY

The lifetime prevalence of schizophrenia (including the closely related disorders of schizoaffective disorder and schizophreniform disorder) is approximately 1% (Keith, Regier, & Rae, 1991). In general, prevalence of schizophrenia is remarkably stable across a wide range of different populations, such as gender, race, religion, or level of industrialization (Jablensky, 1999). However, schizophrenia is more common in urban areas of industrialized countries (Peen & Dekker, 1997; Takei, Sham, O'Callaghan, Glover, & Murray, 1995; Torrey, Bowler, & Clark, 1997). Such increased risk is related to the likelihood that people with schizophrenia will drift to urban areas and also that they are born in urban areas (Torrey et al., 1997).

Because schizophrenia frequently has an onset during early adulthood, persons who have the illness are less likely to marry or remain married, particularly males (Eaton, 1975; Munk-Jørgensen, 1987), and are less likely to complete higher levels of education (Kessler, Foster, Saunders, & Stang, 1995). It has long been known that there is an association between poverty and schizophrenia. People who belong to lower socioeconomic classes are more likely to develop the disorder (Hollingshead & Redlich, 1958; Salokangas, 1978). Historically, two theories have been advanced to account for this association. The *social drift* hypothesis postulates that the debilitating effects of schizophrenia on the capacity to work result in a lowering of socioeconomic means and hence poverty (Aro, Aro, & Keskimäki, 1995). The *environmental stress* hypothesis proposes that high levels of stress associated with poverty precipitate schizophrenia in some individuals who would not otherwise develop the illness (Bruce, Takeuchi, & Leaf, 1991). Both of these explanations may be partly true, and longitudinal research on changes in socioeconomic class status and schizophrenia provide conflicting results. For example, Fox (1990) reanalyzed data from several longitudinal studies and found that after controlling for initial levels of socioeconomic class, downward drift was not evident. However, Dohrenwend et al. (1992) did find evidence for social drift, even after controlling for socioeconomic class. Thus, more work is needed to sort out the relationships between socioeconomic status and schizophrenia.

CLINICAL PICTURE

Most studies on the dimensions of schizophrenia agree on at least three major groups of symptoms (Liddle, 1987; Mueser, Curran, & McHugo, 1997; Van Der Does, Dingemans, Linszen, Nugter, & Scholte, 1993). Schizophrenia is characterized by three broad classes of symptoms: positive symptoms, negative symptoms, and cognitive impairments. *Positive symptoms* refer to thoughts, sensory experiences, and behaviors that patients have, but are ordinarily absent in persons who do not have the illness. Common examples of positive symptoms include hallucinations (e.g., hearing voices), delusions (e.g., believing that people are persecuting you), and bizarre behavior (e.g., maintaining a peculiar posture for no apparent reason). *Negative symptoms*, on the other hand, are the absence or diminution of cognitions, feelings, or behaviors that persons ordinarily have who do not have the illness. Common negative symptoms include blunted or flattened affect (e.g., diminished facial expressiveness), poverty of speech (i.e., diminished verbal communication), anhedonia (i.e., inability to experience pleasure), apathy, psychomotor retardation (e.g., slow rate of speech), and physical inertia. *Cognitive impairments* are difficulties in memory, attention, abstract reasoning (i.e., understanding a concept), and executive functions (e.g., ability to anticipate or plan). These impairments may interfere with patients' ability to focus for sustained periods on work or recreational pursuits, interact effectively with others, perform basic activities of daily living, or participate in conventional psychotherapeutic interventions (Bellack, Gold, & Buchanan, 1999; Brekke, Raine, Ansel, Lencz, & Bird, 1997; Sevy & Davidson, 1995; Velligan, Mahurin, Diamond, Hazleton, Eckert, & Miller, 1997). Cognitive impairments also result in difficulties in generalizing training or knowledge to other areas (i.e., transfer of training problems). Thus, many rehabilitative efforts focus on training the patient directly in the environment in which skills will be used.

Positive symptoms of schizophrenia tend to fluctuate over the course of the disorder and are often in remission between episodes of the illness. In addition, positive symptoms tend to be responsive to the effects of antipsychotic medication (Kane & Marder, 1993). In contrast, negative symptoms and cognitive impairments tend to be stable over time and are less responsive to antipsychotic medications (Greden & Tandon, 1991). However, there is some evidence that atypical antipsychotic medications such as clozapine, risperidone, and olanzapine have a beneficial impact on negative symptoms and cognitive functioning (Green et al., 1997; Tollefson & Sanger, 1997; Wahlbeck et al., 1999).

Aside from the core symptoms of schizophrenia, many patients with schizophrenia experience negative emotions (e.g., depression, anxiety, and anger) as a consequence of their illness. Depression is very common among people with schizophrenia and has been associated with poor outcomes (e.g., increased hospital use and lower employment rates) and suicidal tendencies (Sands & Harrow, 1999). In addition, it is generally estimated that approximately 10 percent of persons with schizophrenia die from suicide (Drake, Gates, Whitaker, & Cotton, 1985; Roy, 1986). However, recent data and modeling techniques show lifetime rates of suicide for schizophrenia at 4%, compared to 6% for affective disorders and 7% for alcohol dependence (Inskip, Harris, & Barraclough, 1998). Difficulties with anxiety are common and are often due to positive symptoms, such as hallucinations or paranoid delusions (Argyle, 1990; Penn, Hope, Spaulding, & Kucera, 1994). Finally, anger and hostility may also be present, especially when the patient is paranoid.

In addition to the symptoms and negative emotions commonly present in schizophrenia, individuals who have this diagnosis often have comorbid substance use disorders. Epidemiological surveys have repeatedly found that persons who have psychiatric disorders are at increased risk of alcohol and drug abuse (Mueser, Yarnold, et al., 1990; Mueser, Yarnold, & Bellack, 1992). This risk is highest for persons who have the most severe psychiatric disorders, including schizophrenia and bipolar disorder. For example, individuals with schizophrenia are more than four times as likely to have a substance abuse disorder than individuals in the general population (Regier et al., 1990). In general, approximately 50% of all patients with schizophrenia have a lifetime history of substance use disorder, and 25 to 35% have a recent history of such a disorder (Mueser, Bennett, & Kushner, 1995).

Presence of comorbid substance use disorders in schizophrenia has consistently been associated with a worse course of the illness, including increased vulnerability to relapses and hospitalizations, housing instability and homelessness, violence, economic family burden, and treatment noncompliance (Drake & Brunette, 1998). For these reasons, recognition and treatment of substance use disorders in patients with schizophrenia is crucial to the overall management of the illness.

Another important clinical feature of schizophrenia is lack of insight and compliance with treatment (Amador & Gorman, 1998; Amador, Strauss, Yale, & Gorman, 1991). Many patients with schizophrenia have little or no insight into the fact that they have a psychiatric illness, or even that they have any problems at all. This denial of illness can lead to noncompliance with recommended treatments, such as psychotropic medications and psychosocial therapies (McEvoy et al., 1989). Furthermore, fostering patients' insight into the illness is a difficult and often impossible task.

Noncompliance with treatment is a related problem but can also occur due to the severe negativity often present in the illness, independent of poor insight. Problems of paranoia and distrust may contribute to noncompliance, in that some patients may believe medications or treatment providers are dangerous to them. Further, side effects of some medications, particularly the typical antipsychotics, are unpleasant and can also lead to noncompliance. Medication noncompliance increases the risk of patients to relapse and is therefore a major concern to clinical treatment providers (Buchanan, 1992). Strategies for enhancing compliance involve helping patients become more active participants in their treatment and identifying personal goals of treatment that are highly relevant for that individual (Corrigan, Liberman, & Engle, 1990; Kemp, Hayward, Applewhaite, Everitt, & David, 1996; Kemp, Kirov, Everitt, Hayward, & David, 1998).

People with schizophrenia are sometimes assumed to be violent or otherwise dangerous. Indeed, rates of violence are higher in people who have schizophrenia and other severe mental illnesses compared to the general population (Hodgins, Mednick, Brennan, Schulsinger, & Engberg, 1996; Swanson, Holzer, Ganju, & Jono, 1990). Actual rates of violence are difficult to ascertain. Rates can vary widely depending upon the source of information (e.g., self-report vs. collateral reports), the definition of violence, and the population studied (e.g., inpatients vs. outpatients). However, the majority of people who have schizophrenia and other mental illnesses are not violent (Swanson, 1994). When violence does occur, it is often associated with substance abuse (Steadman et al., 1998) or the combination of substance abuse and medication noncompliance (Swartz, Swanson, Hiday, Borum, Wagner, & Burns, 1998). Other factors such as psychopathy (Nolan, Volavka, Mohr, & Czobor, 1999) or antisocial personality disorder

(Hodgins & Côté, 1993, 1996) have also been implicated. Finally, targets of violence tend to be family members or friends rather than strangers (Steadman et al., 1998).

Although there is an increased rate of violence in schizophrenia, people with schizophrenia are much more likely to be the victims of violence. For example, in a recent survey of a large number of people who have severe mental illness, one-third of the men and women with schizophrenia reported severe physical or sexual assault in the past year (Goodman, Salyers, Mueser, & Rosenberg, submitted). These numbers are striking compared to estimates of the general population, in which 0.3% of women and 3.5% of men reported assault in the past year (Tjaden & Thoennes, 1998). Similarly, people who have severe mental illness (SMI) are more likely than a community sample to be the victims of violent crime (Hiday, Swartz, Swanson, Borum, & Wagner, 1999). In addition, between 34 and 53% of patients who have severe mental illness report childhood sexual or physical abuse (Greenfield, Strakowski, Tohen, Batson, & Kolbrener, 1994; Jacobson & Herald, 1990; Rose, Peabody, & Stratigeas, 1991; Ross, Anderson, & Clark, 1994), and 43 to 81% report some type of victimization during their lives (Carmen, Rieker, & Mills, 1984; Hutchings & Dutton, 1993; Jacobson, 1989; Jacobson & Richardson, 1987; Lipschitz et al., 1996). Studies of the prevalence of interpersonal trauma in women who have SMI indicate especially high vulnerability to victimization, and rates range as high as 77 to 97% for episodically homeless women (Davies-Netzley, Hurlburt, & Hough, 1996; Goodman, Dutton, & Harris, 1995). Thus, interpersonal violence is so common in the SMI population that it can be considered to be a normative experience (Goodman, Dutton, & Harris, 1997).

Exposure to traumatic events may lead to posttraumatic stress disorder (PTSD), a condition characterized by reliving the traumatic experience (e.g., nightmares and intrusive memories); avoidance of people, places, and things that remind the person of the event; and increased arousal symptoms (e.g., irritability and sleep problems). Prevalence of PTSD among people who have schizophrenia and other SMIs ranges from 29 to 43% (Cascardi, Mueser, DeGirolomo, & Murrin, 1996; Craine, Henson, Colliver, & MacLean, 1988; Mueser, Goodman et al., 1998; Switzer et al., 1999). These rates of current PTSD are far in excess of the lifetime prevalence of PTSD in the general population, and estimates range between 8 and 12% (Breslau, Davis, Andreski, & Peterson, 1991; Kessler, Sonnega, Bromet, Hughes, & Nelson, 1995; Resnick, Kilpatrick, Dansky, Saunders, & Best, 1993). Exposure to trauma and presence of PTSD are likely to worsen the course of schizophrenia and complicate treatment. For example, research shows that both discrete stressors (e.g., life events) and exposure to a stressful environment can worsen psychotic disorders (Butzlaff & Hooley, 1998). PTSD is also associated with substance abuse (Chilcoat & Breslau, 1998), which, as described earlier, can have severe consequences for people with schizophrenia.

Case Study

Jamie is a 25-year-old man who was diagnosed with schizophrenia 5 years ago. During the summer before his junior year in college, he was working in a busy office. He became progressively more concerned that his office mates were "out to get him" and that there was an intricate plot to discredit him. He also believed that his co-workers were secretly communicating with each other about him through certain facial expressions, choice of clothing, and the configuration of items on their desks. As his paranoia escalated, he became more disorganized in his thinking and behavior, was less able to take care of his daily activities, and could no longer come to work. He began to believe he was dying from a variety of sources, including being poisoned by indoor air pollution. These symptoms led to psychiatric hospitalization where he was first diagnosed with provisional schizophreniform disorder and treated with antipsychotic medication. At that time, he had to leave his job, quit school, and move back home with his parents. After 6 months of impairment, his diagnosis was changed to schizophrenia.

Today Jamie continues to struggle with schizophrenia. Even in the absence of psychotic symptoms, he maintains poor eye contact and shows little facial expression. For example, he rarely smiles spontaneously. His hygiene is generally good, but when his psychotic symptoms increase, he becomes more disheveled, smokes more cigarettes, and becomes agitated. He is prescribed medications which he admits help him feel better, less paranoid, and decrease his ideas of reference (that things around him have special meaning for him). However, he does not believe he has a mental illness and does not like the idea of having to rely on medications. He also does not like the weight gain he has experienced. He periodically stops taking his medications when he feels better; however, these breaks from medication have resulted in dramatic increases in his symptoms and have led to several rehospitalizations.

Jamie is currently trying to complete his bachelor's degree, one class at a time. He still lives with his parents, and although he would like to move out, he is unsure about his ability to live on his own. He does not have close friends but has become involved with a peer support center and sometimes volunteers there. Jamie hopes to finish his degree and eventually go on to graduate school in some area of psychology.

COURSE AND PROGNOSIS

Schizophrenia usually has an onset in late adolescence or early adulthood, most often between ages 16 and 25. Because schizophrenia usually occurs during early adulthood, many developmental tasks are disrupted, including forming close interpersonal or dating relationships, pursuing higher education, career development, separating from parents, and identity formation. Increased attention to first break or early onset psychosis may potentially avoid some of the long-term problems in these areas (Lincoln & McGorry, 1995). It is extremely rare for the first onset of schizophrenia to occur before adolescence (e.g., before age 12), and most diagnostic systems consider childhood-onset schizophrenia a disorder different from adolescent or adult onset (American Psychiatric Association, 1994). More common than childhood schizophrenia, but nevertheless rare in the total population of persons with schizophrenia, are individuals who develop the illness later in life, such as after age 45 (Cohen, 1990). Late-onset schizophrenia is characterized by positive symptoms but is less likely to involve formal thought disorder and negative symptoms (Bartels, Mueser, & Miles, 1998). Late-onset schizophrenia is further complicated by the lack of clear-cut distinguishing characteristics that discriminate this disorder from a variety of other disorders that develop later in old age (Howard, Almeida, & Levy, 1994).

Before onset of schizophrenia, some, but not all, persons have impairments in their premorbid social functioning (Zigler & Glick, 1986). For example, some people who later develop schizophrenia were more socially isolated, passed fewer social-sexual developmental milestones, and had fewer friends in childhood and adolescence. Aside from problems in social functioning, before developing schizophrenia, some children display a maladaptive pattern of behaviors, including disruptive behavior, problems in school, and impulsivity (Baum & Walker, 1995; Hans, Marcus, Henson, Auerbach, & Mirsky, 1992). Similarly, symptoms of conduct disorder in childhood, such as repeated fighting, truancy, and lying, have been found predictive of the later development of schizophrenia (Asarnow, 1988; Cannon, Mednick, Parnas, Schulsinger, Praestholm, & Vestergaard 1993; Neumann, Grimes, Walker, &

Baum 1995; Robins, 1966; Robins & Price, 1991; Rutter, 1984; Watt, 1978). However, other patients display no unusual characteristics in their premorbid functioning.

A second moderating factor related to the prognosis of schizophrenia is patient gender. Women tend to have a later age of onset of the illness, spend less time in hospitals, and demonstrate better social competence and social functioning than men who have the illness (Goldstein, 1988; Häfner et al., 1993; Mueser, Bellack, Morrison, & Wade, 1990). The benefits experienced by women are not explained by societal differences in tolerance for deviant behavior. Several different hypotheses have been advanced to account for the superior outcome of women with schizophrenia (e.g., biological differences and interactions with socioenvironmental stressors; Castle & Murray, 1991; Flor-Henry, 1985), but no single theory has received strong support.

In general, onset of schizophrenia can be described as either gradual or acute. The gradual onset of schizophrenia can take place over many months, and it may be difficult for family members and others to clearly distinguish the onset of the illness. In cases of acute onset, symptoms develop rapidly during a period of a few weeks, and dramatic and easily observed changes occur during this time. People who have acute onset of schizophrenia have a somewhat better prognosis than those who have a more insidious illness (Fenton & McGlashan, 1991; Kay & Lindenmayer, 1987).

Although schizophrenia is a long-term and severe psychiatric illness, there is considerable interindividual variability in the course of illness (Marengo, 1994). Generally, though, once schizophrenia has developed, the illness usually continues at varying degrees of severity throughout most of the person's life. Schizophrenia is usually an episodic illness, and periods of acute symptom severity require more intensive, often inpatient, treatment interspersed by periods of higher functioning between episodes. Despite the fact that most patients with schizophrenia live in the community, it is comparatively rare, at least in the short term, for patients to return to their premorbid levels of functioning between episodes.

Some general predictors of the course and outcome of schizophrenia have been identified, such as premorbid functioning, but overall, the ability to predict outcome is rather poor (Avison & Speechley, 1987; Tsuang, 1986). The primary reason is that symptom severity and functioning are determined by the dynamic interplay between biological vulnerability, environmental factors, and coping skills (Nuechterlein & Dawson, 1994; Liberman et al., 1986). Factors such as compliance with medication (Buchanan, 1992), substance abuse (Drake, Osher, & Wallach, 1989), exposure to a hostile or critical environment (Butzlaff & Hooley, 1998), the availability of psychosocial programming (Bellack & Mueser, 1993), and assertive case management and outreach (Mueser, Bond, Drake, & Resnick, 1998; Mueser, Drake, & Bond, 1997; Quinlivan et al., 1995) are all environmental factors that in combination play a large role in determining outcome.

The importance of environmental factors and rehabilitation programs in determining the outcome of schizophrenia is illustrated by two long-term outcome studies conducted by Harding and her associates (DeSisto, Harding, McCormick, Ashikaga, & Brooks, 1995; Harding, Brooks, Ashikaga, Strauss, & Breier, 1987a,b). The first study was conducted in Vermont, which had a highly developed system of community-based rehabilitation programs for persons who have severe mental illness. Patients in this study demonstrated surprisingly positive outcomes during the 20- to 40-year follow-up period. In contrast, similar patients in Maine, where more traditional hospital-based treatment programs existed, fared substantially worse during the long-term course of their illnesses. Thus, the outcome of most cases of schizophrenia is not predetermined by specific biological factors but rather is influenced by the interaction between biological and environmental factors.

In summary, the prognosis for schizophrenia is usually considered fair, and there is general agreement that it is worse than for other major psychiatric disorders, such as bipolar disorder or major depression. Despite widespread acceptance that schizophrenia is usually a lifelong disability, recent research on the long-term outcome of schizophrenia has challenged this assumption. Several long-term studies which have followed up patients 20 to 40 years after developing schizophrenia suggest that previous estimates of recovery from schizophrenia are overly conservative (Harding & Keller, 1998). Although definitions of "recovery" vary from one study to the next, some studies suggest as many as 20 to 50% of patients fully recover from schizophrenia later in life (Ciompi, 1980; Harding et al., 1987a,b).

FAMILIAL AND GENETIC CONSIDERATIONS

The etiology of schizophrenia has been a topic of much debate during the past one hundred years. Kraepelin (1919/1971) and Bleuler (1911/1950) clearly thought that the illness had a biological origin. However, from the 1920s to the 1960s, alternative theories gained prominence, speculating that the disease resulted from disturbed family interactions (Bateson, Jackson, Haley, & Weakland, 1956). Psychogenic theories of the etiology of schizophrenia, positing that the illness was psychological in nature, rather than biological, played a dominant role in shaping the attitudes and behavior of professionals toward patients with schizophrenia and their relatives (Fromm-Reichmann, 1950; Searles, 1965). These theories have not been supported empirically (Jacob, 1975; Waxler & Mishler, 1971). Moreover, in many cases, psychogenic theories fostered poor relationships between mental health professionals and relatives (Terkelsen, 1983), which have only begun to mend in recent years (Mueser & Glynn, 1999).

For more than a century, clinicians have often noted that schizophrenia tends to "run in families." However, the clustering of schizophrenia in family members could reflect learned behavior that is passed on from one generation to the next, rather than predisposing biological factors. In the 1950s and 1960s, two paradigms were developed for evaluating the genetic contributions to the illness. The first approach, the *high-risk* paradigm involves examining the rate of schizophrenia in adopted-away offspring of mothers with schizophrenia. If the rate of schizophrenia in children of biological parents with schizophrenia is higher than in the general population, even in the absence of contact with those parents, a role for genetic factors in developing the illness is supported. The second approach, the *monozygotic/dizygotic twin* paradigm involves comparing the concordance rate of schizophrenia in identical twins (monozygotic) compared to fraternal twins (dizygotic). Because monozygotic twins share the exact same gene pool, whereas dizygotic twins share only approximately half of their genes, a higher concordance rate of schizophrenia among monozygotic twins than dizygotic twins, even reared in the same environment, would support a role for genetic factors in the etiology of schizophrenia.

During the past thirty years, numerous studies employing either the high-risk or twin paradigm have examined the role of genetic factors in schizophrenia. Almost uniform agreement across studies has indicated that the risk of developing schizophrenia in biological relatives of persons with schizophrenia is greater than in the general population, even in the absence of any contact between the relatives (Kendler & Diehl, 1993). Thus, strong support exists for the role of genetic factors in the etiology of at least some cases of schizophrenia. For example, the risk that a woman with schizophrenia will give birth to a child who later develops schizophrenia is approximately 10%, compared to only 1% in the general population (Gottesman, 1991). Similarly, the risk that one identical twin will develop schizophrenia if his or her co-twin also has schizophrenia is between 25 and 50%, compared to a risk of about 10% for fraternal twins (Walker, Downey, & Caspi, 1991).

The fact that identical twins do not have a 100% concordance rate of schizophrenia, as might be expected if the disorder were purely genetic, has raised intriguing questions about the etiology of schizophrenia. Some have proposed that development of schizophrenia might be the consequence of an interaction between genetic and environmental factors. The results of one study suggest this might be the case. Tienari (1991; Tienari et al., 1987) compared the likelihood of developing schizophrenia in three groups of children raised by adoptive families. Two groups of children had biological mothers with schizophrenia and the third group had biological mothers who had no psychiatric disorder. The researchers divided the adoptive families of the children into two broad groups based on the level of disturbance in the family: healthy adoptive families and disturbed adoptive families. Follow-up assessments were conducted to determine presence of schizophrenia and other severe psychiatric disorders in the adopted children raised in all three groups. The researchers found that children of biological mothers with schizophrenia who were raised by adoptive families that had high levels of disturbance were significantly more likely to develop schizophrenia or another psychotic disorder (46%) than either similarly vulnerable children raised in families that had low levels of disturbance (5%) or children who had no biological vulnerability raised in either disturbed (24%) or healthy (3%) adoptive families. This study raises the intriguing possibility that some cases of schizophrenia develop as a result of the interaction between biological vulnerability and environmental stress.

Although there is strong evidence that genetic factors can play a role in the development of schizophrenia, there is also a growing body of evidence pointing to the critical influence of other biological, nongenetic factors. For example, obstetric complications, maternal exposure to the influenza virus, and other environmental insults to a developing fetus (e.g., maternal starvation) are all associated with an increased risk of developing schizophrenia (Geddes & Lawrie, 1995; Kirch, 1993; Rodrigo, Lusiardo, Briggs, & Ulmer, 1991; Susser & Lin, 1992; Susser et al., 1996; Takei et al., 1996; Torrey, Bowler, Rawlings, & Terrazas, 1993). Thus, there is a growing consensus that the etiology of schizophrenia may be heterogeneous; genetic factors play a role in the development of some cases, and early environmental factors play a role in the development of other cases. This heterogeneity may account for the fact that the genetic contribution to schizophrenia has consistently been lower than the genetic contribution to bipolar disorder (Goodwin & Jamison, 1990).

Although families do not cause schizophrenia, there are important interactions between the family and patient that deserve consideration. First, it has repeatedly been found that critical attitudes and high levels of emotional overinvolvement (Expressed Emotion—EE) on the part of the relatives toward the patient strongly predict the likelihood that patients will relapse and be rehospitalized (Butzlaff & Hooley, 1998). The importance of family factors is underscored by the fact that the severity of patients' psychiatric illness or their social skill impairments are not related to family EE (Mueser et al., 1993). Rather, family EE acts as a stressor that increases the vulnerability of patients with schizophrenia to relapse.

A second important family consideration is the amount of burden on relatives who care for a mentally ill person. Family members of patients with schizophrenia typically experience a wide range of negative emotions related to coping with the illness, such as anxiety, depression, guilt, and anger (Hatfield & Lefley, 1987, 1993; Oldridge & Hughes, 1992). Burden is even associated with negative health consequences for relatives (Dyck, Short, & Vitaliano, 1999). Family burden may be related to levels of expressed emotion, ability to cope with the illness, and ultimately the ability of the family to successfully monitor and manage the schizophrenia in a family member (Mueser & Glynn, 1999). Thus, Expressed Emotion and family burden are important areas for assessment and intervention (see Family Assessment later).

DIAGNOSTIC CONSIDERATIONS

The diagnostic criteria for schizophrenia are fairly similar across a variety of different diagnostic systems. In general, the diagnostic criteria specify some degree of social impairment, combined with positive and negative symptoms that last for a significant period (e.g., six months or more). The diagnostic criteria for schizophrenia according to DSM-IV (American Psychiatric Association, 1994) are summarized in Table 1.

The diagnosis of schizophrenia requires a clinical interview with the patient, a thorough review of all available records, and standard medical evaluations to rule out the possible role of organic factors (e.g., CAT scan to rule out a brain tumor). In addition, because many patients are poor historians or may not provide accurate accounts of their behavior, information from significant others, such as family members, is often critical in establishing a diagnosis of schizophrenia. Because of the wide variety of symptoms characteristic of schizophrenia and variations in interviewing style and format across different clinical interviewers, the use of structured clinical interviews, such as the Structured Clinical Interview for DSM-IV (First, Spitzer, Gibbon, & Williams, 1996) can greatly enhance the reliability and validity of psychiatric diagnosis.

Structured clinical interviews have two main advantages over more open clinical inter-

---

TABLE 1. DSM-IV Criteria for the Diagnosis of Schizophrenia

A. Presence of at least two of the following characteristic symptoms in the active phase for at least 1 month (unless the symptoms are successfully treated):
   1. Delusions
   2. Hallucinations
   3. Disorganized speech (e.g., frequent derailment or incoherence)
   4. Grossly disorganized or catatonic behavior
   5. Negative symptoms (i.e., affect flattening, alogia, or avolition)
      Note: only one of these symptoms is required if delusions are bizarre or hallucinations consist of a voice keeping a running commentary on the person's behavior or thoughts, or two or more voices conversing with each other.
B. Social/occupational dysfunction: For a significant proportion of the time from the onset of the disturbance, one or more areas of functioning, such as work, interpersonal relationships, or self-care, are markedly below the level achieved prior to the onset (or, when the onset is in childhood or adolescence, failure to achieve expected level of interpersonal, academic, or occupational achievement).
C. Duration: Continuous signs of the disturbance persist for at least 6 months. This 6-month period must include at least 1 month of symptoms that meet criterion A (i.e., active-phase symptoms) and may include periods of prodromal or residual symptoms. During these prodromal or residual periods, the signs fo the disturbance may be manifested only by negative symptoms or by two or more symptoms listed in criterion A present in an attenuated form (e.g., odd beliefs, unusual perceptual experiences).
D. Schizoaffective and mood disorders exclusion: Schizoaffective disorder and mood disorder with psychotic features have been ruled out because either (1) no major depressive or manic episodes have occurred concurrently with the active-phase symptoms or (2) if mood episodes have occurred during active-phase symptoms, their total duration has been brief relative to the duration of the active phase and residual periods.
E. Substance/general medical condition exclusion: The disturbance is not due to the direct effects of a substance (e.g., drugs of abuse, medication) or a general medical condition.

views. First, structured interviews provide definitions of the key symptoms agreed upon by experts, thus making explicit the specific symptoms required for diagnosis. Second, by conducting the interview in a standardized format, including a specific sequence of asking questions, variations in interviewing style are minimized, thus enhancing the comparability of diagnostic assessments across different clinicians. The second point is especially crucial considering that most research studies of schizophrenia employ structured interviews to establish diagnoses. If the findings of clinical research studies are to be generalized into clinical practice, efforts must be made to ensure the comparability of the patient populations and the assessment techniques employed.

The symptoms of schizophrenia overlap those of many other psychiatric disorders. Establishing a diagnosis of schizophrenia requires particularly close consideration of three other overlapping disorders: substance use disorders, affective disorders, and schizoaffective disorder. We discuss here issues related to each of these disorders and the diagnosis of schizophrenia.

Substance Use Disorders

Substance use disorder, such as alcohol dependence or drug abuse, can be either a differential diagnosis to schizophrenia or a comorbid disorder (i.e., the patient can have both schizophrenia *and* a substance use disorder). With respect to differential diagnosis, substance use disorders can interfere with a clinician's ability to diagnosis schizophrenia and can lead to misdiagnosis if the substance abuse is covert (Corty, Lehman, & Myers, 1993; Kranzler et al., 1995). Psychoactive substances, such as alcohol, marijuana, cocaine, and amphetamine, can produce symptoms that mimic those found in schizophrenia, such as hallucinations, delusions, and social withdrawal (Schuckit, 1995). Because diagnosis of schizophrenia requires the presence of specific symptoms in the absence of identifiable organic factors, schizophrenia can only be diagnosed in persons who have a history of substance use disorder by examining the individual's functioning during sustained periods of abstinence from drugs or alcohol. When such periods of abstinence can be identified, a reliable diagnosis of schizophrenia can be made. However, patients who have a long history of substance abuse and few or no periods of abstinence are more difficult to assess. For example, in a sample of 461 patients admitted to a psychiatric hospital, a psychiatric diagnosis could not be confirmed nor ruled out due to history of substance abuse in 71 patients (15%) (Lehman, Myers, Dixon, & Johnson, 1994).

Substance use disorder is the most common comorbid diagnosis for persons with schizophrenia. Because substance abuse can worsen the course and outcome of schizophrenia, recognition and treatment of substance abuse in schizophrenia is a critical goal of treatment. The diagnosis of substance abuse in schizophrenia is complicated by several factors. Substance abuse, as in the general population, is often denied due to social and legal sanctions (Stone, Greenstein, Gamble, & McLellan, 1993; Galletly, Field, & Prior, 1993), a problem that may be worsened in this population because of a fear of losing benefits. Denial of problems associated with substance abuse, a core feature of primary substance use disorders, may be further heightened by psychotic distortions and cognitive impairments present in schizophrenia. Furthermore, the criteria used to establish a substance use disorder in the general population are less useful for diagnosis in schizophrenia (Corse, Hirschinger, & Zanis, 1995). For example, the common consequences of substance abuse in the general population are loss of employment, driving under the influence of alcohol, and relationship problems. Those are less often experienced by people with schizophrenia, who are often unemployed, do not own cars, and have limited interpersonal relationships. Rather, patients with schizophrenia more often experience increased symptoms and rehospitalizations, legal problems, and housing instability secondary to substance abuse (Drake & Brunette, 1998).

Patients with schizophrenia tend to use smaller quantities of drugs and alcohol (Cohen & Klein, 1970; Crowley, Chesluk, Dilts, & Hart, 1974; Lehman et al., 1994) and rarely develop the full physical dependence syndrome that is often present in persons who have a primary substance use disorder (Corse et al., 1995; Drake et al., 1990; Test, Wallisch, Allness, & Ripp, 1989) or show other physical consequences of alcohol such as stigmata (Mueser, Rosenberg et al., 1999). Even very low scores on instruments developed for the primary substance use disorder population, such as the Addiction Severity Inventory, indicate substance use disorder in patients who have SMI (Appleby, Dyson, Altman, & Luchins, 1997; Corse et al., 1995; Lehman, Myers, Dixon, & Johnson, 1996). Because of the difficulties in using existing measures of substance abuse for people who have schizophrenia and other severe mental illnesses, a new screening tool was developed specifically for these populations: the Dartmouth Assessment of Lifestyle Instrument (DALI; Rosenberg et al., 1998). The DALI is an 18-item questionnaire that has high classification accuracy for current substance use disorders of alcohol, cannabis, and cocaine for people who have severe mental illness.

Despite difficulties involved in assessing comorbid substance abuse in patients with schizophrenia, recent developments in this area indicate that if appropriate steps are taken, reliable diagnoses can be made (Drake, Rosenberg, & Mueser, 1996). The most critical recommendations for diagnosing substance abuse in schizophrenia include (1) maintain a high index of suspicion of substance abuse, especially if a patient has a past history of substance abuse; (2) use multiple assessment techniques, including self-report instruments, interviews with patients, clinician reports, reports of significant others, and biological assays; and (3) be alert to signs that may be subtle indicators of a substance use disorder, such as unexplained symptom relapses, familial conflict, money management problems, and depression or suicidality. Once a substance use disorder has been diagnosed, integrated treatment that addresses both the schizophrenia and the substance use disorder is necessary to achieve a favorable clinical outcome (Drake, Mercer-McFadden, Mueser, McHugo, & Bond, 1998).

Affective Disorders

Schizophrenia overlaps the major affective disorders more prominently than any other psychiatric disorder. The differential diagnosis of schizophrenia from affective disorders is critical because the disorders respond to different treatments, particularly pharmacological interventions. Two different affective disorders, bipolar disorder and major depression, can be especially difficult to distinguish from schizophrenia. The differential diagnosis of these disorders from schizophrenia is complicated by the fact that affective symptoms (e.g., depression and grandiose delusions) are frequently present in persons with schizophrenia, and psychotic symptoms (e.g., hallucinations and delusions) may be present in persons who have major affective disorders (American Psychiatric Association, 1994; Pope & Lipinski, 1978).

The crux of making a differential diagnosis between schizophrenia and a major affective disorder is to determine whether psychotic symptoms are present *in the absence of* affective symptoms. If there is strong evidence that psychotic symptoms persist even when the person is not experiencing symptoms of mania or depression, then the diagnosis is either schizophrenia or the closely related disorder of schizoaffective disorder (discussed later). However, if symptoms of psychosis are present during an affective syndrome, but disappear when the person's mood is stable, the appropriate diagnosis is either major depression or bipolar disorder. For example, it is common for people who have bipolar disorder to have hallucinations and delusions during the height of a manic episode, but for these psychotic symptoms to subside when the person's mood becomes stable again. Similarly, persons who have major depression often experience hallucinations or delusions during a depressive episode, which subside as their moods improve. If the patient experiences chronic mood problems, meeting criteria for manic, depressive, or mixed episodes, it may be difficult or impossible to establish a diagnosis of schizophrenia because there are no sustained periods of stable mood.

Schizoaffective Disorder

Schizoaffective disorder is a diagnostic entity that overlaps the affective disorders and schizophrenia (American Psychiatric Association, 1994). As shown in Table 2, the following conditions must be met for a person to be diagnosed with schizoaffective disorder: (1) the person must meet criteria for an affective syndrome (i.e., a 2-week period in which manic, depressive, or mixed affective features are present to a significant degree), (2) the person must meet criteria for the symptoms of schizophrenia during a period when they are not experiencing an affective syndrome (e.g., hallucinations or delusions in the absence of manic or depressive symptoms), and (3) the affective syndrome must be present for a substantial period of the person's psychiatric illness (i.e., a patient who experiences brief affective syndromes and who is chronically psychotic and has other long-standing impairments would be diagnosed with schizophrenia, rather than schizoaffective disorder). Finally, (4) these three conditions must not be due to medical conditions or substances.

Schizoaffective disorder and major affective disorder are frequently mistaken for one another because it is incorrectly assumed that schizoaffective disorder simply requires the presence of both psychotic and affective symptoms. Rather, as described in the preceding section, if psychotic symptoms always coincide with affective symptoms, the person has an affective disorder, whereas if psychotic symptoms are present in the absence of an affective syndrome, the person meets criteria for either schizoaffective disorder or schizophrenia. Distinguishing between schizophrenia and schizoaffective disorder can be more difficult because judgment must be made whether affective symptoms have been present for a substantial part of the person's illness. Decision rules for determining the extent to which affective symptoms must be present to diagnose a schizoaffective disorder have not been established.

Although the differential diagnosis between schizophrenia and schizoaffective disorder is difficult, clinical implications of this distinction are less important than between the affective disorders and either schizophrenia or schizoaffective disorder. Research on family history and treatment response suggest that schizophrenia and schizoaffective disorder are similar disorders and respond to the same interventions (Mattes & Nayak, 1984; Levinson & Levitt, 1987; Kramer et al., 1989; Levinson & Mowry, 1991). In fact, many studies of schizophrenia

TABLE 2. DSM-IV Criteria for the Diagnosis of Schizoaffective Disorder

A. An uninterrupted period of illness which at some time there is either a major depressive episode (which must include depressed mood) or manic episode concurrent with symptoms that meet criterion A of schizophrenia.

B. During the same period of illness, there have been delusions or hallucinations for at least 2 weeks in the absence of prominent mood symptoms.

C. Symptoms meeting the criteria for a mood disorder are present for a substantial portion of the total duration of the active and residual periods of the illness.

D. The disturbance is not due to the direct effects of a substance (e.g., drugs of abuse, medication) or a general medical condition.

routinely include patients who have schizoaffective disorder and find few differences. Therefore, the information provided in this chapter on schizophrenia also pertains to schizoaffective disorder, and the differential diagnosis between the two disorders is not of major importance from a clinical perspective.

PSYCHOLOGICAL AND BIOLOGICAL ASSESSMENT

Diagnostic assessment provides important information about the potential utility of interventions for schizophrenia (e.g., antipsychotic medications). However, assessment does not end with a diagnosis. It must be supplemented with additional psychological and biological assessments.

Psychological Assessment

A wide range of different psychological formulations has been proposed for understanding schizophrenia. For example, there are extensive writings about psychodynamic and psychoanalytic interpretations of schizophrenia. Although this work has made contributions to the further development of these theories, these formulations have not improved the ability of clinicians to understand patients who have this disorder or led to more effective interventions (Mueser & Berenbaum, 1990). Therefore, use of projective assessment techniques based on psychodynamic concepts of personality, such as the Rorschach and Thematic Apperception Test, are not considered here.

As noted earlier, schizophrenia is often associated with impairments in memory, attention, abstract reasoning, and executive functioning. These impairments result in difficulties in generalizing new knowledge to different situations (i.e., transfer of training problems). Thus, assessment needs to be conducted in the environments in which the skills are to be used. For example, successful employment interventions incorporate ongoing assessment on the job, rather than extensive prevocational testing batteries that do not generalize to real-world settings (Bond, 1998; Drake & Becker, 1996). Similarly, when assessing independent living skills, these need to be measured directly in the patient's living environment or in simulated tests (Wallace, Liberman, Tauber, & Wallace, in press).

A great deal of research has been done on the functional assessment of social skills in people with schizophrenia. Social skills are individual behavioral components, such as eye contact, voice loudness, and the specific choice of words, which in combination are necessary for effective communication with others (Mueser & Bellack, 1998). As previously described, poor social competence is a hallmark of schizophrenia. Although not all problems in social functioning are the consequence of poor social skill, many social impairments are related to skill deficits (Bellack, Morrison, Wixted, & Mueser, 1990).

A number of different strategies can be used to assess social skill. Direct interviews with patients is a good starting place for identifying broad areas of social dysfunction. These interviews can focus on answering questions, such as, Is the patient lonely? Would the patient like more or closer friends? Is the patient able to stand up for his or her rights? Is the patient able to get others to respond positively? Patient interviews are most informative when combined with interviews with significant others, such as family members and clinicians who are familiar with the nature and quality of the patient's social interactions, as well as natural observations of the patient's social interactions. The combination of these sources of information is useful for identifying specific areas in need of social skills training.

One strategy for assessing social skills that yields the most specific type of information is role-play assessments. Role plays involve brief simulated social interactions between the patient and a confederate who takes the role of an interactive partner. During role plays, patients are instructed to act as though the situation were actually happening in real life. Role plays can be as brief as 15 to 30 seconds to assess skill areas such as initiating conversations or can be as long as several minutes to assess skills such as problem-solving ability. Role plays can be audiotaped or videotaped and later rated on specific dimensions of social skill. Alternatively, role playing can be embedded into procedures of social skills training, in which patients practice targeted social skills in role plays, followed by positive and corrective feedback and additional role play rehearsal. In the latter instance, the assessment of social skills is integrated into the training of new skills, rather than proceeding skills training.

Recent research on the reliability and validity of social skill assessments and benefits of social skills training for patients with schizophrenia has demonstrated the utility of the social skills construct. Patients with schizophrenia, it has been consistently found, have worse social skills than patients who have other psychiatric disorders (Bellack, Morrison, Wixted, & Mueser, 1990; Bellack, Mueser, Wade, Sayers, & Morrison, 1992; Mueser, Bellack, Douglas, & Wade, 1991), and approximately half of the patients with schizophrenia demonstrate stable deficits in basic social skills compared to the nonpsychiatric population (Mueser, Bellack, Douglas, & Morrison, 1991). In the absence of skills training, social skills tend to be stable over periods of time as long as six months to one year (Mueser, Bellack, Douglas, & Morrison, 1991). Social skill in patients with schizophrenia is moderately correlated with the level of premorbid social functioning, current role functioning, and quality of life (Mueser, Bellack, Morrison, & Wixted, 1990). Social skills tend to be associated with negative symptoms (Appelo et al., 1992; Bellack, Morrison, Wixted, & Mueser, 1990; Lysaker, Bell, Zito, & Bioty, 1995; Penn, Mueser, Spaulding, Hope, & Reed, 1995) but not with positive symptoms (Mueser, Douglas, Bellack, & Morrison, 1991; Penn et al., 1995). Furthermore, role-play assessments of social skill are also strongly related with social skill in more natural contexts, such as interactions with significant others (Bellack, Morrison, Mueser, Wade, & Sayers, 1990). Patients with schizophrenia show a wide range of impairments in social skill, including areas such as conversational skill, conflict resolution, assertiveness, and problem solving (Bellack, Sayers, Mueser, & Bennett, 1994; Douglas & Mueser, 1990). Thus, ample research demonstrates that the social skills of patients with schizophrenia are impaired, tend to be stable over time in the absence of intervention, and are strongly related to other measures of social functioning. Furthermore, there is growing evidence that supports the efficacy of social skills training for schizophrenia (Dilk & Bond, 1996; Liberman, Wallace, Blackwell, Kopelowicz, Vaccaro, & Mintz, 1998; Marder et al., 1996).

Family Assessment

Assessment of family functioning is highly relevant in schizophrenia for two reasons. As discussed earlier, EE is an important stressor that can increase the chance of relapse and rehospitalization. In addition, family burden has its own negative consequences and can be related to EE and the ability of the family to care for the person with schizophrenia. Thus, a thorough assessment of these family factors is important to identify targets for family intervention.

A number of specific methods can be used to assess a negative emotional climate in the family and the burden of the illness. Interviews of individual family members, including the patient and the entire family, coupled with observation of more natural family interactions, can provide invaluable information about the quality of family functioning. The vast majority of research on family EE has employed semistructured interviews of individual family members, the Camberwell Family Interview (Leff & Vaughn, 1985). This is primarily a research instrument, and it is too time-consuming for clinical practice. Alternatives to the Camberwell Family Interview have been proposed (e.g., Magaña et al., 1986), although none has yet gained widespread acceptance. Several studies have successfully employed the Family Environment Scale (Moos & Moos, 1981), a self-report instrument completed by family members, which it has been found, is related to symptoms and outcome in patients with schizophrenia (Halford, Schweitzer, & Varghese, 1991).

Many instruments have been developed for assessing family burden. The most comprehensive instrument that has well-established psychometric properties is the Family Experiences Interview Schedule (Tessler & Gamache, 1995). This measure provides information regarding both the dimensions of the subjective burden (e.g., emotional strain) and the objective burden (e.g., economic impact), as well as specific areas in which the burden is most severe (e.g., household tasks).

The importance of evaluating family functioning is supported by research demonstrating clinical benefits of family intervention for schizophrenia. More than 10 long-term controlled studies of family treatment for schizophrenia have shown that family intervention has a significant impact on reducing relapse rates and rehospitalizations (Baucom, Shoham, Mueser, Daiuto, & Stickle, 1998). The critical elements shared across different models of family intervention are education about schizophrenia, the provision of ongoing support, improved communication skills, and a focus on helping all family members improve the quality of their lives (Dixon & Lehman, 1995; Glynn, 1992; Lam, 1991).

Biological Assessment

Biological assessments are becoming more common in the clinical management of schizophrenia. For diagnosis, biological assessments may be used to rule out possible organic factors such as a tumor, stroke, or covert substance abuse. Urine and blood specimens are sometimes obtained to evaluate the presence of substance abuse. Similarly, blood samples may be obtained to determine whether the patient is compliant with the prescribed antipsychotic medication, although the specific level of medication in the blood has not been conclusively linked to clinical response. Blood levels may also be monitored to ensure appropriate levels of mood stabilizers (e.g., lithium). Some newer medications also require ongoing blood tests to detect very rare but potentially lethal blood disorders (Alvir, Lieberman, & Safferman, 1995; Young, Bowers, & Mazure, 1998).

Biological measures are sometimes used to characterize impairments in brain functioning that are associated with schizophrenia, although these assessments do not have clear implications for treatment of the illness at this time. For example, CAT scans of the brain indicate that between one-half and two-thirds of all patients with schizophrenia have enlarged cerebral ventricles, indicative of cortical atrophy (Liddle, 1995). Similarly, magnetic resonance imaging (MRI) studies show reduced brain volume in several brain structures for people with schizophrenia (Lawrie & Abukmeil, 1998). In addition, MRI studies, positron emission tomography (PET), and single photon emission computerized tomography (SPECT) have shown reduced metabolism and blood flow in several cortical and subcortical areas (Kindermann, Karimi, Symonds, Brown, & Jeste, 1997; Liddle, 1997; McClure, Keshaven, & Pettegrew, 1998). Gross structural impairments in brain functioning, such as enlarged ventricles, tend to be associated with a wide range of neuropsychological impairments and negative symptoms often present in schizophrenia (Andreasen, Flaum, Swayze, Tyrrell, & Arndt, 1990; Buchanan et al., 1993; Merriam, Kay, Opler, Kushner, & van Praag, 1990).

To date, most of the advances in treating schizophrenia have been in psychopharmacology. Biological assessments are still not useful for diagnosing the illness or for guiding treatment. However, the clinical utility of biological assessment is likely to increase in the years to come as advances continue in understanding the biological roots of schizophrenia.

GENDER, ETHNIC, AND CULTURAL ISSUES

A number of issues related to gender are important for understanding the psychopathology in the course of schizophrenia. As described in the section on course and prognosis, women tend to have a milder overall course of schizophrenia than men. The net consequence of this is that, although similar numbers of men and women have schizophrenia, men are more likely to receive treatment for the disorder. In fact, most research on the treatment of schizophrenia is conducted on samples ranging from 60 to 100% male.

Because treatment studies usually sample patients who are currently receiving treatment, often inpatient treatment, the efficacy of widely studied psychosocial interventions, such as social skills training and family therapy has been less adequately demonstrated for women. For example, some research suggests that social skills training may be more helpful to men than to women (Mueser, Levine, Bellack, Douglas, & Brady, 1990; Schaub, Behrendt, Brenner, Mueser, & Liberman, 1998; Smith et al., 1997). There is need for more research on the effects of treatments for women with schizophrenia. At the same time, further consideration needs to be given to the different needs of women who have this illness. For example, women with schizophrenia are much more likely to marry and have children then men. Therefore, it is crucial that psychosocial interventions be developed to address the relationship, family planning, and parenting needs of women with schizophrenia (Apfel & Handel, 1993; Coverdale & Grunebaum, 1998).

Another issue related to gender that is in need of further consideration is exposure to trauma. As described earlier, people with schizophrenia are at risk of being victims of violence. Although both men and women with schizophrenia report histories of abuse and assault, women report more sexual assault (Mueser, Goodman, et al., 1998). Further, in the general population, women are more likely to be abused than men, are more likely to sustain injuries, and are more likely to be economically dependent upon perpetrators of domestic violence. Thus, there is particular need to recognize and address trauma in the lives of women with schizophrenia. Accurate detection of trauma is further complicated by the fact that most severely mentally ill persons who have been physically or sexually assaulted deny that they have been "abused" (Cascardi et al., 1996). Development of programs that address the cause of domestic violence and their sequelae, especially for women with schizophrenia, is a priority in this area (see Harris, 1996).

Research on the relationships between race, ethnicity, and severe psychiatric disorders demonstrates that cultural factors are critical to understanding how persons with schizophrenia are perceived by others in their social milieu, as well as the course of the illness. Although prevalence of schizophrenia is comparable across different cultures, several studies have shown that course of the illness is more benign in developing countries compared to industrialized nations (Lo & Lo, 1977; Murphy & Raman, 1971; Sartorius et al., 1986). Westermeyer (1989) has raised questions about the comparability of patient samples in cross-cultural studies, but a consensus remains that the course of schizophrenia tends to be milder in nonindustrialized countries (Jablensky, 1989).

Several different interpretations have been offered to account for the better prognosis of schizophrenia in some cultures (Lefley, 1990). It is possible that the strong stigma and social rejection that results from severe mental illness and poses an obstacle to patient's ability to cope effectively with their disorders and assimilate into society (Fink & Tasman, 1992) is less prominent in some cultures (Parra, 1985). Greater cultural and societal acceptance of the social deviations in schizophrenia may enable patients to live less stressful and more productive lives. Family ties, in particular, may be stronger in developing countries or in certain ethnic minorities and less vulnerable to the disorganizing effects of mental illness (Lin & Kleinman, 1988). For example, Liberman (1994) has described how the strong functional ties of severely mentally ill persons to their families and work foster the reintegration of patients back into Chinese society following psychiatric hospitalization. In contrast, until recently, families of patients with schizophrenia in many Western societies were viewed by mental health professionals as either irrelevant, or worse, as causal agents in the development of the illness (Lefley, 1990; Mueser & Glynn, 1999), thus precluding them from a role in psychiatric rehabilitation. Furthermore, the use of other social supports such as importance of the church to the African-American community and its potential therapeutic benefits may vary across different ethnic groups or cultures (Griffith, Young, & Smith, 1984; Lincoln & Mamiya, 1990).

Some have hypothesized that different cultural interpretations of the individual's role in society and of the causes of mental illness may interact to determine course and outcome. Estroff (1989) has suggested that the emphasis on the "self" in Western countries, compared to a more family or societally based identification, has an especially disabling effect on persons with schizophrenia, whose sense of self is often fragile or fragmented. Another important consideration is the availability of adaptive concepts for understanding mental illness. For example, *espiritsmo* in Puerto Rican culture is a system of beliefs that involve interactions between the invisible spirit world and the visible world in which spirits can attach themselves to persons (Comas-Díaz, 1981; Morales-Dorta, 1976). Spirits are hierarchically ordered in terms of their moral perfection, and the practice of espiritismo is guided by helping individuals who are spiritually ill to achieve higher levels of this perfection. Troubled persons are not identified as "sick" nor are they blamed for their difficulties; in some cases, symptoms such as hallucinations may be interpreted favorably as signs that the person is advanced in spiritual development, resulting in some prestige (Comas-Díaz, 1981). Thus, certain cultural interpretations of schizophrenia may promote more acceptance of persons who display the symptoms of schizophrenia, as well as avoiding the common assumption that these phenomenological experiences are the consequence of a chronic, unremitting condition.

Understanding different cultural beliefs, values, and social structures can have important implications for the diagnosis of schizophrenia. Religious practices and beliefs may complicate diagnosis. For example, high levels of religiosity have been found in people with schizophrenia (Brewerton, 1994). Without a clear understanding of their religious and cultural backgrounds, patients may be misdiagnosed (May, 1997). Ethnic groups may differ in their willingness to report symptoms, as illustrated by one study which reported that African-American patients were less likely to report symptoms than Hispanics or non-Hispanic Whites (Skilbeck, Acosta, Yamamoto, & Evans, 1984). Other studies have found that African-Americans are more likely to be diagnosed with schizophrenia than other ethnic groups (e.g., Adams, Dworkin, & Rosenberg, 1984). Knowledge of cultural norms appears critical to avoid the possible misinterpretation of culturally bound beliefs and practices when arriving at a diagnosis. Several studies have shown that ethnic differences in diagnosis vary as a function of both the patient's and the interviewer's ethnicity (Baskin, Bluestone, & Nelson, 1981; Loring & Powell, 1988). Misdiagnosis of affective disorders as schizophrenia is the most common problem with the diagnosis of ethnic minorities in the United States (e.g., Jones, Gray, & Parsons, 1981, 1983).

Cultural differences are also critical in treating schizophrenia, both with respect to service utilization and the nature of treatment provided. There is a growing body of information documenting the fact that ethnic groups differ in their use of psychiatric services. A number of studies have indicated that Hispanics and Asian-Americans use fewer psychiatric services than non-Hispanic Whites, whereas Blacks utilize more emergency and inpatient services (Cheung & Snowden, 1990; Hough et al., 1987; Hu, Snowden, Jerrell, & Nguyen, 1991; Padgett, Patrick, Burns, & Schlesinger, 1994; Sue, Fujino, Hu, Takeuchi, & Zane, 1991). Aside from culturally based practices that may cause some individuals to seek assistance outside the mental health system (e.g., practitioners of *santeria*; González-Wippler, 1992), access to and retention in mental health services may be influenced by the proximity of mental health services (Dworkin & Adams, 1987) and by the ethnicity of treatment providers. Sue et al. (1991) reported that matching clinician and client ethnicity resulted in higher retention of ethnic minorities in mental health services. Increasing access to needed services for racial/ ethnic minorities may require a range of strategies, including ensuring that services are available in the communities where clients live, working with the natural social supports in the community, awareness of relevant cultural norms, and adequate representation of ethnic minorities as treatment providers.

Cultural factors may have an important bearing on psychotherapeutic treatments provided for schizophrenia. Sue and Sue (1990) described the importance of providing psychotherapy driven by goals that are compatible with clients' cultural norms. This requires both knowledge of subcultural norms and familiarity with the other social support mechanisms typically available to those clients. Interventions developed for one cultural group may need substantial modification to be effective in other groups. For example, Telles et al. (1995) reported that behavioral family therapy, which has been found effective in reducing relapse in schizophrenia for samples of non-Hispanic White and African American patients (Mueser & Glynn, 1999), was significantly less effective for Hispanic-Americans (of Mexican, Guatemalan, and Salvadoran descent) who had low levels of acculturation than for more acculturated patients. However, adaptations of the same family model were effective for samples of Chinese patients (Xiong et al., 1994; Zhang, Wang, Li, & Phillips, 1994). These findings underscore the importance of tailoring psychosocial interventions to meet the unique needs of clients from different cultural backgrounds.

A final cultural factor is stigma, that is, negative attitudes that lead to prejudice and discrimination against people with schizophrenia. Although a stigma can be present for a variety of disabilities, attitudes towards people who have severe mental illness tend to be more negative (Corrigan & Penn, 1999). Stigma may stem from the characteristics of the disorder itself, such as poor social skills, bizarre behavior, and unkempt appearance, and stigma may develop and be maintained through negative media portrayals and myths (e.g., dangerousness, unpredictability) (Farina, 1998). Stigma and discrimination can greatly undermine the person's ability to recover from the effects of schizophrenia and integrate into society. For example, people who have severe mental illness identify role functioning, such as employment, developing and maintaining friendships and intimate relationships, and regular activities as critical to their recovery (Uttaro & Mechanic, 1994). However, many studies have shown that these are the very areas most affected by stigma (Farina, 1998). Much is being done to try to reduce the stigma associated with schizophrenia and other mental illness. In particular, strategies that involve active education and increased contact with people with mental illness may be most effective in eradicating this serious problem (Corrigan & Penn, 1999).

SUMMARY

Schizophrenia is a severe, long-term psychiatric illness characterized by impairments in social functioning, the ability to work, self-care skills, positive symptoms (hallucinations, delusions), negative symptoms (social withdrawal, apathy), and cognitive impairments. Schizophrenia is a relatively common illness that afflicts approximately 1% of the population. It tends to have an episodic course over the lifetime, and symptoms gradually improve over the long term. Most evidence indicates that schizophrenia is a biological illness that may be caused by a variety of factors, such as genetic contributions and early environmental influences (e.g., insults to the developing fetus). Despite the biological nature of schizophrenia, environmental stress can either precipitate the onset of the illness or symptom relapses. Schizophrenia can be reliably diagnosed with structured clinical interviews, and particular attention must be paid to the differential diagnosis of affective disorders. There is a high comorbidity of substance use disorders in persons with schizophrenia, which must be treated if positive outcomes are to occur. The psychological assessment of schizophrenia is most useful when it focuses on the behavioral, rather than the dynamic dimensions of the illness. Thus, assessments and interventions focused on social skill deficits and family functioning have yielded promising treatment results. Biological assessments are useful at this time primarily for descriptive, rather than clinical purposes. Finally, a great many issues related to gender and racial or ethnic factors remain unexplored. Although schizophrenia remains one of the most challenging psychiatric illnesses to treat, substantial advances have been made in recent years in developing reliable diagnostic systems, understanding the role of various etiological factors, developing effective pharmacological and psychosocial treatments, and identifying factors that mediate the long term outcome of the illness, such as stress and substance abuse. These developments bode well for the ability of researchers and clinicians to continue making headway in treating this serious illness.

REFERENCES

Adams, G. L., Dworkin, R. J., & Rosenberg, S. D. (1984). Diagnosis and pharmacotherapy issues in the care of Hispanics in the public sector. *American Journal of Psychiatry, 141*, 970–974.

Alvir, J. M. J., Lieberman, J. A., & Safferman, A. Z. (1995). Do white-cell count spikes predict agranulocytosis in clozapine recipients? *Psychopharmacology Bulletin, 31*, 311–314.

Amador, X. F., & Gorman, J. M. (1998). Psychopathologic domains and insight in schizophrenia. *Psychiatric Clinics of North America, 21*, 27–42.

Amador, X., Strauss, D., Yale, S., & Gorman, J. M. (1991). Awareness of illness in schizophrenia. *Schizophrenia Bulletin, 17*, 113–132.

American Psychiatric Association. (1994). *Diagnostic and statistical manual of mental disorders*, 4th ed. (DSM-IV). Washington, DC: Author.

Andreasen, N. C., Flaum, M., Swayze, V. W., II, Tyrrell, G., & Arndt, S. (1990). Positive and negative symptoms in schizophrenia: A critical reappraisal. *Archives of General Psychiatry, 47*, 615–621.

Apfel, R. J., & Handel, M. H. (1993). *Madness and loss of motherhood: Sexuality, reproduction, and long-term mental illness*. Washington, DC: American Psychiatric Press.

Appelo, M. T., Woonings, F. M. J., van Nieuwenhuizen, C. J., Emmelkamp, P. M. G., Sloof, C. J., & Louwerens, J. W. (1992). Specific skills and social competence in schizophrenia. *Acta Psychiatrica Scandinavica, 85*, 419–422.

Appleby, L., Dyson, V., Altman, E., & Luchins, D. (1997). Assessing substance use in multiproblem patients: Reliability and validity of the Addiction Severity Index in a mental hospital population. *Journal of Nervous and Mental Disease, 185*, 159–165.

Argyle, N. (1990). Panic attacks in chronic schizophrenia. *British Journal of Psychiatry, 157*, 430–433.

Aro, S., Aro, H., & Keskimäki, I. (1995). Socio-economic mobility among patients with schizophrenia or major affective disorder: A 17-year retrospective follow-up. *British Journal of Psychiatry, 166*, 759–767.

Asarnow, J. R. (1988). Children at risk for schizophrenia. Converging lines of evidence. *Schizophrenia Bulletin, 14*, 613–631.

Avison, W. R., & Speechley, K. N. (1987). The discharged psychiatric patient: A review of social, social-psychological, and psychiatric correlates of outcome. *American Journal of Psychiatry, 144*, 10–18.

Bartels, S. J., Mueser, K. T., & Miles, K. M. (1998). Schizophrenia. In M. Hersen & V. B. Van Hasselt (Eds.), *Handbook of clinical geropsychology* (pp. 173–194). New York: Plenum.

Baskin, D., Bluestone, H., & Nelson, M. (1981). Ethnicity and psychiatric diagnosis. *Journal of Clinical Psychology, 37*, 529–537.

Bateson, G., Jackson, D. D., Haley, J., & Weakland, J. (1956). Toward a theory of schizophrenia. *Behavioral Science, 1*, 251–264.

Baucom, D. H., Shoham, V., Mueser, K. T., Daiuto, A. D., & Stickle, T. R. (1998). Empirically supported couple and family interventions for adult mental health problems. *Journal of Consulting and Clinical Psychology, 66*, 53–88.

Baum, K. M., & Walker, E. F. (1995). Childhood behavioral precursors of adult symptom dimensions in schizophrenia. *Schizophrenia Research, 16*, 111–120.

Bellack, A. S., Gold, J. M., & Buchanan, R. W. (1999). Cognitive rehabilitation for schizophrenia: Problems, prospects, and strategies. *Schizophrenia Bulletin, 25*, 257–274.

Bellack, A. S., Morrison, R. L., Mueser, K. T., Wade, J. H., & Sayers, S. L. (1990). Role play for assessing the social competence of psychiatric patients. *Psychological Assessment, 2*, 248–255.

Bellack, A. S., Morrison, R. L., Wixted, J. T., & Mueser, K. T. (1990). An analysis of social competence in schizophrenia. *British Journal of Psychiatry, 156*, 809–818.

Bellack, A. S., & Mueser, K. T. (1993). Psychosocial treatment for schizophrenia. *Schizophrenia Bulletin, 19*, 317–336.

Bellack, A. S., Mueser, K. T., Wade, J. H., Sayers, S. L., & Morrison, R. L. (1992). The ability of schizophrenics to perceive and cope with negative affect. *British Journal of Psychiatry, 160*, 473–480.

Bellack, A. S., Sayers, M., Mueser, K. T., & Bennett, M. (1994). An evaluation of social problem solving in schizophrenia. *Journal of Abnormal Psychology, 103*, 371–378.

Bleuler, E. (1950). *Dementia praecox or the group of schizophrenias* (J. Zinkin, Trans.). New York: International Universities Press. (Original work published 1911).

Bond, G. R. (1998). Principles of the individual placement and support model: Empirical support. *Psychiatric Rehabilitation Journal, 22*, 11–23.

Brekke, J. S., Raine, A., Ansel, M., Lencz, T., & Bird, L. (1997). Neuropsychological and psychophysiological correlates of psychosocial functioning in schizophrenia. *Schizophrenia Bulletin, 23*, 19–28.

Breslau, N., Davis, G. C., Andreski, P., & Peterson, E. (1991). Traumatic events and posttraumatic stress disorder in an urban population of young adults. *Archives of General Psychiatry, 48*, 216–222.

Brewerton, T. D. (1994). Hyperreligiosity in psychotic disorders. *Journal of Nervous and Mental Disease, 182*, 302–304.

Bruce, M. L., Takeuchi, D. T., & Leaf, P. J. (1991). Poverty and psychiatric status: Longitudinal evidence from the New Haven epidemiologic catchment area study. *Archives of General Psychiatry, 48*, 470–474.

Buchanan, A. (1992). A two-year prospective study of treatment compliance in patients with schizophrenia. *Psychological Medicine, 22*, 787–797.

Buchanan, R. W., Breier, A., Kirkpatrick, B., Elkashef, A., Munson, R. C., Gellad, F., & Carpenter, W. T. (1993). Structural abnormalities in deficit and nondeficit schizophrenia. *American Journal of Psychiatry, 150*, 59–65.

Butzlaff, R. L., & Hooley, J. M. (1998). Expressed emotion and psychiatric relapse: A meta-analysis. *Archives of General Psychiatry, 55*, 547–552.

Cannon, T. D., Mednick, S. A., Parnas, J., Schulsinger, F., Praestholm, J., & Vestergaard, A. (1993). Developmental brain abnormalities in the offspring of schizophrenic mothers. *Archives of General Psychiatry, 50*, 551–564.

Carmen, E., Rieker, P. P., & Mills, T. (1984). Victims of violence and psychiatric illness. *American Journal of Psychiatry, 141*, 378–383.

Cascardi, M., Mueser, K. T., DeGirolomo, J., & Murrin, M. (1996). Physical aggression against psychiatric inpatients by family members and partners: A descriptive study. *Psychiatric Services, 47*, 531–533.

Castle, D. J., & Murray, R. M. (1991). Editorial: The neurodevelopmental basis of sex differences in schizophrenia. *Psychological Medicine, 21*, 565–575.

Cheung, F. K., & Snowden, L. R. (1990). Community mental health and ethnic minority populations. *Community Mental Health Journal, 26*, 277–289.

Chilcoat, H. D., & Breslau, N. (1998). Posttraumatic stress disorder and drug disorders: Testing causal pathways. *Archives of General Psychiatry, 55*, 913–917.

Ciompi, L. (1980). Catamnestic long-term study of life and aging in chronic schizophrenic patients. *Schizophrenia Bulletin, 6*, 606–618.

Cohen, C. I. (1990). Outcome of schizophrenia into later life: An overview. *The Gerontologist, 30*, 790–797.

Cohen, M., & Klein, D. F. (1970). Drug abuse in a young psychiatric population. *American Journal of Orthopsychiatry, 40*, 448–455.

Comas-Díaz, L. (1981). Puerto Rican espiritismo and psychotherapy. *American Journal of Orthopsychiatry, 51,* 636–645.

Corrigan, P. W., Liberman, R. P., & Engle, J. D. (1990). From noncompliance to collaboration in the treatment of schizophrenia. *Hospital and Community Psychiatry, 41,* 1203–1211.

Corrigan, P. W., & Penn, D. L. (1999). Lessons from social psychology on discrediting psychiatric stigma. *American Psychologist, 54,* 765–776.

Corse, S. J., Hirschinger, N. B., & Zanis, D. (1995). The use of the Addiction Severity Index with people with severe mental illness. *Psychiatric Rehabilitation Journal, 19,* 9–18.

Corty, E., Lehman, A. F., & Myers, C. P. (1993). Influence of psychoactive substance use on the reliability of psychiatric diagnosis. *Journal of Consulting and Clinical Psychology, 61,* 165–170.

Coverdale, J. H., & Grunebaum, H. (1998). Sexuality and family planning. In K. T. Mueser & N. Tarrier (Eds.), *Social functioning in schizophrenia* (pp. 224–237). Boston: Allyn & Bacon.

Craine, L. S., Henson, C. E., Colliver, J. A., & MacLean, D. G. (1988). Prevalence of a history of sexual abuse among female psychiatric patients in a state hospital system. *Hospital and Community Psychiatry, 39,* 300–304.

Crowley, T. J., Chesluk, D., Dilts, S., & Hart, R. (1974). Drug and alcohol abuse among psychiatric admissions. *Archives of General Psychiatry, 30,* 13–20.

Davies-Netzley, S., Hurlburt, M. S., & Hough, R. (1996). Childhood abuse as a precursor to homelessness for homeless women with severe mental illness. *Violence and Victims, 11,* 129–142.

DeSisto, M. J., Harding, C. M., McCormick, R. V., Ashikaga, T., & Brooks, G. W. (1995). The Maine and Vermont three-decade studies of serious mental illness: I. Matched comparison of cross-sectional outcome. *British Journal of Psychiatry, 167,* 331–342.

Dilk, M. N., & Bond, G. R. (1996). Meta-analytic evaluation of skills training research for individuals with severe mental illness. *Journal of Consulting and Clinical Psychology, 64,* 1337–1346.

Dixon, L. B., & Lehman, A. F. (1995). Family interventions for schizophrenia. *Schizophrenia Bulletin, 21,* 631–643.

Dohrenwend, B. R., Levav, I., Shrout, P. E., Schwartz, S., Naveh, G., Link, B. G., Skodol, A. E., & Stueve, A. (1992). Socioeconomic status and psychiatric disorders: The causation-selection issue. *Science, 255,* 946–952.

Douglas, M. S., & Mueser, K. T. (1990). Teaching conflict resolution skills to the chronically mentally ill: Social skills training groups for briefly hospitalized patients. *Behavior Modification, 14,* 519–547.

Drake, R. E., & Becker, D. R. (1996). The individual placement and support model of supported employment. *Psychiatric Services, 47,* 473–475.

Drake, R. E., & Brunette, M. F. (1998). Complications of severe mental illness related to alcohol and drug use disorders. In M. Galanter (Ed.), *Recent developments in alcoholism,* Vol. 14: *The consequences of alcoholism* (pp. 285–299). New York: Plenum.

Drake, R. E., Gates, C., Whitaker, A., & Cotton, P. G. (1985). Suicide among schizophrenics: A review. *Comprehensive Psychiatry, 26,* 90–100.

Drake, R. E., Mercer-McFadden, C., Mueser, K. T., McHugo, G. J., & Bond, G. R. (1998). Review of integrated mental health and substance abuse treatment for patients with dual disorders. *Schizophrenia Bulletin, 24,* 589–608.

Drake, R. E., Osher, F. C., Noordsy, D. L., Hurlbut, S. C., Teague, G. B., & Beaudett, M. S. (1990). Diagnosis of alcohol use disorders in schizophrenia. *Schizophrenia Bulletin, 16,* 57–67.

Drake, R. E., Osher, F. C., & Wallach, M. A. (1989). Alcohol use and abuse in schizophrenia: A prospective community study. *Journal of Nervous and Mental Disease, 177,* 408–414.

Drake, R. E., Rosenberg, S. D., & Mueser, K. T. (1996). Assessment of substance use disorder in persons with severe mental illness. In R. E. Drake & K. T. Mueser (Eds.), *Dual diagnosis of major mental illness and substance abuse disorder II: Recent research and clinical implications. New directions in mental health services,* Vol. 70 (pp. 3–17). San Francisco: Jossey-Bass.

Dworkin, R. J., & Adams, G. L. (1987). Retention of Hispanics in public sector mental health services. *Community Mental Health Journal, 23,* 204–216.

Dyck, D. G., Short, R., & Vitaliano, P. P. (1999). Predictors of burden and infectious illness in schizophrenia caregivers. *Psychosomatic Medicine, 61,* 411–419.

Eaton, W. W. (1975). Marital status and schizophrenia. *Acta Psychiatrica Scandinavica, 52,* 320–329.

Estroff, S. E. (1989). Self, identity, and subjective experiences of schizophrenia: In search of the subject. *Schizophrenia Bulletin, 15,* 189–196.

Farina, A. (1998). Stigma. In K. T. Mueser & N. Tarrier (Eds.), *Handbook of social functioning in schizophrenia* (pp. 247–279). Boston: Allyn & Bacon.

Fenton, W. S., & McGlashan, T. H. (1991). Natural history of schizophrenia subtypes: II. Positive and negative symptoms and long term course. *Archives of General Psychiatry, 48,* 978–986.

Fink, P. J., & Tasman, A. (Eds.). (1992). *Stigma and mental illness*. Washington, DC: American Psychiatric Press.

First, M. B., Spitzer, R. L., Gibbon, M., & Williams, J. B. W. (1996). *Structured clinical interview for Axes I and II DSM-IV disorders-patient ed.* New York: Biometrics Research Department, New York State Psychiatric Institute.

Flor-Henry, P. (1985). Schizophrenia: Sex differences. *Canadian Journal of Psychiatry, 30*, 319–322.

Fox, J. W. (1990). Social class, mental illness, and social mobility: The social selection-drift hypothesis for serious mental illness. *Journal of Health and Social Behavior, 31*, 344–353.

Fromm-Reichmann, F. (1950) *Principles of intensive psychotherapy*. Chicago: University of Chicago Press.

Galletly, C. A., Field, C. D., & Prior, M. (1993). Urine drug screening of patients admitted to a state psychiatric hospital. *Hospital and Community Psychiatry, 44*, 587–589.

Geddes, J. R., & Lawrie, S. M. (1995). Obstetric complications and schizophrenia: A meta-analysis. *British Journal of Psychiatry, 167*, 786–793.

Glynn, S. M. (1992). Family-based treatment for major mental illness: A new role for psychologists. *The California Psychologist, 25*, 22–23.

Glynn, S. M. (1998). Psychopathology and social functioning in schizophrenia. In K. T. Mueser & N. Tarrier (Eds.), *Handbook of social functioning in schizophrenia* (pp. 66–78). Boston: Allyn & Bacon.

Goldman, H. H. (1982). Mental illness and family burden: A public health perspective. *Hospital and Community Psychiatry, 33*, 557–560.

Goldstein, J. M. (1988). Gender differences in the course of schizophrenia. *American Journal of Psychiatry, 146*, 684–689.

González-Wippler, M. (1992). *Powers of the Orishas: Santeria and the worship of saints*. New York: Original Publications.

Goodman, L. A., Dutton, M. A., & Harris, M. (1995). Physical and sexual assault prevalence among episodically homeless women with serious mental illness. *American Journal of Orthopsychiatry, 65*, 468–478.

Goodman, L. A., Dutton, M. A., & Harris, M. (1997). The relationship between violence dimensions and symptom severity among homeless, mentally ill women. *Journal of Traumatic Stress, 10*, 51–70.

Goodman, L. A., Salyers, M. P., Mueser, K. T., & Rosenberg, S. D. (submitted). Recent victimization in women and men with severe mental illness: Prevalence and correlates.

Goodwin, F. K., & Jamison, K. R. (1990). *Manic-depressive illness*. New York: Oxford University Press.

Gottesman, I. I. (1991). *Schizophrenia genesis: The origins of madness*. New York: Freeman.

Greden, J. F., & Tandon, R. (Eds.). (1991). *Negative schizophrenic symptoms: Pathophysiology and clinical implications*. Washington, DC: American Psychiatric Press.

Green, M. F., Marshall, B. D., Jr., Wirshing, W. C., Ames, D., Marder, S. R., McGurk, S., Kern, R. S., & Mintz, J. (1997). Does Risperidone improve verbal working memory in treatment-resistant schizophrenia? *American Journal of Psychiatry, 154*, 799–804.

Greenfield, S. F., Strakowski, S. M., Tohen, M., Batson, S. C., & Kolbrener, M. L. (1994). Childhood abuse in first-episode psychosis. *British Journal of Psychiatry, 164*, 831–834.

Griffith, E. E. H., Young, J. L., & Smith, D. L. (1984). An analysis of the therapeutic elements in a Black church service. *Hospital and Community Psychiatry, 35*, 464–469.

Häfner, H., Riecher-Rössler, A., An Der Heiden, W., Maurer, K., Fätkenheuer, B., & Löffler, W. (1993). Generating and testing a causal explanation of the gender difference in age at first onset of schizophrenia. *Psychological Medicine, 23*, 925–940.

Halford, W. K., Schweitzer, R. D., & Varghese, F. N. (1991). Effects of family environment on negative symptoms and quality of life on psychotic patients. *Hospital and Community Psychiatry, 42*, 1241–1247.

Hans, S. L., Marcus, J., Henson, L., Auerbach, J. G., & Mirsky, A. F. (1992). Interpersonal behavior of children at risk for schizophrenia. *Psychiatry, 55*, 314–335.

Harding, C. M., Brooks, G. W., Ashikaga, T., Strauss, J. S., & Breier, A. (1987a). The Vermont longitudinal study of persons with severe mental illness, I: Methodology, study sample, and overall status 32 years later. *American Journal of Psychiatry, 144*, 718–726.

Harding, C. M., Brooks, G. W., Ashikaga, T., Strauss, J. S., & Breier, A. (1987b). The Vermont longitudinal study of persons with severe mental illness, II: Long-term outcome of subjects who retrospectively met DSM-III criteria for schizophrenia. *American Journal of Psychiatry, 144*, 727–735.

Harding, C. M., & Keller, A. B. (1998). Long-term outcome of social functioning. In K. T. Mueser and N. Tarrier (Eds.), *Handbook of social functioning in schizophrenia* (pp. 134–148). Boston: Allyn & Bacon.

Harris, M. (1996). Treating sexual abuse trauma with dually diagnosed women. *Community Mental Health Journal, 32*, 371–385.

Hatfield, A. B., & Lefley, H. P. (Eds.). (1987). *Families of the mentally ill: Coping and adaptation*. New York: Guilford.

Hatfield, A. B., & Lefley, H. P. (Eds.). (1993). *Surviving mental illness: Stress, coping, and adaptation.* New York: Guilford.

Hiday, V. A., Swartz, M. S., Swanson, J. W., Borum, R., & Wagner, H. R. (1999). Criminal victimization of persons with severe mental illness. *Psychiatric Services, 50,* 62–68.

Hodgins, S., & Côté, G. (1993). Major mental disorder and antisocial personality disorder: A criminal combination. *Bulletin of the American Academy of Psychiatry Law, 21,* 155–160.

Hodgins, S., & Côté, G. (1996). Schizophrenia and antisocial personality disorder: A criminal combination. In L. B. Schlesinger (Ed.), *Explorations in criminal psychopathology: Clinical syndromes with forensic implications* (pp. 217–237). Springfield, IL: Charles C. Thomas.

Hodgins, S., Mednick, S. A., Brennan, P. A., Schulsinger, F., & Engberg, M. (1996). Mental disorder and crime: Evidence from a Danish birth cohort. *Archives of General Psychiatry, 53,* 489–496.

Hollingshead, A. B., & Redlich, F. C. (1958). *Social class and mental illness: A community study.* New York: Wiley.

Hough, R. L., Landsverk, J. A., Karno, M., Burnam, A., Timbers, D. M., Escobar, J. I., & Regier, D. A. (1987). Utilization of health and mental health services by Los Angeles Mexican-Americans and non-Hispanic whites. *Archives of General Psychiatry, 44,* 702–709.

Howard, R., Almeida, O., & Levy, R. (1994). Phenomenology, demography and diagnosis in late paraphrenia. *Psychological Medicine, 24,* 397–410.

Hu, T., Snowden, L. R., Jerrell, J. M., & Nguyen, T. D. (1991). Ethnic populations in public mental health: Services choices and level of use. *American Journal of Public Health, 81,* 1429–1434.

Hutchings, P. S., & Dutton, M. A. (1993). Sexual assault history in a community mental health center clinical population. *Community Mental Health Journal, 29,* 59–63.

Inskip, H. M., Harris, E. C., & Barraclough, B. (1998). Lifetime risk of suicide for affective disorder, alcoholism, and schizophrenia. *British Journal of Psychiatry, 172,* 35–37.

Jablensky, A. (1989). Epidemiology and cross-cultural aspects of schizophrenia. *Psychiatric Annals, 19,* 516–524.

Jablensky, A. (1999). Schizophrenia: Epidemiology. *Current Opinion in Psychiatry, 12,* 19–28.

Jacob, T. (1975). Family interaction in disturbed and normal families: A methodological and substantive review. *Psychological Bulletin, 82,* 33–65.

Jacobson, A. (1989). Physical and sexual assault histories among psychiatric outpatients. *American Journal of Psychiatry, 146,* 755–758.

Jacobson, A., & Herald, C. (1990). The relevance of childhood sexual abuse to adult psychiatric inpatient care. *Hospital and Community Psychiatry, 41,* 154–158.

Jacobson, A., & Richardson, B. (1987). Assault experiences of 100 psychiatric inpatients: Evidence of the need for routine inquiry. *American Journal of Psychiatry, 144,* 508–513.

Jones, B. E., Gray, B. A., & Parsons, E. B. (1981). Manic-depressive illness among poor urban Blacks. *American Journal of Psychiatry, 138,* 654–657.

Jones, B. E., Gray, B. A., & Parsons, E. B. (1983). Manic-depressive illness among poor urban Hispanics. *American Journal of Psychiatry, 140,* 1208–1210.

Kane, J. M., & Marder, S. R. (1993). Psychopharmacologic treatment of schizophrenia. *Schizophrenia Bulletin, 19,* 287–302.

Kay, S. R., & Lindenmayer, J. (1987). Outcome predictors in acute schizophrenia: Prospective significance of background and clinical dimensions. *Journal of Nervous and Mental Disease, 175,* 152–160.

Keith, S. J., Regier, D. A., & Rae, D. S. (1991). Schizophrenic disorders. In L. N. Robins & D. A. Regier (Eds.), *Psychiatric disorders in America: The epidemiologic catchment area study* (pp. 33–52). New York: Free Press.

Kemp, R., Hayward, P., Applewhaite, G., Everitt, B., & David, A. (1996). Compliance therapy in psychotic patients: Randomised controlled trial. *British Medical Journal, 312,* 345–349.

Kemp, R., Kirov, G., Everitt, B., Hayward, P., & David, A. (1998). Randomised controlled trial of compliance therapy. Eighteen-month follow-up. *British Journal of Psychiatry, 173,* 271–272.

Kendler, K. S., & Diehl, S. R. (1993). The genetics of schizophrenia. *Schizophrenia Bulletin, 19,* 261–285.

Kessler, R. C., Foster, C. L., Saunders, W. B., & Stang, P. E. (1995). Social consequences of psychiatric disorders, I: Educational attainment. *American Journal of Psychiatry, 152,* 1026–1032.

Kessler, R. C., Sonnega, A., Bromet, E., Hughes, M., & Nelson, C. B. (1995). Posttraumatic stress disorder in the national comorbidity survey. *Archives of General Psychiatry, 52,* 1048–1060.

Kindermann, S. S., Karimi, A., Symonds, L., Brown, G. G., & Jeste, D. V. (1997). Review of functional magnetic resonance imaging in schizophrenia. *Schizophrenia Research, 27,* 143–156.

Kirch, D. G. (1993). Infection and autoimmunity as etiologic factors in schizophrenia: A review and reappraisal. *Schizophrenia Bulletin, 19,* 355–370.

Kraepelin, E. (1971). *Dementia praecox and paraphrenia* (R. M. Barclay, Trans.). New York: Krieger. (Original work published 1919).

Kramer, M. S., Vogel, W. H., DiJohnson, C., Dewey, D. A., Sheves, P., Cavicchia, S., Litle, P., Schmidt, R., & Kimes, I. (1989). Antidepressants in "depressed" schizophrenic inpatients. *Archives of General Psychiatry, 46,* 922–928.

Kranzler, H. R., Kadden, R. M., Burleson, J. A., Babor, T. F., Apter, A., & Rounsaville, B. J. (1995). Validity of psychiatric diagnoses in patients with substance use disorders: Is the interview more important than the interviewer? *Comprehensive Psychiatry, 36,* 278–288.

Lam, D. H. (1991). Psychosocial family intervention in schizophrenia: A review of empirical studies. *Psychological Medicine, 21,* 423–441.

Lawrie, S. M., & Abukmeil, S. S. (1998). Brain abnormality in schizophrenia: A systematic and quantitative review of volumetric magnetic resonance imaging studies. *British Journal of Psychiatry, 172,* 110–120.

Leff, J., & Vaughn, C. (1985). *Expressed emotion in families: Its significance for mental illness.* New York: Guilford.

Lefley, H. P. (1990). Culture and chronic mental illness. *Hospital and Community Psychiatry, 41,* 277–286.

Lehman, A. F., Myers, C. P., Dixon, L. B., & Johnson, J. L. (1994). Defining subgroups of dual diagnosis patients for service planning. *Hospital and Community Psychiatry, 45,* 556–561.

Lehman, A. F., Myers, C. P., Dixon, L. B., & Johnson, J. L. (1996). Detection of substance use disorders among psychiatric inpatients. *The Journal of Nervous and Mental Disease, 184,* 228–233.

Levinson, D. F., & Levitt, M. M. (1987). Schizoaffective mania reconsidered. *American Journal of Psychiatry, 144,* 415–425.

Levinson, D. F., & Mowry, B. J. (1991). Defining the schizophrenia spectrum: Issues for genetic linkage studies. *Schizophrenia Bulletin, 17,* 491–514.

Liberman, R. P. (1994). Treatment and rehabilitation of the seriously mentally ill in China: Impressions of a society in transition. *American Journal of Orthopsychiatry, 64,* 68–77.

Liberman, R. P., Mueser, K. T., Wallace, C. J., Jacobs, H. E., Eckman, T., & Massel, H. K. (1986). Training skills in the psychiatrically disabled: Learning coping and competence. *Schizophrenia Bulletin, 12,* 631–647.

Liberman, R. P., Wallace, C. J., Blackwell, G., Kopelowicz, A., Vaccaro, J. V., & Mintz, J. (1998). Skills training versus psychosocial occupational therapy for persons with persistent schizophrenia. *American Journal of Psychiatry, 155,* 1087–1091.

Liddle, P. F. (1987). Schizophrenic syndromes, cognitive performance and neurological dysfunction. *Psychological Medicine, 17,* 49–57.

Liddle, P. F. (1995). Brain imaging. In S. R. Hirsch & D. R. Weinberger (Eds.), *Schizophrenia* (pp. 425–439). Cambridge, MA: Blackwell Science.

Liddle, P. F. (1997). Dynamic neuroimaging with PET, SPET or fMRI. *International Review of Psychiatry, 9,* 331–337.

Lin, K.-M., & Kleinman, A. M. (1988). Psychopathology and clinical course of schizophrenia: A cross-cultural perspective. *Schizophrenia Bulletin, 14,* 555–567.

Lincoln, E. C., & Mamiya, L. H. (1990). *The Black church in the African-American experience.* Durham, NC: Duke University Press.

Lincoln, C. V., & McGorry, P. (1995). Who cares? Pathways to psychiatric care for young people experiencing a first episode of psychosis. *Psychiatric Services, 46,* 1166–1171.

Lipschitz, D. S., Kaplan, M. L., Sorkenn, J. B., Faedda, G. L., Chorney, P., & Asnis, G. M. (1996). Prevalence and characteristics of physical and sexual abuse among psychiatric outpatients. *Psychiatric Services, 47,* 189–191.

Lo, W. H., & Lo, T. (1977). A ten-year follow-up study of Chinese schizophrenics in Hong Kong. *British Journal of Psychiatry, 131,* 63–66.

Loring, M., & Powell, B. (1988). Gender, race, and DSM-III: A study of the objectivity of psychiatric diagnostic behavior. *Journal of Health and Social Behavior, 29,* 1–22.

Lysaker, P. H., Bell, M. D., Zito, W. S., & Bioty, S. M. (1995). Social skills at work: Deficits and predictors of improvement in schizophrenia. *Journal of Nervous and Mental Disease, 183,* 688–692.

Magaña, A. B., Goldstein, M. J., Karno, M., Miklowitz, D. J., Jenkins, J., & Falloon, I. R. H. (1986). A brief method for assessing expressed emotion in relatives of psychiatric patients. *Psychiatry Research, 17,* 203–212.

Marder, S. R., Wirshing, W. C., Mintz, J., McKenzie, J., Johnston, K., Eckman, T. A., Lebell, M., Zimmerman, K., & Liberman, R. P. (1996). Two-year outcome for social skills training and group psychotherapy for outpatients with schizophrenia. *American Journal of Psychiatry, 153,* 1585–1592.

Marengo, J. (1994). Classifying the courses of schizophrenia. *Schizophrenia Bulletin, 20,* 519–536.

Mattes, J. A., & Nayak, D. (1984). Lithium versus fluphenazine for prophylaxis in mainly schizophrenic schizoaffectives. *Biological Psychiatry, 19,* 445–449.

May, A. (1997). Psychopathology and religion in the era of "enlightened science": A case report. *European Journal of Psychiatry, 11,* 14–20.

McClure, R. J., Keshavan, M. S., & Pettegrew, J. W. (1998). Chemical and physiologic brain imaging in schizophrenia. *Psychiatric Clinics of North America, 21*, 93–122.

McEvoy, J. P., Freter, S., Everett, G., Geller, J. L., Appelbaum, P., Apperson, L. J., & Roth, L. (1989). Insight and the clinical outcome of schizophrenic patients. *The Journal of Nervous and Mental Disease, 177*, 48–51.

Merriam, A. E., Kay, S. R., Opler, L. A., Kushner, S. F., & van Praag, H. M. (1990). Neurological signs and the positive-negative dimension in schizophrenia. *Biological Psychiatry, 28*, 181–192.

Moos, R. H., & Moos, B. S. (1981). *Family environment scale manual.* Palo Alto, CA: Consulting Psychologists Press.

Morales-Dorta, J. (1976). *Puerto Rican espiritismo: Religion and psychotherapy.* New York: Vantage Press.

Mueser, K. T., & Bellack, A. S. (1998). Social skills and social functioning. In K. T. Mueser & N. Tarrier (Eds.), *Handbook of social functioning in schizophrenia* (pp. 79–96). Boston: Allyn & Bacon.

Mueser, K. T., Bellack, A. S., Douglas, M. S., & Morrison, R. L. (1991). Prevalence and stability of social skill deficits in schizophrenia. *Schizophrenia Research, 5*, 167–176.

Mueser, K. T., Bellack, A. S., Douglas, M. S., & Wade, J. H. (1991). Prediction of social skill acquisition in schizophrenic and major affective disorder patients from memory and symptomatology. *Psychiatry Research, 37*, 281–296.

Mueser, K. T., Bellack, A. S., Morrison, R. L., & Wade, J. H. (1990). Gender, social competence, and symptomatology in schizophrenia: A longitudinal analysis. *Journal of Abnormal Psychology, 99*, 138–147.

Mueser, K. T., Bellack, A. S., Morrison, R. L., & Wixted, J. T. (1990). Social competence in schizophrenia: Premorbid adjustment, social skill, and domains of functioning. *Journal of Psychiatric Research, 24*, 51–63.

Mueser, K. T., Bellack, A. S., Wade, J. H., Sayers, S. L., Tierney, A., & Haas, G. (1993). Expressed emotion, social skill, and response to negative affect in schizophrenia. *Journal of Abnormal Psychology, 102*, 339–351.

Mueser, K. T., Bennett, M., & Kushner, M. G. (1995). Epidemiology of substance use disorders among persons with chronic mental illnesses. In A. Lehman & L. Dixon (Eds.), *Double jeopardy: Chronic mental illness and substance abuse* (pp. 9–25). Chur, Switzerland: Harwood Academic.

Mueser, K. T., & Berenbaum, H. (1990). Psychodynamic treatment of schizophrenia: Is there a future? *Psychological Medicine, 20*, 253–262.

Mueser, K. T., Bond, G. R., Drake, R. E., & Resnick, S. G. (1998). Models of community care for severe mental illness: A review of research on case management. *Schizophrenia Bulletin, 24*, 37–74.

Mueser, K. T., Curran, P. J., & McHugo, G. J. (1997). Factor structure of the Brief Psychiatric Rating Scale in schizophrenia. *Psychological Assessment, 9*, 196–204.

Mueser, K. T., Drake, R. E., & Bond, G. R. (1997). Recent advances in psychiatric rehabilitation for patients with severe mental illness. *Harvard Review of Psychiatry, 5*, 123–137.

Mueser, K. T., Douglas, M. S., Bellack, A. S., & Morrison, R. L. (1991). Assessment of enduring deficit and negative symptom subtypes in schizophrenia. *Schizophrenia Bulletin, 17*, 565–582.

Mueser, K. T., & Glynn, S. M. (1999). *Behavioral family therapy for psychiatric disorders,* 2nd ed. Oakland, CA: New Harbinger.

Mueser, K. T., Goodman, L. B., Trumbetta, S. L., Rosenberg, S. D., Osher, F. C., Vidaver, R., Aucielo, P., & Foy, D. W. (1998). Trauma and posttraumatic stress disorder in severe mental illness. *Journal of Consulting and Clinical Psychology, 66*, 493–499.

Mueser, K. T., Levine, S., Bellack, A. S., Douglas, M. S., & Brady, E. U. (1990). Social skills training for acute psychiatric patients. *Hospital and Community Psychiatry, 41*, 1249–1251.

Mueser, K. T., Rosenberg, S. D., Drake, R. E., Miles, K. M., Wolford, G., Vidaver, R., & Carrieri, K. (1999). Conduct disorder, antisocial personality disorder, and substance use disorders in schizophrenia and major affective disorders. *Journal of Studies on Alcohol, 60*, 278–284.

Mueser, K. T., Yarnold, P. R., & Bellack, A. S. (1992). Diagnostic and demographic correlates of substance abuse in schizophrenia and major affective disorder. *Acta Psychiatrica Scandinavica, 85*, 48–55.

Mueser, K. T., Yarnold, P. R., Levinson, D. F., Singh, H., Bellack, A. S., Kee, K., Morrison, R. L., & Yadalam, K. Y. (1990). Prevalence of substance abuse in schizophrenia: Demographic and clinical correlates. *Schizophrenia Bulletin, 16*, 31–56.

Munk-Jørgensen, P. (1987). First-admission rates and marital status of schizophrenics. *Acta Psychiatrica Scandinavica, 76*, 210–216.

Murphy, H. B. M., & Raman, A. C. (1971). The chronicity of schizophrenia in indigenous tropical peoples. *British Journal of Psychiatry, 118*, 489–497.

Nuechterlein, K. H., & Dawson, M. E. (1984). A heuristic vulnerability/stress model of schizophrenic episodes. *Schizophrenia Bulletin, 10*, 300–312.

Neumann, C. S., Grimes, K., Walker, E., & Baum, K. (1995). Developmental pathways to schizophrenia: Behavioral subtypes. *Journal of Abnormal Psychology, 104*, 558–566.

Nolan, K. A., Volovka, J., Mohr, P., & Czobor, P. (1999). Psychopathy and violent behavior among patients with schizophrenia or schizoaffective disorder. *Psychiatric Services, 50*, 787–792.

Oldridge, M. L., & Hughes, I. C. T. (1992). Psychological well-being in families with a member suffering from schizophrenia. *British Journal of Psychiatry, 161*, 249– 251.

Padgett, D. K., Patrick, C., Burns, B. J., & Schlesinger, H. J. (1994). Women and outpatient mental health services: Use by Black, Hispanic, and White women in a national insured population. *The Journal of Mental Health Administration, 21*, 347–360.

Parra, F. (1985). Social tolerance of the mentally ill in the Mexican-American community. *International Journal of Social Psychiatry, 31*, 37–47.

Peen, J., & Dekker, J. (1997). Admission rates for schizophrenia in The Netherlands: An urban/rural comparison. *Acta Psychiatrica Scandinavica, 96*, 301–305.

Penn, D., Hope, D. A., Spaulding, W. D., & Kucera, J. (1994). Social anxiety in schizophrenia. *Schizophrenia Research, 11*, 277–284.

Penn, D. L., Mueser, K. T., Spaulding, W. D., Hope, D. A., & Reed, D. (1995). Information processing and social competence in chronic schizophrenia. *Schizophrenia Bulletin, 21*, 269–281.

Pope, H. G., & Lipinski, J. F. (1978). Diagnosis in schizophrenia and manic-depressive illness. *Archives of General Psychiatry, 35*, 811–828.

Quinlivan, R., Hough, R., Crowell, A., Beach, C., Hofstetter, R., & Kenworthy, K. (1995). Service utilization and costs of care for severely mentally ill clients in an intensive case management program. *Psychiatric Services, 46*, 365–371.

Regier, D. A., Farmer, M. E., Rae, D. S., Locke, B. Z., Keith, S. J., Judd, L. L., & Goodwin, F. K. (1990). Comorbidity of mental disorders with alcohol and other drug abuse. *Journal of the American Medical Association, 264*, 2511–2518.

Resnick, H. S., Kilpatrick, D. G., Dansky, B. S., Saunders, B. E., & Best, C. L. (1993). Prevalence of civilian trauma and post-traumatic stress disorder in a representative national sample of women. *Journal of Consulting and Clinical Psychology, 61*, 984–991.

Robins, L. N. (1966). *Deviant children grown up*. Huntington, NY: Krieger.

Robins, L. N., & Price, R. K. (1991). Adult disorders predicted by childhood conduct problems: Results from the NIMH Epidemiologic Catchment Area project. *Psychiatry, 54*, 116–132.

Rodrigo, G., Lusiardo, M., Briggs, G., & Ulmer, A. (1991). Differences between schizophrenics born in winter and summer. *Acta Psychiatrica Scandinavica, 84*, 320–322.

Rose, S. M., Peabody, C. G., & Stratigeas, B. (1991). Undetected abuse among intensive case management clients. *Hospital and Community Psychiatry, 42*, 499–503.

Rosenberg, S. D., Drake, R. E., Wolford, G. L., Mueser, K. T., Oxman, T. E., Vidaver, R. M., Carrieri, K. L., & Luckoor, R. (1998). Dartmouth assessment of lifestyle instrument (DALI): A substance use disorder screen for people with severe mental illness. *The American Journal of Psychiatry, 155*, 232–238.

Ross, C. A., Anderson, G., & Clark, P. (1994). Childhood abuse and the positive symptoms of schizophrenia. *Hospital and Community Psychiatry, 45*, 489–491.

Roy, A. (Ed.). (1986). *Suicide*. Baltimore: Williams and Wilkins.

Rutter, M. (1984). Psychopathology and development: I. Childhood antecedents of adult psychiatric disorder. *Australian and New Zealand Journal of Psychiatry, 18*, 225–234.

Salokangas, R. K. R. (1978). Socioeconomic development and schizophrenia. *Psychiatria Fennica*, 103–112.

Sands, J. R., & Harrow, M. (1999). Depression during the longitudinal course of schizophrenia. *Schizophrenia Bulletin, 25*, 157–171.

Sartorius, N., Jablensky, A., Korten, A., Ernberg, G., Anker, M., Cooper, J. E., & Day, R. (1986). Early manifestations and first-contact incidence of schizophrenia in different cultures. *Psychological Medicine, 16*, 909–928.

Schaub, A., Behrendt, B., Brenner, H. D., Mueser, K. T., & Liberman, R. P. (1998). Training schizophrenic patients to manage their symptoms: Predictors of treatment response to the German version of the Symptom Management Module. *Schizophrenia Research, 31*, 121–130.

Schuckit, M. A. (1995). *Drug and alcohol abuse: A clinical guide to diagnosis and treatment (critical issues in psychiatry)*, 4th ed. New York: Plenum.

Searles, H. (1965) *Collected papers on schizophrenia and related subjects*. New York: International Universities Press.

Sevy, S., & Davidson, M. (1995). The cost of cognitive impairment in schizophrenia. *Schizophrenia Research, 17*, 1–3.

Skilbeck, W. M., Acosta, F. X., Yamamoto, J., & Evans, L. A. (1984). Self-reported psychiatric symptoms among Black, Hispanic, and White outpatients. *Journal of Clinical Psychology, 40*, 1184–1189.

Smith, T. E., Hull, J. W., Anthony, D. T., Goodman, M., Hedayat-Harris, A., Felger, T., Kentros, M. K., MacKain, S. J., & Romanelli, S. (1997). Post-hospitalization treatment adherence of schizophrenic patients: Gender differences in skill acquisition. *Psychiatry Research, 69*, 123–129.

Steadman, H. J., Mulvey, E. P., Monahan, J., Robbins, P. C., Appelbaum, P. S., Grisso, T., Roth, L. H., & Silver, E. (1998). Violence by people discharged from acute psychiatric inpatient facilities and by others in the same neighborhoods. *Archives of General Psychiatry, 55*, 393–401.

Stone, A., Greenstein, R., Gamble, G., & McLellan, A. T. (1993). Cocaine use in chronic schizophrenic outpatients receiving depot neuroleptic medications. *Hospital and Community Psychiatry, 44*, 176–177.

Sue, S., Fujino, D. C., Hu, L.-T., Takeuchi, D. T., & Zane, N. W. S. (1991). Community mental health services for ethnic minority groups: A test of the cultural responsiveness hypothesis. *Journal of Consulting and Clinical Psychology, 59*, 533–540.

Sue, D. W., & Sue, D. C. (1990). *Counseling the culturally different: Theory and practice*, 2nd ed. New York: Wiley-Interscience.

Susser, E., & Lin, S. (1992). Schizophrenia after prenatal exposure to the Dutch Hunger Winter of 1944–1945. *Archives of General Psychiatry, 49*, 983–988.

Susser, E., Neugebauer, R., Hoek, H. W., Brown, A. S., Lin, S., Labovitz, D., & Gorman, J. M. (1996). Schizophrenia after prenatal famine: Further evidence. *Archives of General Psychiatry, 53*, 25–31.

Susser, E., Struening, E. L., & Conover, S. (1989). Psychiatric problems in homeless men: Lifetime psychosis, substance use, and current distress in new arrivals at New York City shelters. *Archives of General Psychiatry, 46*, 845–850.

Swanson, J. W. (1994). Mental disorder, substance abuse, and community violence: An epidemiological approach. In J. Monahan & H. Steadman (Eds.), *Violence and mental disorder: Developments in risk assessment* (pp. 101–136). Chicago: University of Chicago Press.

Swanson, J. W., Holzer, C. E., Ganju, V. K., & Jono, R. T. (1990). Violence and psychiatric disorder in the community: Evidence from the Epidemiologic Catchment Area Surveys. *Hospital and Community Psychiatry, 41*, 761–770.

Swartz, M. S., Swanson, J. W., Hiday, V. A., Borum, R., Wagner, H. R., & Burns, B. J. (1998). Violence and severe mental illness: The effects of substance abuse and nonadherence to medication. *The American Journal of Psychiatry, 155*, 226–231.

Switzer, G. E., Dew, M. A., Thompson, K., Goycoolea, J. M., Derricott, T., & Mullins, S. D. (1999). Posttraumatic stress disorder and service utilization among urban mental health center clients. *Journal of Traumatic Stress, 12*, 25–39.

Takei, N., Mortensen, P. B., Klaening, U., Murray, R. M., Sham, P. C., O'Callaghan, E., & Munk-Jorgensen, P. (1996). Relationship between in utero exposure to influenza epidemics and risk of schizophrenia in Denmark. *Biological Psychiatry, 40*, 817–824.

Takei, N., Sham, P. C., O'Callaghan, E., Glover, G., & Murray, R. M. (1995). Schizophrenia: Increased risk associated with winter and city birth—a case-control study in 12 regions within England and Wales. *Journal of Epidemiology and Community Health, 49*, 106–109.

Telles, C., Karno, M., Mintz, J., Paz, G., Arias, M., Tucker, D., & Lopez, S. (1995). Immigrant families coping with schizophrenia: Behavioral family intervention vs. case management with a low-income Spanish-speaking population. *British Journal of Psychiatry, 167*, 473–479.

Terkelsen, K. G. (1983) Schizophrenia and the family: II. Adverse effects of family therapy. *Family Process, 22*, 191–200.

Tessler, R., & Gamache, G. (1995). *Evaluating family experiences with severe mental illness: To be used in conjunction with The Family Experiences Interview Schedule (FEIS): The Evaluation Center @ HSRI toolkit.* Cambridge, MA: The Evaluation Center @ HSRI.

Test, M. A., Wallisch, L. S., Allness, D. J., & Ripp, K. (1989). Substance use in young adults with schizophrenic disorders. *Schizophrenia Bulletin, 15*, 465–476.

Tienari, P. (1991). Interaction between genetic vulnerability and family environment: The Finnish adoptive family study of schizophrenia. *Acta Psychiatrica Scandinavica, 84*, 460–465.

Tienari, P., Sorri, A., Lahti, I., Naarala, M., Wahlberg, K., Moring, J., Pohjola, J., & Wynne, L. C. (1987). Genetic and psychosocial factors in schizophrenia: The Finnish adoptive family study. *Schizophrenia Bulletin, 13*, 477–484.

Tjaden, P., & Thoennes, N. (1998). Prevalence, incidence, and consequences of violence against women: Findings from the national violence against women survey. Washington, DC: U.S. Department of Justice, National Institute of Justice, Research in Brief.

Tollefson, G. D., & Sanger, T. M. (1997). Negative symptoms: A path analytic approach to a double-blind, placebo- and haloperidol-controlled clinical trial with olanzapine. *American Journal of Psychiatry, 154*, 466–474.

Torrey, E. F. (1995). *Surviving schizophrenia: A manual for families, consumers, and providers*, 3rd ed. New York: HarperCollins.

Torrey, E. F., Bowler, A. E., & Clark, K. (1997). Urban birth and residence as risk factors for psychoses: An analysis of 1880 data. *Schizophrenia Research, 25,* 169–176.

Torrey, E. F., Bowler, A. E., Rawlings, R., & Terrazas, A. (1993). Seasonality of schizophrenia and stillbirths. *Schizophrenia Bulletin, 19,* 557–562.

Torrey, E. F., Stieber, J., Ezekiel, J., Wolfe, S. M., Sharfstein, J., Noble, J. H., & Flynn, L. M. (1992). Criminalizing the seriously mentally ill: The abuse of jails as mental hospitals. Joint report of the National Alliance of the Mentally Ill, Arlington, VA, and Public Citizen's Health Research Group, Washington, DC.

Tsuang, M. T. (1986). Predictors of poor and good outcome in schizophrenia. In L. Erlenmeyer-Kimling & N. E. Miller (Eds.), *Life-span research on the prediction of psychopathology.* Hillsdale, NJ: Erlbaum.

Uttaro, T., & Mechanic, D. (1994). The NAMI consumer survey analysis of unmet needs. *Hospital and Community Psychiatry, 45,* 372–374.

Van Der Does, A. J. W., Dingemans, P. M. A. J., Linszen, D. H., Nugter, M. A., & Scholte, W. F. (1993). Symptom dimensions and cognitive and social functioning in recent-onset schizophrenia. *Psychological Medicine, 23,* 745–753.

Velligan, D. I., Mahurin, R. K., Diamond, P. L., Hazleton, B. C., Eckert, S. L., & Miller, A. L. (1997). The functional significance of symptomatology and cognitive function in schizophrenia. *Schizophrenia Research, 25,* 21–31.

Wahlbeck, K., Cheine, M., Essali, A., & Adams, C. (1999). Evidence of clozapine's effectiveness in schizophrenia: A systematic review and meta-analysis of randomized trials. *American Journal of Psychiatry, 156,* 990–999.

Walker, E., Downey, G., & Caspi, A. (1991). Twin studies of psychopathology: Why do the concordance rates vary? *Schizophrenia Research, 5,* 211–221.

Wallace, C. J., Liberman, R. P., Tauber, R., & Wallace, J. (in press). The independent living skills survey: A comprehensive measure of the community functioning of severely and persistently mentally ill individuals. *Schizophrenia Bulletin.*

Watt, N. F. (1978). Patterns of childhood social development in adult schizophrenics. *Archives of General Psychiatry, 35,* 160–165.

Waxler, N. E., & Mishler, E. G. (1971). Parental interaction with schizophrenic children and well siblings. *Archives of General Psychiatry, 25,* 223–231.

Westermeyer, J. (1989). Psychiatric epidemiology across cultures: Current issues and trends. *Transcultural Psychiatric Research Review, 26,* 5–25.

Xiong, W., Phillips, M. R., Hu, X., Ruiwen, W., Dai, Q., Kleinman, J., & Kleinman, A. (1994). Family-based intervention for schizophrenic patients in China: A randomised controlled trial. *British Journal of Psychiatry, 165,* 239–247.

Young, C. R., Bowers, M. B., & Mazure, C. M. (1998). Management of the adverse effects of clozapine. *Schizophrenia Bulletin, 24,* 381–390.

Zhang, M., Wang, M., Li, J., & Phillips, M. R. (1994). Randomised-control trial of family intervention for 78 first-episode male schizophrenic patients: An 18-month study in Suzhou, Jiangsu. *British Journal of Psychiatry, 165,* 96–102.

Zigler, E., & Glick, M. (1986). *A developmental approach to adult psychopathology.* New York: Wiley.

17

Substance Abuse Disorders

Timothy J. O'Farrell

Description of the Disorder

Introduction

This chapter discusses serious psychological problems that can arise in relation to the use of certain substances. These substances are called psychoactive substances because they can be used to affect moods, thinking, and behavior. In most societies, use of certain substances to modify mood or behavior is regarded as normal and appropriate, and such use may be a valued part of the culture. Customary and social drinking of alcohol as a beverage with meals or to enhance interaction at social gatherings is one example. The ritual use of peyote (a drug obtained from the mescal cactus that produces a variety of vivid visual hallucinations) for religious purposes by Indians in Mexico and the southwestern United States is another example. Further, some psychoactive substances are used for medical purposes under a physician's prescription to relieve pain, decrease anxiety, or for other appropriate medical purposes. Therefore, this chapter is concerned not with these and other normal and appropriate uses of psychoactive substances, but rather with the use of such substances that is considered pathological largely due to the negative behavioral effects of the substance's use. Table 1 lists major classes of psychoactive substances that are commonly subject to problematic use. The criteria for determining problematic use of such substances are considered next.

Criteria for Diagnosing a Substance Use Disorder

The most frequently used and most widely accepted clinical description of substance abuse disorders is contained in the fourth edition of the *Diagnostic and Statistical Manual of Mental Disorders* (DSM-IV) published by the American Psychiatric Association (APA, 1994). In DSM-IV, substance abuse problems are classified under the general heading of Substance-Related Disorders, which includes problems with alcohol and with other drugs.

The essential feature of substance-related disorders, as described in DSM-IV, is a

Timothy J. O'Farrell • Department of Psychiatry, Harvard Medical School, Boston, Massachusetts; and Veterans Affairs Medical Center, Brockton, Massachusetts 02301.

Advanced Abnormal Psychology, Second Edition, edited by Hersen and Van Hasselt. Kluwer Academic/Plenum Publishers, New York, 2001.

TABLE 1. Classes of Psychoactive Substances

1. Alcohol
2. Amphetamine (e.g., "speed")
3. Cannabis (e.g., marijuana)
4. Cocaine
5. Hallucinogens (e.g., LSD)
6. Inhalants (e.g., glue sniffing)
7. Nicotine
8. Opioids (e.g., heroin, morphine)
9. Phenylcyclidine (PCP, e.g., "angel dust")
10. Sedatives, hypnotics (e.g., barbiturates), or anxiolytics (e.g., Valium, Xanax)

maladaptive pattern of substance use, leading to clinically significant impairment or distress (APA, 1994). In DSM-IV, problems with substance use can be described as *substance dependence* or *substance abuse* depending on the seriousness of the problem and on specific diagnostic criteria. Although, in most cases, a separate diagnosis is made for each specific problematic substance (e.g., alcohol dependence, cocaine abuse), DSM-IV diagnostic criteria are stated in general terms that apply to all of the substances listed in Table 1.

SUBSTANCE DEPENDENCE

At least three of the seven symptoms listed in Table 2 must be present for the diagnosis of substance dependence. To qualify for the diagnosis, at least three of these symptoms must have occurred in the same 12-month period (APA, 1994).

A final point is that DSM-IV further specifies substance dependence as occurring (1) *with physiological dependence*, if there is evidence of tolerance or withdrawal (i.e., either item 1 or item 2 in Table 2 is present); or (2) *without physiological dependence*, if there is no evidence of

TABLE 2. DSM-IV Diagnostic Criteria for Substance Dependence[a]

1. Tolerance, as defined by either of the following:
    a. a need for markedly increased amounts of the substance to achieve intoxication or desired effect;
    b. markedly diminished effect with continued use of the same amount of the substance.
2. Withdrawal, as manifested by either of the following:
    a. the characteristic withdrawal syndrome for the substance (as specified in DSM-IV);
    b. the same (or closely related) substance is taken to relieve or avoid withdrawal symptoms.
3. The substance is often taken in larger amounts or over a longer period than was intended.
4. A persistent desire or unsuccessful efforts to cut down or control substance use.
5. A great deal of time is spent in activities necessary to obtain the substance (e.g., visiting multiple doctors or driving long distances), use the substance (e.g., chain-smoking), or recover from its effects.
6. Important social, occupational, or recreational activities are given up or reduced because of substance use.
7. The substance use is continued despite knowledge of having a persistent or recurrent physical or psychological problem that is likely to have been caused or exacerbated by the substance (e.g., recurrent cocaine use despite recognition of cocaine-induced depression, or continued drinking despite recognition that an ulcer was made worse by alcohol consumption).

[a]Reprinted with permission from the *Diagnostic and Statistical Manual of Mental Disorders*, 4th Ed. Copyright 1994, American Psychiatric Association.

tolerance or withdrawal (i.e., neither item 1 or item 2 in Table 2 is present). Because the results of withdrawing from substance use vary according to the substance (e.g., alcohol versus heroin), DSM-IV also provides specific criteria for the characteristic withdrawal syndrome and symptoms that occur after stopping or sharply reducing substance intake after a period of prolonged and heavy use.

SUBSTANCE ABUSE

Less severe substance use problems that do not meet the criteria for substance dependence may be classified as substance abuse problems. In DSM-IV, substance abuse is a residual category for noting maladaptive patterns of substance use that have never met the criteria for substance dependence for the specific substance under consideration. The maladaptive pattern of use is indicated by at least one of the following: "(1) recurrent substance use resulting in a failure to fulfill major role obligations at work, school, or home (e.g., repeated absences or poor work performance related to substance use; substance-related absences, suspensions, or expulsions from school; neglect of children or household); (2) recurrent substance use in situations in which it is physically hazardous (e.g., driving an automobile or operating a machine when impaired by substance use); (3) recurrent substance-related legal problems (e.g., arrests for substance-related disorderly conduct); (4) continued substance use despite having persistent or recurrent social or interpersonal problems caused or exacerbated by the effects of the substance (e.g., arguments with spouse about consequences of intoxication, physical fights)" (APA, 1994). Examples of situations in which a diagnosis of substance abuse would be appropriate (APA, 1987, p.169) include

1. A college student binges on cocaine every few weekends. These periods are followed by a day or two of missing school because of "crashing." There are no other symptoms.
2. A middle-aged man repeatedly drives his car when intoxicated with alcohol. There are no other symptoms.
3. A woman keeps drinking alcohol even though her physician has told her that it is responsible for exacerbating the symptoms of a duodenal ulcer. There are no other symptoms.

PROBLEMS WITH MORE THAN ONE SUBSTANCE

Among patients seeking help for substance use disorders, many individuals have problems that involve the use of more than one substance. When an individual's problems meet the criteria for more than one substance-related disorder, multiple diagnoses are made. The case of Jack Smith described later in this chapter provides an example of an individual who has multiple substance-related disorders.

Another type of case involving problems with multiple substances is diagnosed as *polysubstance dependence*. This diagnosis is reserved to denote a period of at least six months during which the person was repeatedly using substances from at least three of the categories (not including nicotine) listed in Table 1, but no single substance predominated. During this period, the dependence criteria of Table 2 were met for substances as a group but not for any specific substance (APA, 1994).

Table 3 summarizes important and key points about the definitions and characteristics of substance-related disorders.

TABLE 3. Important and Key Points about Definitions of Substance-Related Disorders

1. Psychoactive substances can be used to affect moods, thinking, and behavior. When serious negative behavioral effects occur from the use of such substances, these serious psychological problems are called *substance-related disorders.*
2. Ten classes of substances that can lead to psychoactive substance disorders are (1) alcohol; (2) amphetamines (e.g., "speed"); (3) cannabis (e.g., marijuana); (4) cocaine; (5) hallucinogens (e.g., LSD); (6) inhalants (e.g., glue sniffing); (7) nicotine; (8) opioids (e.g., heroin, morphine); (9) phencyclidine (PCP, e.g., "angel dust"); (10) sedatives, hypnotics (e.g., barbiturates), or anxiolytics (e.g., Valium, Xanax).
3. Essential features of the disorder are a maladaptive pattern of substance use leading to clinically significant impairment or distress.
4. *Substance dependence* is diagnosed if the person has had at least three of seven specific symptoms which must have occurred in the same 12-month period.
5. *Substance abuse* is diagnosed for less severe problems that have never met the criteria for substance dependence but involve recurrent substance use that results in failure to fulfill major role obligations (at work, school, or home), recurrent physically hazardous use (e.g., driving while intoxicated), *or* recurrent legal problems *or* continued use despite adverse social or interpersonal consequences.

EPIDEMIOLOGY

Epidemiology data on substance use disorders presented here come from the National Comorbidity Study (NCS; Kessler et al., 1994). The NCS was a large-scale study of a nationally representative sample of Americans sponsored by the U.S. National Institute of Mental Health to determine the prevalence of and extent of co-occurrence of different psychiatric disorders in the United States and the factors that are associated with elevated risk for and co-occurrence of different disorders. The NCS study data on substance use disorders were chosen because they provide an estimate of the prevalence of diagnosed disorders, not just a description of the patterns and problems of substance use. Although the NCS data are based on interviews conducted in 1990-1992 and on diagnostic criteria from DSM-III-R (i.e., *Diagnostic and Statistical Manual of Mental Disorders*, 3rd ed., revised; APA, 1987) rather than the DSM-IV, they represent some of the best data available. Other sources will be cited when NCS estimates may be misleading or when data are not available in the NCS. An earlier study, the Epidemiologic Catchment Area study (ECA; Robins & Regier, 1991), will serve as a frequent source to supplement NCS information.

Prevalence of Substance Use Disorders

OVERALL PREVALENCE RELATIVE TO OTHER PSYCHIATRIC DISORDERS

Table 4 presents NCS data from Kessler et al. (1994) on the prevalence of substance use disorders in the United States throughout the lifetimes of persons interviewed in the NCS study and for the year before being interviewed. Alcoholism, as indicated by a diagnosis of alcohol abuse or alcohol dependence, is the most frequent psychiatric disorder and has a lifetime prevalence of 24%, a full 10% higher than the next most frequent disorder (i.e., social phobia, lifetime prevalence = 13.3%). When alcohol and drug problems are considered together, substance use disorders are the most frequent (27% lifetime prevalence) psychiatric disorders followed by anxiety disorders (25% lifetime prevalence) and affective disorders (19% lifetime prevalence).

Due to methodological concerns, some have questioned whether the prevalence rates for

TABLE 4. Prevalence of Substance-Related Disorders in the United States[a]

	Total sample		Men		Women	
	Lifetime	Past year	Lifetime	Past year	Lifetime	Past year
Alcohol abuse/dependence	23.5%	9.7%	32.6%	14.1%	14.6%	5.3%
Drug abuse/dependence	11.9%	3.6%	14.6%	5.1%	9.4%	2.2%
Any substance use disorders[b]	26.6%	11.3%	35.4%	16.1%	17.9%	6.6%

[a]These prevalence data are taken from the National Comorbidity Study data presented by Kessler et al. (1994).
[b]Includes individuals with alcohol abuse/dependence or drug abuse/dependence. Prevalence for combined substance use disorder category is less than combined prevalence for alcohol and drug problems because some individuals had both alcohol and drug problems.

alcoholism in the past year might be overly high estimates. These "past year" figures are important because they estimate the number of people who are affected by alcoholism during any year. As indicated in Table 4, each year nearly 10% of U.S. adults, it was estimated, have a problem with alcohol, and 14% of men and about 5% of women are affected (Kessler et al., 1994). More conservative methods showed that 6.9% overall (11.0% of men and 3.8% of women) had an alcoholism problem in the past year (Kessler et al., 1997). By either estimate, alcoholism is a major problem in the United States, and 7% to 10% of the population (11 to 14% of men and 4 to 5% of women) were actively symptomatic in the past year.

RELATIVE PREVALENCE OF DIFFERENT TYPES OF SUBSTANCE USE DISORDERS

What types of lifetime substance use disorders were experienced by those in the NCS sample who had such a disorder? Considering the 35.4% of men in the NCS sample who had a substance use disorder, Table 5 indicates that more than 20% had only alcohol problems, about 3% had only drug problems, and about 12% had problems that involved both alcohol and drugs. Another way to look at this same question is presented in Figure 1. Nearly 60% of men who had substance use disorders suffered only from alcohol problems, a third had both alcoholism and drug problems, and the remaining 8% had only drug problems.

Among those who had drug problems, lifetime prevalence rates of drug dependence disorder varied considerably in the NCS study, depending on the type of drug (Anthony, Warner, & Kessler, 1994). Figure 2 shows that 7.5% of adults experienced at least one drug dependence disorder. Cannabis (marijuana) dependence was the most frequently diagnosed disorder that affected an estimated 4.2%. Other disorders affected less than 3% of the population. Two points must be considered when evaluating the prevalence rates in Figure 2. First, these rates which apply to all adults do not reflect the rates of disorder in specific subgroups of the U.S. population. For example, among those age 25–34, the lifetime odds of experiencing a drug dependence disorder is three and one-half times that for the general

TABLE 5. Lifetime Prevalence of Alcohol and/or Drug Disorders among Men

Alcohol abuse/dependence only	20.7%
Drug abuse/dependence only	2.8%
Both alcohol abuse/dependence and drug abuse/dependence	11.9%

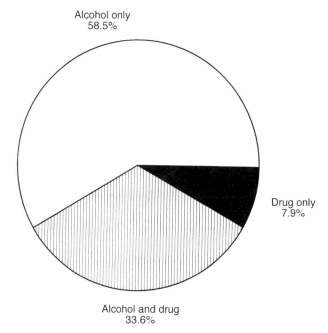

Alcohol only
58.5%

Drug only
7.9%

Alcohol and drug
33.6%

FIGURE 1. Relative proportion of alcohol, drug, and combined problems for those who have a lifetime diagnosis of substance use disorder.

population. Second, these rates are for drug dependence and do not consider the less severe diagnosis of drug abuse; the prevalence of either drug abuse or drug dependence is nearly 12% as reported in Table 4.

Factors Related to Higher Risk of Substance Use Disorders

The NCS data (Kessler et al., 1994, 1997) presented in Table 4 showed that substance use disorders were more common among men than women. More than twice as many men as women experience alcohol abuse or dependence and one and a half times as many men as women experience drug disorders. Although men continue to exceed women in the prevalence of substance use disorders, the gap between men and women is less than it was in earlier studies (e.g., Robins & Regier, 1991). People who have completed fewer years of education and the unmarried—particularly those who have experienced more than one separation or divorce—are more likely than more educated and married persons to experience alcoholism or drug problems. Age is also a significant risk factor; younger people are more likely to experience alcoholism or drug problems (ages 25–34). It should be remembered that the association between these factors and higher rates of substance use disorder does not necessarily mean that they cause or are caused by the substance use disorder.

Another type of risk factor, the extent of use of the substance, was also examined in an earlier study, the Epidemiologic Catchment Area study (ECA; Robins & Regier, 1991). Substance exposure is a prerequisite for developing a substance use disorder (Helzer, Burnham, & McEvoy, 1991), so it is interesting to examine alcohol consumption patterns and the frequency of illicit drug use in relation to the prevalence of substance use disorders. Figure 3

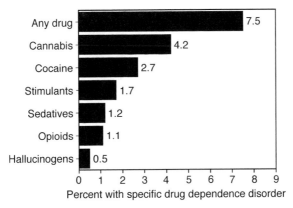

FIGURE 2. Lifetime prevalence of specific drug dependence disorders.

presents ECA study data on lifetime patterns of alcohol use. Lifelong abstainers account for about 10% of the U.S. population. Another 60% are social drinkers who deny both heavy consumption and alcohol-related problems. The most interesting group is *heavy or problem drinkers* defined in the ECA study as "those who reported seven or more drinks at least one evening a week for several months (or daily for two weeks or more) and/or one or more lifetime drinking problems" (Helzer et al., 1991). The prevalence rate of alcohol abuse or dependence among these heavy drinkers was 48.5%, nearly four times the rate in the general population. Regarding drug problems, people who have ever used illicit drugs have a three times greater chance of having a drug disorder. Further, 54% of those who used illicit drugs daily for two weeks or more had a lifetime diagnosis of drug abuse/dependence that was nearly nine times the rate for the general population.

Table 6 summarizes important and key points about the epidemiology of substance-related disorders.

CLINICAL PICTURE

The clinical picture of substance use disorders seen in treatment centers has become more varied and complicated in the past decade. Patients in their forties who have primarily alcohol problems are still seen in treatment centers. Such patients used to comprise the largest segment of the treatment population. More recently a greater number of younger patients have sought help, and these patients tend to have problems with multiple substances. Therefore, two cases from the author's experience are described briefly to illustrate these different types of patients.

The Case of Frank Johnson

Case Identification. Frank Johnson was a 45-year-old, unemployed, white, male accountant. He was the father of six children, ages 13 to 21. He had been separated from his wife for five months when admitted to the medical service of a large veterans' hospital.

Presenting Complaints. Mr. Johnson's complaints were difficulty in sleeping, tenseness, depression, chest pains, and excessive alcohol use of from one to two quarts of rum daily for 4½ months before admission. Given his history of serious cardiac problems, he

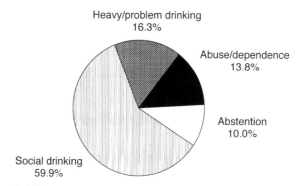

FIGURE 3. Lifetime drinking pattern in the Epidemiologic Catchment Area study.

was admitted to the medical service for detoxification from alcohol and close monitoring of his cardiac status.

Events Leading to Hospitalization. These were (1) his oldest son had a court hearing following an arrest for theft; (2) after a heated argument with his wife about the son's difficulties, the wife had initiated a court petition for legal separation; and (3) thoughts of suicide, including an idea of purchasing a gun for this purpose.

Earlier History. Frank began drinking at age 15 at parties during high school but did not feel it was a problem then or later during military service and college. Around age 30, his work as an accountant began to involve increased drinking with clients and associates. At age 36 when the patient had his first heart attack, his physician advised him to stop drinking, a warning that went unheeded. During the next six years, he suffered more cardiac problems and a ruptured disk that required a spinal fusion. Drinking continued to increase. Despite the extensive history of heavy drinking, both Frank and his wife dated onset of what they considered a drinking problem to the period when at age 42, after suffering the health problems, he lost his job due to company reorganization, and his oldest son was arrested. Frank's drinking escalated to a quart or more of rum per day. On occasion, he became verbally abusive and threatening to his wife, especially when they argued about the oldest son's problems or Frank's excessive drinking.

About 18 months before the present hospital admission, Frank again suffered serious chest pain. When his physician diagnosed possible alcoholic cardiomyopathy, he entered a

---

TABLE 6. Important and Key Points about the Epidemiology of Substance-Related Disorders

1. Substance-related disorders are the most prevalent type of psychiatric disorder in the United States; 27% of adults in the National Comorbidity Study experienced this disorder in their lifetimes.
2. This same study indicated that in the past year, 7 to 10% of the U.S. population (11 to 14% of men and 4 to 5% of women) experienced alcohol abuse or dependence.
3. Of men in the general population who have substance use disorders, nearly 60% have problems of alcoholism, while a third have both alcoholism and drug problems, and the remaining 8% had only drug problems. Many treatment centers have a higher proportion of patients who have both alcoholism and drug problems.
4. The following factors are related to higher risk for substance use disorders:
   a. male gender
   b. less education, drop out from high school or college
   c. unmarried, separated or divorced more than once
   d. younger age
5. Heavy and repeated use of the substance is a controllable risk factor for substance use disorders.

seven-day detoxification program. He did not drink and attended Alcoholics Anonymous (AA) sporadically for six weeks after this first alcoholism treatment but resumed drinking after an argument with his wife. The patient found a new job and resumed heavy drinking. After an incident in which the patient became extremely abusive and threatening, the couple separated just before their twenty-fifth wedding anniversary and remained living apart for two months. Six months after their reconciliation and approximately 5 months before the present admission, Mr. Johnson quit his job after his boss told him he should get help for his drinking problem. The couple again separated. The patient continued to drink up to two quarts of rum daily on many days. He became increasingly depressed over the separation from his wife and children, worked at a new job, and continued drinking very heavily, until the events (described above) that immediately preceded his admission to the hospital.

Assessment. Medical evaluation revealed elevated liver enzymes without liver pathology and a history of coronary artery disease complicated by alcoholic cardiomyopathy. The Time-Line Follow-Back drinking interview (TLFB; Sobell & Sobell, 1996) showed that he had spent 80% of the days in the previous year drinking from one to two quarts of rum daily. He had experienced blackouts and severe shakes and sweats when trying to stop drinking on his own. On the Michigan Alcoholism Screening Test (MAST; Selzer, 1971), he received a very elevated score of 47, indicating multiple and serious consequences from alcohol abuse. A diagnostic interview was conducted by a psychiatrist in response to the patient's complaints of depression, sleep disturbance, and suicidal ideation and his request for antidepressant medication. The psychiatrist concluded that *Alcohol Dependence* was the primary diagnosis and that the "depression" and other complaints were caused by the alcohol problem and did not represent an affective disorder for which an antidepressant would be helpful. Finally, an evaluation of the marital relationship was conducted.

Reviewing the assessment and historical materials indicated a number of antecedents that had been associated with alcohol consumption. For each antecedent, the short-term consequence of the drinking had brought some temporary improvement but the longer-term consequences had been to create or exacerbate serious life problems. The following analysis was presented to Mr. Johnson and he concurred with this formulation of factors involved in his drinking:

1. He was a rigid, perfectionist who experienced considerable anxiety and both mental and physical (muscular) tension in response to daily life events. After his first episode of chest pain, he became fearful when he experienced muscular tension that this might lead to a heart attack. Alcohol relieved the tension and his fears about a heart attack in the short run but exacerbated his heart problem leading to alcoholic cardiomyopathy in the long run.

2. Business-related social drinking with clients and associates seemed to help these relationships initially. As time went on, he developed a reputation as a heavy drinker that contributed to his loss of two jobs. Drinking helped relieve his distress over this job instability but cost him his current job when he had to enter the hospital for alcoholism treatment.

3. Marital conflict clearly contributed to the drinking, which brought temporary escape from feelings of frustration, anger, and loss associated with these conflicts. Eventually, drinking led to increasingly more frequent and severe outbursts at his wife that led to police intervention, marital separation, and finally a legal separation.

4. The losses experienced led to feelings of depression, sadness, and guilt, at first relieved by, and later seriously increased by, the alcohol. When intoxicated, he had made one suicidal gesture, and serious suicidal ideas continued to frighten the patient when he was abstinent.

5. He had become physically dependent on alcohol and some of his drinking was done to ward off withdrawal symptoms.

Treatment. After detoxification from alcohol and repeated testing to ensure that his cardiac condition was stable, Frank entered an inpatient alcoholism treatment program.

This was followed by outpatient aftercare treatment that included couples counseling. At five years after hospital discharge, the patient remained continuously abstinent and employed with stable cardiac functioning. The couple's marriage had stabilized. No separations had occurred.

The patient's high degree of motivation for change certainly was an important factor in the success of the treatments used. He had lost his job, seriously risked his health, considered suicide, and nearly lost his family when he entered the hospital for detoxification, all because of his drinking. The inpatient treatment bolstered his desire for change and increased his motivation by providing specific methods he could use to cope with his drinking and other problems. The outpatient treatment reinforced sobriety directly and indirectly by reducing marital conflicts that had been one threat for continued sobriety. The interested reader is referred to the handbook by Hester and Miller (1995) for more information on current methods for treating alcoholism.

The Case of Jack Smith

Case Identification. Jack Smith was a 36-year-old, unemployed, white, male surveyor technician. He was the father of two preschool-age children. He had been separated from his wife for four months at the time of his admission to the alcohol and drug treatment program of a large veterans' hospital.

Presenting Complaints. Mr. Smith's complaints at the time of admission were that he had been drinking up to a quart of vodka daily for the past four months and taking morphine, 200 milligrams intravenously, daily for the past two and a half months. Given the quantity of his substance intake and past history of blackouts and severe tremors, he was judged physically dependent on both alcohol and morphine. Therefore, he was admitted for a 5-day medical detoxification program to withdraw safely from his alcohol and morphine.

Events Leading to Hospitalization. These were (1) he had been unemployed due to a job layoff for over a year; (2) his house had been foreclosed on by a bank due to nonpayment of his mortgage; (3) his wife had insisted he leave due to his substance abuse; and (4) when feeling depressed about the loss of his family, job, and house, he had tried unsuccessfully to kill himself by drinking a large amount of vodka and inhaling paint solvent until he passed out.

Early History. Jack began drinking at age 15 in high school when he drank heavily on weekends and smoked marijuana. On a number of occasions, he and some friends inhaled paint solvent together. On one occasion, he blacked out briefly when he deeply inhaled the solvent. This experience scared him and his friends. He stopped the inhalant abuse and did not return to it until the incident just before admission described before.

Jack had been a very nervous child and adolescent who experienced periods of strong anxiety when confronted with new social or achievement situations. His father was a recovering alcoholic. His parents had been separated during his preschool years, a time of marked financial and emotional insecurity for Jack and his mother and brother.

When Jack graduated from high school, he enrolled at the local community college. The new social and academic challenges made him very anxious, and his weekend drinking increased to nearly daily drinking to make him feel more comfortable. Eventually, he began missing classes, got behind in his school work, and dropped out of school.

He joined the Army and decided not to drink. He remained abstinent through basic training. When sent to an Army technical school far from home for training as a surveyor technician, he began drinking heavily on a daily basis. It was not long before he entered a 28-day Army alcohol rehabilitation program, after which he resumed drinking fairly soon. Two years later, he again requested substance abuse treatment. This time in addition to drinking he also had been involved in intravenous heroin use for six months. For his remaining two years in the Army, he limited his drinking to beer in barrooms, no hard drugs, and occasional marijuana.

Upon return to civilian life, his drinking escalated. After an embarrassing incident while drunk, he entered an inpatient treatment program, joined Alcoholics Anonymous (AA), and remained substance-free for two years. During this sober period, he met and married his wife and got a stable job as a surveyor technician in a large company. During the next nine years, he was mostly abstinent but drank for a few weeks on three occasions, generally to relieve intense states of anxiety, each of which was followed by a brief treatment center admission.

About 18 months before the present hospital admission, Jack began occasional use of morphine obtained from a co-worker. A few months later Jack's employer of seven years had large scale layoffs due to an economic downturn. He returned to drinking at first only occasionally and then to bouts of heavy drinking that lasted for many days. He also increased his frequency of morphine use. Financial stress and marital conflict increased as he continued without steady employment. When Jack lost a temporary job due to drinking about the same time as the bank began foreclosure proceedings on his home, Jack's wife insisted that he leave. After the separation, Jack quickly progressed to daily heavy drinking and regular morphine use.

Assessment. In terms of drinking and drug-taking behavior, the Time Line Follow-Back interview showed that he had spent 65% of the days in the previous year drinking a pint to a quart of vodka daily and 35% of these days taking morphine. On the Michigan Alcoholism Screening Test, he received a score of 49, a very elevated score indicating multiple and serious adverse consequences of substance use. Jack's score of 30 on the Alcohol Dependence Scale (Skinner & Allen, 1982), his experience of severe shakes and sweats when trying to stop drinking on his own, and the fact that he had gone to a detox center whenever he stopped drinking in the prior 10 years, all indicated a substantial physical dependence on alcohol. He had also become dependent on morphine.

Jack's current and previous behavior warranted multiple diagnoses. Substance-related disorders included current Alcohol Dependence and Morphine Dependence and a lifetime diagnosis for Heroin Dependence, Marijuana Abuse, and Inhalant Abuse. In addition, he suffered from a longstanding generalized anxiety disorder. Both the early family dysfunction and instability and his father's alcoholism probably contributed to the development of Jack's problems. The challenges of late adolescence and young adulthood led to increased anxiety largely dealt with by drinking and drug use. After the Army when he joined AA, got married and had a steady job, he remained mostly abstinent except for brief relapses when he felt extremely anxious. When faced with the emotional, financial, and marital stresses of extended unemployment during a recession, Jack increased his substance use. Once separated from his wife and children, his substance use increased even further leading to admission to the treatment center.

Treatment. After medical detoxification, Jack continued his alcohol and drug treatment program. During this inpatient stay, he renewed his involvement with AA but complained that anxiety made it difficult for him to feel comfortable and get involved in the AA meetings the way he should. To deal with the anxiety disorder, Jack received a prescription from the treatment center's psychiatrist for BuSpar (generic name buspirone), an anxiety medication that has very low potential for psychological or physical addiction. Jack also was referred to an anxiety management therapy group when he was discharged from the treatment center. He went to live in a substance-free halfway house upon discharge from the treatment center because his wife was reluctant to take him back at that time.

As of this writing it has been nine months since Jack's discharge from the treatment center. He has remained alcohol-free and drug-free. He attends AA three to four times a week and is actively involved. His anxiety is much improved. Jack and his wife are continuing in outpatient couples therapy having reconciled three months after his hospital discharge. Although still unemployed, he has enrolled in a job retraining program.

COURSE AND PROGNOSIS

The course and prognosis for substance-related disorders are somewhat complex. These vary from one substance to another, as well as within one type of substance use problem. Further, information drawn from clinical samples seeking treatment often is not applicable to the large numbers of people who do not seek treatment.

Evidence from Epidemiological Studies of the General Population

The picture that emerges from epidemiological studies of the course and progression of alcohol and drug problems is relatively clear. Data from the Epidemiologic Catchment Area study (ECA; Robins & Regier, 1991) already described earlier are presented because the information from the ECA study is more complete than that currently available from the National Comorbidity Study (Kessler et al., 1994) and are relatively consistent with other epidemiological studies in terms of results on the course of the disorders.

In general, alcohol and drug problems, viewed from the perspective of the ECA general population epidemiological study, begin by about age 20, and more than half of the cases who ever experienced the disorder were in remission (i.e., had no problems related to substance use in the past year) at the time of the ECA interview. Substance use disorders had among the highest rates of remission of any of the psychiatric disorders assessed in the ECA study.

When examined in more detail, some differences were noted between drug and alcohol problems. Drug problems, compared with alcohol problems, have a consistently more youthful onset, a shorter period of risk, and a shorter duration for cases that enter remission. The first drug problem occurs at a median age of 18 years, the age of risk for the onset of most drug problems occur between ages 16 and 21, and onset is rare *before* age 15. For those whose drug problems were in remission at the time of the interview, the period of active problems had lasted a mean of 2.7 years. Alcohol problems are more variable in course and progression than drug problems. Although almost 40% of those who develop alcoholism have their first alcohol-related problems between ages 15 to 19, cases of alcoholism continue to develop in the 20s, 30s, and 40s. The age of risk for developing alcoholism extends through the late 30s when 90% of those who develop alcohol-related problems will have done so. The duration of alcoholism for those in the ECA study who were in remission (i.e., had no alcohol related problems in the last year) was 9 years, on average, and three-quarters were in remission within 11 years.

Robins, Locke, and Regier (1991) remark that the high rates of remission for alcohol and drug disorders in the ECA study differ from results for clinical samples where relapse rates are traditionally very high. Nonetheless, the ECA data agree with previous follow-up studies in the general population, which also show high rates of remission and high rates of instability in the reporting of current problems between interviews a few years apart (Taylor & Helzer, 1983).

Helzer et al. (1991), commenting on these ECA findings, note the differences between alcoholics in treatment samples and in general population studies:

> These results (of high remission rates and short duration of the disorder) are very different from those seen in patients, who frequently come to treatment for the first time only after many years of alcohol

problems. Our findings may help to explain why so few persons with alcohol problems in the general population seek care. Many appear to be able to reduce their drinking sufficiently to terminate their difficulties quite early in the course of their disorder. It is those who try and fail that appear for treatment. (Helzer et al., 1991, pp. 97–98)

From the vantage point of epidemiological studies of the general population, substance use disorders show considerable change over time and many cases are in remission at any given time. This is in marked contrast with substance use treatment experience in which substance use disorders are seen as very difficult to treat, unlikely to have good and enduring remission after treatment, and (in the case of alcoholism) as a progressively deteriorating disease that inevitably gets worse and leads either to death or abstinence (Jellinek, 1960). A number of factors may explain the differing perspectives. As already indicated, the general population studies may contain many more substance abusers who have less severe problems than treatment populations that consist mostly of the more severe cases. General population studies generally are cross-sectional and retrospective; they interview individuals at one time and ask them about their current and former problems. Those who have the worst substance abuse outcome—death—are eliminated from consideration. Further, the future course of the disorder in those who have active substance use disorders at the time of the interview cannot be determined. Longitudinal studies of treatment samples provide an additional perspective on the course and prognosis of substance use disorders.

Evidence from Longitudinal Studies of Treatment Samples

Before the mid-1970s, the course and progression of substance use disorders, especially alcoholism, was considered relatively straightforward and simple. Alcoholism was seen as a progressively deteriorating disease that has a natural progression of symptoms that became increasingly severe over time ending inevitably in death or disability unless the disease was arrested through lifelong abstinence, generally achieved by regular attendance at Alcoholics Anonymous meetings (Jellinek, 1960).

Currently the course and progression of alcoholism among those whose problems are serious enough to seek treatment are seen as much more complex than had been thought heretofore. First, no one course applies to all or most of the cases seen in treatment centers. Clearly, the belief that all or most alcoholics show a progressive, deteriorating course is not supported by current evidence. Alcoholics have a variety of outcomes to their disorder. Second, although this finding has caused considerable controversy, it also is clear that some alcoholics can drink without experiencing problems, suggesting that total abstinence may not be the only way for all alcoholics to resolve their problems. A well-known study that illustrates these two important changes is described next.

OUTCOMES FOUR YEARS AFTER ALCOHOLISM TREATMENT

Table 7 describes the outcomes of more than 600 alcoholics four years after they were treated at one of eight Alcoholism Treatment Centers (Polich, Armor, & Braiker, 1981). The sample was chosen to be representative of all males admitted to treatment at the eight designated centers. The centers' patient populations were very similar to all patients treated in a U.S. government network of treatment centers at the time of the study. Therefore, the results come from a large, fairly representative sample of alcoholics in U.S. treatment centers. Although this classic study is now a bit old, its findings are still quite relevant.

Before considering Table 7, we must note that 15% of the patients were dead, more than

TABLE 7. Outcome during Four Years after Alcoholism Treatment[a]

1. Continuously abstinent	7%
2. Long-term abstainers	6%
3. Nonproblem drinkers	9%
4. Either abstainer or nonproblem drinker	6%
5. Alternated between drinking with serious problems and short-trem abstinence	52%
6. Consistently drinking with serious problems	20%

[a]This table was constructed from information in Polich, Armor, & Braiker (1981, p. 216). The percentages given are for the patients still alive four years after treatment.

half of these from alcohol-related causes, four years after treatment. This represents more than two and a half times the expected death rate for men whose demographic characteristics are similar to those in the sample. This subgroup seems to fit the progressive deteriorating course described by Jellinek and other disease model proponents. The 20% in Group 6 who drank fairly consistently and had drinking related problems might also be considered to have had a continuing if not progressive course after treatment. Those who stayed abstinent the entire 4 years, a small minority of 7%, also could fit the progression through abstinence. Group 3, the 9%, who had no problems, provided the greatest challenge to the disease model and the most controversy. Drinking without problems meant that the patient did not experience any serious, alcohol-related, adverse consequences (e.g., health problems, legal problems, work or family problems) or dependence symptoms (e.g., tremors, morning blackouts). These patients tended to be younger and have fewer signs of physical dependence (i.e., tolerance and withdrawal symptoms) on alcohol when they entered treatment, indicating they had less severe, less chronic problems. Group 4, the 6% who had periods of abstinence and of nonproblem drinking, also do not appear to fit the progressive disease model. The largest group of patients, 52% of the sample in Group 5, consisted of those who alternated between periods of problem drinking and short-term abstinence.

The Polich et al. data provide a different picture of the course of alcoholism than seen in epidemiological general population studies where about half are in remission. Only 28% of the treatment sample are in remission (Groups 1 to 4 of Table 7) four years after treatment. For the most part, these data do not fit the progressive deteriorating disease concept of alcoholism, because the majority do not show such a progressive course and some obtain remission without abstinence.

The picture that emerges from the Polich et al. data is that the course of alcoholism and paths to remission and recovery vary considerably. Some alcoholics do show a progressively deteriorating course in which they continue to drink heavily and consistently and have serious alcohol-related problems, including death. Others improve and enter remission either via long-term abstinence or a return to nonproblem drinking (the latter generally among younger, less severe cases). About half continue to alternate between periods of short-term abstinence and continued problem drinking.

Table 8 summarizes important and key points in the course and prognosis of substance-related disorders.

FAMILIAL AND GENETIC PATTERNS

Familial and genetic patterns of substance use disorders have been studied extensively for alcoholism and to a somewhat lesser extent for drug abuse/dependence. As we shall see,

TABLE 8. Important and Key Points about the Course and Prognosis of Substance-Related Disorders

1. The course and prognosis for substance use disorders differ in studies of the general population compared to treatment center patients who have a higher proportion of more severe problems.
2. In the general population, drug problems have a youthful onset from age 16 to 25. More than half enter remission (i.e., at least one year without problems) within three years of the onset of the disorder.
3. In the general population, alcoholism onset occurs by age 20 for 40% of alcoholism problems, but the age of risk extends through the late 30s and early 40s. About half of the cases of alcoholism go into remission within 11 years of their onset.
4. In treatment center patients, alcoholism is no longer seen has having a uniformly progressive deteriorating course that ends in death or is "arrested" by abstinence. This view has been called the unitary disease model.
5. A large scale study of the course of alcoholism over the four years after treatment showed that:
    a. some alcoholics (20 to 35%) do not improve or progressively deteriorate from continued heavy drinking and serious alcohol related problems, including death.
    b. a little more than a quarter have a stable remission either via long-term abstinence or a return to nonproblem drinking.
    c. The remaining cases continue to alternate between periods of short-term abstinence and problem drinking.

findings of familial and genetic patterns for alcoholism vary considerably based on the type of sample studied, the gender, and the type and severity of alcoholism.

Alcoholism

FAMILIAL PATTERNS FOR ALCOHOLISM

In a widely cited early paper, Cotton (1979) reviewed 39 studies of the familial incidence of alcoholism. Most of the studies reviewed by Cotton focused on samples of alcoholics drawn from inpatient and outpatient psychiatric settings. Cotton concluded that alcoholics were approximately four to five times more likely to have an alcoholic parent than control groups not seen in psychiatric settings.

In representative community and U.S. national samples, the risk for offspring to experience a problem with alcoholism if their parent was an alcoholic was only 1.4 to 1.7 times greater than for those without parental alcoholism (Russell, 1990). This increased risk is not nearly as great as noted by Cotton (1979) in her review of family patterns of alcoholics from treatment settings. These differences in findings from treatment and community samples are not surprising. Alcoholics who seek treatment are more likely to have severe alcoholism problems and to suffer from concomitant psychopathology (Helzer & Pryzbeek, 1988; Kessler et al., 1999). Thus, it appears that familial patterns for alcoholism differ as a function of the severity of the alcoholism.

GENETIC STUDIES OF ALCOHOLISM

As already indicated, alcoholism runs in families. Such a familial pattern can be caused by genetic inheritance of a predisposition to alcoholism, shared environmental factors within families (e.g., modeling of expectancies and patterns of use for alcohol), or both. Based on a sizable literature examining genetic factors in alcoholism, most researchers would, no doubt, agree that genetic factors influence the risk of alcoholism among men (e.g., Prescott & Kendler, 1999) and women (e.g., Kendler, Neale, Heath, Kessler, & Eaves, 1994). There is some evidence that the strength of the genetic influence is greater for a more severe than a less severe type of alcoholism (e.g., Cloninger, 1987; Johnson, Van Den Bree, & Pickens, 1996;

McGue, Pickens, & Svikis, 1992) and for men than for women (e.g., McGue et al., 1992). However, the specific nature and the practical implications of a genetic predisposition to alcoholism remain unresolved. Schuckit (1999) addresses both of these issues.

In terms of the specific nature of a genetic predisposition to alcoholism, Schuckit (1999) presents the general consensus in the field that genetic influences on alcoholism probably do not represent one specific gene but rather these influences may involve multiple genes or incomplete expression of several genes along with environmental influences. Schuckit (1999) summarizes four major areas that are being studied: (1) genetic variation in alcohol metabolizing enzymes, an example of which are some Asian men and women who have adverse reactions (e.g., skin flushing, nausea) to ingesting alcohol and thus have a low risk of alcoholism, (2) genetic variation in the level of response to alcohol such that some individuals can consume large quantities of alcohol with relatively little effect and thus are more likely to develop alcoholism, (3) genetically influenced brain wave characteristics that are more common in alcohol-dependent people and their children than expected from chance alone, and (4) genes controlling the brain's dopamine neurochemical system.

Schuckit (1999) also discusses the practical implications of a genetic predisposition to alcoholism for prevention and treatment. "Regarding prevention, the genetic data reinforce the wisdom of teaching children of alcoholics that they carry a heightened vulnerability toward a serious disorder, which can be avoided by abstinence or diminished by adhering to limited levels of alcohol intake" (Schuckit, 1999, p. 1876). Specific implications for treatment are more complex and await further research given the multiple, and as yet not fully confirmed, genetic pathways of influence to increased risk of alcoholism.

Drug Abuse and Dependence

Familial and genetic influences on the development of drug abuse/dependence have not been investigated as extensively as for alcoholism, but some important studies are being conducted that have recently reported initial results. Drug problems run in families and there is elevated familial risk of drug abuse or dependence disorders involving cannabis, cocaine, hallucinogenics, and opioids (Bierut et al., 1998; Croughan, 1985; Merikangas et al., 1998). A genetic influence has been found for abuse or dependence on cannabis, stimulants, cocaine, opioids, sedatives, and hallucinogenics among men (Tsuang et al., 1996; Van Den Bree, Johnson, Neale, & Pickens, 1998) and cannabis, cocaine, and stimulants among women (Kendler, Karkowski, & Prescott, 1999; Kendler & Prescott, 1998a,b), and genetic influences are somewhat stronger among men than women. Despite these interesting initial findings, further studies are required to elucidate the relative contribution of genetic and environmental factors to the development of drug abuse and dependence.

Table 9 summarizes important and key points about familial and genetic patterns pertaining to substance-related disorders.

DIAGNOSTIC CONSIDERATIONS

Diagnostic criteria for the substance-related disorders of dependence and abuse based on DSM-IV were described at the start of this chapter. Other diagnostic issues are considered here. These include substance-induced disorders of intoxication and withdrawal, other substance-induced disorders, other frequently observed coexisting psychopathology, and identification and treatment of substance use disorders and problems.

Table 9. Important and Key Points
about Familial and Genetic Patterns of Substance-Related Disorders

1. Children of alcoholics consistently have higher rates of alcoholism than children whose parents are not alcoholic. However, the extent of increased risk of alcoholism varies considerably and is greater when the parents' alcoholism is more severe.
2. Children of treatment center alcoholics (who generally have more severe problems) were four to five times more likely to be alcoholic themselves, whereas in representative population samples the risk was 1.4 to 1.7 times greater if the child had an alcoholic parent.
3. A genetic influence on the risk of alcoholism is generally accepted. The specific nature and the practical implications of a genetic predisposition to alcoholism remain unresolved.
4. Prevention efforts should teach children of alcoholic parents that they carry a heightened vulnerability to a serious disorder, which can be avoided by abstinence or reduced by keeping alcohol intake to limited levels.
5. Drug problems run in families also, and initial studies support a genetic influence on drug abuse/dependence disorders. Further studies are required to elucidate the relative contribution of genetic and environmental factors to the development of drug abuse and dependence.

Substance-Related Disorders of Intoxication and Withdrawal

DSM-IV lists and describes substance-induced disorders associated with *states of alcohol or drug intoxication or withdrawal*. Complications from the specific intoxication states, such as traffic accidents and physical injury due to Alcohol Intoxication or potential for serious violence due to PCP Intoxication, are also described in DSM-IV for each of the substances. Although intoxication is frequent in those who have substance use disorders, it does not necessarily occur in all cases of the disorder, and intoxication can occur without the person suffering from a substance use disorder. Characteristic withdrawal syndromes that occur after regular heavy use when a person stops or reduces intake of the substance are also described for each substance in DSM-IV. Marked physical signs of withdrawal are common for alcohol, opioids, sedatives, hypnotics, and anxiolytics. Such physical signs are less obvious for amphetamines, cocaine, nicotine, and cannabis, but intense subjective emotional symptoms can occur upon withdrawal from heavy use of these substances. No significant withdrawal is seen even after repeated use of hallucinogens, and PCP withdrawal has not been documented in humans (APA, 1994).

Other Substance-Induced Disorders

Eight substance-induced disorders, described in DSM-IV, are behavioral disorders that can be associated with chronic heavy use of the various psychoactive substances. These include delirium, dementia, amnestic disorder, psychotic disorder, mood disorder, anxiety disorder, sex dysfunction, and sleep disorder. Such mental symptoms that occur as a result of chronic, heavy substance use are diagnosed under the substance that induced the symptoms (e.g., alcohol delirium, cocaine psychotic disorder).

Other Coexisting Psychopathology

Persons who have substance use disorders often experience additional types of psychopathology. These additional types of psychopathology are generally described as "coexisting," "co-occurring," or "comorbid" disorders. We have already seen that two or more types

TIMOTHY J. O'FARRELL

of substance use disorder frequently co-occur. For example, approximately half of those who have a drug abuse/dependence problem also experience a problem with alcoholism.

Nearly three-fourths (73%) of those with abuse alcohol or dependence in the NCS study received another diagnosis; additional disorders were more common among female (80%) than among male (70%) alcoholics (Kessler et al., 1997). In the NCS, the most common additional diagnoses for both alcoholic men and women were drug abuse/dependence, antisocial personality, anxiety disorders, and affective disorders. Among alcoholics hospitalized for treatment, antisocial personality disorder and depression are the most frequent co-occurring disorders (Hesselbrock, Meyer, & Keener, 1985). Helzer et al. (1991) argue that treatment-seeking alcoholics have higher rates of coexisting depression than community samples because the occurrence of depression may motivate alcoholics to seek treatment.

Comorbidity results for drug abuse/dependence have not been published yet for the NCS. However, based on the earlier ECA study, persons who have drug abuse/dependence problems are quite likely to have other disorders; 71% overall (75% in men, 65% in women) had at least one additional disorder in the ECA study. The most common additional disorder is alcoholism which was experienced by nearly half, followed by antisocial personality disorder, mania, schizophrenia, and phobic disorder.

When alcohol or drug disorders coexist with other disorders, it often is difficult to know whether or not one disorder caused the other. For example, it is possible that alcohol or drug use makes already existing problems (e.g., depression, phobic symptoms, antisocial behaviors) worse. Alternatively, the alcohol or drug use may have been made worse by the other disorder when the person drank or used drugs in an effort at self-medication to reduce the symptoms of the other disorder (Anthony & Helzer, 1991). At times, a "vicious cycle" can occur in which alcohol or drug use leads to other emotional problems which are temporarily relieved by more alcohol or drug use only to reappear as more serious problems once the temporary escape provided by substance use is over. The case of Frank Johnson described earlier is a good example. This case also illustrates the important clinical point that diagnosis and treatment of coexisting psychopathology requires considerable expertise and a degree of patience because some disorders (e.g., depression) that coexist with substance use problems can be accurately diagnosed only after a period of abstinence.

Identification and Treatment of Substance Use Disorders and Problems

Even though substance use disorders are the most common mental or behavioral disorder in the United States, 85–90% of people who have substance use disorders never receive treatment for these problems (Kessler et al., 1999; Robins & Regier, 1991). Consider also that a large number of individuals do not meet diagnostic criteria for substance use disorder, but nonetheless are heavy substance users who may have problems related to their substance use. These individuals are the heavy problem drinkers noted in Figure 3, and the individuals who have mild to moderate alcohol problems noted in Figure 4. Due to their large numbers, these individuals who have mild to moderate alcohol problems place a great burden of costs on themselves and on society for alcohol-related traffic accidents, injuries, lost productivity from work, etc. Still, as we have already discussed, only those who have severe problems receive treatment. Finally, even among the more severe cases seen in treatment settings, there is considerable variability in the nature of the substance use symptoms experienced, the type and extent of additional life problems and coexisting psychopathology, the age of onset, the course of illness and the prognosis for recovery, and in the extent to which genetic and environmental influences are important.

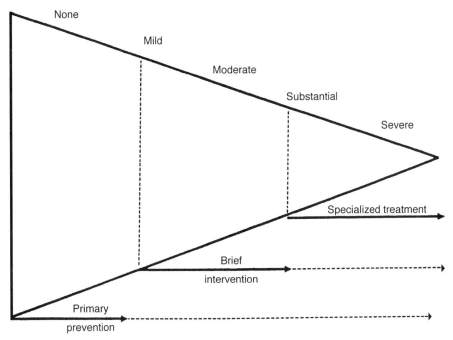

FIGURE 4. Alcohol problems and a proposal for their treatment (reprinted with permission from p. 212 of Institute of Medicine (1990). *Broadening the base of treatment for alcohol problems.* Washington, DC: National Academy Press).

In 1990, the U.S. National Academy of Sciences released a report of a committee on treatment of alcohol problems. Figure 4, taken from the committee's report, conveys the vision of expanded identification and treatment of alcohol problems that flowed from the committee's judgments and recommendations. The *committee's* judgments that efforts to treat alcohol problems in the United States have been too narrowly focused on those people who have the most severe problems and that treatment should be matched to a patient's needs even among the more severe cases produced recommendations for a number of significant additions and changes in treating alcohol problems.

First, a greatly expanded role for community agencies and settings is proposed. These include health-care settings, schools, courts, social welfare agencies and so forth. This role involves identifying individuals who have alcohol problems, providing brief interventions (six or fewer sessions) to reduce or eliminate alcohol consumption by those who have mild or moderate alcohol problems, and referring those who have substantial or severe problems to the specialized alcoholism treatment sector. The varied professionals in community settings would need considerable additional training for these roles.

Second, the specialist treatment of alcohol problems also would be considerably broadened. Specialist treatment refers to public and private inpatient and outpatient centers that specialize in treating alcohol problems. As envisioned, treatment would begin with a comprehensive assessment by which the person would be matched to the most appropriate type of intervention (e.g., inpatient or residential vs. outpatient). Follow-up data would be gathered after treatment to determine outcomes, and feedback of outcome information would be used to improve the matching guidelines used in assessment and treatment assignment. Although all of the components of the recommended treatment system have been the subject of consider-able research and scholarly effort, currently,

> most treatment programs do not offer more than a single treatment option ... neither do most offer ... comprehensive assessment ... With only a single treatment option, matching can not be carried out ... few treatment programs engage in comprehensive outcome monitoring, and without monitoring, there can be no feedback. (Institute of Medicine, 1990, pp. 334–335)

Third, an explicit goal of all treatment would be to eliminate problems due to alcohol consumption, suggesting that the goal for drinking behavior also might be matched to the type and severity of the person's alcohol problem. Thus, reduced drinking rather than abstinence might be sufficient to eliminate problems, particularly among persons who have mild to moderate alcohol problems.

Finally, the report recommends establishing a few pilot programs to test the feasibility of expanded and comprehensive treatment systems. The committee concludes that, although methods of financing would have to be developed, the social costs saved by appropriate intervention would likely offset the financial costs of a broadened national commitment to treating alcohol problems.

The widespread nature of substance use disorders and their associated societal costs have moved those concerned with treating these problems beyond the diagnostic issues of abnormal psychology into the public health arena where screening and identifying problems replaces diagnosis of disorders. Clearly, this is the thrust of the Institute of Medicine report on alcohol problems just discussed. No similar report exists for drug abuse problems. Efforts beyond treatment in the drug abuse area have focused on preventing illicit drug use among school-age youth and young adults. Given the decline in the frequent use of illicit drugs by U.S. youth (U.S. HHS, 1992), these prevention efforts, along with more negative societal attitudes about drug use have been at least partially successful. Suburban youth have shown the greatest reductions in drug use, which remains a significant problem among inner city youth.

Table 10 summarizes important and key points about diagnostic considerations pertaining to substance-related disorders.

Summary

Psychoactive substances can be used to affect moods, thinking, and behavior. The serious negative behavioral effects that occur from using such substances are called *substance-related disorders*. The essential features of the disorders are a maladaptive pattern of substance use leading to clinically significant impairment or distress.

Substance-related disorders are the most common psychiatric disorder in the United States. A recent study found lifetime prevalence of 27%, and in the past year, 7 to 10% of the U.S. population (11 to 14% of men and 4 to 5% of women) experienced a substance use disorder.

The course and prognosis for substance use disorders differ in studies of the general population compared to treatment center patients who have a higher proportion of more severe problems. In the general population, drug problems have a youthful onset from age 16 to 25, and more than half enter remission within 3 years of onset of the disorder. In the general population, alcoholism onset occurs by age 20 for 40% of problems, but the age of risk extends through the late 30s and early 40s, and about half go into remission within 11 years of their onset. In treatment center patients, the course of treatment varies. Some alcoholics (20 to 35%) do not improve or progressively deteriorate, a little more than a quarter have stable remissions,

TABLE 10. Important and Key Points
about Diagnostic Considerations for Substance-Related Disorders

1. Substance-induced disorders associated with substance use include
   a. states of alcohol or drug intoxication or withdrawal;
   b. Other behavioral disorders (e.g., memory loss, hallucinations, delusions) associated with chronic heavy substance use.
2. Persons who have substance use disorders often experience additional types of psychopathology. Antisocial personality, anxiety, and affective disorders are the most common additional coexisting psychopathologies.
3. Most (85–90%) of these who have substance use disorders never receive treatment. Active disorders and heavy substance use that does not meet diagnostic criteria produce substantial costs to society for traffic accidents, injuries, and lost productivity related to substance use.
4. A government panel urged *expanded identification and treatment of alcohol problems* in which
   a. community settings (health clinics, courts, etc.) would
      —identify individuals who have alcohol problems,
      —provide brief interventions (six or fewer sessions) for those who have mild or moderate alcohol problems, and
      —refer more severe problems to specialized alcoholism treatment centers.
   b. alcoholism treatment centers would
      —conduct a comprehensive assessment,
      —match person to appropriate type of intervention, and
      —gather follow-up data to measure the outcome and to improve the success of the treatment matching process.

and the remaining cases continue to alternate between periods of short-term abstinence and problems.

Children of alcoholics consistently have higher rates of alcoholism than children whose parents are not alcoholic. However, the extent of increased risk for alcoholism varies considerably. Children of treatment center alcoholics were four to five times more likely to be alcoholic themselves, whereas in representative population samples, the risk was 1.4 to 1.7 times greater if the child had an alcoholic parent. A genetic influence on risk for alcoholism is generally accepted. The specific nature and the practical implications of a genetic predisposition to alcoholism remain unresolved. Drug problems also run in families, and initial studies support a genetic influence on drug abuse/dependence disorders.

Substance-related disorders include states of alcohol or drug intoxication or withdrawal, and substance-induced disorders (e.g., dementia, mood disorder) are associated with chronic heavy substance use. Persons who have substance use disorders often have additional psychopathology, of which antisocial personality, affective disorders, and anxiety disorders are most common.

Most (85–90%) substance use disorders are never treated. Recent U.S. government reports have recommended expanded identification and treatment of substance use problems.

ACKNOWLEDGMENTS.   Preparation of this chapter was supported by the National Institute on Alcohol Abuse and Alcoholism (grant K02AA00234) and by the Department of Veterans Affairs.

REFERENCES

American Psychiatric Association. (1987). *Diagnostic and statistical manual of mental disorders*, 3rd ed., rev. Washington, DC: Author.

American Psychiatric Association. (1994). *Diagnostic and statistical manual of mental disorders*, 4th ed. Washington, DC: Author.

Anthony, J. C., & Helzer, J. E. (1991). Syndromes of drug abuse and dependence. In L. N. Robins & D. A. Regier (Eds.), *Psychiatric disorders in America: The Epidemiologic Catchment Area study* (pp. 116–154). New York: Free Press.

Anthony, J. C., Warner, L. A., & Kessler, R. C. (1994). Comparative epidemiology of dependence on tobacco, alcohol, controlled substances, and inhalants: Basic findings from the National Comorbidity Study. *Experimental and Clinical Psychopharmacology, 2*, 244–268.

Bierut, L. J., Dinwiddie, S. H., Begleiter, H., Crowe, R. R., Hesselbrock, V., Nurnberger, J. I., Porjesz, B., Schuckit, M. A., & Reich, T. (1998). Familial transmission of substance dependence: Alcohol, marijuana, cocaine, and habitual smoking. *Archives of General Psychiatry, 55*, 982–988.

Cloninger, C. R. (1987). Neurogenetic adaptive mechanisms in alcoholism. *Science, 236*, 410–416.

Cotton, N. S. (1979). The familial incidence of alcoholism. *Journal of Studies on Alcohol, 40*, 89–116.

Croughan, J. L. (1985) The contributions of family studies to understanding drug abuse. In L. N. Robins (Ed.), *Studying drug abuse*. New Brunswick, NJ: Rutgers University Press.

Helzer, J. E., Burnham, A., & McEvoy, L. T. (1991). Alcohol abuse and dependence. In L. N. Robins & D. A. Regier (Eds.), *Psychiatric disorders in America: The Epidemiologic Catchment Area study* (pp. 81–115). New York: Free Press.

Helzer, J. E., & Pryzbeck, T. R. (1988). The co-occurrence of alcoholism with other psychiatric disorders in the general population and its impact on treatment. *Journal of Studies on Alcohol, 49*, 219–224.

Hesselbrock, M. N., Meyer, R. E., & Keener, J. J. (1985). Psychopathology in hospitalized alcoholics. *Archives of General Psychiatry, 42*, 1050–1055.

Hester, R. K., & Miller, W. R. (Eds.). (1995). *Handbook of alcoholism treatment approaches: Effective alternatives*, 2nd ed. New York: Pergamon.

Institute of Medicine. (1990). *Broadening the base of treatment for alcohol problems*. Washington, DC: National Academy Press.

Jellinek, E. M. (1960). *The disease concept of alcoholism*. Highland Park, NJ: Hillhouse Press.

Johnson, E. O., Van Den Bree, M. B., & Pickens, R. W. (1996). Subtypes of alcohol-dependent men: A typology based on relative genetic and environmental loading. *Alcoholism: Clinical and Experimental Research, 20*, 1472–1480.

Kendler, K. S., Karkowski, L., & Prescott, C. A. (1999). Hallucinogen, opiate, sedative and stimulant use and abuse in a population-based sample of female twins. *Acta Psychiatrica Scandanavica, 99*, 368–376.

Kendler, K. S., Neale, M. C., Heath, A. C., Kessler, R. C., & Eaves, L. J. (1994). A twin-family study of alcoholism in women. *American Journal of Psychiatry, 151*, 707–715.

Kendler, K. S., & Prescott, C. A. (1998a). Cannabis use, abuse, and dependence in a population-based sample of female twins. *American Journal of Psychiatry, 155*, 1016–1022.

Kendler, K. S., & Prescott, C. A. (1998b). Cocaine use, abuse, and dependence in a population-based sample of female twins. *British Journal of Psychiatry, 173*, 345–350.

Kessler, R. C., McGonagle, K. A., Zhao, S., Nelson, C. B., Hughes, M., Eshleman, S., Wittchen, H. U., & Kendler, K. S. (1994). Lifetime and 12-month prevalence of DSM-III-R psychiatric disorders in the United States: Results from the National Comorbidity Study. *Archives of General Psychiatry, 51*, 8–19.

Kessler, R. C., Zhao, S., Katz, S. J., Kouzis, A. C., Frank, R. G., Edlund, M., & Leaf, P. (1999). Past year use of outpatient services for psychiatric problems in the National Comorbidity Study. *American Journal of Psychiatry, 156*, 115–123.

Kessler, R. C., Crum, R. M., Warner, L. A., Nelson, C. B., Schulenberg, J., & Anthony, J. C. (1997). Lifetime co-occurrence of DSM-III-R alcohol abuse and dependence with other psychiatric disorders in the National Comorbidity Study. *Archives of General Psychiatry, 54*, 313–321.

McGue, M., Pickens, R. W., & Svikis, D. S. (1992). Sex and age effects on the inheritance of alcohol problems: A twin study. *Journal of Abnormal Psychology, 101*, 3–17.

Merikangas, K. R., Stolar, M., Stevens, D. E., Goulet, J., Preisig, M. A., Fenton, B., Zhang, H., O'Malley, S. S., & Rounsaville, B. J. (1998). Familial transmission of substance use disorders. *Archives of General Psychiatry, 55*, 973–979.

National Institute on Drug Abuse. (NIDA). (1989). National household survey on drug abuse: 1988 population estimates (DHHS Publication No. ADM 89-1636). Rockville, MD: Author.

Polich, J. M., Armor, D. J., & Braiker, H. B. (1981). *The course of alcoholism: Four years after treatment*. New York: Wiley.

Prescott, C. A., & Kendler, K. S. (1999). Genetic and environmental contributions to alcohol abuse and dependence in a population-based sample of male twins. *American Journal of Psychiatry, 156*, 34–40.

Robins, L. N., Locke, B. A., & Regier, D. A. (1991). An overview of psychiatric disorders in America. In L. N. Robins & D. A. Regier (Eds.), *Psychiatric disorders in America: The Epidemiologic Catchment Area study* (pp. 328–386). New York: Free Press.

Robins, L. N., & Regier, D. A. (Eds.). (1991). *Psychiatric disorders in America: The Epidemiologic Catchment Area study*. New York: Free Press.

Russell, M. (1990). Prevalence of alcoholism among children of alcoholics. In M. Windle & J. S. Searles (Eds.), *Children of alcoholics: Critical perspectives* (pp. 9–38). New York: Guilford.

Schuckit, M. A. (1999). New findings in the genetics of alcoholism. *Journal of the American Medical Association, 281*, 1875–1876.

Selzer, M. L. (1971). The Michigan Alcoholism Screening Test: The quest for a new diagnostic instrument. *American Journal of Psychiatry, 127*, 1653–1658.

Skinner, H. A., & Allen, B. A. (1982). Alcohol dependence syndrome: Measurement and validation. *Journal of Abnormal Psychology, 91*, 199–209.

Sobell, L. C., & Sobell, M. B. (1996). *Timeline followback user's guide: A calendar method for assessing alcohol and drug use*. Toronto, Canada: Addiction Research Foundation.

Taylor, J. R., & Helzer, J. E. (1983). The natural history of alcoholism. In B. Kissin & H. Begleiter (Eds.), *The biology of alcoholism*, Vol. 6. New York: Plenum.

Tsuang, M. T., Lyons, M. J., Eisen, S. A., Goldberg, J., True, W., Lin, N., Meyer, J. M., Toomey, R., Faraone, S. V., & Eaves, L. (1996). Genetic influences on DSM-III-R drug abuse and dependence. *American Journal of Medical Genetics, 67*, 472–477.

U.S. Department of Health and Human Services. (1992). National Household Survey on Drug Abuse. *ADAMHA News*, January–February, 18–19.

Van Den Bree, M. B., Johnson, E. O., Neale, M. C., & Pickens, R. W. (1998). Genetic and environmental influences on drug use and abuse/dependence in male and female twins. *Drug and Alcohol Dependence, 52*, 231–241.

18

Sexual Disorders

William O'Donohue, Tamara Penix, and Lisa Regev

Sexual functioning is important for many reasons. Biologically, of course, it is critical for the propagation of the species. And speaking less biologically, it can be the source of one of life's greatest treasures—children. It can be a source of great physical pleasure. It can also result in becoming close to another person in a very special way. One can experience and give comfort, closeness, and intimacy in sexual contact. Finally, sexual functioning can be an important component of a positive self-image—most of us like to think of ourselves as sexually desirable and sexually skilled. Thus, when sexual functioning becomes a problem, these benefits may also be jeopardized. Partners may leave, self-esteem may plummet, and one can feel lonely and estranged from others.

Sexual behavior is also one of the most evaluated domains of human functioning. Most of us have fairly strong ideas about what is appropriate sexual behavior and what is not. Masturbation, premarital sex, extramarital sex, having a large number of sexual partners, homosexual contact, use of prostitutes, pornography use, sex with children, viewing strippers, nudity, spanking, and cross-dressing are all possible sexual behaviors and are all behaviors about which we usually have strong views regarding how "good" or "bad" they are. Thus, some sexual behavior is considered disordered because we judge that the object choice—the goal—of the behavior is problematic. Exposing oneself to strangers, rubbing up against strangers for sexual satisfaction, and sexual attraction to children are examples of object choices that are regarded as *paraphilic* ("para"—outside; and "philia"—to love; thus literally to love something that is abnormal).

In this chapter we discuss these two types of sexual disorders. *Sexual dysfunctions* can occur when someone has a normal object choice but has some problems performing or acting on this normal orientation. *Paraphilias* are sexual disorders because the person is sexually interested and aroused by inappropriate stimuli.

William O'Donohue, Tamara Penix, and Lisa Regev • Department of Psychology, University of Nevada-Reno, Reno, Nevada 89557-0062.

Advanced Abnormal Psychology, Second Edition, edited by Hersen and Van Hasselt. Kluwer Academic/Plenum Publishers, New York, 2001.

Sexual Dysfunctions

Description of the Disorder

The model often used to classify the sexual dysfunctions is found in the *Diagnostic and statistical manual of mental disorders*, 4th ed. (DSM-IV; APA, 1994). This model is based on Masters and Johnson's (1966) postulations of a sexual response cycle, as well as Kaplan's (1977) addition of an initial desire phase. The model consists of a four-phase sexual response cycle: desire, excitement, orgasm, and resolution. The first phase, desire, is characterized by sexual fantasies and urges to engage in sexual activity. The excitement phase is characterized by subjective feelings of sexual arousal, as well as characteristic physiological changes. During this phase, nondisordered men experience penile tumescence (swelling) and erection, and women experience vasocongestion in the pelvis, as well as vaginal lubrication and swelling. The third phase, orgasm, consists of a peaking of sexual pleasure and release of sexual tension. Males experience a sensation of ejaculatory inevitability, which is followed by ejaculation of semen, accompanied by a sensation of extreme pleasure. Females experience contractions of the wall of the outer third of vagina and a sensation or multiple sensations of pleasure. During this phase, the anal sphincter also rhythmically contracts in both genders. The final phase, resolution, consists of a sense of muscular relaxation. During this phase, males are not able to obtain an erection for a period of time, which varies with factors such as age, health, and the attractiveness of the partner. Females, on the other hand, may be able to respond to further sexual stimulation almost immediately.

Sexual dysfunction is described in the DSM-IV as a disruption in one or more of the first three phases of the sexual response cycle described before, or pain associated with sexual activity. The DSM-IV lists four general categories of sexual dysfunctions; two to three dysfunctions are within each category, resulting in a total of nine specific sexual dysfunctions. These include: Sexual Desire Disorders (Hypoactive Sexual Desire Disorder, Sexual Aversion Disorder), Sexual Arousal Disorders (Female Sexual Arousal Disorder, Male Erectile Disorder), Orgasmic Disorders (Female Orgasmic Disorder, Male Orgasmic Disorder, Premature Ejaculation), and Sexual Pain Disorders (Dyspareunia, Vaginismus). Other sexual dysfunctions include Sexual Dysfunction due to a General Medical Condition, where the disorder is caused by the direct physiological effects of a general medical condition; Substance Induced Sexual Dysfunction, where substance or medication use causes the disorder, and Sexual Dysfunction Not Otherwise Specified. Each disorder is defined by three criteria, the first of which is the distinguishing criterion among the sexual dysfunctions. The remaining two criteria are similar for all sexual dysfunctions, as will be discussed.

Hypoactive Sexual Desire Disorder

Clients who present with this disorder report persistent or recurrent low levels of desire or interest in engaging in sexual activity, including a complete deficiency or absence of sexual fantasies. When diagnosing this disorder, factors that affect sexual functioning such as age and the context of the person's life should be taken into account. For example, relationship satisfaction and cultural setting should be considered before making a diagnosis. Generally, the client who has Hypoactive Sexual Desire Disorder does not initiate sexual activity and may engage in it only reluctantly when a partner initiates sexual activity.

SEXUAL AVERSION DISORDER

Clients presenting with this disorder report persistent or recurrent aversion to and active avoidance of genital sexual contact with a sexual partner. The client generally reports moderate to extreme anxiety, fear, or disgust when genital sexual activity is initiated by a partner. This aversion may generalize to other sexual behaviors, such as kissing and nongenital touching.

FEMALE SEXUAL AROUSAL DISORDER

Females who present with this disorder report a persistent or recurrent inability to attain or maintain sufficient vaginal lubrication until the sexual activity is complete. This may result in ending the sexual activity prematurely or in pain during sexual intercourse.

MALE ERECTILE DISORDER

Males who present with this dysfunction report a persistent or recurrent inability to attain or maintain an adequate erection. This can occur in a number of patterns. Some males report an inability to attain an erection from the onset of a sexual encounter. Others first experience an adequate erection and then lose penile tumescence when attempting penetration. Still others can attain an adequate erection through penetration, but lose tumescence during thrusting. Some males experience an erection only during self-masturbation or upon awakening. Males who suffer from this disorder tend to be particularly concerned with monitoring their erectile response, thereby resulting in distracting, anxiety-provoking, nonarousing thoughts.

FEMALE ORGASMIC DISORDER

Females presenting with this problem report a persistent or recurrent delay in, or absence of, orgasm following normal sexual excitement. In diagnosing this disorder, the clinician must take into account the woman's age, sexual experience, and the adequacy of stimulation she receives.

MALE ORGASMIC DISORDER

Just as in female orgasmic disorder, males presenting with this problem report a persistent or recurrent delay in, or absence of, orgasm following normal sexual excitement. Again, the clinician must take into account factors that affect orgasmic functioning including the man's age, as well as the focus, intensity, and duration of the sexual stimulation. Most commonly, the male cannot reach orgasm during intercourse but can ejaculate from manual or oral stimulation. Others can reach orgasm during intercourse, but only after prolonged, intense stimulation prior to intercourse.

PREMATURE EJACULATION

Males who present with this disorder report persistent or recurrent ejaculation with minimal sexual stimulation before, on, or shortly after penetration and before the person wishes it. When diagnosing this disorder, the clinician must take into account factors that affect the duration of the excitement phase, such as age, novelty of the sexual partner or situation, and recent frequency of sexual activity. Generally, males who suffer from this disorder can delay orgasm during self-masturbation for a longer period of time than during sexual intercourse.

DYSPAREUNIA

Males and females who present with this disorder report persistent or recurrent genital pain during sexual intercourse. This pain is usually experienced during intercourse, but it may also occur before or after intercourse. Females describe the pain as either superficial during insertion or deep during thrusting.

VAGINISMUS

Women who present with this dysfunction report recurrent or persistent involuntary contractions of the perineal muscles surrounding the outer third of the vagina when vaginal penetration with penis, finger, tampon, or speculum is attempted. In some women, anticipation of vaginal insertion may result in muscle spasms. The contractions may range from mild, resulting in some tightness, to severe, preventing penetration.

The other two criteria required for diagnosing each of these disorders are similar across the sexual dysfunctions. The second criterion for each of these disorders is that the problem causes marked distress or interpersonal difficulty. Some clients presenting with these disorders indicate that they are distressed by the sexual difficulty. Others indicate that their partners are finding their sexual difficulty problematic. However, if neither partner is distressed by the sexual "inadequacy," a diagnosis is not warranted.

The third criterion for each of these disorders includes one or more of the following: ruling out another psychological problem, a medical problem, or the use of a medication or drug of abuse that may have negatively impacted sexual functioning. Psychological problems that may affect sexual functioning include Posttraumatic Stress Disorder as a result of a sexual assault, Obsessive Compulsive Disorder, and Major Depressive Disorder. Medical problems that may affect sexual functioning include a chronic or acute medical condition, medication use, and previous surgery.

The sexual dysfunctions are also categorized within subtypes by the onset, context, and etiological factors associated with them. To indicate the nature of the onset of the disorder, it is necessary to determine whether the dysfunction is lifelong or acquired. The lifelong subtype indicates that the sexual problem has been present from the start of sexual functioning. The acquired diagnosis applies if the problem develops after a period of normal sexual functioning. To indicate the context in which the sexual dysfunction occurs, it is necessary to indicate whether the dysfunction is generalized or situational. The generalized type applies if the dysfunction occurs during all types of stimulation, situations, or partners. If the dysfunction is limited to specific types of stimulation, situations, or partners, the dysfunction is of the situational type. To indicate etiological factors associated with sexual dysfunction, it is necessary to specify whether the problem is due to psychological factors or due to combined factors, including psychological factors and either a general medical condition and/or substance use.

Epidemiology

Recent research suggests that sexual dysfunction is common. In a survey of adult sexual behavior in the United States in which 1749 women and 1410 men ages 18 to 59 participated, 43% of women and 31% of men were suffering from sexual dysfunction (Laumann, Paik, & Rosen, 1999). For women, 22% suffered from low sexual desire, 14% suffered from arousal problems, and 7% experienced sexual pain disorders. For men, 21% suffered from premature ejaculation, 5% suffered from erectile dysfunction, and 5% suffered from low sexual desire. For females, the prevalence of sexual problems generally decreases as they age, whereas the opposite is true for males. Males report more erectile problems and less desire for sexual activity with increasing age. Males ages 50–59 were three times as likely to experience these difficulties compared to males ages 18–29.

Clinical Picture

The following are case examples of actual patients. Identifying information has been changed so as to protect the confidentiality of the clients.

> J.P. is a 27-year-old waiter who sought treatment for an erectile dysfunction. He reported an inability to maintain an erection intravaginally. He reported being able to reach orgasm when stimulated orally or manually by his partner. He also reported no erectile problems during masturbation. His problem has resulted in depression, which is what led him to seek treatment. J.P. consulted with a urologist who determined that there was no organic basis for his dysfunction. A detailed sexual history revealed that he has attempted intercourse with seven women, and the first interaction was at age 15. He was unable to maintain an erection his first time. Since then he has been able to maintain an erection intravaginally approximately five times. Successful coital attempts resulted from sexual interactions consisting of extended foreplay, when he was relaxed, and when his partner communicated understanding of his problem. Factors contributing to failure to reach orgasm include not knowing the woman well, skipping foreplay, drinking seven to eight beers, and having sexually inhibiting thoughts including that he wished it were over. He reported that he did not want to disappoint women, "but then the big disappointment" occurs when he cannot maintain an erection for intercourse. Assessment of relationship factors reveals that he has never been in a long-term relationship. He reported that for him to have a girlfriend, he would first need to be able to satisfy her sexually. According to J.P., women expect sex on the first or second date, which is why he has refrained from dating for the past 2 months.
>
> J.P. suffered from Male Erectile Disorder. Treatment is discussed in the following section.
>
> S.L. is a 32-year-old housewife who reported suffering from very low sexual desire. She has been married eight years, and six months ago she gave birth to their first child. She and her husband have not had intercourse for nine months before seeking therapy. During the initial interview, S.L. reported she was date raped at the age of 15. She also reported that since that time she has had little desire for either physical or sexual intimacy. She was treated for Posttraumatic Stress Disorder two years before seeking sex therapy. She reported that when she completed this previous therapy, she no longer blamed herself for the incident and her nightmares had subsided. Currently, S.L. does not derive pleasure from her sexual experiences with her husband. This began during her pregnancy. When she and her husband attempted intercourse during pregnancy, she never reached orgasm. When her husband would reach orgasm and she did not, she felt used by her husband because he was pleasured by the experience and she was not. For the last six months, her husband has initiated

sexual activity approximately once per week and she refused each time. One week before seeking therapy, her husband threatened to leave her if she does not seek treatment, so he can have his wife back.

S.L. meets diagnostic criteria for both Hypoactive Sexual Desire Disorder and Female Orgasmic Disorder. Treatment is discussed in the following section.

Course and Prognosis

To date, there are relatively few controlled psychotherapeutic treatment outcome studies to attest to the efficacy of treating sexual dysfunction. O'Donohue, Dopke, and Swingen (1997) and O'Donohue, Swingen, Dopke, and Regev (1999) provide comprehensive reviews of them. Some of the following are effective psychological treatments for sexual dysfunctions.

HYPOACTIVE SEXUAL DESIRE DISORDER

Orgasm consistency training produced positive outcomes for women suffering from this disorder. Orgasm consistency training for the couple consists primarily of teaching directed masturbation, sensate focus, techniques to improve the timing of male orgasm, and the coital alignment technique (Hurlbert, 1993). These techniques focus on increasing sexual satisfaction, thereby enhancing the individual's desire for sexual activity. Directed masturbation involves teaching skills for reaching orgasm through masturbation. Sensate focus involves teaching the couple to focus on sensations that accompany sexual activities instead of focusing on performance as a goal (Masters & Johnson, 1970). This technique is used to reduce the anxiety some experience when trying to reach the performance goal of orgasm, which may result in failure. The man also learns to control the timing of his ejaculation, so as to prolong the sexual activity. The couple learns the coital alignment technique so as to increase the possibility that the woman reaches orgasm during intercourse by teaching the couple to position themselves so that the penis shaft consistently contacts the clitoris (Eichel, Eichel, & Kule, 1988). These sexual techniques are more likely to result in the woman achieving orgasm and thereby produce a more satisfying experience. Little is known concerning what would be an effective strategy for males suffering from this disorder. Other strategies may involve medications or treating another psychological disorder, such as depression or couples problems, assuming such factors have not been ruled out.

SEXUAL AVERSION DISORDER

Systematic desensitization (Wolpe, 1958) is effective for women suffering from this disorder (Wincze, 1971). This technique assumes that the dysfunction results from anxiety produced by sexual stimuli. By exposing the client gradually to anxiety-provoking sexual stimuli, according to their anxiety hierarchy during a relaxed state, the client learns to experience less anxiety when presented with sexual stimuli. This can then lead to improved sexual interactions. Little is known about what would be an effective strategy for males who suffer from this disorder.

MALE ERECTILE DISORDER

Men who suffer from this disorder are different from sexually functional men in a number of ways (Barlow, 1986). They experience negative affect in sexual contexts, they underreport their level of arousal, they are not distracted by nonsexual-performance-related stimuli, they are distracted by performance-related sexual stimuli, and anxiety inhibits their sexual arousal. For sexually functional men, the opposite is true. Men who suffer from this disorder are generally preoccupied with interfering thoughts during sexual encounters. These thoughts may include spectatoring, whereby the individual monitors his arousal, thinking about the firmness of his penis, or about disappointing his sexual partner. To overcome this problem, it is important to reduce these interfering thoughts. This can be achieved by replacing these thoughts with sexually stimulating thoughts. Other strategies include systematic desensitization (Auerbach & Kilman, 1977), rational-emotive therapy designed to correct cognitive distortions (Munjack et al., 1984), and providing information concerning sexuality (Goldman & Carroll, 1990). Some of these strategies may also be effective for women who are experiencing arousal problems; more research is needed to determine what is an effective strategy for women who suffer from Female Sexual Arousal Disorder.

FEMALE ORGASMIC DISORDER

Directed masturbation has been effective for women who present with this problem (Kohlenberg, 1974). This technique involves education and self-exploration, directed masturbation, sexual fantasy and imagery, and sensate focus. Women then share the effective masturbation techniques with their partners. Another effective strategy is bibliotherapy using the self-help book *Becoming orgasmic* (Heiman, LoPiccolo, & LoPiccolo, 1976). This book describes various techniques women can use to help them reach orgasm, individually and with a partner. These include targeting psychological inhibitions as well as teaching sexual education and skills. More research on the strategies that would be useful for males who suffer from Male Orgasmic Disorder is needed.

PREMATURE EJACULATION

An effective treatment strategy for men who present with this disorder includes teaching the couple sensate focus, the squeeze technique, and intravaginal ejaculatory control (Lowe & Milkulas, 1975). The squeeze technique (Masters & Johnson, 1970) involves teaching the male ejaculatory control by squeezing the head of his penis firmly when he is on the verge of ejaculating. Practicing this repeatedly while sexually stimulated will generally result in the ability to control ejaculatory latency.

VAGINISMUS AND DYSPAREUNIA

To date, there are no controlled psychotherapeutic treatment outcome studies to attest to the efficacy of treatment for these disorders. The primary strategy used for women suffering from vaginismus is instructing the woman to gradually insert a finger or dilator into her vagina. This procedure begins with inserting her smallest finger or thinnest dilator until the involuntary spasms subside. Once she is comfortable, she moves on to a larger finger or thicker dilator. This strategy provides the woman with complete control over the insertions, which may act to reduce tension surrounding insertion. Once she becomes comfortable with this procedure, her partner can be included while the woman still maintains complete control of inserting the finger or dilator and eventually the penis.

Diagnostic Considerations

Sexual functioning is multivariate. Many variables influence human sexual behavior. Before beginning treatment for a client presenting with sexual dysfunction, it is necessary to assess the individual's sexual functioning, medical history, psychological functioning, and relationship factors comprehensively. Where possible, a comprehensive assessment of the individual's sexual partner along these dimensions may vastly contribute to a fuller understanding of the problem.

Sexual problems and strengths can be assessed in a number of ways. These include a diagnostic interview, questionnaires, self-report behavioral records, and physiological measures. Each of these assessment devices provide invaluable information to the clinician when making diagnostic decisions. Conte (1986) and Avina and O'Donohue (1999) provided a useful review of various devices used when assessing sexual functioning. Currently, there is little consensus concerning what constitutes a sexual dysfunction. Many different interpretations of the DSM diagnostic criteria have led to numerous distinct formulations. Readers interested in sexuality-related measures and their psychometric properties are referred to Davis, Yarber, Bauserman, Schreer, and Davis (1998).

To make diagnostic decisions, the clinician must take into account the individual's medical history. Sexual problems can be psychological, may be due to a general medical condition or substance use, or a combination. Generally, it is important for the client first to undergo a gynecological or urological examination by a physician so as to rule out an organic basis for the disorder. Other medical aspects that must be assessed are the individual's acute and chronic medical conditions, medication use, and surgical history. Any one of these may contribute to sexual problems. Medical conditions that are linked to sexual dysfunction include cardiovascular disease, cancer, neurological disease, diabetes, end-stage renal disease, chronic obstructive pulmonary disease, and chronic pain (Schover & Jensen, 1988). Medications that may affect sexual functioning include certain antipsychotic, antidepressant, and antihypertensive drugs. Abusing alcohol or illicit drugs may also negatively impact sexual functioning.

Psychological functioning is another important variable to assess when making diagnostic decisions concerning sexual dysfunctions. Psychological disorders such as Major Depressive Disorder, Posttraumatic Stress Disorder, and Obsessive–Compulsive Disorder may account for the sexual dysfunction and should be ruled out before making a diagnosis of sexual dysfunction. Similarly, relationship dissatisfaction may account for the sexual dysfunction, particularly among individuals experiencing low desire for sexual activity. Consequently, successful couples therapy might allay the sexual problem. The Dyadic Adjustment Scale (Spanier, 1976) is a frequently used measure to determine relationship satisfaction.

PARAPHILIAS

Description of the Disorder

In contrast with the sexual dysfunctions, conceptualizations of paraphilias are made on legal and social grounds, as well as on the medical and psychological bases of the disorders. Therefore, paraphilia is a blanket term that covers a group of disorders that are characterized by an abnormal sexual component. Because what is abnormal is socially determined, the line at which sexual behavior is deemed "deviant" has shifted with the times. What is considered deviant in 2000 is different from what was termed deviant in 1980. For example, homo-sexuality was a paraphilia in the first two versions of the Diagnostic and Statistical Manual (APA, 1952, 1968). Later, it was included in the taxonomy only if it was ego-dystonic (unwanted) for the individual (APA, 1980). In the current version, it is no longer considered a disorder (APA, 1994). The current roster of paraphilias includes a variety of behaviors and attitudes that comprise the most recent American Psychiatric Association view of abnormal sexuality.

Paraphilias are characterized by recurrent and strong sexually arousing fantasies, sexual urges, or sexual behaviors that involve objects, nonconsenting partners, or the suffering and/or humiliation of oneself or one's partner during sexual activity. These fantasies, urges, or behaviors must last at least six months and cause clinically significant distress or impairment in social, occupational, or other important areas of functioning. There are endless variations of these broad criteria, however, only the most prevalent combinations are discussed in this chapter.

EXHIBITIONISM

Involves exposing the genitals to an unsuspecting stranger. Masturbation during the exposure sometimes occurs.

FETISHISM

Involves the use of inanimate objects to achieve sexual arousal. Sometimes these objects are necessary to achieve sexual gratification. The fetishist may hold or wear the preferred object while masturbating or may ask his sexual partner to wear the object during sexual encounters. When the object is unattainable, some individuals report sexual dysfunction.

FROTTEURISM

Involves becoming sexually aroused by rubbing against or touching a nonconsenting person. This most often occurs in crowded places such as public transportation or elevators.

PEDOPHILIA

Involves an adult fantasizing about or engaging in sexual activity with a prepubescent child of either sex. Some are attracted only to boys, some only to girls, and some to both. The pedo-phile must be at least sixteen years old and five years older than the child to receive this diagnosis.

SEXUAL MASOCHISM

Involves being sexually stimulated by experiencing humiliation, bondage, or physical suffering such as a beating. These behaviors may occur with or without a sexual partner.

SEXUAL SADISM

Involves deriving sexual pleasure from the psychological and/or physical suffering of the sexual partner or victim. Partners may be consenting or nonconsenting. The severity of the suffering often escalates over time.

Transvestic Fetishism

Involves achieving sexual gratification by dressing in clothes of the opposite gender. Individuals may masturbate while they are dressed in these garments to heighten the sexual satisfaction.

Voyeurism

Involves observing another person(s) who is taking off his/her clothes or engaging in sexual activity. Most often the voyeur's presence is unknown. Masturbation may occur while watching the victim or later, based on the memory of what was seen.

Paraphilia Not Otherwise Specified

These are diverse and sometimes unique paraphilias in which an individual achieves sexual arousal or gratification through a more uncommon object or activity. Included are

Necrophilia. Having or fantasizing about sexual relations with corpses.
Coprophilia. Involving feces in sexual activities.
Zoophilia. Involving animals in sexual activities.
Telephone scatalogia. Making obscene telephone calls.

Achieving sexual gratification from fantasies or the act of raping or sexually assaulting an adult is not a specific disorder according to the DSM, but it is included in the sexual sadism category if the assailant obtains sexual gratification from these activities.

Epidemiology

The prevalence of paraphilias is unknown due to the secretive nature of most aberrant *sexual* behavior. Researchers must use imperfect indicators to find out how prevalent these behaviors are. For example, the commercial distribution of paraphilic materials is a multi-billion dollar industry and growing, particularly through the invention of the World Wide Web. These figures indicate a substantial market, though the specific number of consumers is unknown. Many paraphilias involve illegal activities such as having sex with children. It is often only through contact with the legal system that these disorders are revealed. However, although legal involvement may disclose the presence of a paraphilia, the criminal status and personal nature of the activities impede accurate reports of the history of its development, specific activities, and frequencies of the behaviors. As a result, the field relies on incomplete evidence in its attempts to understand the epidemiology of these disorders.

Most individuals who have a paraphilia are men, though women exhibit the full range of disorders in much smaller numbers. It is estimated now that women account for at least 5% of the cases of sexual molestation against females and 20% of molestations of males (Finkelhor, 1984). However, these figures demonstrate that it is primarily males who engage in inappropriate sexual fantasizing and behaviors and if there is a victim, it is almost always a woman or child. Those who are interested in paraphilic behavior in females are encouraged to review Hunter and Mathews (1998).

The onset of these disorders tends to be in adolescence. Newly pubescent children develop sexual fantasies that involve the objects, persons, or activities of choice. It may be either during adolescence or later in adulthood that individuals begin to act on these fantasies if they do act on them. There is great variation in the frequency and magnitude of these behaviors across individuals. Once again it is difficult to know if the information about paraphilic behaviors is accurate because researchers must rely on the self-reports of sometimes unwilling subjects. However, some paraphilics limit their fantasies and activities to their homes and may never escalate into more public behaviors that may be discovered by other people. Others start with fantasies and activities that they engage in at home and then progress to increasingly risky behaviors. For example, a man may begin by wearing his wife's lingerie when she is out of town. He might then introduce his cross-dressing into their sexual activities. Later, he may begin cross-dressing on the weekends in public, thereby increasing the risk of social costs. The risk may become a component of the sexual arousal in these cases.

More than one paraphilia may be exhibited by the same person. There are patterns of relatedness amongst the paraphilias, particularly for certain disorders (Freund & Watson, 1990). Those who exhibit one problem will often report other paraphilic activities as well. Some studies have found the co-occurrence of voyeurism, exhibitionism, rape, and frotteurism in many of their subjects, but the number and types of paraphilias are unique to each individual. The most recent study is Bradford, Boulet, and Pawlak (1992). In their sample of 443 men undergoing a forensic assessment, they found that of the 115 men who reported voyeurism, 66% had engaged in frotteurism, 52% had engaged in exhibitionism, and 47% admitted having raped someone (Freund, Seto, & Kuban, 1998). In addition, for those individuals who have co-occurring paraphilias, there is a pattern of escalation from "hands-off" activities to those that are "hands-on."

It is not uncommon for voyeurs to report having escalated to frotteurism. For example, a young man of 25 who was incarcerated for a date rape reported that he began as a "peeping tom" at his university. He would sneak around the women's dormitories late in the evening when he expected co-eds to be undressing. Later, he added masturbation to his nightly prowling. After about six months, he no longer found simply watching the women as arousing as it had been and he began to fantasize about touching a woman that did not know he was there. His first visit to jail occurred when he went into the women's locker room at the gym and touched a woman who was showering.

Some people who have paraphilias report only deviant sexual arousal, but others report arousal to both paraphilic and nonparaphilic objects and activities. This includes pedophiles who may be varied in their sexual interests. Some prefer a particular age-group and gender, and others are nonspecific in their interests. They may abuse children of either gender and of any age. Others are also sexually attracted to adult partners.

There are a variety of theories that attempt to explain the development of the array of paraphilias. What these biological and psychological theories have in common is that none entirely explains the development and maintenance of these behaviors.

Biological theories have focused mainly on the relationship of hormone levels to sexual behaviors. It was hypothesized that the hormone levels of paraphilics are different from nonparaphilics. However, research has shown that this is not the case (Hucker & Bain, 1990). What has been demonstrated is that if a male's level of testosterone is reduced to prepubescent levels, his sexual drive and fantasies are reduced (Maletzky, 1991). This produces a reduction in paraphilic behavior for some people (Bradford, 1998). Other physiological theories include central nervous system damage or a genetic predisposition to express sexuality in an unusual manner. However, no research supports these theories at this time.

Psychological theories have been somewhat more revealing, although none offers a full and empirically supportable view of the development and maintenance of undesirable sexual behaviors. There are numerous and similar versions of many of these theories, and they may be grouped into several broad categories. The major theories that are being investigated today include the cognitive-behavioral models, the social learning models, the addiction models, the abused abuser models, and the courtship disorder models.

COGNITIVE-BEHAVIORAL MODELS

Sexual behavior follows behavioral principles. Deviant sexual arousal can be conditioned and maintained through environmental stimuli including one's thoughts (O'Donohue & Plaud, 1991).

SOCIAL LEARNING MODELS

Sexual behavior is influenced by the environment in which the paraphilic was raised. Early sexual behavior is modeled and shaped by parents. It is also affected by other factors in the family including neglect, violence, overtly sexual behavior in the family, or aggressive sexual behavior in the family.

ADDICTION MODELS

Paraphilics, it is assumed, engage in deviant sexual behavior as a soothing or avoidance measure to meet some need that is not being met in their lives.

ABUSED-ABUSER MODELS

The paraphilic was sexually abused by someone as a child and having had this as an early sexual experience, the later sexual expression takes the same form.

COURTSHIP DISORDER MODELS

Normal human sexual interaction (courtship) is characterized by preferences for a certain sequence of sexual activities. Paraphilics become entrenched in one phase of the sequence and do not fully engage the entire courtship sequence.

None of these theories has been adequately tested. It will take many more studies to refine them to discover the roots of these disorders and possible points of early intervention.

Clinical Picture

The following is a case example of an actual patient. Identifying information has been changed to protect client confidentiality.

> H.B. is a 28-year-old male accountant who self-referred for evaluation and treatment following his wife's discovery of his paraphilic behavior. He had kept his exhibitionism a secret for the first two years of their marriage. He had never been arrested for his behavior but had recently increased the risk of criminal charges by exposing himself in more populated public areas. He told his wife of his disorder after exposing himself to an adult woman in the bathroom of a train. He could no longer keep the secret because the train conductor chastised him in front of his wife. She reported that she had no idea that he engaged in these fantasies and activities. She was puzzled because she thought their sex life was satisfying for both of them and never suspected her model husband of any deviant activities. H.B. is a highly intelligent man who is employed by a distinguished accounting

firm. He has many friends and is a respected member of his community. The following sexual history was obtained.

H.B. reported that he began masturbating around age nine or ten when he accidentally discovered the pleasurable sensations of doing so alone in his room. He said that his parents began to argue more frequently when he was eleven and that masturbation became a way to block out the fighting. It was a way to ignore what was happening at home and to soothe himself. He reports that he would masturbate several times daily to produce these positive feelings. His first sexual activity with a partner occurred in a dating relationship when he was seventeen. He reported a natural progression of sexual activities from kissing to sexual touching to intercourse over a period of months. His private masturbation behavior continued.

He attended an Ivy League school where he experienced both academic and financial stressors. As the stressors increased, so did the frequency of the masturbation. He began to feel abnormal compared with his friends. He isolated himself more and more from them and was not getting the same soothing feeling from his sexual behavior. He began to have more satisfying fantasies in which he was watching people get undressed or have sexual relations. He began watching females undress in situations in which he knew he would not get caught. Later, he incorporated voyeurism into his sexual activities with his girlfriend through role-playing. Despite the frequency with which he was experiencing sexual release, he was not feeling fully satisfied.

His fantasies took on a new dimension when he thought of exposing his genitals to an unsuspecting person. He imagined how powerful he would feel at her embarrassment or fear. His fantasies always ended with the woman wanting to have sex with him because she found him so desirable. He began to go out of town on the weekends to find isolated places where he could experiment with exposing himself. Each time he felt both powerful during the act and shameful afterwards. He believed that if one of the victims would just accept him and want to have sex with him, he could stop. He increased the frequency of his exhibitionism in his search for the perfect victim and felt he was leading a double life. After his participation in an Introductory Psychology class, he went for counseling for the problem, but dropped out after a few weeks. He said that he really did not want to stop because it was the only comforting thing in his life at the time. He was able to keep the behavior a secret from all of his friends and family until the train incident. He reported that he was exhausted from trying to appear to be the model citizen while cruising for potential victims and covering up his activities. He said he was afraid of his new fantasies because they included thoughts of exposing himself to teenagers instead of adult women.

Diagnostic Considerations

Diagnosing paraphilias is rarely straightforward due to several interfering factors, including accessing the disordered individuals, inaccurate self-reports of sexual behaviors, particularly those with a criminal aspect, the ethical and practical problems of naturally studying sexual behavior, and the inadequacy of physiological and psychological measures in revealing the true nature and extent of these behaviors. Beyond these problems of gaining access to the phenomena, engaging in paraphilic behavior is reinforcing for the individual. These are pleasurable activities that the individual does not want to give up just for the sake of giving them up. The only reason paraphilics would want to be treated for their behavior is to reduce the negative consequences. The motivation for accurate assessment and treatment is often in conflict with the desire to continue the behaviors. This often keeps paraphilics from being diagnosed and treated.

A second broad classification issue relates to the diagnosis of pedophilia. This diagnosis follows the same structure as those of other paraphilias. The person must have fantasies, urges, or behaviors that involve sexual activity with a prepubescent child. The person must be at least 16 years old and five years older than the child. The diagnosis is complicated by the third criterion, that the fantasies or behaviors cause clinically significant distress or impairment in social, occupational, or other important areas of functioning. Often, adults who have sex with children report that they are not distressed by their behavior and that it does not create impairments in any areas of their lives. As a result, there are individuals who engage in disturbing sexual behaviors with children, but who do not fit the diagnostic system. Researchers in the field have attempted to solve this problem to make the classifications more functional.

One approach has been to distinguish between pedophilic and nonpedophilic offenders; those who are pedophilic are attracted primarily to children whereas nonpedophilics are primarily attracted to adults. A distinction is also made between intrafamilial (incestuous) offenders and extrafamilial offenders. Other schemas attempt to make distinctions based strictly on the ages of the offender and victim, an aspect which is included in the DSM-IV taxonomy. However, this strategy does not address relevant variables such as the level of sexual functioning of the participants. Strict age criteria also functionally remove adolescence from the taxonomy, a time during which many paraphilias develop. Other researchers have used the words "child molester" versus "pedophile" to distinguish between those who are remorseful for their actions and those who are not. Whether this is useful remains to be seen. A classification system that has demonstrated some utility is based on the context in which the offense occurs. In this model, distinctions are made between situational offenders, preferential offenders, and predatory offenders. Offenders who prefer children and are predatory are the most treatment-resistant (Maletzky, 1993).

Further complicating the process of diagnosis is that inappropriate sexual behaviors sometimes result from problems other than deviant sexual arousal. A number of cognitive and psychological problems apart from the paraphilias may produce unusual sexual behavior in some patients. People who have developmental disabilities may have deficits in their knowledge of what is appropriate sexual behavior or in their impulse control and may consequently engage in unwelcome activities. At other times, there may be a decline in the appropriate sexual behavior of an individual. Psychoses typically develop years after a person has become sexually active. At times, as part of the break with some aspects of reality, the individual may exhibit aberrant sexual behavior. For example, someone might develop the delusion that he is really a woman and might begin to dress in women's clothing. However, when the delusion is treated with a psychotropic medication, the idea and the cross-dressing may cease. Dementia is another situation in which sexual behavior may become dysfunctional. A demented patient may rub up against or touch a stranger in an elevator thinking that the person is his girlfriend, for example.

Therefore, the first step in making a thorough and useful diagnosis is to rule out any cognitive deficits or alternative psychological disorders that might be producing the unusual sexual behaviors. This may involve a medical examination to rule out things like a brain injury, a more general clinical interview to determine the individual's psychiatric and psychological history, and/or psychological testing to determine the presence of cognitive deficits. Substance abuse must also be assessed, though it is important to understand exactly how it impacts the individual's sexual behavior. Some paraphilics who engage in criminal behavior use substances purposively to be less cognizant of the consequences of the behavior, and it is possible that others may not be cognizant of their actions if they are in a blackout state of drug or alcohol intoxication. Some predatory offenders drink before cruising for a victim to lessen anxiety, whereas others engage in an offense situationally after having abused substances. The offenders are at fault in either case, but the diagnosis and treatment approach may be different.

After alternative diagnoses have been ruled out, it is important to conduct a thorough interview covering the individual's sexual history. This includes the onset of puberty and sexual behavior, fantasies and activities including paraphilic and nonparaphilic behaviors, the objects or subjects by which the person is sexually aroused, any presence of sexual dysfunction, and sexuality-related knowledge and beliefs. The person's ability to attract an appropriate sexual partner may also be assessed through a discussion of a broad range of social skills. Several paper-and-pencil tests have been developed that may assist in gathering the most useful information quickly.

Psychophysiological methods are another assessment tool that some researchers find useful. These are assessment devices that attempt to learn about a person's sexual arousal patterns and sexual behaviors without relying on the verbal report of the client. Included in these approaches are penile plethysmography and vaginal photoplethysmography and polygraph tests.

Penile plethysmography is a procedure that attempts to get information about sexual arousal patterns through physiological measurement. The procedure is conducted in the privacy of a laboratory. A mercury-in-rubber strain gauge is placed around the penis. This device detects changes in the circumference of the penis and these changes are recorded as the individual views explicit material that includes a variety of subjects in sexual and nonsexual activities. Currently, the use of nonexplicit, ambiguous materials is being tested in this procedure with similar changes in penile tumescence. Limitations to the procedure include the ability of some men to control their physiological responses to all stimuli, objections to the use of explicit materials, and that the procedure has been tested mainly in research settings and its use for clinical purposes has not been validated.

Similar to this procedure is the use of vaginal photoplethysmography in women. Four dependent measures of sexual arousal are provided by this device which is attached to the vagina of the patient. It measures blood volume, pulse rate, vaginal pulse amplitude, and response duration in response to slides of people of different ages and genders engaged in sexual and nonsexual scenarios.

A third psychophysiological approach that is used with both genders is the polygraph. The procedure involves asking questions of the paraphilic while measuring pulse, blood pressure, EKG, and galvanic skin response. Changes in the readings are observed, and those that differ from baseline may be interpreted as indications of dishonesty for the question that is being asked. The validity of polygraphy has been questioned for many uses including questions of sexual deviancy (Abrams, 1991). In addition, ethical concerns have been raised in relation to its use with alleged sexual offenders. The concerns are that it cannot assist the offender, but can only hurt him, that it is intrusive, and that unfounded conclusions are reached due to its misuse. In addition, myths about the polygraph may lead to confessions about sexual offenses that might not be given without the use of deception, whether the deception is intended or because the limits of the polygraph are not fully explained to the client. There are cases in which offenders admit more fully to crimes and to the extent of crimes when the polygraph is used.

Another useful diagnostic tool is corroborating information from people who are involved with the paraphilic or from official record reviews. Romantic partners, friends, and family members are often good sources of valuable information about the habits of those who have sexual disorders. Differences in their accounts and those of the patient may provide opportunities to gain a fuller picture of the behaviors.

Official records may also provide insight into the parameters of the problematic sexual behaviors. Police and court records, past medical records, and psychological records may be obtained by interviewers with the consent of the client. These may provide information that has been forgotten or was deliberately hidden by the client.

Clinical Course and Prognosis

Just as there are biological and psychological theories of the etiology of paraphilias, both perspectives also apply to treatment. There has been some controversy over the efficacy of various treatment approaches. The overall efficacy of any one program of treatment has not been proved due to ethical concerns about having a nontreatment group included in studies. The thought has been that it is unethical to withhold a treatment, even if its efficacy has not been shown. As a result, though many of the approaches are effective in reducing paraphilic behaviors for some people, they are not conclusively supported by evidence. In addition, because these treatment outcome studies are new and techniques are being refined, it is not yet clear which parts of the treatment are effective and which are not. This leaves programs that may have components that are costly and ineffective or are even harmful to effective aspects of the work or to the clients. More research is being conducted at this time to make stronger determinations about what works under what conditions for whom in the reduction of unwanted sexual behaviors.

Physiological interventions focus on castration, both chemical and surgical to reduce the physical ability of a person to engage in paraphilic behavior. The focus of these treatments is to reduce sexual drive in males by reducing circulating testosterone. This may be done surgically or by using antiandrogen medications or other hormonal agents. Surgical procedures are not commonly used to treat paraphilias in the United States. Most paraphilics are unwilling to consent to surgery because it is painful and permanent.

Pharmacological treatments include the use of antiandrogens and new investigations into the use of certain psychotropic medications that have decreased sexual drive as a side effect in many of the patients who have taken them. Antiandrogens, including Androcur (CPA) and hormonal agents including Depo-Provera (MPA), have demonstrated utility in reducing the sexual drive of men (Bradford, 1998). Frequency of erections is reduced as are sexual behaviors, fantasies, masturbation, and intercourse. This makes them useful in treating harmful paraphilic behaviors, but there are problems associated with their use. First, there are side effects that interfere with patient compliance. These include weight gain, headaches, tiredness, muscle cramps, and rarely, blood clots. CPA is not approved for use in the United States due to severe reactions in the liver in some people who use the drug. An additional problem is that the drugs work only to decrease sexual fantasies and behaviors when they are in the system. They have no lasting or permanent effects. Thus, the decrease in sexual drive hinges on patient compliance with the medication regimen. Motivation to continue this regimen throughout the life span is low because of the unpleasant side effects and the consequences of taking the medication.

Using the sexual side effects of some neuroleptic and SSRI medications is an avenue that is currently being investigated in treating paraphilias. These drugs have appealed to some researchers because they may produce less severe side effects than the antiandrogens and may therefore increase patient compliance. However, they may produce nausea and agitation and they are not as powerful as the hormonal treatments in reducing sexual drive. Medications are commonly used at this time during critical periods when paraphilics are trying to learn other ways of controlling their paraphilic behaviors.

An additional problem of using medications to reduce sexual drive is that sexual satisfaction is not always the motivating factor in paraphilic activity. Sadists may rape a woman out of anger and not as a result of a high sex drive. Even if sexual drive is reduced, a motivated individual can harm someone in a sexual way without needing an erection. Furthermore, the effects of these drugs may be bypassed by a motivated individual. Hormone replacement drugs are available to counteract the effects of the other drugs if compliance is being monitored.

Psychological treatments for paraphilias are evolving. Those that have the most evidence that they work in reducing unwanted sexual behaviors are those that are based on the cognitive and behavioral traditions. Cognitive therapy takes the general stance that external behavior can be changed if thoughts are altered. Therapists take the clients' beliefs about themselves as hypotheses that may be tested. Therapy is a process of challenging established beliefs to promote more effective applications in everyday life. Cognitive therapy focuses on two components of paraphilic behavior, cognitive distortions and lack of empathy. Cognitive distortions include distorted beliefs, false assumptions about situations, and rationalizations or justifications for inappropriate sexual behaviors. The focus of this therapy is altering beliefs such as, "that little girl wanted sex. She seduced me." A second area that gets the attention of cognitive therapists is the paraphilics' empathy for others who might be harmed by their behavior. This training brings the paraphilics into contact with the way their behavior affects other people by using videotapes, stories of victims, and role-plays in which the paraphilic portrays the other person.

Behavior therapy involves applying behavioral principles to human problems. The focus in behavior therapy is to use the principles of classical and operant conditioning to find points of intervention such that behavioral patterns may be changed toward more favorable consequences. To treat paraphilias, these approaches include positive conditioning, aversive conditioning, and satiation techniques. Positive conditioning procedures address behaviors that are assumed to be missing in the behavioral repertoire of the paraphilic and that interfere with appropriate expressions of sexuality. These techniques include training a variety of social skills that are related to attracting an appropriate sexual partner and learning to achieve sexual gratification in more socially appropriate ways. Alternative behavior completion is another skills-based approach in which the client learns how to substitute new behaviors for old ones earlier in the behavioral sequence that normally leads to a display of paraphilic behavior.

Aversion therapy pairs something aversive with a deviant sexual behavior to reduce the likelihood that the sexual behavior will result in the future. Aversive items that are used include electric shock, ammonia, and other strongly scented items that induce nausea, such as rotting meat. A close relative of aversion therapy is covert sensitization. It is similar to simple aversion therapy in that an aversive item is paired with the deviant sexual arousal. The difference in this case is that the conditioning process is more complex and does not involve the use of noxious substances. Intensely repellent results are imagined and paired with typical sexual fantasies or scenes that the paraphilic likes to replay in his or her mind. For example, a pedophile might imagine a detailed fantasy in which he entices a young girl to take off her underwear.

When he touches her genitals, he begins to smell something. He discovers that she has not cleaned herself and that he has feces all over his hand. He retracts his hand, but the smell will not go away. He hears her mother coming and the smell is overwhelming. He is sure he is going to get caught this time. He runs to the bathroom and washes his hands repeatedly to get rid of the smell. He realizes that away from the child, he can breathe freely and without the fear of getting caught.

The scenario is rehearsed repeatedly in great detail. Vicarious conditioning is a related strategy that presents aversive results of inappropriate sexual behaviors in video form for paraphilics to watch. Each of these procedures works with some paraphilics; however, others report that these strategies are not powerful enough.

Satiation techniques have been some of the most promising for aiding paraphilics in controlling their deviant sexual arousal. These approaches are based on the premise that deviant sexual arousal is reinforced through both sexual fantasies and masturbation. Verbal satiation involves repeatedly verbalizing every available sexual fantasy in detail while masturbating to orgasm. The scenes are repeated until they are no longer sufficiently arousing. This procedure seems to have a small inoculation effect in that new fantasies do not have the same power to elicit an erection. However, with this procedure, there is some concern that sexual arousal may be extinguished altogether, which may also be an unhealthy state for the paraphilic. Other procedures address this problem. In masturbatory satiation, the client is instructed to masturbate to verbalized deviant sexual fantasies. At the moment that he is about to ejaculate, he must switch to nondeviant sexual fantasies and to continue those through the rest of the sexual act. A reversal of this procedure is also used. In this approach, the client is asked to masturbate to orgasm using only nondeviant fantasies. After orgasm occurs, he is then instructed to masturbate to deviant fantasies for about half an hour in a flaccid state. In all of these procedures the verbalizations are monitored by a tape recorder to ensure that the appropriate instructions are being followed so that the deviant arousal is not being strengthened.

Relapse prevention is a cognitive-behavioral program of treatment that incorporates most of the aforementioned strategies. It is a treatment model that was developed to treat drug and alcohol addiction that has since been modified to be applied to paraphilias, including exhibitionism, voyeurism, sexual sadism, and pedophilia. The major premise of relapse prevention is that these behaviors cannot be cured, only controlled through a program of conscious monitoring of the many, linked behaviors and conditions in the environment that could lead to engaging in a paraphilic act. This monitoring is learned in conjunction with other cognitive and behavioral strategies that focus on increasing empathy, alleviating cognitive distortions, and controlling deviant sexual arousal. A complete program addresses the motivating factors such as arousal and faulty cognitions, and also teaches the client to monitor aspects of his environment (including thoughts and behaviors) that typically lead to paraphilic activities. Homework and review sessions are an important part of this treatment as reminders of the techniques that have been learned and how they apply to daily life. Relapse prevention programs are not uniform, yet they all tend to incorporate some of the cognitive and behavioral strategies discussed before. Similar cognitive-behavioral treatment strategies are being used with adolescents who exhibit sexually inappropriate behaviors, though they do not classify as paraphilics in the current system. Relapse prevention theory is currently under revision toward an increased understanding of the relapse process and an expansion of the precision and scope of the treatment.

For a complete review of treatment rationales, techniques, and outcomes, readers are referred to the Maletzky chapter on paraphilias in *A guide to treatments that work* by Peter Nathan and Jack Gorman (Maletzky, 1998).

SUMMARY

Paraphilias are better understood than ever before. However many important questions remain unanswered, questions that can be addressed only through new theory development and research. A comprehensive theory is lacking to guide the studies that are being conducted. Without an organizing theory, it is difficult to know how the pieces of information that are being gathered about sexual offending fit together. Beyond theory, the field needs measurement instruments that are psychometrically sound to better study the phenomena of interest. Without adequate measurement, it becomes increasingly difficult to conduct strong tests to clarify sexual behaviors. The field also needs ardent proponents who work to disseminate accurate information about the impact of paraphilias and the needs of researchers and clinicians if that impact is to be changed. This includes academics who are willing to speak publicly about findings, lobbyists to promote funding and interest in government, and administrators who support strong research proposals so that appropriate programs of prevention and treatment can be developed.

REFERENCES

Abrams, S. (1991). The use of polygraphy with sex offenders. *Annals of Sex Research, 4,* 239–263.

American Psychiatric Association. (1952). *Diagnostic and statistical manual of mental disorders,* 1st ed. Washington, DC: Author.

American Psychiatric Association. (1968). *Diagnostic and statistical manual of mental disorders,* 2nd ed. Washington, DC: Author.

American Psychiatric Association. (1980). *Diagnostic and statistical manual of mental disorders,* 3rd ed. Washington, DC: Author.

American Psychiatric Association. (1994). *Diagnostic and statistical manual of mental disorders,* 4th ed. Washington, DC: Author.

Anderson, B. L. (1981). A comparison of systematic desensitization and directed masturbation in the treatment of primary orgasmic dysfunction in females. *Journal of Consulting and Clinical Psychology, 49,* 568–570.

Auerbach, R., & Kilmann, P. R. (1977). The effects of group systematic desensitization on secondary erectile failure. *Behavior Therapy, 8,* 330–339.

Avina, C., & O'Donohue, W. (1999). The measurement of sexual behavior. Manuscript in preparation.

Barlow, D. H. (1986). Causes of sexual dysfunction: The role of anxiety and cognitive interference. *Journal of Consulting and Clinical Psychology, 54,* 140–148.

Bradford, J. (1998). Medical interventions in sexual deviance. In D. R. Laws & W. O'Donohue (Eds.), *Sexual deviance: Theory, assessment, and treatment.* New York: Guilford.

Bradford, J., Boulet, J., & Pawlak, A. (1992). The paraphilias: A multiplicity of deviant behaviours. *Canadian Journal of Psychiatry, 37,* 104–108.

Conte, H. R. (1986). Multivariate assessment of sexual dysfunction. *Journal of Consulting and Clinical Psychology, 5,* 149–157.

Davis, C., Yarber, W., Bauserman, R., Schreer, G., & Davis, S. (Eds.). (1998). *Handbook of sexuality-related measures.* Thousand Oaks, CA: Sage.

Eichel, E. W., Eichel, J. D., & Kule, S. (1988). The technique of coital alignment and its relation to female orgasmic response and simultaneous orgasm. *Journal of Sex and Marital Therapy, 14,* 129–141.

Finkelhor, D. (1984). *Child sexual abuse: New theory and research.* New York: Free Press.

Freund, K., Seto, M., & Kuban, M. (1998). Frotteurism and the theory of courtship disorder. In D. R. Laws & W. O'Donohue (Eds.), *Sexual deviance: Theory, assessment, and treatment.* New York: Guilford.

Freund, K., & Watson, R. (1990). Mapping the boundaries of courtship disorder. *Journal of Sex Research, 27,* 589–606.

Goldman, A., & Carroll, J. L. (1990). Educational intervention as an adjunct to treatment of erectile dysfunction in older couples. *Journal of Sex and Marital Therapy, 19,* 127–141.

Heiman, J., LoPiccolo, L., & LoPiccolo, J. (1976). *Becoming orgasmic: A sexual growth program for women.* Englewood Cliffs, NJ: Prentice-Hall.

Hucker, S., & Bain, J. (1990). Androgenic hormones and sexual assault. In W. L. Marshall, D. R. Laws, & H. E. Barbaree (Eds.), *Handbook of sexual assault: Issues, theories, and treatment of the offender* (pp. 93–102). New York: Plenum.

Hunter, J., & Mathews, R. (1998). Sexual deviance in females. In D. R. Laws & W. O'Donohue (Eds.), *Sexual deviance: Theory, assessment, and treatment.* New York: Guilford.

Hurlbert, D. F. (1993). A comparative study using orgasm consistency training in the treatment of women reporting hypoactive sexual desire. *Journal of Sex and Marital Therapy, 19*, 41–55.

Kaplan, H. S. (1977). Hypoactive sexual desire. *Journal of Sex and Marital Therapy, 3*, 3–9.

Kohlenberg, R. J. (1974). Directed masturbation and the treatment of primary orgasmic dysfunction. *Archives of Sexual Behavior, 3*, 349–356.

Laumann, E. O., Paik, A., & Rosen, R. C. (1999). Sexual dysfunction in the United States: Prevalence and predictors. *Journal of the American Medical Association, 281*, 537–544.

Lowe, J. C., & Mikulas, W. L. (1975). Use of written material in learning self-control of premature ejaculation. *Psychological Reports, 37*, 295–298.

Maletzky, B. (1991). The use of medroxyprogesterone acetate to assist in the treatment of sexual offenders. *Annals of Sex Research, 4*, 117–129.

Maletzky, B. (1993). Factors associated with success and failure in the behavioral and cognitive treatment of sexual offenders. *Annals of Sex Research, 6*, 241–258.

Maletzky, B. (1998). The paraphilias: Research and treatment. In P. Nathan & J. Gorman (Eds.), *A guide to treatments that work*. New York: Oxford University Press.

Masters, W. H., & Johnson, V. E. (1966). *Human sexual response*. Boston: Little/Brown.

Masters, W. H., & Johnson, V. E. (1970). *Human sexual inadequacy*. Boston: Little/Brown.

Munjack, D. J., Schlaks, A., Sanchez, V. C., Usigli, R., Zulueta, A., & Leonard, M. (1984). Rational-emotive therapy in the treatment of erectile failure: An initial study. *Journal of Sex and Marital Therapy, 10*, 170–175.

O'Donohue, W. T., Dopke, C., & Swingen, D. (1997). Psychotherapy for female sexual dysfunction: A review. *Clinical Psychology Review, 17*, 537–566.

O'Donohue, W. T., & Plaud, J. (1991). The long-term habituation of sexual arousal in the human male. *Journal of Behavior Therapy and Experimental Psychiatry, 22*, 87–96.

O'Donohue, W. T., Swingen, D., Dopke, C., & Regev, L. (1999). Psychotherapy for male sexual dysfunction: A review. *Clinical Psychology Review, 19*, 519–530.

Schover, L. R., & Jensen, S. B. (1988). *Sexuality and chronic illness: A comprehensive approach*. New York: Guilford.

Spanier, G. B. (1976). Measuring dyadic adjustment: New scales for assessing the quality of marriage and similar dyads. *Journal of Marriage and the Family, 38*, 15–28.

Wincze, J. P. (1971). A comparison of systematic desensitization and "vicarious extinction" in a case of frigidity. *Journal of Behavior Therapy and Experimental Psychiatry, 2*, 285–289.

Wolpe, J. (1958). *Psychotherapy by reciprocal inhibition*. Stanford, CA: Stanford University Press.

19

Personality Disorders

Brian P. O'Connor and Jamie A. Dyce

Descriptions of the Disorders

We all have our moments. We all occasionally seem peculiar and perhaps even annoying to those around us. For individuals who have personality disorders (PDs), these are not isolated episodes, but chronic, central, defining, and dysfunctional aspects of who they are. PDs are characteristic, maladaptive patterns of thoughts, feelings, perceptions, and behaviors that begin early and last long; that are displayed in a wide range of situations; that affect many spheres of the individual's life; and that involve notable departures from the standards of normal living and interpersonal behavior in the individual's sociocultural group. They are often described as extreme and inflexible manifestations of personality characteristics that can be found in normal populations.

The heterogeneous set of DSM-IV PDs (American Psychiatric Association [APA], 1994) exists in the region between psychological health and illness. Social and occupational functioning may be impaired, but contact with reality is generally maintained. People do not suddenly become "ill" with a PD and seek help. Rather, these people feel normal and at home with their conditions, presumably because their disordered personalities and self-concepts are all they know and remember. They often value the very habits and features in themselves that are troublesome for those around them. PDs are thus "ego-syntonic," whereas most other DSM disorders are ego-dystonic conditions that feel unfamiliar and undesirable. PDs are more closely tied to cultural expectations than other DSM disorders, and they require that judgments of personality deviance be made about persons who often value their maladaptive beliefs and habits. Although the individuals are typically not distressed by their lack of adjustment or by their warped personalities, they are often unhappy people and distress can be found in their lives. PDs often co-occur with, and contribute to, other difficulties, such as academic problems, work problems, family and relationship problems, substance abuse, violence and criminality, suicide, mortality, accidents, emergency room visits, child custody battles, and therapy failures, dropouts, and referrals. They may affect the course of Axis I disorders, as well as the

Brian P. O'Connor • Department of Psychology, Lakehead University, Thunder Bay, Ontario, Canada P7B SE1. **Jamie A. Dyce** • Department of Psychology, Concordia University College of Alberta, Edmonton, Alberta, Canada T5B 4E4.

Advanced Abnormal Psychology, Second Edition, edited by Hersen and Van Hasselt. Kluwer Academic/Plenum Publishers, New York, 2001.

nature and degree of response to psychological and pharmacological treatments. They occasionally foreshadow the developments of psychoses. They also tend to have a self-fulfilling, vicious cycle aspect, wherein the rigid ways of responding to life events result in experiences that ultimately maintain and deepen the problematic patterns. Individuals who have PDs are often reluctant to accept professional help, and they tend to blame others for their difficulties.

There are ten PDs in the DSM-IV, and they are grouped into three clusters on the basis of descriptive similarities. Cluster A includes the paranoid, schizoid, and schizotypal personality disorders that involve withdrawn, suspicious, odd, or eccentric behavior. Cluster B includes the antisocial, borderline, histrionic, and narcissistic personality disorders that involve dramatic, emotional, or erratic behavior, often accompanied by labile and shallow moods and intense interpersonal conflicts. Cluster C includes the avoidant, dependent, and obsessive–compulsive personality disorders that involve anxiety and fearfulness. In the DSM-IV, PDs are categorical, "you-have-it-or-you-don't" phenomena. However, many researchers now suspect that PDs, instead, are dimensions on which different people have disparate scores. In either case, it is remarkable and puzzling that particular constellations of otherwise normal personality characteristics become rigid and extreme and coalesce to form the recurring distinctive patterns of personality maladjustment that clinicians often encounter in their work.

The individual PDs will now be described in more detail. The descriptions below end with examples of popular film characters who displayed important PD features (Hyler, 1988). The examples are not all prototypical PDs, and they were not formally diagnosed using the DSM-IV criteria, but they nevertheless provide memorable illustrations. Interested readers are referred to Gunderson and Phillips (1995), Livesley (1995), Stone (1993a), Sutker and Adams (1993), and Widiger and Sanderson (1997) for excellent, more detailed descriptions of the individual PDs.

The *paranoid* PD involves unjustified suspiciousness and distrust of others, who are assumed to be malicious and deceitful. Cognitive impairment is reflected in tendencies to interpret even trivial events as having hidden, threatening meanings; to perceive attacks from others when none have been made; to bear grudges; and to be preoccupied with doubts about the loyalty and trustworthiness of friends, co-workers, and relationship partners. Speech is coherent, although often based on faulty premises. Individuals who have the paranoid PD scrutinize others for signs of threat, manage to find evidence for their concerns, and feel persecuted. They are guarded and have a need to be self-sufficient. They are often concerned with rank and power, experience occupational difficulties, blame others for their problems, become involved in hostile disputes, and may threaten lawsuits. They tend to be secretive and avoid intimacy, self-disclosure, and dependency because they fear vulnerability and exploitation. They have few friends and eventually distrust their occasional allies. Suspicions about emotional and sexual infidelities result in ongoing arguments, complaints, sarcasm, vigilance, discomfort, and conflict in close relationships. Film example: Humphrey Bogart's character in *The Caine Mutiny*.

The defining features of the *schizoid* PD include disinterest in and detachment from social relationships; inappropriate, flat, or restricted emotional responses to others; a consistent preference for solitary activities; indifference to praise and criticism; and generally low levels of pleasure in life, including minimal interest in sensory and sexual experiences. Schizoid individuals may appear slightly uncomfortable, may give short answers to queries, and may display little eye contact and humor. They appear eccentric, aloof, and unaffected by the everyday interests and concerns of others. They appear unable to experience and express emotions, especially anger and aggression. They are oblivious and indifferent to the emotional lives of others and to the rewards, punishments, and subtleties of social interactions. They are often lifelong loners who may develop attachments to animals or objects, but not people. Plans they may have for developing relationships are generally never carried out, and opportunities are not pursued. They may have contact with first-degree relatives, but they usually do not have close friends or confidants, and they rarely marry. They are passive and indecisive in the face of life events and lack ambition. They may succeed at solitary occupations and develop stable, distant relationships in these contexts. They may develop interests in fads and intellectual movements, but without social involvement. They prefer solitary intellectual activities and gadgets, and their imaginations and fantasy lives may be slightly richer than their real lives. Their thought and speech may by odd, but not incoherent, and they retain contact with reality. Film examples: Batman and Sandra Bullock's character in *The Net*, although these examples contain only some schizoid PD elements and are not prototypical.

The *schizotypal* PD is a mild, schizophrenia-like disorder that is characterized by cognitive and interpersonal deficits. The individuals display odd thinking patterns, vocabulary, and use of words. They may have ideas of reference, peculiar superstitions, beliefs in magical powers, bizarre fantasies, mystical experiences, paranoid thoughts, and perceptual distortions. They are typically withdrawn, socially inept, sensitive to anger, and lack close contacts, apart from relatives. They experience persistent social anxiety that is associated with their paranoid thoughts about others and that contributes to their relationship deficits. Their behavior and appearance may be odd, and they are restricted in their emotional expressions. They may be drifters and are at risk of becoming involved in cults. They rarely date or marry. They prefer their own eccentric cognitive worlds, and they lead empty lives. They may display psychotic symptoms when stressed, but the cognitive distortions are not severe enough to warrant a diagnosis of schizophrenia. Film example: Robert DeNiro's character in *Taxi Driver*.

People who have the *antisocial* PD were previously labeled psychopaths, sociopaths, and "morally insane." The DSM-IV criteria for diagnosing this disorder focus on irresponsible and harmful behaviors. There is consistent disregard for and violation of the rights of others, as manifested in a wide range of criminal-type behaviors (assault, theft, vandalism, child and spouse abuse, substance abuse, sadism). There is repeated lying for personal gain; impulsiveness, irritability, and aggressiveness; disregard for safety; inconsistent work behavior; failure to honor financial and interpersonal commitments; and a lack of remorse for harmful actions. Antisocial personalities can be superficially charming and ingratiating. They may have relationships, but they cannot maintain stable, mutually satisfying, intimate relationships. Their inner lives are flat and emotionally empty. The social world is hostile and self-serving in their eyes, and other people are objects to be used and abused. Antisocial personalities are egocentric manipulators and swindlers who rarely feel shame or empathy. Their expressions of emotion do not seen genuine. Although usually of average or above average intelligence, there is nevertheless a failure to plan, a disregard for truth, a lack of insight, and a failure to learn from past problems. They are impulsive, reckless, and concerned with immediate gratification. They act as if codes of conduct do not apply to them and as if they are immune to the negative consequences of their actions. Harmful and criminal behaviors are performed for thrills and not just personal gain. Antisocial personalities occur in high concentrations in prison populations, but they can be found in many segments of society and are a major drain on social resources. Film examples: Malcolm McDowell's character in *A Clockwork Orange*, Anthony Hopkins's character (Hannibal Lecter) in *Silence of the Lambs*, Robert DeNiro's character in *Cape Fear*, Michael Douglas's character in *Wall Street*, and the main characters in Truman Capote's *In Cold Blood*. Other famous examples are Bonnie and Clyde and killers Ted Bundy and Gary Gilmore.

The *borderline* PD is characterized by intense and chaotic relationships; extreme and unstable self-images and perceptions of significant others that vary from idealization to strong devaluation; and potentially self-damaging impulsivity (e.g., substance abuse, promiscuity, overspending, gambling, shop-lifting, reckless driving), especially in times of crisis. There is strong concern with feelings of abandonment, chronic feelings of emptiness, difficulty controlling anger, and occasional paranoid or dissociative symptoms. There is little sense of identity or meaning in life. The person feels bad, evil, and there is often an underlying depression. The individual forms intense attachments but then becomes nervous and upset over imagined slights. People who have the borderline PD cannot bear to be alone and want support from others (not materialistic gains). They are quick to view others as cruel persecutors and they become argumentative and sarcastic. They display destructive behavior toward others, experience frequent rejections, and search for quick fixes for their pain. Self-mutilation and suicidal behavior may occur, especially in response to interpersonal conflicts and losses. The person's values, career choices, and long-term goals are unstable, and their crisis-filled lives may create difficulties at work and school. They may occasionally seem to improve and get their lives back on track, but they soon fall into further crises. Film example: Glenn Close's character in *Fatal Attraction*.

The *histrionic* PD involves excessive emotionally and attention-seeking behavior. These persons are unsure of their value, and they are uncomfortable when they are not the center of attention. They are flamboyant in their dress and speech, and they are often inappropriately flirtatious in social interactions, all apparently stemming from a need for social approval. Emotional responses are shallow, shifting, and exaggerated. They talk about themselves and are concerned with physical appearance. They are excitable; they crave novelty and sensational experiences; they are trusting, easily frustrated, overly reactive; and they may throw temper tantrums. They display interest in others and are eager to please. They may be quick to form new relationships, but they have problems forming lasting attachments. After initially positive impressions, others may eventually perceive that they are shallow and insincere. Histrionic persons become dependent, demanding, manipulative, and needy with others, and their relationships are not as intimate as they may claim. They are not in-depth or critical thinkers, but they may do well in positions that require creativity and imagination. Their speech is vague, impressionistic, and replete with exaggerated descriptions of people and events. Film examples: Blanche Dubois and Stanley Kowalski in *A Streetcar Named Desire*, and Gloria Swanson's character in *Sunset Boulevard*. Another popular example is pianist/celebrity Liberace.

The *narcissistic* PD involves grandiose self-importance, a strong need for admiration, and a lack of empathy. These individuals believe that they are special, unique, and a cut above the masses. They require and feel entitled to high levels of admiration and special treatment. They envy the accomplishments of others and believe that others are envious of them. They have fantasies of unbounded success, beauty, brilliance, or fame and may engage in displays of superiority. They draw attention to and exaggerate their accomplishments and extract compliments from others. They may appear distant and self-sufficient, but they are also shallow and attention-seeking. Their self-esteem is fragile, and they are sensitive to criticism. They often feel inadequate, undeserving, and empty, even when they are successful. Impression management victories feel hollow, perhaps because they are so strongly sought, and the hollowness may soon fuel further efforts to impress. Narcissistic persons may become outraged in response to minor slights and rejections and then become preoccupied with revenge. Depression may soon follow. They are sensitive to their own feelings but oblivious to the needs and feelings of others, and they often treat others as objects to be exploited. Their relationships are erratic and strained, and they have difficulty remaining in love. They alternate between idealization and contempt for close others. Other people are potentially admiring audiences, not full human beings. Narcissistic individuals may be motivated to excel on the job, but often have troubled relationships with co-workers. They expect high levels of dedication from subordinates but have little regard for their well-being and give little in return. Narcissists also tend to lack the levels of talent needed to reach their aspired levels of fame. Film example: Jack Nicholson's character in *A Few Good Men.*

The *avoidant* PD is characterized by anxious social inhibition, feelings of social and personal inferiority, and sensitivity to criticism and rejection. In first encounters, avoidant persons appear uncertain, self-effacing, and eager to please. Internally, they are preoccupied with negative thoughts about assertiveness and appearing foolish, and they are prone to interpret statements from others as criticism. They are creatures of habit whose activities are limited by feelings of incompetence and fears of embarrassment. The risks associated with new activities are exaggerated. Unlike the schizoid PD, avoidant persons desire social contacts, but they have difficulty initiating relationships because they are too shy and insecure to seek them out. They become involved with others only when they are certain of being liked. The fear of shame and ridicule may restrain the development of more intimate relationships, and they may be clinging and fearful of losing the few close contacts they do establish. Avoidant persons are often isolated, lonely, and bored, and they have few close relationships apart from immediate relatives. They may marry and work, although their adjustment is tenuous and fragile. They tend to hold marginal jobs in which they may function adequately, especially when the positions do not require social skills. However, there is minimal career advancement. The social inhibition is more pervasive and chronic in the avoidant PD than it is in social phobia. Film example: Woody Allen's character in *Zelig.*

Persons who have the *dependent* PD have a strong, pervasive need to be cared for. There is excessive fear of separation, clinging behavior, and submissiveness. They are unassertive, unwilling to make demands on others, reluctant to disagree with others, and they accommodate to others excessively, all out of a fear of disapproval and loss of support. They lack confidence in their abilities and have difficulties initiating new activities. They seek advice and reassurance from others before making decisions and would prefer to have others assume responsibility for most aspects of their lives. They feel anxious and helpless when alone, and are preoccupied with fears of being left to care for themselves. However, they can be self-sacrificing in the degree to which they care for others. They will seek out relationships, despite fear of being rejected. They will tolerate mistreatment and perform undesirable tasks to maintain affection. They give priority to the needs of others, yet others may lose respect, take advantage, and reject them. The development of intimacy may be adversely affected by the preoccupation with maintaining relationships. They respond to threatened interpersonal losses with submission and appeasement, in contrast to the rage displayed in the borderline PD. They also quickly seek replacements when important relationships end. They tend to avoid positions of responsibility and become anxious and seek reassurance when placed in leadership positions. They consider other people to be stronger and more competent, and they tend to have jobs that involve doing tasks for others. Film example: Bill Murray's character in *What About Bob*, and Jean Stapleton's character in the television show, "All In The Family."

Persons who have the *obsessive–compulsive* PD are perfectionists who are preoccupied with orderliness and mental and interpersonal control. They tend to be concerned with rules, lists, and schedules, even at the expense of efficiency. Work and productivity seem more important than friendships and good times, which are likely to be planned. They are preoccupied with "shoulds" and are overly conscientious and moral. They are rigid, stubborn, serious, neat, formal, and punctual. They are unwilling to compromise or let themselves be convinced by others. They may procrastinate over even small decisions and become anxious in the face of uncertainty; yet, they can also be hard-driving, do-it-now types. They tend to be intellectualizers who have little spontaneity. They are emotionally restricted and have trouble expressing affection. Anger may be the most common and visible emotion, although it is rarely expressed strongly. They may become depressed as they realize the emptiness of their lifelong preoccupation with order, rules, and performance at the expense of enriching leisure activities and relationships. They enjoy routines, insist on doing things their own way, and are reluctant to delegate. They are stingy in their spending on both themselves and others and tend to hoard money and possessions. They often marry and often have good careers, but few friends. Unlike people who have obsessive–compulsive disorder (OCD), these individuals generally do not have obsessions or compulsions and the obsessive–compulsive PD is not a diathesis for OCD (Black & Noyes, 1997). They are excessively conscientious but not necessarily anxious and nervous. Film examples: Jack Nicholson's character in *As Good As It Gets*, although this character also displayed features of OCD, and Dan Aykroyd's character in *Dragnet*.

Obviously, many PD features can be found in well-adjusted individuals and are not inherently dysfunctional. Extremity, rigidity, pervasiveness, chronicity, and centrality are what make constellations of these features abnormal and problematic. "Why these PDs and not others?" For example, why is there a dependent PD, but no "independent" PD (Tavris, 1992). Psychologists currently do not have good answers to this question because there is no encompassing theory of personality that accounts for the development of the various PDs. Experts have also debated the existence of other PDs besides the ten described in the DSM-IV. These include the depressive, self-defeating, sadistic, and passive–aggressive PDs. Descriptions can be found in the DSM-III-R (APA, 1987), in the appendix of the DSM-IV (APA, 1994), and in Widiger and Sanderson (1997). The DSM-IV also permits clinicians to use the diagnosis of "PD Not Otherwise Specified" for individuals who meet the general criteria for PDs, but not the criteria for specific PDs.

EPIDEMIOLOGY

Estimates of the prevalence of PDs in the general population have long been somewhat variable. Many of the primary epidemiological studies did not use DSM criteria or standard measures for diagnosing PDs. In some of the larger investigations, such as the Epidemiological Catchment Area study (Robins & Regier, 1991), most PDs were simply not assessed. The criteria for diagnosing PDs have also changed across versions of the DSM, and sometimes there were dramatic effects on prevalence estimates. For example, modification to the DSM-III criteria (APA, 1980) resulted in an eightfold increase in the number of people categorized with the schizoid PD when using the DSM-III-R criteria (APA, 1987; Morey, 1988). Further, little epidemiological research has been conducted using the DSM-IV PD criteria. The existing data, based primarily on North American and European samples, indicate that between 10% and 13% of persons in the general population meet the criteria for a PD at any given time (Weissman, 1993). The rates are slightly higher in urban populations and in lower socioeconomic groups. Estimates of the prevalence of PDs among inpatients and outpatients are based on more extensive data. Between one-half and two-thirds of these people typically meet the criteria for at least one PD.

Prevalence rates for the individual PDs, derived from the DSM-IV (APA, 1994), Weissman (1993), and Widiger and Sanderson (1997), are reported in Table 1. The estimates from all three sources are based on reviews of the literature. The estimates for clinical populations are

TABLE 1. Prevalence (in percentages) of Personality Disorder

| | Weissman (1993) | Widiger & Sanderson (1997) | | DSM-IV | | |
	General population	General population	Clinical population	General population	Clinical population	Sex differences
Paranoid	0.4–0.8	0.5–2.5	2–30	0.5–2.5	2–30	M > F
Schizoid	0.7–1.8	<1	NA[a]	NA[a]	NA[a]	M > F
Schizotypal	0.5–5.6	3	NA[a]	3	NA[a]	M > F
Antisocial	2.0–3.0	2	20–30	2	3–30	M > F
Borderline	0.0–4.6	2	8–15	2	10–20	F > M
Histrionic	2.1–3.0	1–3	NA[a]	2–3	10–15	F > M
Narcissistic	0.0–2.1	NA	2–20	1	2–16	M > F
Avoidant	0.0–5.1	1	5–25	0.5–1	10	M = F
Dependent	1.7–6.7	2–4	5–30	NA[a]	NA[a]	F > M
Obs.–comp.	1.6–6.4	1–3	5	1	3–10	M > F

[a]NA = estimate not available.

based on both inpatient and outpatient samples and have wider ranges. Prevalences for the "PD not otherwise specified" diagnostic category do not appear in Table 1, although this is the most common PD diagnosis (Morey, 1988; Widiger & Sanderson, 1997, p. 1313).

A finding that remains hidden in the summary estimates in Table 1 is that the relative frequencies of PDs are quite consistent across studies, despite the varying prevalence estimates. The most commonly diagnosed PD is borderline, followed by the histrionic, schizotypal, and dependent PDs. Higher concentrations of individuals who have particular PDs or PD symptoms are also found in particular segments of society. For example, higher concentrations of the paranoid PD (or its symptoms) can be found among prisoners, elderly people, hearing-impaired people, refugees and immigrants, and delusional disorder patients (Bernstein, Useda, & Siever, 1995). Higher concentrations of the borderline PD occur among people who seek help for substance-abuse, eating disorders, and mood disorders. Avoidant PDs can be found among people who seek help for anxiety disorders, and dependent PDs can be found among those who seek help for mood disorders and relationship counseling. High concentrations of the antisocial PD occur in forensic populations, although this PD may be overdiagnosed in these groups and underdiagnosed in nonclinical samples (Widiger & Corbitt, 1995). The obsessive–compulsive PD may occur in higher concentrations among first-borns and in professions that require perseverance and attention to detail (Gunderson & Phillips, 1995).

Sex differences are also relatively consistent in PD diagnoses, as summarized in Table 1. Males receive more diagnoses of the antisocial, paranoid, schizoid, schizotypal, narcissistic, and obsessive–compulsive PDs. Women receive more diagnoses of the borderline, histrionic, and dependent PDs. The sex differences in PD prevalence rates have at least a rough correspondence with the masculine and feminine sex-role orientations and are thereby consistent with the claim that PDs are maladaptively extreme manifestations of normal personality traits. However, there is ongoing controversy (Widiger, 1998) over the relative frequencies with which females are diagnosed with the borderline, histrionic, and dependent PDs (the sex ratio in these diagnosis is approximately 3:1). Do men and women vary in how susceptible they are to these PDs, or do clinicians merely perceive their male and female patients differently? There are also emerging indications of cultural differences in the conceptualization of PDs and in prevalence rates (Paris, 1998a; Tang & Huang, 1995).

CLINICAL PICTURE

Case Description: Paranoid Personality Disorder

Gary is a 50-year-old millworker who was referred for counseling by his employer because of chronic difficulties in getting along with others. Gary has little insight into his own role in a variety of interpersonal conflicts and claims that co-workers regularly plot against him to make his job more difficult. Transfers to other jobs within the mill did not solve the problems. Co-workers describe Gary as defensive, cold, and humorless. In counseling, he was reluctant to discuss personal matters and the therapist had difficulty developing an alliance. Gary believes that psychologists and psychiatrists cannot be trusted because "they are in the mind-f____ing business." He has filed a number of small claims suits against his neighbors, whom he also firmly believes have been trying to take advantage of him for years.

Case Description: Schizoid Personality Disorder

Jerry is a 25-year-old male who was referred for counseling by his parents. Although Jerry did not understand why he was going for counseling, his parents believed he was depressed and not well adjusted. Jerry finished college, but he is unemployed and has never kept a steady job. He has never dated, has no friends, and appears unconcerned about his impoverished social life. He lives with his parents and spends his time reading, watching television, and playing computer games. In counseling, he mumbles and tends to give yes or no answers. Outsiders describe Jerry as a colorless person who prefers to be alone.

Case Description: Schizotypal Personality Disorder

Helen is a single, 46-year-old library worker who was urged to seek help for depression and anxiety by her relatives and family doctor. She has few close friends and is uncomfortable with her younger co-workers, whom she believes are critical of her. Her older sister was diagnosed with undifferentiated schizophrenia 20 years ago. Helen prefers to stay home because she feels anxious around others. She also says that she can sometimes make things happen by just willing them to happen. She believes that she has some special purpose, although she has difficulty articulating what this might be. Helen sometimes laughs inappropriately during conversations, and she is described by others as odd and eccentric.

Case Description: Antisocial Personality Disorder

Max is a 31-year-old male who was recently released from prison. He has an extensive and varied criminal record (including convictions for car theft, assault, and rape) that began when he was 13. He was ordered to undergo counseling as part of his parole but views it as "a lot of bullshit." Max can be entertaining in conversations, and he often brags about his encounters with the law. He talks as if he is a multitalented overachiever. When questioned about the truthfulness of his claims, he either changes the topic or becomes angry. The counselor noted that although Max had fathered three children, he does not seem concerned about them and does not pay child support. However, he is quite critical of his own alcoholic father's treatment of him when he was young. Max previously had a number of jobs at construction sites, but he tended to drift from place to place after quickly becoming tired of the grind.

Case Description: Borderline Personality Disorder

Jennifer is 28 years old, currently unemployed, and was recently hospitalized after attempting suicide. She had cuts and slashes on both arms. After her release from hospital emergency, she spent two weeks in a psychiatric unit. Her psychologist there discovered that the suicide attempt occurred after a fight with her boyfriend. She reported that mutilating her body usually somehow made her feel better. It was also discovered that she had been repeatedly sexually abused by her older brother, was bulimic in her late teens and early twenties, and sometimes takes drugs. In her adult life, Jennifer has had numerous impulsive relationships with both men and women, although she does not consider herself bisexual. Jennifer admits being moody, emotional, and often hostile with others. She also wonders about her meaning in life, feels unloved, and frequently finds herself staring into space.

Case Description: Histrionic Personality Disorder

Nancy is a 32-year-old part-time actress who has been involved in stage productions since she was a child. She entered counseling after separating from her second husband. She reported that she was her father's little princess. She had many boyfriends in her adolescence and often dated several at a time. She never had many close female friends and prefers the company of men because she considers that women are too competitive. She wears tight-fitting clothes, light blue nail polish, and platinum blond hair, which she often plays with while talking. She is friendly, agreeable, and sometimes even flirtatious with her counselor. She is surprised that so many men are interested in her and perplexed that her relationships never work out. Nancy sometimes comes to counseling sessions with a host of emotional issues to unload, but these seem to evaporate soon after they are presented.

Case Description: Narcissistic Personality Disorder

Lance is a 53-year-old, apparently successful, university professor who sought help for depression and lingering feelings of emptiness. Lance could not understand why he was refused a promotion because he claimed to be respected and liked by almost everyone. However, his colleagues, who admire his accomplishments, consider him self-centered, arrogant, annoying, and inconsiderate. Lance's wife said that he had urged her to have breast implants because her breasts were too small, and that he seemed unconcerned with the way his statements might hurt her. Lance is a lonely person who has shifting, marginal acquaintances and few close friends.

Case Description: Avoidant Personality Disorder

Susie is a quiet, 22-year-old student who was unable to give required classroom presentations. Her instructor recommended that she seek the services of the school counselor. It was soon discovered that her social anxieties are chronic, pervasive, and not restricted to public speaking. Susie claims that she has always been very shy, had few friends as a child, and was often teased. She has few friends now and spends much of her time alone. She had one boyfriend in high school, but felt rejected when they broke up, and has not dated since. She says she likes people and feels lonely but does not have the confidence to strike up conversations or friendships. She believes she is not very smart or competent, although she usually does well in her courses. She attributed a recent scholarship to being lucky. The counselor noted that Susie is sensitive to criticism and tends to brood about social encounters and the reactions of others. Susie claims that "if people really knew me, they would not like me."

Case Description: Dependent Personality Disorder

Debbie is a 38-year-old, devoted housewife who has four children. She was urged to seek counseling by her husband, and she admits feeling increasingly stressed, depressed, and nervous during the last couple of years. Debbie describes her husband in almost idyllic terms, but she is worried that their marriage may seem stale in her husband's eyes, and she suspects that he is thinking about leaving her. Her husband expressed frustration with Debbie's "whiny-ness," with her difficulty in making every-day decisions on her own, and with her inability to tolerate being alone. He admits having a busy job, but he claims he is a normal loving husband who spends as much time with his family as other men. The psychologist was initially impressed with Debbie's cooperative attitude in counseling sessions. She seemed eager to please and was a model patient. However, the counselor soon noticed that he was giving Debbie too much advice and that the apparent progress in the therapeutic relationship was not generalizing to the outside world.

Case Description: Obsessive–Compulsive Personality Disorder

Kathy is a 52-year-old college administrator who is married and has two children. She sought counseling for feelings of depression, emptiness, and for anxiety over recent events at work. Kathy has long been one of the college's best employees and often works 50 hours a week. However, she is reluctant to delegate tasks because she believes others cannot be trusted to do things properly. She recently insisted that an employee be fired for immoral behavior, but the decision was overturned by one of her superiors, and she feels anxious about the whole experience. It was also discovered that her family environment has long been lifeless and full of routines. Kathy is a committed wife and mother, but she is stingy, humorless, and excessively concerned with order, cleanliness, and proper behavior. Her marriage is dull, and she has trouble with one of her children, who seems intent on maintaining the habits and lifestyle that she despises.

COURSE AND PROGNOSIS

Very little is known about the natural histories of PDs. High-quality longitudinal data are simply not available (Perry, 1993). The DSM-IV specifies that PDs must appear, or (in retrospect) must *have* appeared, in adolescence or early adulthood to make a PD diagnosis. However, personality distortions do not suddenly flare up at this time. The various personality characteristics often emerge earlier in life, and perhaps they merely crystallize and stabilize in young adulthood. The fact that PDs are also chronic, pervasive in their influence on many life domains, and ego-syntonic, make it hardly surprising that their courses are generally steady and their prognoses bleak (Perry, 1993; Stone, 1993b). Resistance to treatment is typically high. PDs are often most intense when individuals are in their twenties, and some PDs slowly fade with time, notably the antisocial, borderline and narcissistic PDs. However, there is much variability in outcomes even in these cases (e.g., from suicides to satisfactory recoveries in the case of borderline PDs). The existence of comorbid conditions, such as depression or substance abuse, and the absence of treatment can make prognoses particularly poor. If there is a comorbid Axis I condition, then the prognosis may be poor for both the Axis I condition and the PD (see Reich & Vasile, 1993, and Tyrer, Gunderson, Lyons, & Tohen, 1997, for reviews). A meta-analysis of studies on PDs in people more than 50 years of age revealed an overall prevalence rate of 10% (Abrams & Horowitz, 1996). This estimate is in the same range as the PD prevalence estimates for the general population, suggesting no major drop-off with age. In fact, PDs may be underdiagnosed in older adults (Segal, Hersen, Van Hasselt, Silberman, & Roth, 1996).

Frances (1982) noted that diagnosing a PD does not provide an informative starting point for deciding how to treat a PD. This remains true today, although some progress has been made. Enthusiastic descriptions of particular treatment methods for particular disorders are readily found in the literature (e.g., Clarkin, Yeomans, & Kernberg, 1999), but there have been few high-quality, controlled outcome studies. There has been much recent interest in (and use of) pharmacological treatments for PDs (Kapfhammer & Hippius, 1998; Links, Heslegrave, & Villella, 1998). However, currently, no medications are remarkably effective, although breakthroughs are anticipated. Drugs are most effective for PDs that resemble Axis I disorders (e.g., the schizotypal, borderline, and avoidant PDs) and for reducing distress in time of crises. For example, low doses of antipsychotic medication can be effective for borderline and schizotypal people during these times, and borderline and avoidant persons may respond to antidepressants. Medication is most effective when there are comorbid conditions, although little is known about the long-term effects of medication, and the existing prescription guidelines are tentative.

It is unreasonable to expect brief drug or psychotherapy treatments to have immediate, substantial, and enduring effects on long-standing, ingrained personality structures. The habits of a lifetime are not easily lost. It is partly for these reasons that relatively in-depth, psychodynamically oriented techniques have traditionally been the most commonly used therapeutic approaches. The current therapeutic literature for many PDs retains a psychodynamic flavor. However, there has recently been interest in applying other therapeutic modalities in the treatment of PDs, including cognitive therapy, dialectical behavioral therapy, brief psychodynamic therapy, social skills and assertiveness training, and psychoeducation (Beck & Freeman, 1990; Dowson & Grounds, 1995; Sperry, 1995; Stone, 1993b). Although these techniques await careful empirical evaluation, the relevant literatures and case studies are nevertheless replete with good descriptions of the therapeutic obstacles that arise when dealing with clients who have particular PDs. There is more clinical knowledge about managing the often problematic therapeutic relationships with PD clients (Clarkin et al., 1999; Gunderson & Phillips, 1995; Perry & Valliant, 1989) than there is knowledge about the relative effectiveness of competing, formal therapeutic modalities. However, treatment goals should be modest, perhaps involving reductions in symptoms in times of crisis and slow, slight improvements in relationships, living habits, thinking styles, and emotional reactions. Most personality disordered individuals will never reach normal levels of functioning. Social skill training may seem desirable in many cases, but the changes may be only superficial.

FAMILIAL AND GENETIC PATTERNS

The fact that PDs begin early and last long suggests to many experts that both genes and early family experiences may be important to their etiology. Direct, high-quality data on genetic and environmental influences are sparse, but the conclusions that have been reached from the available research are consistent. For most PDs, genetic and environmental influences are equally important, and neither can be ignored.

There have been relatively few twin and adoption studies that focus specifically on PDs, and confounds with Axis I conditions are common in the available data sets (Bouchard, 1997; Dahl, 1993; Nigg & Goldsmith, 1994). The most extensive and supportive genetic evidence currently available is for paranoid, schizoid, schizotypal, borderline, and antisocial PDs. Cluster A PDs have been studied because of their membership in the schizophrenia spectrum, but they have not always been carefully measured and distinguished from one another in research. These PDs are also significantly more common in the biological relatives of diagnosed schizophrenics than in the general population (Nigg & Goldsmith, 1994), suggesting a common diathesis. Also suggestive are similarities between these PDs and schizophrenia in responses to antipsychotic medication, especially for the schizotypal PD. However, the risk of developing schizophrenia is higher for the schizotypal PD than for the schizoid PD (Siever, Bernstein, & Silverman, 1995). Also, behavior genetic research indicates that the paranoid PD may be more closely related to the Axis I delusional disorder than to schizophrenia (Bernstein et al., 1995). Twin research on the antisocial PD, as well as research on the adopted children of criminals and antisocial parents, has been relatively consistent in providing evidence for the importance of genetic influences (Sutker, Bugg, & West, 1993). Investigations of the borderline PD also typically confirm the importance of genetic influences on the PD (Widiger & Trull, 1993). Few data are available for the histrionic, narcissistic, and Cluster C PDs.

The sparseness of quality data on the heritability of PDs has focused attention on the heritability of general personality characteristics, for which more extensive data are available (Bouchard, 1997; Nigg & Goldsmith, 1994). Obvious similarities exist between PDs and "normal" personality dimensions (e.g., aggressiveness, emotionality, shyness, impulsivity). Research on identical twins reared together and apart, on fraternal and identical twins, and on adopted and nonadopted siblings, indicates that most personality characteristics have heritability coefficients in the 40 to 50% range. Environmental factors (and error) account for the remaining 50 to 60% of the variation. The heritability estimates for PDs and for normal personality characteristics are also very similar (Livesley, Schroeder, Jackson, & Jang, 1994). Genetic influences are thus substantial, although it is currently not known exactly what is inherited. Recent speculations have focused on neurotransmitters and brain systems (Silk, 1998). It has also been suggested that PDs are characterological versions of Axis I disorders (Siever & Davis, 1991) that possess a similar biological basis.

Speculations about the early familial experiences of individuals who have PDs have been numerous, varied, and often heavily flavored with psychoanalytic and object relations concepts. The primary speculations in the literature for the individual PDs are summarized in Table 2. The empirical evidence is most extensive for the antisocial PD. The entries for most of the other PDs in Table 2 are relatively untested. Though the speculations are varied, there is consensus on the assumption that early experiences with significant others leave enduring marks on the individuals who eventually develop PDs. Psychodynamic models focus on affective reactions, separation-individuation difficulties, and on problems in developing an adaptive sense of self. Cognitive theorists (e.g., Beck & Freeman, 1990) focus on exaggerated, distorted, core beliefs about self and others that are held by individuals who have particular PDs. For example, schizoid persons may have an ingrained belief that "close relationships with others are unrewarding and messy." Maladaptive beliefs are acquired through learning and modeling, and they become overly powerful and rigidly held. Behavioral explanations focus on rewards and punishments for inappropriate behaviors and on the early lack of affectionate responsiveness that lead to deficiencies in acquiring social skills.

The twin and adoption studies that have produced evidence for the importance of environmental influences also indicate that such influences are "specific" and not shared. For

TABLE 2. Early Family Experiences

Personality disorder	Early family experiences
Paranoid	Parental rage; modeling of suspicion, distrust, and prejudice; humiliation by others
Schizoid	Cold, neglectful, ungratifying early relationships; social isolation; encouragement and modeling of withdrawal and indifference
Schizotypal	Shame and humiliation; irrational and overwhelming parental rage
Antisocial	Absent, assaultive, hostile, rejecting, inconsistent parenting; poverty and unsettled family circumstances; abuse
Borderline	Maternal frustration and difficulty tolerating negative emotions; withdrawal of parental affection in response to separation/individuation; threats of abandonment; familial conflict; neglect; abuse; nurturance in response to wounded feelings
Histrionic	Eroticized and conflictual attachments to opposite sex parent; authoritarian, puritanical parental attitudes
Narcissistic	Disdain and neglect of childhood fears, failures, dependency, and vulnerability; parental rejection, control, and low empathy; conditional regard and high expectations; excessive idealization combined with inconsistent interest and devaluation
Avoidant	Parental rejection, control, overprotectiveness, and excessive cautiousness; minimal parental community involvement; experiences of embarrassment, humiliation, and rejection
Dependent	Parental overprotectiveness, authoritarianism, premature demands for independence and reinforcement of dependence
Obs.-comp.	Parental pressure, disapproval, and high expectations; overemphasis on social and cultural standards

[a]Sources: Bornstein (1993), Gunderson & Phillips (1995), Perry & Valliant (1989), Sutker et al. (1993), Widiger & Sanderson (1997), Widiger & Trull (1993).

example, identical twins who are reared together are as similar to one another, across a variety of traits, as identical twins who are reared apart (Bouchard, 1997). Environmental influences are substantial, but shared experiences in the same family environment do not increase similarities in personality characteristics. The implication of this finding is that the family experiences that are summarized in Table 2, if accurate, are not shared and are unique to specific individuals within family environments. This possibility may be difficult to imagine, but it is strongly suggested by the best available data. At this point, researchers often speak of numerous, complex, as-yet-unknown gene-environment interactions (Paris, 1998b). Biological and neurological predispositions presumably combine with problematic early attachment histories to create warped personality structures.

Diagnostic Considerations

The literature on PD assessment, diagnosis, and classification is voluminous (see Clark, Livesley, & Morey, 1997; Strupp, Horowitz, & Lambert, 1997, for recent reviews). There is more consensus on the nature of the problems and challenges than there is on solutions. The diagnostic challenges are greater for PDs than for many other DSM-IV disorders. PDs are, by definition, broad patterns that involve a wider domain of behavior than other disorders. Selected traits or behaviors may not seem problematic when viewed in isolation, but their overall constellations may be maladaptive. Clinicians must somehow identify the broad constellations and must then determine whether the characteristics are stable across time and situations. Single interviews and single sources of information are not likely to be sufficient, yet there is often little time for the necessary in-depth assessments. The challenges are compounded by the fact that a variety of traits appear in the criteria for each PD, and not all of the criteria are necessary for diagnoses. This can result in remarkable differences among people who qualify for diagnoses of the same PDs. Clinicians who formulate working diagnoses must then deal with clients who are often unwilling to see their personalities as disordered. Clinicians must remain sensitive to the way their own personality characteristics and values may act as distorting lenses that influence the degree to which they perceive particular traits in others as deviant and maladaptive. Problems in differential diagnosis are also likely to be encountered because of the possible co-occurrence of a PD with an Axis I disorder or because of the co-occurrence of a PD with other PDs. Finally, the DSM criteria for PDs are sometimes vague, which can make it difficult for clinicians to distinguish actual comorbidities from conceptual comorbidities.

The realization that PDs may coexist with currently active psychiatric conditions is what led to the placement of PDs on a separate axis in the DSM-III (APA, 1980). Empirical research since this change confirms that people who have PDs are significantly more likely to have Axis I disorders than people without PDs (e.g., Tyrer et al., 1997; Zimmerman & Coryell, 1989). A review of the literature by Van Velzen and Emmelkamp (1996) revealed that approximately 50% of patients who have anxiety disorders, depressive disorders, or eating disorders also receive a PD diagnosis. Yet, the DSM criteria require differentiating PDs from such common disorders, which is no small task for clinicians. The differences between social phobia and the avoidant PD, between depression and the borderline PD, or between schizophrenia and the schizotypal PD are sometimes difficult to perceive when dealing with real people. Clinicians must also differentiate PDs from the symptoms that result from situational crises, medical conditions, brain trauma, medication, and substance abuse. Problems associated with immigration or with the expression of cultural values can also make personalities seem deviant and maladjusted. Attention must be focused on whether PD-like symptoms are chronic, stable, and early developing, or whether they flare up exclusively during times of stress and active mental illness. The lack of insight into personality problems and the apparent ego-syntonic nature of the difficulties may also suggest a PD instead of an Axis I condition.

During the past 15 years, several semistructured interviews and self-report measures have been developed to improve the reliability and validity of PD assessments (see Widiger & Sanderson, 1995, and Van Velzen & Emmelkamp, 1996, for reviews). Some of these assessment tools consist of questions that precisely match DSM criteria, whereas others focus on thematic content areas (e.g., work, social relationships). The structured interviews can be time-consuming, sometimes requiring up to four hours. However, the self-report measures are typically considered screening devices that merely provide suggestive evidence that should be carefully investigated using structured interviews.

One frustrating problem with PD interviews, self-report tests, and clinical judgments is their low levels of diagnostic agreement. A review of the literature by Clark et al. (1997) revealed that agreement indices (kappas) for structured interviews varied between .35 and .51. The agreement between clinical interviews and structured interviews was slightly lower (values ranged between .21 and .38), and the agreement between structured interviews and self-report measures was lower still (kappas ranged between .08 and .42). The median degrees of agreement for studies that reported correlation coefficients varied between .39 and .51. These modest values are not scientifically or clinically acceptable (Perry, 1992, p. 1645). Another measurement problem is that people in anxious, depressed, or psychotic-like states sometimes obtain high scores on particular PD scales, once again highlighting the need to distinguish between states and traits. Also problematic is the fact that though PDs are defined as enduring patterns (APA, 1994, p. 629), PD diagnoses are not stable over time. For example, Zimmerman (1994) found an average stability (kappa) of .56 for less than one-week periods and an average stability of .51 for longer periods (see Clark et al., 1997, and McDavid & Pilkonis, 1996, for reviews). A gold standard for PD assessment is obviously not yet available.

High comorbidity between PDs is another diagnostic phenomenon frequently noted in the literature (Stuart, Pfohl, Battaglia, Bellodi, Grove, & Cadoret, 1998). Between 67 and 85% of patients who meet the criteria for one PD also meet the criteria for at least one other PD. More than 90% of people who receive the borderline diagnosis qualify for other PD diagnoses (Clark et al., 1997). It is estimated that the mean number of potential PD diagnoses in people who have at least one PD falls somewhere between 1.5 and 5.6 PDs according to Dolan, Evans, and Norton (1995), and between three and four PDs according to Widiger and Sanderson (1995). These comorbidities are peculiar and disturbing, but fortunately, not random (e.g., the obsessive–compulsive and antisocial PDs rarely co-occur, as do the schizoid and histrionic PDs; Clark et al., 1997). PD comorbidities are recognized in the DSM-IV manual (APA, 1994); however, the levels are clearly excessive, and there are no clinical guidelines for dealing with these occurrences. In practice, clinicians often provide only one PD diagnosis in their clients' charts. Table 3 contains brief descriptions for differentiating individual PDs from other conditions that they sometimes resemble. Readers should consult the references in the note to Table 3 for more extensive discussions of differential diagnosis.

According to Clark et al. (1997), the various problems in PD assessment stem from both faulty instrumentation and from deficiencies in the DSM descriptions of PDs. If the conceptualizations of PDs are crude and inaccurate, then the psychometric properties of measures designed to assess PD constructs will also be poor. PD criteria are often ambiguous trait adjectives that require inferences of pathological deviation by clinicians. For example, behavioral indicators for "clinically significant impairment," for "excessive social anxiety," for "shallow expression of emotions," and for "requires excessive admiration" are not provided. The inferential leaps required for Axis II diagnoses are generally greater than those for Axis I diagnoses. The consequences are lower levels of diagnostic agreement, lower levels of stability over time, and higher comorbidities. The descriptions and conceptualizations of PDs in the DSM have been evolving and improving, but many challenges remain (see the review by Coolidge & Segal, 1998). The DSM was designed as a descriptive, heuristic, filing system for psychiatric diagnoses (Clark et al., 1997), and it is likely to become more scientifically based with time. Researchers may easily find faults with the DSM, but it is also true that the deliberations of DSM committees would be facilitated and their conceptualizations of disorders would be enhanced if the data from researchers were more clear and informative. Descriptions of PDs can also be found in the International Statistical Classification of Diseases-10. There are many similarities and some differences between the DSM-IV and the ICD-10 with regard to PDs and many of the same diagnostic problems.

One final diagnostic peculiarity should be mentioned at this point. Normal personality trait language is used to describe PDs in the DSM-IV. Personality pathology is apparently a matter of extremeness on commonly found trait dimensions. However, a categorical system is used in diagnosis. This model of qualitatively distinct clinical syndromes is seriously challenged by the extensive comorbidity evidence and by the heterogeneity of PD phenomena (Clark et al., 1997). There are also no signs of sharp demarcations between individuals with and without PDs in their scores on personality trait dimensions (Clark et al., 1997; Livesley et al., 1994). A dimensional model of PDs is likely to appear in the DSM some day, but only if and when personality psychologists themselves agree on the basic dimensions of personality (APA, 1994; Frances, 1993).

TABLE 3. Differential Diagnosis[a]

PD	Differentiate from	Differentiate by
Paranoid	Schizophrenia	Delusions less psychotic and bizarre; absence of hallucinations
	Schizotypal PD	Absence of cognitive and perceptual distortions; less eccentric behavior
	Antisocial PD	No long history of social deviance or motivation to exploit others
	Borderline PD	Is not self-destructive; fewer intense relationships
Schizoid	Paranoid PD	Fewer social contacts and interactions; less paranoia and verbal aggression
	Schizotypal PD	Absence of social anxiety; cognitive-perceptual distortions; and eccentricities
	Avoidant PD	Weak desire to intimate relationships; indifference to others
	Obs.-comp. PD	Lacks underlying capacity for intimacy
Schizotypal	Schizophrenia	No enduring overt psychosis; less deterioration in functioning
	Borderline PD	Cognitive-perceptual distortions more enduring; weak desire for relationships; less impulsive and manipulative
	Avoidant PD	Cognitive-perceptual distortions and eccentricities; weak desire for relationships
Antisocial	Borderline PD	More distant relationships; no desire for nurturance or fears of abandonment; less depression and self-destructiveness; early history of conduct disorder
	Histrionic PD	More calculated aggression and exploitation; less emotional dependence on others; less exaggerated emotions; early history of conduct disorder
	Narcissistic PD	Less need for admiration; more reckless and impulsive; concern with material gains, not superiority; early history of conduct disorder
Borderline	Mood disorders	Moods shift in response to interpersonal events; anger and deliberate self-destructiveness
	Posttraumatic stress	Early and chronic seeking of nurturance and fears of exploitation
	Narcissistic PD	Feels bad or evil; more impulsivity and instability in identity and emotions
	Histrionic PD	Self-destructiveness; chronic emptiness; feels evil or bad; enduring feelings of mistreatment
	Dependent PD	Reacts to feelings of emptiness and abandonment with rage and demands; unstable relationships
Histrionic	Dependent PD	More flamboyant, emotional, and uninhibited; less docile
	Narcissistic PD	Willing to be perceived as weak or dependent; greater warmth; more emotional outbursts; more juvenile, flirtatious, and melodramatic attention-seeking
Narcissistic	Obs.-comp. PD	Less guilt and rigid conscientiousness; more exhibitionism; less self-criticism
Avoidant	Social phobia	More pervasive difficulties relating to others and with intimacy; greater social skill deficits and interpersonal sensitivities; early onset
	Dependent PD	Fear of others, of closeness, and of rejection; cautious in forming new relationships; less emotionally expressive and demanding; social anxiety and mistrust; social withdrawal
Obs.-comp.	Obs.-comp. disorder	Absence of repetitive intrusive thoughts and ritualistic behaviors; egosyntonic

[a]Sources: APA (1994); Gunderson & Phillips (1995); Perry & Valliant (1989); Widiger & Sanderson (1997).

Some clinicians (e.g., Butcher & Rouse, 1996) doubt that models of normal personality characteristics are sufficiently comprehensive to incorporate clinical phenomena such as PDs. However, recent findings by O'Connor and Dyce (1998) indicate that the five-factor model of general personality traits (Costa & Widiger, in press) might be adequate for this purpose. O'Connor and Dyce (1998) first conducted a joint analysis of scores on PD scales and scores on the five factors (neuroticism, extraversion, openness of experience, agreeableness, and conscientiousness) in a large sample of university students. Factor analyses revealed that the dimensions in the PD scores were well defined by the five "normal" factors in this nonclinical sample. Then, data from 14 previously published large-scale studies of PDs using clinical samples were reanalyzed in relation to the university student data. These analyses revealed that the PD configurations in the clinical data were well captured by the five-factor model and were highly congruent with the PD configuration in the student data. Further, competing models of PD configuration, which were often based on clinical speculation, provided lower levels of fit to the PD data than the five-factor model. These findings imply that the same personality dimensions underlie scores on PDs in both clinical and nonclinical populations and that the dimensions are those from the familiar five-factor model. Normal and abnormal personalities (and normal and abnormal personality characteristics) exist in the same universe of basic psychological dimensions. The differences between clinical and nonclinical populations are matters of extremity and degree, at least in the case of PDs.

Summary

There are ten heterogeneous, categorical PDs in the DSM-IV. PDs are maladaptive, extreme, rigid, pervasive, and chronic manifestations of otherwise normal and common personality characteristics. Individuals who have PDs often value their peculiarities and lack insight into the way their social and occupational difficulties are self-generated. PDs occur in 10 to 13% of the general population and in 50 to 67% of individuals who receive treatment for psychological difficulties. PDs must be evident by adolescence or young adulthood to make a diagnosis, but developmental trends may be obvious before then. PDs also last long and are resistant to change, although psychotherapeutic and pharmacological treatments are becoming more specialized. PDs, it is believed, complicate the courses of Axis I disorders and are associated with a variety of costly personal and social consequences. Behavioral genetic research on PDs and normal personality traits, although sometimes sparse, consistently provides evidence for both genetic and specific environmental influences. There is a widespread assumption that early experiences leave enduring marks on individuals who subsequently develop PDs. Speculations about significant early family experiences are common, varied, and often untested. The diagnostic challenges faced by clinicians are considerable because PDs are complex and the criteria are sometimes vague. PD assessment instruments do not show high levels of diagnostic agreement, the stabilities for diagnoses of supposedly enduring traits are too low, and comorbidities with Axis I disorders and other PDs are often very high. A swell of research interest in PDs has developed during the past 15 years, which bodes well for the knowledge base of an important but previously neglected psychiatric phenomenon.

References

Abrams, R. C. & Horowitz, S. V. (1996). Personality disorders after age 50: A meta-analysis. *Journal of Personality Disorders, 10,* 271–281.

American Psychiatric Association. (1980). *Diagnostic and statistical manual of mental disorders,* 3rd ed. Washington, DC: Author.

American Psychiatric Association. (1987). *Diagnostic and statistical manual of mental disorders,* 3rd ed., rev. Washington, DC: Author.

American Psychiatric Association. (1994). *Diagnostic and statistical manual of mental disorders,* 4th ed. Washington, DC: Author.

Beck, A. T., & Freeman, A. (1990). *Cognitive therapy of personality disorders.* New York: Guilford.

Bernstein, D. P., Useda, D., & Siever, L. J. (1995). Paranoid personality disorder. In W. J. Livesley (Ed.), *The DSM-IV personality disorders* (pp. 45–57). New York: Guilford.

Black, D. W., & Noyes, R. (1997). Obsessive–compulsive disorder and Axis II. *International Review of Psychiatry, 9,* 111–118.

Bornstein, R. F. (1993). *The dependent personality.* New York: Guilford.

Bouchard, T. J. (1997). The genetics of personality. In K. Blum, E. P. Noble, R. S. Sparkes, T. H. J. Chen, & J. G. Cull (Eds.), *Handbook of psychiatric genetics* (pp. 273–296). Boca Raton, FL: CRC Press.

Butcher, J. N., & Rouse, S. V. (1996). Personality: Individual differences and clinical assessment. *Annual Review of Psychology, 47,* 87–111.

Clark, L. A., Livesley, W. J., & Morey, L. (1997). Personality disorder assessment: The challenge of construct validity. *Journal of Personality Disorders, 11,* 205–231.

Clarkin, J. F., Yeomans, F. E., & Kernberg, O. F. (1999). *Psychotherapy for borderline personality.* New York: Wiley.

Coolidge, F. L., & Segal, D. L. (1998). Evolution of personality disorder diagnosis in the diagnostic and statistical manual of mental disorders. *Clinical Psychology Review, 18,* 585–599.

Costa, P. T., & Widiger, T. A. (in press). *Personality disorders and the five-factor model of personality,* 2nd ed. Washington, DC: American Psychological Association.

Dahl, A. A. (1993). The personality disorders: A critical review of family, twin, and adoption studies. *Journal of Personality Disorders, 7,* 86–99.

Dolan, B., Evans, C., & Norton, K. (1995). Multiple Axis-II diagnoses of personality disorder. *British Journal of Psychiatry, 166,* 107–112.

Dowson, J. H., & Grounds, A. T. (1995). *Personality disorders: Recognition and clinical management.* New York: Cambridge University Press.

Frances, A. (1982). Categorical and dimensional systems of personality diagnosis: A comparison. *Comprehensive Psychiatry, 23,* 516–527.

Frances, A. (1993). Dimensional diagnosis of personality: Not whether, but when and which. *Psychological Inquiry, 4,* 110–111.

Gunderson, J. G., & Phillips, K. A. (1995). Personality disorders. In H. I. Kaplan & B. J. Sadock (Eds.), *Comprehensive textbook of psychiatry,* 6th ed. (pp. 1425–1461). Baltimore: Williams and Wilkins.

Hyler, S. E. (1988). DSM-III at the cinema: Madness in the movies. *Comprehensive Psychiatry, 29,* 195–206.

Kapfhammer, H. P., & Hippius, H. (1998). Pharmacotherapy in personality disorders. *Journal of Personality Disorders, 12,* 277–288.

Links, P. S., Heslegrave, R., Villella, J. (1998). Psychopharmacological management of personality disorders: An outcome-focused model. In K. R. Silk (Ed.), *Biology of personality disorders* (pp. 93–127). Washington, DC: American Psychiatric Press.

Livesley, W. J. (1995). *The DSM-IV personality disorders.* New York: Guilford.

Livesley, W. J., Schroeder, M. L., Jackson, D. N., & Jang, K. L. (1994). Categorical distinctions in the study of personality disorder: Implications for classification. *Journal of Abnormal Psychology, 103,* 6–17.

Livesley, W. J., Schroeder, M. L., Lang, K. L., Jackson, D. N., & Vernon, P. A. (1993). Genetic and environmental contributions to dimensions of personality disorder. *American Journal of Psychiatry, 150,* 1826–1831.

McDavid, J. D., & Pilkonis, P. A. (1996). The stability of personality disorder diagnoses. *Journal of Personality Disorders, 10,* 1–15.

Morey, L. C. (1988). Personality disorders in DSM-III and DSM-III-R: Convergence, coverage, and internal consistency. *American Journal of Psychiatry, 145,* 573–577.

Nigg, J. T., & Goldsmith, H. H. (1994). Genetics of personality disorders: Perspectives from personality and psychopathology research. *Psychological Bulletin, 115,* 346–380.

O'Connor, B. P., & Dyce, J. A. (1998). A test of models of personality disorder configuration. *Journal of Abnormal Psychology, 107,* 3–16.

Paris, J. (1998a). Personality disorders in sociocultural perspective. *Journal of Personality Disorders, 12,* 289–301.

Paris, J. (1998b). Anxious traits, anxious attachment, and anxious-cluster personality disorders. *Harvard Review of Psychiatry, 6,* 142–148.

Perry, J. C. (1992). Problems and considerations in the valid assessment of personality disorders. *American Journal of Psychiatry, 149,* 1645–1653.

Perry, J. C. (1993). Longitudinal studies of personality disorders. *Journal of Personality Disorders, 7,* 63–85.

Perry, J. C., & Valliant, G. E. (1989). Personality disorders. In H. I. Kaplan & B. J. Sadock (Eds.), *Comprehensive textbook of psychiatry,* 5th ed. (pp. 1352–1395). Baltimore: Williams and Wilkins.

Reich, J. H., & Vasile, R. G. (1993). Effect of personality disorders on the treatment outcome of Axis I conditions: An update. *Journal of Nervous and Mental Disease, 181,* 475–484.

Robins, L. N., & Regier, D. (1991). *Psychiatric disorders in America: The Epidemiologic Catchment Area study.* New York: Free Press.

Segal, D. L., Hersen, M., Van Hasselt, V. B., Silberman, C., & Roth, L. (1996). Diagnosis and assessment of personality disorders in older adults: A critical review. *Journal of Personality Disorders, 10,* 384–399.

Siever, L. J., Bernstein, D. P., & Silverman, J. M. (1995). Schizotypal personality disorder. In W. J. Livesley (Ed.), *The DSM-IV personality disorders* (pp. 71–90). New York: Guilford.

Siever, L. J., & Davis, K. L. (1991). A psycho-biological perspective on the personality disorders. *American Journal of Psychiatry, 148,* 1647–1658.

Silk, K. R. (1998). *Biology of personality disorders.* Washington, DC: American Psychiatric Press.

Sperry, L. (1995). *Handbook of diagnosis and treatment of the DSM-IV personality disorders.* New York: Brunner/ Mazel.

Stone, M. H. (1993). *Abnormalities of personality: Within and beyond the realm of treatment.* New York: W. W. Norton.

Stone, M. H. (1993b). Long-term outcome in personality disorders. *British Journal of Psychiatry, 162,* 299–313.

Strupp, H. H., Horowitz, L. M., & Lambert, M. J. (1997). *Measuring patient changes in mood, anxiety, and personality disorders: Toward a core battery.* Washington, DC: American Psychological Association.

Stuart, S., Pfohl, B., Battaglia, M., Bellodi, L., Grove, W., & Cadoret, R. (1998). The co-occurrence of DSM-III-R personality disorders. *Journal of Personality Disorders, 12,* 302–315.

Sutker, P. B., & Adams, H. E. (1993). *Comprehensive handbook of psychiatry.* New York: Plenum.

Sutker, P. B., Bugg, F., & West, J. A. (1993). Antisocial personality disorder. In P. B. Sutker & H. E. Adams (Eds.), *Comprehensive handbook of psychiatry* (pp. 337–369). New York: Plenum.

Tang, S., & Huang, Y. (1995). Diagnosing personality disorders in China. *International Medical Journal, 2,* 291–297.

Tavris, C. (1992). *The mismeasure of woman.* New York: Simon & Schuster.

Tyrer, P., Gunderson, J., Lyons, M., & Tohen, M. (1997). Extent of comorbidity between mental state and personality disorders. *Journal of Personality Disorders, 11,* 242–259.

Van Velzen, C. J. M., & Emmelkamp, P. M. G. (1996). The assessment of personality disorders: Implications for cognitive and behavior therapy. *Behavior Research and Therapy, 34,* 655–668.

Weissman, M. M. (1993). The epidemiology of personality disorders: A 1990 update. *Journal of Personality Disorders, 7,* 44–62.

Widiger, T. A. (1998). Sex biases in the diagnosis of personality disorders. *Journal of Personality Disorders, 12,* 95–118.

Widiger, T. A., & Corbitt, E. M. (1995). Antisocial personality disorder. In W. J. Livesley (Ed.), *The DSM-IV personality disorders* (pp. 103–126). New York: Guilford.

Widiger, T. A., & Sanderson, C. J. (1995). Assessing personality disorders. In J. N. Butcher (Ed.), *Clinical personality assessment* (pp. 380–394). New York: Oxford University Press.

Widiger, T. A., & Sanderson, C. J. (1997). Personality disorders. In A. Tasman, J. Kay, & J. A. Lieberman (Eds.), *Psychiatry,* Vol. 2 (pp. 1291–1317). Philadelphia: W.B. Saunders.

Widiger, T. A., & Trull, T. J. (1993). Borderline and narcissistic personality disorders. In P. B. Sutker & H. E. Adams (Eds.), *Comprehensive handbook of psychiatry* (pp. 371–394). New York: Plenum.

Zimmerman, M. (1994). Diagnosing personality disorders: A review of issues and research methods. *Archives of General Psychiatry, 51,* 225–245.

Zimmerman, M., & Coryell, W. (1989). DSM-III personality disorder diagnoses in a nonpatient sample. *Archives of General Psychiatry, 46,* 682–689.

20

Individual Factors Influencing Medical Conditions

KRISTINE L. BRADY AND PATRICIA L. FIERO

INTRODUCTION

This chapter is concerned with actual medical conditions that are significantly influenced by psychological, behavioral, and/or environmental factors. Psychological factors that contribute to medical conditions include personality variables such as negative stress appraisal styles or excessive worrying. Contributing maladaptive behaviors or coping strategies can include smoking, overeating, or working excessively. Environmental factors (e.g., job stress and divorce) are typically unrelated to individuals, yet can interact with their physiology, behaviors, and personality type. Medical conditions that are mediated by individual and environmental factors include (but are not limited to) cardiovascular disorders, gastritis, headache, insomnia, irritable bowel syndrome, asthma, cancer, diabetes, and skin problems. Unlike somatoform disorders for which no physical cause can be detected, these disorders present themselves *as real medical problems* which have been caused or exacerbated by individual and environmental factors.

When people engage in health-compromising behaviors (e.g., poor diet and smoking), they are more likely to develop medical diseases (Bernard & Krupat, 1994). For example, stress and anxiety can bring on bouts of dermatological conditions such as eczema and psoriasis (Gupta, Gupta, Kirkby, Schork, Corr, Ellis, & Voorhees, 1989). Researchers do not necessarily agree on the direction of causality or the degree of influence that individual factors can have on medical conditions, and there is no consensus on the actual cause of some disorders (e.g., headaches and ulcers). Nevertheless, there is strong empirical support for the position that many medical problems are mediated and/or exacerbated by stress and psychological responses to stress. The authors of this chapter embrace a transactional perspective (see Eysenck, 1991; Lazarus & Folkman, 1984) in which medical conditions are the product of interactions among physiology, psychology, behavior, and environment.

KRISTINE L. BRADY • California School of Professional Psychology, San Diego, California 92121.   PATRICIA L. FIERO • Medical University of South Carolina, Charleston, South Carolina 29425-0742.

Advanced Abnormal Psychology, Second Edition, edited by Hersen and Van Hasselt. Kluwer Academic/Plenum Publishers, New York, 2001.

Psychophysiological disorders is the term that was previously used in the *Diagnostic and Statistical Manual of Mental Disorders*, 2nd ed. (DSM-II; American Psychiatric Association, 1968) to describe the interaction between psychological and physiological components that result in medical conditions. In the DSM-II, the definition of these disorders was "physical symptoms that are caused by emotional factors and involve a single organ system, usually under autonomic nervous system innervation" (p. 46). However, in subsequent versions of the DSM (American Psychiatric Association, 1980, 1987, 1994), the diagnosis "Psychophysiologic Disorder" was replaced with "Psychological Factors Affecting Physical Condition." According to the American Psychiatric Association (1994), psychological, behavioral, and environmental factors can contribute to the development, maintenance, and/or exacerbation of a patient's medical condition. They can also interfere with a patient's medical treatment or recovery from illness. When a psychological or behavioral factor significantly affects a medical condition, it should be included in the diagnosis and should be a focus of clinical attention. In the DSM-IV, psychological or behavioral factors that negatively affect a medical condition are coded on Axis I whereas the medical condition itself is coded on Axis III. For an example of a multi-axial diagnosis, see Table 1. These disorders are also referred to as "stress-related illnesses" or "psychophysiological disorders."

Health psychology is a field that is dedicated to promoting and maintaining heath, preventing illness, and providing psychological interventions to assist in treating medical conditions. Health psychology has been strongly influenced by the **biopsychosocial model** of illness, which proposes that medical conditions cannot be diagnosed or treated without taking into account the persons and their environmental contexts. Many of the interventions described in this chapter are based on research conducted by health psychologists. As we describe various medical conditions, we will focus on the psychological and behavioral factors that contribute to them because they are most amenable to change. The following disorders are prevalent in the general population and are the focus of this chapter: cardiovascular disorders, headache, diabetes, and insomnia. However, these represent just a portion of the medical disorders influenced by individual factors that are amenable to change via psychological intervention.

CARDIOVASCULAR DISORDERS

Description

A healthy cardiovascular system is one in which the heart pumps regularly, and the linings of the blood vessels and arteries are smooth and free of blockage. Such smooth lining allows blood to move freely throughout the body and to deliver oxygen to the brain and major

TABLE 1. Example of a DSM-IV Diagnosis
of a Psychological Factor that Affects a Medical Condition

Axis I	Maladaptive health behaviors affecting gastritis including alcohol use and poor diet
Axis II	None
Axis III	Gastritis
Axis IV	Moderate (marital separation and trouble with co-workers)
Axis V	70, mild symptoms including transient insomnia and depressed mood

organs. Individuals who experience significant problems with their cardiovascular system can be diagnosed with one or more **cardiovascular disorders (CVD)**. **Hypertension**, or high blood pressure, refers to a condition in which individuals repeatedly display blood pressure readings outside of the normal range (e.g., higher than 140/90). Hypertension, among other factors, can lead to three additional problems involving the heart and arteries: congestive heart failure, atherosclerosis, and arteriosclerosis. **Congestive heart failure (CHF)** is a disorder diagnosed when the heart does not pump efficiently. This results in decreased blood flow to the body and can negatively affect the kidneys, lungs, and ventricles of the heart. Hypertension contributes to this disorder by placing increased demands on the already weakened heart. Seventy-five percent of CHF cases also have a diagnosis of hypertension (Clayman, 1994). **Atherosclerosis** occurs when cholesterol, fat, and calcium deposit along the inner surfaces of the coronary arteries, resulting in decreased blood flow to the heart. These deposits are called an **atheroma** or **plaque**. Atherosclerosis typically results in arteriosclerosis, or hardening of the arteries. In this condition, coronary arteries become narrow and thick and decrease the blood flow to and from the heart. Hypertension also exacerbates these two arterial conditions by damaging the lining of the arteries because of increased force and pressure against the lining. **Coronary heart disease (CHD)** is the most common CVD which is diagnosed when one's heart does not receive enough oxygen due to atherosclerosis and/or arteriosclerosis. When arteriosclerosis and atherosclerosis become extreme, a **thrombus** or blood clot can develop. Partial coronary blood clots can also cause **angina pectoris**, which is the experience of pressing pain that occurs in the chest and into the left shoulder and arm. This pain is caused by a lack of oxygen in the muscular wall of the heart which occurs when the coronary arteries are partially blocked. When one or more coronary arteries become fully blocked, a **myocardial infarction**, or heart attack, occurs. This blockage prevents oxygen from reaching the heart which damages or kills its tissue. Blood clots in the arterial walls can also cause a heart attack or result in a **stroke**, which occurs when the clot moves to the brain and causes a cerebrovascular accident. Hypertension can also increase the likelihood that one can have a stroke by contributing to plaque formation in the arteries and by possibly moving the plaque formations throughout the cardiovascular system and into the brain.

INDIVIDUAL AND ENVIRONMENTAL FACTORS AFFECTING CARDIOVASCULAR DISORDERS

Several factors are strong contributors to cardiovascular disorders. Psychological factors that contribute to these conditions include Type D personality (high emotional distress + emotional and social inhibition; Denollet, 1997), hostility and anger (also associated with Type A personality; Barefoot, Dahlstrom, & Williams, 1983), emotional distress (Denollet, 1997; Kulkarni, O'Farrell, Erasi, & Kochar, 1998), appraising situations as stressful (Lazarus & Folkman, 1984; Segerstrom, Taylor, Kemeny, & Fahey, 1998), pessimism (Räikkönen, Matthews, Flory, Owens, & Gump, 1999; Segerstrom, Taylor, Kemeny, & Fahey, 1998), depression and anxiety (Booth-Kewley & Friedman, 1987), and strong adherence to the masculine gender role (Eisler, Skidmore, & Ward, 1988; Helgeson, 1990). Behavioral contributors include diet (e.g., high percentage of salt and fat), lack of aerobic exercise, smoking, alcohol use, and poor treatment compliance. Environmental factors can include major life stressors, chronic job stress (Kulkarni, O'Farrell, Erasi, & Kochar, 1998), financial problems, poverty, racism (Kulkarni, O'Farrell, Erasi, & Kochar, 1998), trauma, having a sedentary job, working long hours with low job decision latitude (Sorenson, Lewis, & Bishop, 1996), and lack of social support (Kamarck, Annunziato, & Amateau, 1995; Roy, Kirschbaum, & Steptoe, 1998). See Figure 1 for a graphical representation of the relationships among these factors and CVD.

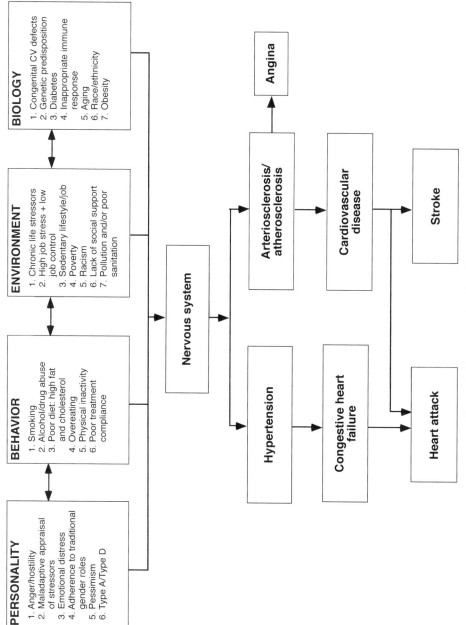

FIGURE 1. The progression of cardiovascular disorders and the role of risk factors.

Epidemiology

Equal numbers of men and women (20%) in this country have been diagnosed with one or more cardiovascular diseases.[1] The combined CVDs are the number one killer of both men and women and account for 41.1% of all deaths in the United States. Before the age of 60, men are more likely to develop serious CVD than women (approximately 33% and 10%, respectively). Yet contrary to popular belief, since 1984 more women have died from CVD than men. For example, in 1996, 47.3% of male deaths were from CVD compared to 52.7% of female deaths. This is likely to be due to the fact that women outlive men by an average of 7 years, giving them more time for the CVD to progress.

Approximately 7% of the general population has CHD. Whites lead at 7.5%, followed by African-Americans at 6.9%, and Mexican-Americans at 5.6%. CHD also accounts for the largest number of CVD deaths, which typically result from fatal heart attacks, and is the primary killer of men and women in the United States. Hypertension is also a significant problem in our society and can lead to many fatal conditions. Twenty-five percent of adults meet the criteria for hypertension, yet more than 30% are not aware that they have it. African-Americans are more likely to develop high blood pressure at an earlier age than Whites and are more likely to suffer from CHD and/or strokes. Hypertension rates are also higher for African-Americans (men 35%; women 34.2%) compared to Native Americans (men 26.8%; women 27.5%), Caucasians (men 24.4%; women 19.3%), and Mexican-Americans (men 25.2%; women 22%). Approximately 1.7% of the population will develop congestive heart failure (CHF), most of whom also have hypertension. Women are more likely to die from CHF than men which is probably due to their longer life span. CHF occurs in similar rates across various racial and ethnic groups.

Clinical Picture

Unfortunately, many of the CVDs do not result in noticeable symptoms and individuals can go on for years without recognizing that they have serious medical conditions. For example, there are no symptoms that occur in hypertension until the disorder has resulted in significant damage to the body (e.g., retinal or kidney damage; Clayman, 1994). CHD can also develop without the knowledge of the patient, and angina pectoris occurs *after* CHD has progressed to a significant level. Therefore, early detection is key, and individuals are encouraged to have their cholesterol and blood pressure readings checked regularly.

Because heart rate and blood pressure are very reactive to external events and stressors, psychologists play an important role in preventing and treating cardiovascular diseases. Behavioral interventions that are particularly promising include stress management, anger management, dietary changes, exercise, and smoking cessation. Relaxation therapy is an effective way to reduce stress level when used regularly (e.g., two 15-minute sessions per day) and can take on many forms such as progressive muscle relaxation, cognitive imagery, meditation, yoga, or even Tai Chi. Regular relaxation reduces psychological tension and anxiety, and it also decreases blood pressure and heart rate (Davison, Williams, Nezami, Bice, & DeQuattro, 1991). Biofeedback also works well to decrease stress and cardiovascular reactivity (Blanchard, 1990; Lee, Kimura, DeQuattro, & Davison, 1989; Patel & Marmot, 1988). However, the best results occur when biofeedback is combined with relaxation training (Hahn, Ro, Song, Kim, Kim, & Yoo, 1993; Aivazyan, Zaitsev, Salenko, Yurenev, & Patrusheva, 1988). For example, long-term effects have been found using biofeedback-based

---

[1]The statistics presented in this section are based on data from the American Heart Association (1999) unless otherwise noted.

relaxation training for up to 3 years for many hypertensive patients (McGrady, Nadsady, & Schumann-Brzezinski, 1991). Anger management and cognitive restructuring can also be used to reduce hostility, anger, and hypertension (Lee, DeQuattro, Allen, Kimura, Aleman, Konugres, & Davison, 1988; Gidron & Davidson, 1996). This may be a particularly relevant avenue to pursue in anger-prone patients because of the strong link between anger, hostility, and CHD.

Case Illustration

Ms. C was a 51-year-old, divorced, African-American woman who lived at home with her 25-year-old son. She worked two full-time jobs as a nurse's assistant and was referred to a behavior therapist for treatment of anxiety and hypertension. She characterized her life as extremely hectic and reported having little time to take care of herself or visit friends and family. Ms. C was diagnosed with borderline diabetes, was on estrogen for menopause, and recently had knee surgery following a work injury. Ms. C presented with many physical and psychological complaints, including weight gain (20 pound increase), nausea, insomnia (trouble falling asleep and early morning awakening), headaches, and lack of assertiveness. She often coped with her stress and daytime fatigue by smoking cigarettes, drinking caffeinated beverages, watching TV, and eating high-fat food. Because Ms. C presented with nearly every risk factor for CHD (hypertension, smoking, low physical activity, overweight, high stress level, poor diet, low social support, and diabetes), a treatment plan was developed that focused on maintaining a healthy diet, increasing physical activity, and using relaxation techniques regularly. All three of these interventions also work well for headaches, insomnia, and anxiety.

Ms. C was seen for a total of seven sessions which she attended every other week. She was very motivated to change her behavior and was compliant with homework assignments. To increase her personal investment in behavioral change and to ensure her participation, she was asked to make a list of the pro's and con's for eating right and exercising which she completed easily in collaboration with her therapist. Examples of her pro-change statements included "better health, more energy, and being happier." Con's for change included "missing fried foods and peer pressure for smoking." After Ms. C demonstrated commitment to behavioral change, treatment began. Self-monitoring and antecedent control procedures (ACP; changing the environment) were used to increase physical activity and maintain her physician-prescribed diabetic meal plan (1500 calories/day). Ms. C monitored her behavior by recording her weight, blood sugar, and food intake daily. ACP involve structuring the environment to maximize the likelihood that positive behaviors will occur while decreasing the likelihood of negative behaviors. Examples of Ms. C's ACP include (1) making healthy meals ahead of time so less work was required when she was tired, (2) developing a scheduled routine for eating and sleeping, (3) removing unhealthy food and leaving healthy foods in sight, (4) leaving an 8-minute exercise tape in the VCR, and (5) finding a "buddy" to walk with, so exercise was more enjoyable. Ms. C often watched TV to relax, while eating, which contributed to her presenting problems. Therefore, she was encouraged to stop turning on the TV after coming home from work and to substitute this with a 20-minute nap. After Ms. C was able to successfully implement the ACP, progressive muscle relaxation was taught to the client in session and was effective in reducing her blood pressure and self-reported anxiety level. She was then given a relaxation tape to use at home and reported engaging in this activity several times a day. Because she responded so well to relaxation training, meditation was also used to stop anxiety-provoking thoughts. She also used a mantra to block worrying thoughts which worked well when she was at work and unable to use her relaxation tape. Ms. C was also a devout Christian, and the therapist incorporated this strength into her treatment. In addition to relaxation training, Ms. C was encouraged to pray silently when she found her anxiety level rising. Finally, she was referred to a vocational training program to help her obtain a less stressful and more rewarding job. At the end of treatment, Ms. C's blood pressure measured

138/60 compared to her pretreatment blood pressure of 170/90, suggesting that treatment was effective for reducing hypertension. Ms. C was able to stick to her 1500-calorie diet and to increase her physical activity somewhat, yet did not lose weight. Her insomnia and cognitive appraisal of stress significantly decreased. Finally, relaxation training and meditation were very effective for headaches, which disappeared after two sessions. Because she was more relaxed, she also decreased the number of cigarettes that she was smoking.

Course and Prognosis

The prognosis for CVD is poor if an individual does not seek treatment and/or make lifelong behavioral changes. For example, in hypertensives, blood pressure will continue to increase as the individual ages. Potential outcomes of untreated hypertension include retinal damage, stroke, heart attack, kidney damage, and/or decreased life-expectancy. According to the American Heart Association (1999), there are five predominant risk factors that contribute to CVD: smoking, high cholesterol, overweight/obesity, physical inactivity, and diabetes mellitus. These factors strongly influence the course and prognosis of CVD.

Smoking cigarettes is a significant predictor of CVD, accounts for 20% of CVD diagnoses, and increases the risk of heart attack and stroke. Women are particularly at risk for CVD if they both smoke and take birth control pills and are two to three times more likely to have high blood pressure if they have been on birth control pills for five or more years. Furthermore, there is evidence that women may have a stronger cardiovascular response to cigarette smoke than men (Stone, Dembroski, Costa, & MacDougall, 1990), further increasing their risk for CVD. Nearly 52% of our population is considered borderline–high in their cholesterol levels (200–239 mg/dL) and 20% have high cholesterol ($\geq$ 240 mg/dL). Because high cholesterol is more common in women than in men, their risk for CVD is further increased. In the United States, individuals are considered overweight if their body mass index (BMI) is 25–29% above the standard BMI range. When this percentage reaches 30% or more, obesity is diagnosed. The prevalence of individuals who are overweight in our country varies between 45.5 and 67.6%, and those who are obese range between 20 and 37.4%. Physical inactivity is especially common in overweight/obese adults and children. Twenty-five percent of adults in this county do not engage in any type of physical activity that increases their heart rate, and only 15% of adults engage in significant physical activity that promotes health and reduces the risk of illness (regular vigorous activity, three times a week, for at least 20 minutes). Finally, those diagnosed with diabetes mellitus are particularly at risk for CVD. Sixty-six percent of individuals who suffer from diabetes will die as a result of a failed cardiovascular system (American Heart Association, 1999).

Many of these risk factors result from maladaptive behaviors that can be reduced or alleviated by appropriate intervention. Smoking cessation and weight-reduction programs that include dietary change are especially beneficial to individuals diagnosed with (or at risk of) CVD. Helping individuals to quit smoking greatly reduces their risk of having heart attacks or strokes. For those exhibiting poor diet and lack of exercise, changing these behaviors significantly decreases atherosclerosis, hypertension, and cholesterol level, thus decreasing the risk for CHD, heart attack, and stroke. Finally, for those with diabetes, promoting medical treatment compliance (e.g., insulin shots), physical activity, and healthy eating are essential for decreasing the risk of CVD (American Heart Association, 1999).

Familial and Genetic Patterns

As reported earlier, there are many race and sex differences across CVDs. However, it is unclear whether these are due to genetic factors or environmental factors (e.g., poverty).

Several cardiovascular disorders are congenital and tend to run in families. Also, several of the contributing risk factors for CVD do have substantial genetic links including obesity, diabetes, and hypertension. Therefore, individuals who have these specific risk factors and/or family members with CVD should be especially vigilant in monitoring their blood pressure and cholesterol levels.

Diagnostic Considerations

When diagnosing a client who has psychological factors that affect a medical condition, it is essential to specify as many of the relevant psychological and behavioral components as possible. This is essential because risk factors are cumulative and a multidimensional intervention plan is the best way to reduce the risk of further health complications. It is also important to take into account potential sex differences in the cognitive appraisal of stress because men and women respond differently to various life events (Barnett, Biener, & Baruch, 1987). For example, women may have much stronger emotional responses (thus increasing cardiovascular reactivity) in certain social events (e.g., a funeral) in which they perceive a need to take care of others, be supportive, and display empathy. Similarly, men may experience greater distress than women in situations of financial distress or job loss. While adherence to traditional gender roles varies greatly across individuals, stronger adherence (for both men and women) increases the likelihood that they will experience emotional distress and increased cardiovascular reactivity when threatened in gender-related situations (Lash, Eisler, & Southard, 1995). Because women are more likely to have confidantes and/or social support networks than men (Helgeson, 1990), it is especially important to determine if male clients are lacking this potential buffer of stress. Measuring the degree of social support is another important factor to consider because of the strong relationship between cardiovascular reactivity and support (Roy, Kirschbaum, & Steptoe, 1998). If clients have strong support systems, this can be taken advantage of in therapy by encouraging them to use their friends and families. If the client has little support in place, measures should be taken to increase and facilitate a positive social support network.

A combination of relaxation training and/or biofeedback, increased exercise, and a healthy diet is recommended for all patients who have CVD. However, the type of relaxation therapy should be chosen on the basis of the individual's preference. Relaxation is effective in decreasing blood pressure and heart rate, but it does not necessarily continue to work once the client leaves the therapist's office. Therefore, if relaxation is used, it is essential that steps are taken to maximize generalization by having the client use relaxation at home and in stressful settings regularly (Southam, Agras, Taylor, & Kraemer, 1982). Relaxation training and biofeedback are also excellent alternatives to pharmacological intervention for pregnant women (Little, Hayworth, Benson, Hall, Beard, Dewhurst, & Priest, 1984) or men/women who have severe side effects from antihypertensive drugs.

HEADACHE

Description

Headache is one of the most common symptoms reported to physicians. Primary headaches are the most frequent (90%) and cannot be explained by brain abnormalities, substance abuse, or medical disease. Secondary headaches are infrequent (10%) and have identifiable structural or metabolic causes. The International Headache Society (Headache Classification Committee of the International Headache Society, 1988) developed a headache classification system for primary headaches that is widely accepted among physicians and researchers. The most common types of recurrent headaches fall into three categories: (1) **migraine headaches** or **vascular headaches**, (2) **tension-type headaches** (sometimes called muscle contraction headaches), or (3) **cluster headaches**. Unique symptoms associated with each type of headache are presented in Table 2. All three types of headaches have been documented in children, adolescents, and adults, and it is possible to be diagnosed with more than one type of recurrent headache.

The pain experienced during a headache does not manifest itself in brain tissue but rather in the membranes that cover the brain and its surrounding muscles, nerves, and blood vessels. Two major factors contributing to headaches are (1) facial, neck, and scalp muscle strain resulting in tension headaches and (2) increased cerebral blood flow and blood vessel swelling that result in migraine headaches. The etiology of cluster headaches is not yet known, but the leading theory is that neuronal injury results in secondary vascular changes which result in headache pain (Sandyk, 1992).

INDIVIDUAL AND ENVIRONMENTAL FACTORS AFFECTING HEADACHES

Migraine and cluster headaches are often triggered by the following: lack of food (e.g., fasting or skipping meals); specific foods (e.g., aged cheeses, red wine, MSG, caffeine, and/or nuts); lack of sleep or too much sleep; before, during, or after menstruation in women; certain odors, lights, or noise; and stress (Holroyd & Penzien, 1994). Tension headaches are often precipitated by neuromuscular strain (e.g., working on a computer without breaks), environmental or perceived stress, and muscular tension. Conversely, cluster headaches occur suddenly, often in the middle of the sleep cycle (Ryan & Ryan, 1989). Some factors that may precipitate cluster headaches include histamine, alcohol, and transition from REM to non-REM sleep (Connors, 1995); however, more research is needed in this area. For children, triggers for migraine and tension headaches are similar. They can include school, fatigue, skipped meals, cold weather, family conflict, or exercising when hot (Finley & Jones, 1992).

TABLE 2. Description of the Three Main Types of Headache Disorders

	Tension-type headache	Migraine headache	Cluster headache
Location	Bilateral	Unilateral	Unilateral
Duration	30 minutes to 7 days	4 to 72 hours	15 minutes to 4 hours
Pain intensity	Mild to moderate, pressing/ tightening (non-pulsating), not aggravated by physical activity	Moderate to severe, pulsating, aggravated by physical activity	Severe to excruciating
Other physical symptoms	Tension in neck; tension in upper back; sensitive temples and scalp	Nausea; vomiting; heightened sensitivity to light, sound, and smells	Nasal congestion; conjunctivitis; drooping eye-lid; irritated and/or watery eyes; facial pain; transient insomnia
Interference with activities	May inhibit daily activities	May prohibit daily activities	Prohibits daily activities
Sex differences	More common in women	More common in women	More common in men

Little is known about environmental factors that affect cluster headaches in children which rarely occur in this group.

Epidemiology

One in ten people in the United States meets the IHS criteria for headaches (American Council for Headache Education, 1996). Recurrent headache accounts for a large percentage of adult outpatient medical visits in the United States (Holroyd & Penzien, 1994) and is on the rise (Solomon, Skobleranda, & Gragg, 1993). According to the National Center for Health Statistics (1995), the number one reason that patients visited a neurologist in 1995 was for headache. Further, 10.3% of the diagnoses made that year were migraines.

For adults, tension headaches are the most common, followed by migraines and cluster headaches, respectively. Prevalence rates for each type of headache vary across studies due to different definitions of headaches. However, since the IHS definitions appeared in the literature, more accurate statistics are available. The lifetime prevalence of migraine headache is about 8%, and significantly more women (12.8%) meet the criteria for diagnosis than men (3.6%; Merikangas, Fenton, Cheng, Stolar, & Risch, 1997). It is estimated that 68% of men and 88% of women have had episodes of tension-type headaches at some point in the their lives. However, 1-year prevalence rates of episodic tension headaches are closer to 25% (Schwartz, Stewart, Simon, & Lipton, 1998). Lifetime prevalence for cluster headaches is approximately 1% (American Council for Headache Education, 1996). One consistent finding across studies is that women are more likely to suffer from tension and migraine headaches, and men are more likely to suffer from cluster headaches.

Less research has been conducted on children, and epidemiological findings are limited. However, headaches are common in children and increase in prevalence during adolescence (Gherpelli, Nagae, Souza, Bosse, Rabello, Diament, & Scoff, 1998). Most of the research on childhood headache has focused on pediatric migraine. Prevalence rates for pediatric migraine vary widely across studies and range between 1 and 8% (Chen, 1993; Congdon & Forsythe, 1979; Labbe & Williamson, 1983). Migraine headaches typically begin between ages 6 to 10, yet have been documented in children as young as 2 years of age (Congdon & Forsythe, 1979). Researchers who have explored tension-type headaches in children note that they may be occurring much more than previously thought (Labbe, 1988). According to Labbe (1988), prevalence rates are not available for tension headaches because of methodological problems and lack of parental reporting. Children who experience tension-type headaches or migraine headaches are likely to present with other physical symptoms in addition to headache, including travel sickness, abdominal pain, and bruxism (Aromaa, Sillanpaa, Rautava, & Helenius, 1998). Cluster headaches are extremely rare in children but can occur prior to age 7 (Maytal, Lipton, Solomon, & Shinnar, 1992).

Clinical Picture

Chronic headache presents differently across individuals. Some can continue to carry out their daily activities, albeit in significant pain, whereas others obtain emergency room care for pain relief. Individuals who have migraines and cluster headaches are more likely to experience severe pain compared to tension headache sufferers. Migraine headaches may appear with or without an aura before their onset. An **aura** is a neurological phenomenon in which individuals see spots or flashing lights in their fields of view before headache onset. They may also experience partial blindness or numbness on one side of their head. Auras do not usually cause pain but may be frightening for the person experiencing them. Contrary to popular belief, most migraine sufferers do not experience an aura before headache onset (Russell & Olesen, 1996). The minority of individuals who do experience an aura report that this symptom disappears within 60 minutes (Holroyd & Penzien, 1994).

Case Illustration

Jason was a 16-year-old adolescent male who suffered from recurrent migraines and was brought to a behavioral medicine clinic by his mother. Headache frequency was two to three times a month, and each headache lasted from 4–8 hours. His headaches were often preceded by rigorous physical activity, such as soccer practice after school. He reported the occurrence of a mild aura before headache onset and described his discomfort as severe with a throbbing pain on one side of his head. During his migraines, he experienced nausea and was sensitive to light and auditory stimuli (e.g., music). Interestingly, his headaches increased in frequency when in San Diego, California during visits to his uncle. He reported that the brightness of the sun caused him to squint his eyes, after which he would develop a migraine. It was hypothesized that squinting resulted in high levels of tension in the muscles around his eyes which triggered the migraine. He typically coped with his migraines by going to his room to lie down. Sleep typically alleviated his migraines, yet interfered with his school work and recreational activities. Jason's mother brought him to a behavioral therapist when his coach threatened to take him off the team if he missed any more practices.

After a medical doctor ruled out a neurological disorder, a thorough history was gathered by Jason's therapist. It was determined that EMG biofeedback,[2] in addition to dietary changes, would be used to treat Jason's headaches. He was also encouraged to decrease his caffeine and chocolate intake. Treatment consisted of 1-hour sessions of biofeedback for a total of 8 weeks. Jason responded well to the treatment and reported that the frequency of his migraine headaches decreased from two to three times a month to approximately one every 6 weeks. Jason was able to continue participating on the soccer team and his school performance improved.

Course and Prognosis

Prognosis for children who experience migraines is good, and a large percentage of children outgrow their diagnosis. However, approximately 20% continue to experience headaches into adolescence and adulthood (Congdon & Forsythe, 1979). Prognosis for tension and migraine headaches is poor for adults and children who do not receive intervention or experience significant life changes (e.g., stress level). Medical interventions include drug therapy either to prevent migraine or treat the symptoms of migraine and tension headaches. Fortunately, both tension and migraine headaches respond well to psychological interventions in both children and adults. Three main behavioral interventions are effective for headache sufferers: biofeedback, stress management, and relaxation training (Holroyd & Penzien, 1994).

---

[2]Biofeedback is the process by which clients learn about their internal physiological events through visual and auditory signals that are transmitted from an electronic device that is attached to the body. Clients learn to manipulate these internal events to decrease maladaptive physical responding. EMG biofeedback is a technique whereby surface electrodes (metallic discs placed on the skin) detect the electrical activity ("signal") in the underlying muscle. The signal is transmitted (via wires) to a computer that amplifies the signal and converts it to an auditory and/or visual signal. By seeing or hearing this signal, the patient obtains "feedback" about the underlying muscle activity and through practice can learn to influence it at will. For example, high muscle tension may produce a high pitched tone, whereas a relaxed muscle might produce a low tone.

Sartory, Mueller, Metsch, and Pothmann (1998) compared progressive muscle relaxation with stress management, biofeedback with stress management, and drug therapy in children aged 8–16. They concluded that both psychological treatments outperformed drug therapy by reducing the frequency and intensity of migraine headaches in these two experimental groups. Furthermore, their analgesic intake was reduced, and their mood increased substantially.

Blanchard, Andrasik, Ahles, Teders, and O'Keefe (1980) conducted a meta-analysis on treatment efficacy and concluded that relaxation training and biofeedback work equally well in decreasing the intensity and duration of both migraine and tension headaches. However, the type of biofeedback that is effective depends on the type of headache. They found that temperature biofeedback works best for migraine headaches and EMG biofeedback works best for tension headaches. Interestingly, both behavioral interventions were superior to pharmaceutical interventions. Because tension headaches are brought on by external stressors and neuromuscular tension, stress management is particularly helpful in decreasing their frequency, duration, and intensity. Holroyd and Penzien (1994) recommend using stress management in combination with relaxation therapy for tension-type headache sufferers.

Prognosis for cluster headaches is not quite as promising as for tension and migraine headaches. There are good preemptive and prophylactic treatments for cluster headaches, but without psychopharmacological treatment, headache frequency and intensity typically increase (Pearce, 1993). However, biofeedback is a promising supplement to drug therapy for decreasing the frequency and severity of cluster headaches (Hoelscher & Lichstein, 1983).

Familial and Genetic Patterns

There is strong evidence in the medical literature regarding familial and genetic links to chronic headaches. Vasomotor instability is hypothesized as the physical trait that is passed on genetically in families. For example, Russell, Iselius, Ostergaard, and Olesen (1998) found that 45.9% of their tension-type headache sample ($n = 122$) had first degree relatives who had chronic tension-type headaches. There is also a strong familial/genetic link for migraine headaches (Russell & Olesen, 1995). Interestingly, migraines that occur without an aura have a higher degree of familial patterning (1.9 times the risk) than migraines experienced with an aura (1.4 times the risk). Cluster headaches are also thought to have a genetic basis and are more likely to occur in individuals who have a family history of cluster headaches (Russell, Andersson, & Iselius, 1996).

Diagnostic Considerations

Before making a primary headache diagnosis, a thorough medical examination should be performed. A head-injury history of the patient should also be conducted as well as a neurological exam to rule out known organic causes. A patient who has sudden headache onset, especially after a head injury, should be seen by a qualified physician (Holroyd & Penzien, 1994). Consultation with a medical doctor is crucial because many medical conditions such as meningitis, Lyme disease, poor vision, and brain tumors can cause headache. To make the proper headache diagnosis, specific questions should be asked about headache onset, pain intensity, the presence of aura, and trigger factors (Marks & Rapoport, 1997). It is also important to assess coping strategies and medication use (over-the-counter and prescription). This is critical because rebound headaches occur when an individual overuses medication. Finally, it is important to consider the role that hormonal influences may have on female patients with headache. It is important to assess each girl/woman individually with regard to her own menstrual cycle and the occurrence of headache. Women who are pregnant or breast feeding may also note changes in their headaches (Wall, 1992).

DIABETES MELLITUS

Description

Diabetes mellitus is a metabolic disorder resulting from inadequate production or utilization of insulin. Insulin is a hormone produced by the pancreas that helps the cells in our body absorb glucose. Insulin is released in response to carbohydrate consumption and enables glucose to be stored in muscles where it is later used for fuel. In the healthy individual, the level of glucose in the blood is tightly regulated within a narrow range by a feedback system. In persons who have diabetes, this feedback system results in two dangerous conditions: hyperglycemia and hypoglycemia. **Hyperglycemia** occurs when glucose levels are higher than the normal range. When glucose cannot be utilized for fuel and accumulates in the bloodstream, the body must turn to proteins and fats for fuel. As a consequence, ketone bodies and free fatty acids rise to toxic levels in the blood. Chronic hyperglycemia is associated with numerous and severe complications such as blindness, nerve damage, kidney disease, and coronary heart disease. By contrast, **hypoglycemia** occurs when blood glucose levels fall below the normal range. This happens in diabetic patients who must take insulin to supplement their own body's production. If they fail to achieve the proper balance between insulin and glucose, too much glucose may be stored in the muscles, leaving insufficient quantities in the bloodstream to feed the brain. If untreated, hypoglycemia is acutely dangerous and can result in cognitive impairment and can even lead to coma and death.

Diabetes can be thought of as three, distinct, related but different disorders. The first disorder, **Type I diabetes**, also called insulin-dependent diabetes mellitus or juvenile onset diabetes, begins in childhood. This is a condition in which the body fails to produce insulin or produces very little insulin. As a result, energy is taken from fat because glucose cannot be used. As the fat is burned, harmful chemicals are released into the body which can become life-threatening. Therefore, individuals who have Type I diabetes require insulin treatments to stay alive and must pay special attention to their diets, the timing of exercise, and food intake. **Type II diabetes**, also called insulin-independent diabetes mellitus or adult-onset diabetes, usually begins in middle adulthood. This condition, it is believed, results from a combination of hyperinsulinemia (excessive levels of insulin) in combination with insulin resistance (failure of the body to respond appropriately to the presence of insulin) or from failure of the pancreas to produce adequate levels of insulin. Persons who have Type II diabetes may or may not take insulin as part of their treatment; often their disease can be controlled with other medications or even with diet and exercise alone. **Gestational diabetes mellitus** (GDM) is a third type of diabetes that occurs in a small number of pregnant women when the mother's insulin output becomes less efficient during pregnancy. In response, her baby produces excess insulin which causes it to gain extra weight. If the mother's insulin is not regulated when GDM develops, the following problems can occur: premature delivery, newborn jaundice, difficult labor, newborn respiratory problems, maternal toxemia, and maternal uterine stretching. GDM is a temporary condition that usually abates postdelivery after proper treatment.

As mentioned, numerous complications can result from diabetes, including kidney disease, retinopathy (damage to the retina of the eye that can cause blindness), neuropathy (nerve damage), stroke, nonhealing wounds and lower extremity amputations, and heart disease. All diabetic patients must pay close attention to the timing and content of their diets and their exercise habits. Moreover, all diabetic patients are susceptible to the complications of diabetes. Most diabetic patients monitor their blood glucose levels several times a day by taking a small sample of their blood and testing it in a machine called a glucometer. Keeping blood glucose levels as close as possible within the normal range has been effective in delaying the onset of these complications and decreasing the chances that they develop at all (DCCT, 1993). **Endocrinologists** and **diabetologists** are medical doctors who specialize in treating diabetic people and work closely with them to find a regimen that will keep their blood glucose levels in a healthy range.

INDIVIDUAL AND ENVIRONMENTAL FACTORS THAT AFFECT DIABETES

Psychological and behavioral factors affect diabetes in many ways. Diabetes is a complicated disorder that requires a behaviorally intensive treatment. For example, it is not unusual for a diabetic patient to have to measure blood glucose levels twice per day and to carefully plan the timing and content of meals, exercise, and insulin dosage. In addition, patients may have to adjust their medical and dietary regimens, according to changes in the environment or glucose levels. As discussed later in the chapter, stress and obesity play a role in controlling diabetes. Psychologists are specialists in behavioral change and can help diabetic people control their weight, cope with stress, and adhere to complex medical and dietetic regimens.

Epidemiology

Approximately 16 million Americans suffer from diabetes, but it is estimated that between 30 and 50% of those afflicted are unaware of their conditions (American Diabetes Association, ADA, 1998; National Health Interview Survey, NHIS, 1993). Diabetic people are two to four times more likely to have heart attacks or strokes and have a 15-year lower life-expectancy than those who are not diabetic. Diabetes is the leading cause of nerve damage, kidney failure, adult blindness, and nontraumatic amputations (Juvenile Diabetes Foundation International, JDFI, 1996).

Five to ten percent of diabetic persons suffer from Type I diabetes. Type I diabetes affects 500,000 to one million people in the United States and varies by race. Prevalence rates are higher for Whites than for African-Americans, and African-Americans have higher rates than Hispanics (National Diabetes Data Group, NDDG, 1995). In contrast, the vast majority of diabetic people (90–95%) have Type II diabetes. Type II diabetes affects more than 14 million people, or about 3% of the population. Prevalence increases with age and is slightly more common in women in the United States than in men (NHIS, 1993). Minorities are more prone to Type II diabetes than Whites; for example, Hispanics are twice as likely as Whites to have Type II diabetes and African-Americans are 1.5 times more likely (NDDG, 1995). Finally, 3 to 5% of pregnant women in the United States suffer from gestational diabetes (USDHHS, 1993).

Clinical Picture

The average age of onset for Type I diabetes is 12 years of age, and the symptoms typically appear suddenly. The following are signs of Type I diabetes: frequent urination, extreme hunger and thirst, dramatic weight loss, weakness and fatigue, irritability and mood swings, nausea and vomiting, and sudden vision changes (JDFI, 1996). Because insulin injections are essential in this group, patients must learn to time their dosages carefully in relation to meals. If insulin is given in the absence of a meal, blood sugar levels can drop dangerously low and lead to hypoglycemia. Patients who have Type II diabetes are usually diagnosed in adulthood, typically after the age of 40. Symptoms of Type II diabetes are similar to those of Type I plus any of the following: drowsiness, numbness in feet and hands, itching, and gum or urinary tract infections (JDFI, 1998). Although not all patients who have Type II diabetes take insulin, keeping blood sugar levels in a controlled range is the aim of interventions for both Type I and Type II diabetic patients.

Case Illustration

Mrs. R, a 65-year-old, moderately obese, African-American woman was referred to a clinical psychologist at a medical center by her endocrinologist who had noted that her blood glucose level had been fluctuating increasingly. The doctor also noted that her self-reported levels of stress had increased and she had cried throughout her last visit. Before treatment by a psychologist, her glycosylated hemoglobin[3] levels were well above the target range. Mrs. R was willing to try psychological intervention but was not convinced that it would help.

During the initial visit to the psychologist, Mrs. R reported that indeed she had been faced with many recent stressors: her husband had died three years earlier; two sisters, a brother, and an aunt had died in the previous eight months; and her only son had recently moved out of the area. She also complained of having more difficulty caring for herself while simultaneously expressing a desire to remain independent (she had just begun receiving the services of a home health nurse at the time of her first visit). She suffered from severe retinopathy and had recently undergone an unsuccessful eye operation, leaving her partially blinded in one eye. Diabetic sensory neuropathy had affected her ability to feel sensations, especially in her hands and feet. Motor neuropathy had damaged the nerves innervating the muscles in her feet and she required special shoes for walking. A further complication of diabetes, intermittent claudication (insufficient blood flow in the legs while walking), gave her debilitating pain and she could walk no more than one city block without stopping to rest. This was problematic because she did not drive and her primary modes of transportation had been walking and taking the bus. Several neighbors and friends from church ran errands for her which, while helpful, left her more and more homebound. In addition, the patient suffered from asthma. She was especially distressed about the fact that she could no longer attend church regularly and that she was home alone so often and not able to socialize.

Mrs. R was seen for twenty-two weekly psychotherapy sessions of 50 minutes each during a 7-month period. Treatment initially focused on helping the patient to recognize that stress was adversely affecting her blood glucose levels which in turn was exacerbating her diabetic complications. The patient appeared to attend to these points and stated that it "must be God's will" for her to be seen by a psychologist, but she had trouble believing that stress could influence her condition. However, she agreed to follow the advice of the psychologist. Mrs. R was taught relaxation strategies to help manage her response to stressors. Diaphragmatic breathing was attempted, but Mrs. R had difficulty because of her asthma, and this approach was abandoned. Instead, she was taught to relax by increasing her

---

[3]Glycosylated hemoglobin is a measure of the amount of glucose that is bound to hemoglobin in the blood. Greater levels of hemoglobin bound to glucose indicate higher levels of glucose in the bloodstream during the past 2–3 months.

hand temperature using biofeedback. As Mrs. R learned to increase her hand temperature, she was reducing the activity of her sympathetic nervous system, the part of the central nervous system that responds to stress. Mrs. R. could see tangible results from the biofeedback (bigger temperature increases across sessions) and kept a log of each day that she practiced at home.

Approximately 6 weeks into treatment, Mrs. R had a second eye surgery which was partially successful. She was encouraged by this modest improvement in her eyesight, and her mood appeared brighter as her vision returned. At this point, Mrs. R was urged to talk about her recent losses to engage in the grieving process. This appeared to be helpful, and she reported an improvement in her mood after expressing feelings of anger, hurt, hopelessness, and even anger toward God. Mrs. R was retested for blood glucose control 3 months after therapy began and showed modest improvement. Mrs. R kept a daily "mood diary" detailing stressful events as well as things that made her feel better. Over time, patterns in her moods and her reactions to them were identified. She appeared to feel best when she was able to get out and walk and when she had social interactions. She fared worst when she did not receive calls or visits and when she did not go outside at all during the day. In response to feeling lonely or stressed, Mrs. R had a habit of deviating from her meal plan. She was also observed deviating when she was at social gatherings and "felt like celebrating." Her favorite foods to eat that were not part of her meal plan were fried foods and desserts which she would consume in large portions. Mrs. R was taught cognitive strategies that helped her take a new perspective when stressors occurred. She learned alternative ways to manage her stress that led her to be less vulnerable to violating her meal plan (e.g., calling friends, getting out to walk, and engaging in relaxation exercises or prayer). She also learned to prepare alternative food choices for herself when she knew she would be going to a social gathering where she would be tempted to "celebrate." At the end of 6 months, Mrs. R reported that her mood was significantly better. She was able to walk three city blocks without leg pain and her glycosylated hemoglobin levels were within the normal range.

Course and Prognosis

Diabetes is a chronic condition for which there is no cure. Diabetes can usually be controlled by appropriate medical treatment and intensive involvement on the part of the patient. Type I diabetic patients require daily insulin doses and are prone to hypoglycemic episodes. Often these episodes come on suddenly without the patient being aware of what is happening. Diet control, exercise, and daily glucose testing is typically required for most Type II diabetic patients, yet only 40% require daily insulin supplements (JDFI, 1996).

Some psychologists have been successful in helping diabetic patients become more in tune with their experiences, so that they can foresee a hypoglycemic episode and take corrective action before it becomes serious (Cox, Gonder-Frederick, Antoun, Cryer, & Clarke, 1993). Psychologists can also offer stress management strategies to help patients cope with their conditions. Stress can cause metabolic changes that affect the body's response to insulin and may necessitate changes in the timing or dosage of insulin. Stress may also lead to changes in eating patterns that disrupt the balance between meals and insulin dosage. For example, like Mrs. R, some people respond to stress by eating sweets in excess which, for a diabetic person, can cause hyperglycemia and can lead to complications during a prolonged period. Conversely, preoccupation with stress might cause a person to forget to eat a planned meal, thereby precipitating a hypoglycemic episode and associated dangers. Relaxation training is often used by psychologists to help people cope with stress, and it has been demonstrated that relaxation training helps people who have Type II diabetes to control their blood glucose levels (Surwit, Ross, & Feinglos, 1991).

Familial and Genetic Patterns

Type I and Type II diabetes are similar in their presentations, but they are independent disorders. There is a 30–50% likelihood that the identical twins of Type I diabetics will also develop the disorder at some point in their lifetimes, much less than would be expected if the disorder were 100% genetically based. Because Type I diabetes usually develops in the winter months and because the genes that confer susceptibility to Type I diabetes are located in a region of chromosome 6 that is responsible for controlling immune response, researchers theorize that a virus may be responsible for triggering the disorder in genetically predisposed individuals (NDDG, 1995). Type II diabetes also has strong genetic and familial links. Having a blood relative with Type II diabetes increases the odds of developing the disorder. Studies show that once one twin is diagnosed, the chance that an identical twin will have the disorder is 60%, twice as high as it is for a fraternal twin. Because identical twins have more shared genes than do fraternal twins, this is evidence that the disorder has a genetic basis (NDDG, 1995). However, stress, age, lower socioeconomic status, and being overweight are environmental risk factors that increase the chances of developing Type II diabetes independent of genetic factors (NDDG, 1995), thus suggesting a gene–environment interaction.

Diagnostic Considerations

The diagnosis of diabetes is made by the referring physician and is determined by a glucose tolerance test. The results are fairly clear-cut, and the health-care professional in charge of psychologically managing the diabetic patient will rarely have to worry about the accuracy of the diagnosis. However, the treating psychologist should know whether the patient suffers from Type I diabetes or Type II diabetes, for how long, the medication regimen, how much exercise is taken, what complications have developed, how the patient feels about the diagnosis, and how well the patient controls blood sugar levels. This information will help guide treatment decisions.

INSOMNIA

Description

Insomnia is difficulty initiating or maintaining sleep and includes one or more of the following symptoms: difficulty in falling asleep, difficulty in maintaining sleep, and early morning awakening. There are two different types of insomnia: primary and secondary. **Primary insomnia** is diagnosed when no biological or psychological cause can be identified. **Secondary insomnia** is diagnosed when a medical or psychological diagnosis is present and results in multiple symptoms, including trouble sleeping. Examples include restless legs syndrome, psychological disorders (e.g., depression), alcohol and drug use (e.g., caffeine), or other medical disorders (e.g., chronic pain). **Chronobiological sleep disorder** refers to instances in which a person is unable to sleep at the appropriate time of day, that is, sleep itself is normal, but the timing of sleep does not coincide with the normal sleep-wake cycle.

Sleep is a behavior, and because psychologists are experts at helping people change their behavior, psychological interventions are often useful for sleep problems, including insomnia. For example, as noted before, depression and anxiety are notorious for causing insomnia (Ford & Kamerow, 1989; Breslau, Roth, Rosenthal, & Andreski, 1996). Poor sleep habits, such as keeping an irregular sleep schedule, using the bed for activities other than sleep, and daytime napping can exacerbate the problem. Dysfunctional thoughts, like worrying about getting enough sleep, may increase physiological arousal and work against the goal of getting to sleep. Some consequences of multiple nights without adequate sleep are poor concentration and irritability which can cause the insomniac to become more distressed, making sleep even harder to achieve.

Epidemiology

Between 30 and 40% of adults experience insomnia within any given year, and 10–15% indicate that the problem is severe or chronic (Mellinger, Balter, & Uhlenhuth, 1985). Insomnia occurs more frequently among women and increases with age (Mellinger et al., 1985; Foley, Monjan, Brown, Simonsick, Wallace, & Blazer, 1995). More than half of the people who are 65 and older and live at home and about two-thirds of those who live in long-term care facilities suffer from sleep problems (NIH Consensus Statement, 1990). Younger adults tend to have difficulty initiating sleep, whereas older adults more often have trouble maintaining sleep.

Clinical Picture

Insomnia may appear at any age and can be sudden or insidious in its onset. Insomnia is typically transient, but chronic insomnia is difficult to ignore because it alters mood and interferes with concentration. Many features of the clinical picture are illustrated in the case of Marsha.

Case Illustration

Marsha, a 22-year-old Caucasian college student, had been experiencing insomnia for the past month, to the extent that she asked her family doctor to prescribe sleep medication for her. This helped temporarily, but she soon ran out of her sleeping pills and ended up back in the doctor's office asking to have her prescription refilled. The doctor had ruled out any medical causes and knew that Marsha had recently broken up with her boyfriend. He referred Marsha to a clinical psychologist for behavioral treatment.

During her initial visit, the psychologist discovered that Marsha was drinking three diet sodas and two cups of coffee a day to keep herself awake for class and often consumed more when she was up late studying for exams. Marsha also reported drinking three to five beers or other alcoholic beverages on weekend evenings when out with friends. Marsha complained that she had trouble falling asleep and would lie awake for up to an hour most nights before falling asleep. In the middle of the night, she often awakened and could not return to sleep. In the morning, she often woke an hour before her alarm and as tired as she was, could not go back to sleep. Therefore, Marsha exhibited all three symptoms of insomnia: difficulty in falling asleep, difficulty in maintaining sleep, and early morning awakening. Difficulty in falling asleep is often associated with excessive worry. Marsha admitted that she often fretted over her breakup with her boyfriend or worried about school after she got in bed. Difficulty in maintaining sleep can be caused by, among other things, ingestion of substances that interfere with sleep architecture (the timing and length of the different stages of sleep normally occur in a specific pattern during the sleep cycle). Marsha's caffeine and alcohol consumption were suspected of playing a role in this part of her sleep problem. Because early morning awakening is a hallmark of clinical depression, Marsha was evaluated for depression and endorsed several symptoms, including frequent crying spells, hopelessness, poor appetite, a 5-pound weight loss, daytime fatigue, and difficulty in concentrating.

Marsha's treatment program was multifaceted. Her depression was treated with anti-depressant medication and cognitive-behavioral therapy (e.g., teaching Marsha to change her negative outlook to a more positive one). Because exercise improves sleep (Sherrill, Kotchou, & Quan, 1998) and is a buffer against stressors, a daily routine of exercising for 20 minutes or more was prescribed for her. She was also instructed to eliminate alcohol and caffeine. She was instructed to reduce her caffeine intake gradually because sudden cessation can result in headaches. She was told that having up to two caffeinated drinks a day (before 4 P.M.) would be acceptable once her insomnia resolved. Marsha also implemented a sleep hygiene program involving stimulus control. She was forbidden to engage in activities other than sleep in the bed (except for sex), was permitted to go to bed only when sleepy, was told to get out of bed if lying awake for more than 15 minutes, and was required to develop a bedtime routine before bed. These instructions were designed to develop an association between the bed and sleep and to decrease the association between her bed and nonsleep activities. Last, Marsha was advised to follow a sleep schedule of regular times for going to bed and waking that did not deviate, even on the weekends. After 1 week, Marsha returned to the psychologist and reported that the first few days had been extremely difficult, especially getting out of bed at 6:30 A.M. on the weekend. However, she reported that she had been getting more sleep during the past several nights. After 4 weeks, Marsha reported that her sleep problems had vanished. She also noted a significant improvement in her mood and concentration.

Course and Prognosis

When sleep disorders are not treated, they often do not abate. Over time, the insomniac's bed becomes associated with the anxiety and frustration of being unable to sleep and getting into bed begins to trigger feelings that exacerbate the problem. Chronic insomnia can lead to fatigue, mood changes (e.g., irritability), difficulty concentrating, poor job performance, and impaired daytime functioning. In extreme cases, falling asleep while driving can occur. Untreated insomniacs have higher rates of automobile crashes than other drivers (Costa e Silva, Chase, Sartorius, & Roth, 1996).

Fortunately, the prognosis for insomnia is very good when treatment is obtained. Secondary insomnia can usually be resolved by treating the primary condition. For those who have transient or acute insomnia, pharmacological sleep aids often work well, especially if combined with behavioral interventions (Morin, Colecchi, Stone, Sood, & Brink, 1999). Behavioral interventions such as stimulus control, relaxation training, sleep scheduling, exercise (as long as it is not vigorous activity occurring within 3–4 hours of bedtime), and sleep restriction are helpful in treating chronic primary insomnia. **Sleep restriction** is an intervention that involves restricting the amount of time in bed to the amount of sleep the patient is currently experiencing and gradually increasing time in bed by 15 minutes per night. This generates sleep debt which is thought to increase propensity to sleep until a regular sleep pattern can be achieved. Adjustments to the environment (e.g., temperature and light) are also helpful. Stimulants (e.g., nicotine and caffeine) and alcohol are best eliminated; if they are used, they should be avoided long before bed. Treating chronobiological sleep disorders, in particular, with bright lights for 30 minutes each morning immediately upon arising has proven effective (Guilleminault, Clerk, Black, Labanowski, Pelayo, & Claman, 1995).

Familial and Genetic Risk Factors

The genetic basis of sleep disorders has not been well studied. One study of more than 2000 twin pairs showed greater likelihood of developing insomnia in monozygotic twins whose twin suffered from insomnia compared to dizygotic twins (McCarren, Goldberg,

Ramakrishnan, & Fabsitz, 1994). This finding suggests that there is a genetic basis for at least some causes of insomnia. Although it is unknown whether primary insomnia has a genetic basis, other researchers have found that genetic makeup has a significant influence on sleep patterns throughout life (Heath, Kendler, Eaves, & Martin, 1990).

Diagnostic Considerations

Insomnia is very often a symptom of another problem, and before it is treated, thorough consideration must be given to the primary cause or causes. Anxiety and depression are often associated with insomnia (Breslau, Roth, Rosenthal, & Andreski, 1996), and many medications (including those used to treat anxiety and depression) can impair good sleep. Insomnia can also be secondary to other sleep disorders, including restless legs syndrome, periodic limb movement disorder, and sleep apnea. Finally, substances such as caffeine, recreational drugs, alcohol, and nicotine can cause insomnia. If no secondary cause can be determined, a diagnosis of primary insomnia can be made.

SUMMARY

Individual factors, the environment, and medical conditions are often intertwined. Maladaptive behaviors and harmful coping strategies clearly contribute to the development and exacerbation of various medical conditions. Fortunately, psychologists have developed many interventions that are successful in promoting more adaptive behaviors. Many treatments can be implemented in a relatively short time with much success. One factor that is relevant to the development of most medical conditions is the experience of stress. Individuals who experience single or chronic stressors *and* evaluate them as "stressful" or "threatening" are much more likely to develop or exacerbate a medical condition compared to those who have low levels of stress. Therefore, stress-reducing interventions such as relaxation training, exercise, and cognitive restructuring can be helpful for many individuals, with or without a medical disorder. In sum, this chapter speaks to the importance of health psychology in integrating psychology and medicine. Hopefully over time, the relationship between these two fields will grow stronger and will provide more opportunities to increase the physical and mental health of patients and clients.

ACKNOWLEDGMENTS.   We thank Ron Acierno, Bonnie Cleaveland, David Fryburg, and Jonathan Karp for their assistance, time, and valuable input.

APPENDIX/ONLINE RESOURCES

Medical Disorders

- Center for Disease Control and Prevention: Statistics
  www.cdc.gov/nchs

Cardiovascular Diseases

- American Heart Association
  www.americanheart.org

- National Heart, Lung and Blood Institute (NHLBI)—High Blood Pressure Information
  www.nhlbi.nih.gov/

Headache

- American Headache Society (AHS)
  http://www.ahsnet.org/
- Journal of the American Medical Association (JAMA)—Migraine Information Center
  http://www.ama-assn.org/special/migraine/
- National Institute of Neurological Disorders and Stroke—Headache
  http://www.ninds.nih.gov/health_and_medical/disorders/

Diabetes

- American Diabetes Association homepage
  http://www.diabetes.org/
- Juvenile Diabetes Foundation
  http://www.jdf.org/
- Centers for Disease Control's Diabetes and Public Health Resource Site
  http://www.cdc.gov/diabetes/
- Arnot Ogden Medical Center: Gestational Diabetes Mellitus
  http://www.aomc.org/gesdiab.html

Insomnia

- National Heart, Lung and Blood Institute (NHLBI): Insomnia
  http://nhlbi.nih.gov/health/prof/sleep
- National Highway Traffic Safety Administration website on Drowsy Driving
  http://www.nhtsa.dot.gov/people/perform/human/Drowsy.html
- National Sleep Foundation homepage
  http://www.sleepfoundation.org/
- American Academy of Sleep Medicine
  http://www.asda.org/
- American Academy of Child and Adolescent Psychiatry: Children's Sleep Problems
  http://www.aacap.org/publications/factsfam/sleep.htm

REFERENCES

Aivazyan, T. A., Zaitsev, V. P, Salenko, B. B., Yurenev, A. P. & Patrusheva, I. F. (1988). Efficacy of relaxation techniques in hypertensive patients. *Health Psychology*, 7, 193–200.

American Council for Headache Education. (1996). *Understanding headache*. Mt. Royal, NJ: Author.

American Diabetes Association. (1998). *Annual report*. Alexandria, VA: Author.

American Heart Association. (1999). *Heart and stroke statistical update*. Dallas, TX: American Heart Association.

American Psychiatric Association. (1968). *Diagnostic and statistical manual of mental disorders*, 2nd ed. Washington, DC: Author.

American Psychiatric Association. (1980). *Diagnostic and statistical manual of mental disorders*, 3rd ed. Washington, DC: Author.

American Psychiatric Association. (1987). *Diagnostic and statistical manual of mental disorders*, 3rd ed., rev. Washington, DC: Author.

American Psychiatric Association. (1994). *Diagnostic and statistical manual of mental disorders*, 4th ed. Washington, DC: Author.

Aromaa, M. A., Sillanpaa, M. L., Rautava, P., & Helenius, H. (1998). Childhood headache at school entry: A controlled clinical study. *Neurology, 50*, 1729–1736.

Barefoot, J. C., Dahlstrom, W. G., & Williams, R. B. (1983). Hostility, CHD incidence, and total mortality: A 25-year follow-up study of 255 physicians. *Psychosomatic Medicine, 45*, 59–63.

Barnett, R. C., Biener, L., & Baruch, G. K. (Eds.). (1987). *Gender and stress*. New York: Macmillan.

Bernard, L. C., & Krupat, E. (1994). *Heath psychology: Biopsychosocial factors in health and illness*. Fort Worth, TX: Harcourt Brace.

Blanchard, E. B. (1990). Biofeedback treatments of essential hypertension. *Biofeedback and Self-Regulation, 15*, 563–579.

Blanchard, E. B., Andrasik, F., Ahles, T. A., Teders, S., & O'Keefe, D. (1980). Migraine and tension headache: A meta-analytic review. *Behavior Therapy, 11*, 613–631.

Booth-Kewley, S., & Friedman, H. S. (1987). Psychological predictors of heart disease: A quantitative review. *Psychological Bulletin, 101*, 343–362.

Breslau, N., Roth, T., Rosenthal, L., & Andreski, P. (1996). Sleep disturbance and psychiatric disorders: A longitudinal epidemiological study of young adults. *Biological Psychiatry, 39*, 411–418.

Chen, A. C. (1993). Headache: Contrast between childhood and adult pain. *International Journal of Adolescent Medicine and Health, 6*(2), 75–93.

Clayman, C. B. (1994). *The American Medical Association Family Medical Guide*, 3rd ed. New York: Random House.

Congdon, P. J., & Forsythe, W. I. (1979). Migraine in childhood. *Clinical Pediatrics, 18*, 353–359.

Connors, M. J. (1995). Cluster headache: A review. *Journal of the American Osteopathology Association, 95*, 533–539.

Costa e Silva, J. A., Chase, M., Sartorius, N., & Roth, T. (1996). Special report from a symposium held by the World Health Organization and the World Federation of Sleep Research Societies: An overview of insomnias and related disorders—recognition, epidemiology and rational management. *Sleep, 19*, 412–416.

Cox, D. J., Gonder-Frederick, L., Antoun, B., Cryer, P. E., & Clarke, W. L. (1993). Perceived symptoms in the recognition of hypoglycemia. *Diabetes Care, 16*, 519–527.

Davison, G. C., Williams, M. E., Nezami, E., Bice, T. L., & DeQuattro, V. L. (1991). Relaxation, reduction in angry articulated thoughts, and improvements in borderline hypertension and heart rate. *Journal of Behavioral Medicine, 14*, 453–468.

Denollet, J. (1997). Personality, emotional distress, and coronary heart disease. *European Journal of Personality, 11*, 343–357.

Diabetes Control and Complications Trial (DCCT) Research Group. (1993). The effect of intensive treatment of diabetes on the development and progression of long-term complications in insulin-dependent diabetes mellitus. *New England Journal of Medicine, 329*, 977–986.

Eisler, R. M., Skidmore, J. R., & Ward, C. H. (1988). Masculine gender-role stress: Predictor of anger, anxiety, and health-risk behaviors. *Journal of Personality Assessment, 52*, 133–141.

Eysenck (1991). Personality as a risk factor in coronary heart disease. *European Journal of Personality, 5*(2), 81–92.

Finley, W. W., & Jones, L. (1992). Biofeedback with children. In C. E. Walker & M. C. Roberts (Eds.), *Handbook of clinical child psychology* (pp. 809–827). New York: Wiley.

Foley, D. J., Monjan, A. A., Brown, S. L., Simonsick, E. M., Wallace, R. B., & Blazer, D. G. (1995). Sleep complaints among elderly persons: An epidemiologic study of three communities. *Sleep, 18*, 425–432.

Ford, D. E., & Kamerow, D. B. (1989). Epidemiologic study of sleep disturbances and psychiatric disorders: An opportunity for prevention? *Journal of the American Medical Association, 262*, 1479–1484.

Gherpelli, J., Nagae Poetscher, L. M., Souza, A. M., Bosse, E. M., Rabello, G. D., Diament, A., & Scoff, M. (1998). Migraine in childhood and adolescence: A critical study of the diagnostic criteria and the influence of age on clinical findings. *Cephalagia, 18*, 333–341.

Gidron, Y., & Davidson, K. (1996). Development and preliminary testing of a brief intervention for modifying CHD predictive hostility components. *Journal of Behavioral Medicine, 19*, 203–220.

Guilleminault C., Clerk, A., Black, J., Labanowski, M., Pelayo, R., & Claman D. (1995). Nondrug treatment trials in psychophysiologic insomnia. *Archives of Internal Medicine, 155*, 838–844.

Gupta, M. A., Gupta, A. K., Kirkby, S., Schork, N. J., Corr, S. K., Ellis, C. N., & Voorhees, J. J. (1989). A psychocutaneous profile of psoriasis patients who are stress reactors. A study of 127 patients. *General Hospital Psychiatry, 11*(3), 166–173.

Hahn, Y. H., Ro, Y. J., Song, H. H., Kim, N. C., Kim, H. S., & Yoo, Y. S. (1993). The effect of thermal biofeedback and progressive muscle relaxation training in reducing blood pressure of patients with essential hypertension. *IMAGE: Journal of Nursing Scholarship, 25*, 204–207.

Headache Classification Committee of the International Headache Society. Classification and diagnostic criteria for headache disorders, cranial neuralgias, and facial pain. *Cephalalgia, 8,* 1–96.

Heath, A. C., Kendler, K. S., Eaves, L. J., & Martin, N. G. (1990). Evidence for genetic influences on sleep disturbance and sleep pattern in twins. *Sleep, 13,* 318–335.

Helgeson, V. S. (1990). The role of masculinity in a prognostic predictor of heart attack severity. *Sex Roles, 22,* 755–774.

Hoelscher, T. J., & Lichstein, K. L. (1983). Blood volume pulse biofeedback treatment of chronic cluster headache. *Biofeedback Self Regulation, 8,* 533–541.

Holroyd, K. A., & Penzien, D. B. (1994). Psychosocial interventions in the management of recurrent headache disorders 1: Overview and effectiveness behavioral medicine synthesis. *Behavioral Medicine, 20*(2), 53–64.

Juvenile Diabetes Foundation International. (1996). *What you should know about diabetes.* New York: Author.

Kamarck, T. W., Annunziato, B. A., & Amateau, B. A. (1995). Affiliation moderates the effects of social threat on stress-related cardiovascular responses: Boundary conditions for a laboratory model of social support. *Psychosomatic Medicine, 57,* 183–194.

Kulkarni, S., O'Farrell, I., Erasi, M., & Kochar, M. S. (1998). Stress and hypertension. *Wisconsin Medical Journal, 11,* 34–38.

Labbe, E. E. (1988). Childhood muscle contraction headache: Current issues in assessment and treatment. *Headache, 28,* 430–434.

Labbe, E. E., & Williamson, D. A. (1983). Temperature biofeedback in the treatment of children with migraine headaches. *Journal of Pediatric Psychology, 8,* 317–326.

Lash, S. J., Eisler, R. M., & Southard, D. R. (1995). Sex differences in cardiovascular reactivity as a function of the appraised gender relevance of the stressor. *Behavioral Medicine, 21*(2), 86–94.

Lazarus, R. S., & Folkman, S. (1984). *Stress, appraisal, and coping.* New York: Springer.

Lee, D. D., DeQuattro, V., Allen, J., Kimura, S., Aleman, E., Konugres, G., & Davison, G. (1988). Behavioral vs beta-blocker therapy in patients with primary hypertension: Effects on blood pressure, left ventricular function and mass, and the pressor surge of social stress anger. *American Heart Journal, 116,* 637–644.

Lee, D. D., Kimura, S., DeQuattro, V., & Davison, G. (1989). Relaxation lowers blood pressure more effectively in hypertensives with raised plasma norepinephrine and blunts pressor response to anger. *Clinical Experiments and Hypertension, 11,* 191–198.

Little, B. C., Hayworth, J., Benson, P., Hall, F., Beard, R. W., Dewhurst, J., & Priest, R. G. (1984). *Lancet, 21*(8382), 865–867.

Marks, D. R., & Rapoport, A. M. (1997). Practical evaluation and diagnosis of headache. *Seminars in Neurology, 17,* 307–312.

Maytal, J., Lipton, R. B., Solomon, S., & Shinnar, S. (1992). Childhood onset cluster headaches. *Headache, 32,* 275–279.

McCarren, M., Goldberg, J., Ramakrishnan, V., & Fabsitz, R. (1994). Insomnia in Vietnam era veteran twins: Influence of genes and combat experience. *Sleep, 17,* 456–461.

McGrady, A., Nadsady, P. A., & Schumann-Brzezinski, C. (1991). Sustained effects of biofeedback-assisted relaxation therapy in essential hypertension. *Biofeedback and Self-Regulation, 16,* 399–411.

Mellinger, G. D., Balter, M. B., & Uhlenhuth, E. H. (1985). Insomnia and its treatment, prevalence and correlates. *Archives of General Psychiatry, 42,* 225–232.

Merikangas, K. M., Fenton, B. T., Cheng, S. H., Stolar, M. J., & Risch, N. 1997. Association between migraine and stroke in a large-scale epidemiological study of the United States. *Journal of the American Medical Association, 54,* 362–368.

Morin, C. M., Colecchi, C., Stone, J., Sood, R., & Brink, D. (1999). Behavioral and pharmacological therapies for late-life insomnia—a randomized controlled trial. *Journal of the American Medical Association, 281,* 991–999.

National Center for Health Statistics. (1994). *Current estimates from the National Health Interview Survey, 1993.* Vital and Health Statistics, Series 10, no. 190. Washington, DC: Centers for Disease Control and Prevention.

National Center for Health Statistics. (1995). *Monitoring health care in America: Quarterly fact sheet, December.* Washington, DC: Centers for Disease Control and Prevention.

National Diabetes Data Group. (1995). *Diabetes in America,* 2nd ed. Washington, DC: National Institutes of Health, National Institute of Diabetes and Digestive and Kidney Diseases. NIH publication No. 95-1468.

National Institutes of Health Consensus Statement. (1990). The treatment of sleep disorders of older people. *March 26–28, 8*(3), 1–22. Washington, DC: National Institutes of Health

Patel, C., & Marmot, M. (1988). Can general practitioners use training in relaxation and management of stress to reduce mild hypertension? *British Medical Journal, 296,* 21–24.

Pearce, J. M. (1993). Natural history of cluster headache. *Headache, 33,* 253–256.

Räikkönen, K., Matthews, K. A., Flory, J. D., Owens, J. F., & Gump, B. B. (1999). Effects of optimism, pessimism, and trait anxiety on ambulatory blood pressure and mood during everyday life. *Journal of Personality and Social Psychology, 76*, 104–113.

Roy, M. P., Kirschbaum, C., & Steptoe, A. (1998). Life events and social support as moderators of individual differences in cardiovascular and cortisol reactivity. *Journal of Personality and Social Psychology, 75*, 1273–1281.

Russell, M. B., Andersson, P. G., & Iselius, L. (1996). Cluster headache is an inherited disorder in some families. *Headache, 36*(10), 138–140.

Russell, M. B., & Olesen, J. (1996). Migrainous disorder and its relation to migraine without aura and migraine with aura. A genetic epidemiological study. *Cephalalgia, 16*, 431–435.

Russell, M. B., Iselius, L., Ostergaard, S., & Olesen, J. (1998). Inheritance of chronic tension-type headache investigated by complex segregation analysis. *Human Genetics, 102*, 138–140.

Ryan, R. E., & Ryan, R. E. (1989). Cluster headaches. *Otolaryngology Clinics of North America, 22*, 1131–1144.

Sandyk, R. (1992). The influence of the pineal gland on migraine and cluster headaches and effects of treatment with picotesla magnetic fields. *International Journal of Neuroscience, 67*, 145–171.

Sartory, G., Mueller, B., Metsch, J., & Pothmann, R. (1998). A comparison of psychological and pharmacological treatment of pediatric migraine. *Behaviour Research and Therapy, 36*, 1155–1170.

Schwartz, B. S., Stewart, W. F., Simon, D., & Lipton, R. B. (1998). Epidemiology of tension-type headache. *Journal of the American Medical Association, 279*, 381–383.

Segerstrom, S. C., Taylor, S. E., Kemeny, M. E., & Fahey, J. L. (1998). Optimism is associated with mood, coping, and immune change in response to stress. *Journal of Personality and Social Psychology, 74*, 1646–1655.

Sherrill, D. L., Kotchou, K., & Quan, S. F. (1998). Association of physical activity and human sleep disorders. *Archives of Internal Medicine, 158*, 1894–1898.

Solomon, G. D., Skobleranda, F. G., & Gragg, L. A. (1993). Quality of life and well-being of headache patients: Measurement by the medical outcomes study instrument. *Headache, 33*, 361–368.

Sorenson, G., Lewis, B., & Bishop, R. (1996). Gender, job factors, and coronary heart disease risk. *American Journal of Health Behavior, 20*, 3–13.

Southam, M. A., Agras, W. S., Taylor, C. B., & Kraemer, H. C. (1982). Relaxation training. Blood pressure lowering during the working day. *Archives of General Psychiatry, 39*, 715–717.

Stone, S. V., Dembroski, T. M., Costa, P. T., & MacDougall, J. M. (1990). Gender differences in cardiovascular reactivity. *Journal of Behavioral Medicine, 13*, 137–156.

Surwit, R. S., Ross, S. L., & Feinglos, M. N. (1991). Stress, behavior, and glucose control in diabetes mellitus. In P. M. McCabe, N. Schneiderman, T. M. Field, & J. S. Skyler (Eds.), *Stress, coping and disease* (pp. 97–117). Hillsdale, NJ: Erlbaum.

U.S. Department of Health and Human Services, Public Health Service, National Institutes of Health, National Institute of Child Health and Human Development. (1993). NIH Pub. No. 93-2788. Washington, DC: Author.

Wall, V. R. (1992). Breastfeeding and migraine headaches. *Human Lactation, 8*, 209–212.

21

Organic Mental Disorders

Gerald Goldstein

Description of the Disorder

There is a traditional distinction made in psychopathology between the so-called organic and functional disorders. The latter type of disorder is generally viewed as a reaction to some environmental or psychosocial stress or as a condition in which the presence of a specific organic etiological factor is strongly suspected, but not proven. The anxiety disorders are examples of the first alternative, and schizophrenia is an example of the second. Organic mental disorders are those conditions that can be more or less definitively associated with temporary or permanent dysfunction of the brain. Thus, individuals who have these illnesses are frequently described as "brain-damaged" patients or patients who have "organic brain syndromes." It is clear that recent developments in psychopathological research and theory have gone a long way toward breaking down this distinction, and it is becoming increasingly clear that many of the schizophrenic, mood, and attentional disorders have their bases in some alteration of brain function. Nevertheless, the clinical phenomenology, assessment methods, and treatment management procedures for patients generally described as brain-damaged are sufficiently unique that the traditional functional versus organic distinction is probably worth retaining. However, the term "organic patient" is rarely used in practice, and characterizations are more often made using the terms dementia, delirium, and amnesia, or specific neurobehavioral syndromes.

Organic mental disorders are basically brain disorders or diseases produced by pathological agents that may impair any organ or system of the body. The brain may be damaged by trauma, or it may become infected. The brain can become cancerous or can lose adequate oxygen through occlusion of the blood vessels that supply it. The brain can be affected through acute or chronic exposure to toxins, such as carbon monoxide or other poisonous substances. Nutritional deficiencies can alter brain function just as they alter the function of other organs and organ systems. Aside from these general systemic and exogenous factors, there are diseases that more or less specifically have the central nervous system as their target. These conditions, generally known as degenerative and demyelinating diseases, include Hunt-

Gerald Goldstein • VA Pittsburgh Healthcare System, Pittsburgh, Pennsylvania 15206.

Advanced Abnormal Psychology, Second Edition, edited by Hersen and Van Hasselt. Kluwer Academic/Plenum Publishers, New York, 2001.

ington's disease, multiple sclerosis, Parkinson's disease, and a number of disorders associated with aging.

It is useful to categorize these various disorders according to temporal and topographical parameters. Thus, certain neuropathological conditions are static and do not change substantially; others are slowly progressive, and some are rapidly progressive. With regard to topography, certain conditions tend to involve focal, localized disease, others multifocal lesions, and still others diffuse brain damage without specific localization. Another very important consideration has to do with morbidity and mortality. Some brain disorders are more or less reversible, some are static and do not produce marked change in the patient over lengthy periods of time, and some are rapidly or slowly progressive, produce increasing morbidity, and eventually lead to death. Thus, some types of brain damage produce a stable condition with minimal changes, some types permit substantial recovery, and other types are in actuality terminal illnesses. Therefore, it is apparent that the kind of brain disorder from which the patient suffers is a crucial clinical consideration in that it has major implications for treatment, management, and planning.

DSM-IV (APA, 1987) has replaced the term "Organic Mental Disorders" with "Delirium, Dementia, and Amnestic and Other Cognitive Disorders." The major disturbance is a deficit in cognition or memory, and the etiology must be a general medical condition, a substance such as alcohol, or a combination of the two. Delirium is a temporary loss of capacity to maintain attention accompanied by correspondingly reduced awareness of the environment. Tremors and lethargy may be accompanying symptoms. Delirium is reversible in most cases but may evolve into a permanent dementia or other neurological disorder. Dementia is a condition in which there is a general loss of intellectual function and typically involves impairment of memory, abstract reasoning, problem-solving ability, and other complex cognitive abilities. Sometimes there is loss of the ability to speak intelligibly. In the amnestic disorders (sometimes known as Korsakoff's syndrome), memory is severely impaired, but other cognitive functions are relatively well preserved. DSM-IV also lists a set of diagnoses that are categorized as "Mental Disorders Due to a General Medical Condition." These disorders are diagnosed when a medical disorder produces symptoms that are not specifically cognitive but may involve personality change, mood disturbance, anxiety, or sleep disturbance. These diagnoses replaced the earlier terms such as "Organic Affective Disorder" which are no longer used.

Within contemporary abnormal psychology, the theoretical approach to these patients is largely neuropsychological in orientation, in that it is based on the assumption that clinical problems associated with brain damage can be understood best in the context of what is known about the relationships between brain function and behavior. Thus, we will expand our presentation beyond the descriptive psychopathology of DSM-IV and attempt to provide some material related to basic brain-behavior mechanisms. There are many sources of brain dysfunction, and the nature of the source has a great deal to do with determining behavioral consequences: morbidity and mortality. Thus, a basic grasp of key neuropathological processes is crucial to understanding the differential consequences of brain damage. Furthermore, it is important to have some conceptualization of the way the brain functions. Research accomplished since the last edition of this book appeared has substantially increased knowledge in this area. For example, we now know a great deal more about the way memories are preserved in brain tissue. New technologies such as functional magnetic resonance imaging have provided important information on the way the brain functions while complex activities are performed.

Clinical neuropsychology is the specialty area within psychology primarily involved in assessing and rehabilitating brain-damaged patients. Clinical neuropsychological research has provided a number of specialized instruments for assessing these patients, as well as a variety of rehabilitative methods aimed at remediating neuropsychological deficits. This research has also pointed out that "brain damage," far from being a single clinical entity, actually represents a wide variety of disorders. Initially, neuropsychologists were strongly interested in the relationship between localization of the brain damage and behavioral outcome. In recent years, however, localization has come to be seen as only one determinant of outcome, albeit often a very important one. Other considerations include such matters as the age of the individual, the individual's age when the brain damage was acquired, the premorbid personality and level of achievement, and the type of pathological process that produced the brain dysfunction.

Dementia

Dementia is probably the most common form of organic mental disorder. There are several types of dementia, but they all involve usually slowly progressive deterioration of intellectual function. The deterioration is frequently patterned, loss of memory generally is the first function to decline, and other abilities deteriorate at later stages of the illness. One major class of dementia consists of those disorders that arise during late life, either during late middle age or old age. In the former case, they are known as presenile dementias, and those that occur during old age are known as senile dementia. As the term is used now, dementia may occur at any age. In children, it is differentiated from mental retardation on the basis of the presence of deterioration from a formerly higher level. Dementia may result from head trauma or essentially any of the neuropathological conditions discussed before. Alcoholism and the nutritional disorders that typically accompany it is one common cause of dementia. A specific type of dementia that generally appears before the presenile period is Huntington's disease. The term dementia, when defined broadly as suggested here, is not particularly useful and does not really provide more information than such terms as "organic brain syndrome" or "chronic brain syndrome." However, when the term is used more specifically, it becomes possible to point out specific characteristics that may be described as syndromes. This specificity may be achieved by defining the dementias as those disorders in which, for no exogenous reason, the brain begins to deteriorate and continues to do so until death. DSM-IV describes these conditions as Dementia of the Alzheimer's Type, because the most common type of progressive degenerative dementia is Alzheimer's disease. Sufficient diagnostic methods are not yet available to diagnose Alzheimer's disease in the living patient, but its presence becomes apparent on examination of the brain at autopsy. Clinically, the course of the illness generally begins with signs of impairment of memory for recent events, followed by deficits in judgment, visual-spatial skills, and language. The language deficit has become a matter of particular interest, perhaps because the communicative difficulties of dementia patients are becoming increasingly recognized. Generally, the language difficulty does not resemble aphasia but can perhaps be best characterized as an impoverishment of speech, word finding difficulties, and progressive inability to produce extended and comprehensible narrative speech. Basically the same finding has been noted in the descriptive writing of Alzheimer's disease patients (Neils, Boller, Gerdeman, & Cole, 1989). The patients wrote shorter descriptive paragraphs than age-matched controls, and also made more handwriting errors of various types.

The end state of dementia is generalized, severe intellectual impairment involving all areas, and the patient sometimes survives for various lengths of time in a persistent vegetative state. The progressive dementia seen in Huntington's disease also involves significant impairment of memory, and other abilities become gradually affected through the course of the illness. However, it differs from Alzheimer's disease in that it is accompanied by choreic movements and by the fact that the age of onset is substantially earlier than for Alzheimer's disease. Because of the chorea, there is also a difficulty in speech articulation frequently seen, which is not the case for Alzheimer's patients. Vascular or multi-infarct dementia is a form of dementia that does not have an unknown etiology but is slowly progressive. This disorder is associated with hypertension and a series of strokes, and the end result is substantial deterioration. However, the course of the deterioration is not considered as uniform as in Alzheimer's disease, but rather is generally described as stepwise and patchy. The patient may remain relatively stable between strokes, and the symptomatology produced may be associated with the site of the strokes. These distinctions between multi-infarct and primary degenerative dementia are clearly described, but it is not always possible to make a definitive differential diagnosis in individual patients. Even such sophisticated imaging methods as the CT scan and MRI do not always contribute to the diagnosis. During the bulk of the course of the illness, the dementia patient will typically appear as confused, possibly disoriented, and lacks the ability to recall recent events. Speech may be very limited, and if fluent, likely to be incomprehensible. The deficit pattern tends to become increasingly global and all functions become more or less involved. Some investigators have attempted to identify syndromal subtypes; some have more deficit in the area of abstraction and judgment, some in the area of memory, and some in affect and personality changes. However, such proposed typology has not been well established, and most patients have difficulties in all three areas. There are some treatable dementias, particularly dementias associated with endocrine disorders or normal pressure hydrocephalus, but there is no curative treatment for Alzheimer's type dementia. Current research offers the hope that pharmacological treatment may eventually ameliorate the course of Alzheimer's disease, but thus far no such effective treatment is available. At this time, extensive efforts are being made to develop medications that slow the progression of Alzheimer's disease. The most promising new drug at present is called Aricept.

There is a type of dementia that is specifically associated with frontal lobe brain damage. The damage may result from a number of processes such as head trauma, tumor, or stroke, but the syndrome produced is more or less the same. Indeed, clinicians speak of a " frontal lobe syndrome." The outstanding features all may be viewed as relating to impaired ability to control, regulate, and program behavior, an ability sometimes described as "executive function." Such impairment is manifested in numerous ways, including poor abstractive ability, impaired judgment, apathy, and loss of impulse control. Language is sometimes impaired, but rather uniquely. Rather than having a formal language disorder, the patient loses the ability to control behavior through language. There is also often a difficulty with narrative speech that has been interpreted as a problem in forming the intention to speak or in formulating a plan for a narrative. Such terms as lack of insight or of the ability to produce goal-oriented behavior are used to describe the frontal lobe patient. In many cases, these activating, regulatory, and programming functions are so impaired that the outcome looks like a generalized dementia with implications for many forms of cognitive, perceptual, and motor activities.

Amnesia

Some degree of impairment of memory is a part of many brain disorders, but there are some conditions in which loss of memory is clearly the most outstanding deficit. When memory loss is particularly severe and persistent, and other cognitive and perceptual functions are relatively intact, the patient can be described as having an amnesic syndrome. Dementia patients are often amnesic, but their memory disturbance is embedded in significant generalized impairment of intellectual and communicative abilities. The amnesic patient generally has normal language and may be of average intelligence. As in aphasia and several other disorders, there is more than one amnesic syndrome. The differences among them revolve around what the patient can and cannot remember. The structures in the brain that are particularly important for memory are the limbic system, especially the hippocampus, and certain brain stem structures, including the mammillary bodies and the dorsomedial nucleus of the thalamus. There are many systems described in the literature for distinguishing among types of amnesia and types of memory. Perhaps the most basic distinction is between anterograde and retrograde amnesia. Anterograde amnesia involves the inability to form new memories from the time of the onset of the illness or trauma that produced the amnesia, whereas retrograde amnesia refers to the inability to recall events that took place before onset. This distinction dovetails with the distinction between recent and remote memory. It also corresponds somewhat with the distinction made between short-term and long-term memory in the experimental literature. However, various theories define these terms somewhat differently and perhaps it is best to use the more purely descriptive terms recent and remote memory in describing amnesic disorders. Then, it can be stated that the most commonly appearing amnesic disorders involve dramatic impairment of recent memory and relative sparing of remote memory. This sparing becomes greater as the events to be remembered become more remote. Thus, most amnesic patients can recall their early lives but may totally forget what occurred during the last several hours. This distinction between recent and remote memory possibly aids in explaining why most amnesic patients maintain normal language function and average intelligence. In this respect, an amnesic disorder is not so much an obliteration of the past as it is an inability to learn new material. Probably the most common type of relatively pure amnesic disorder is alcoholic Korsakoff's syndrome. Although these patients often maintain average levels in a number of areas of cognitive function, they demonstrate a dense amnesia for recent events with relatively well preserved remote memory. Alcoholic Korsakoff's syndrome has been conceptualized by Butters and Cermak (1980) as an information processing defect in which new material is encoded in a highly degraded manner that leads to high susceptibility to interference. Butters and Cermak (1980), as well as numerous other investigators, have accomplished detailed experimental studies of alcoholic Korsakoff's patients in which the nature of their perceptual, memory, and learning difficulties have been described in detail. The results of this research aid in explaining numerous clinical phenomena noted in Korsakoff's patients, such as their capacity to perform learned behaviors without recalling when or if those behaviors were previously executed, or their tendency to confabulate or "fill in" for the events of the past day that they do not recall. Confabulation was once considered a cardinal symptom of Korsakoff's syndrome, but it is seen only in some patients. Another type of amnesic disorder is seen when there is direct, focal damage to the temporal lobes and most importantly to the hippocampus. These temporal lobe or limbic system amnesias are less common than Korsakoff's syndrome but have been well studied because of the light they shed on the neuropathology of memory. These patients share many of the characteristics of Korsakoff's patients but have a much more profound deficit in basic consolidation and storage of new material. When Korsakoff's patients are sufficiently cued and given enough time, they can learn. Indeed, sometimes they can demonstrate normal recognition memory. However, patients who have temporal lobe amnesias may find it almost impossible to learn new material under any circumstances. In some cases, amnesic disorders are modality-specific. If one distinguishes between verbal and nonverbal memory, the translation can be made from the distinction between language and the nonverbal abilities associated with the specialized functions of each cerebral hemisphere. It has in fact been reported that patients who have unilateral lesions involving the left temporal lobe may have memory deficits only for verbal material, whereas right temporal patients have corresponding deficits for nonverbal material. Thus, the left temporal patient may have difficulty in learning word lists, and the right temporal patient may have difficulty with geometric forms. In summary, there are several amnesic syndromes, but they all have in common the symptom of lack of ability to learn new material following the onset of the illness. Sometimes the symptom is modality-specific and involves only verbal or nonverbal material, but more often than not it involves both modalities. There are several relatively pure types of amnesia, notably Korsakoff's syndrome, but memory difficulties are cardinal symptoms of many other brain disorders, notably the progressive dementias and certain disorders associated with infection. For example, people who have herpes encephalitis frequently have severely impaired memories, but they have other cognitive deficits as well.

Other Cognitive Disorders

It is useful to view these disorders in the form of identified patterns of behavioral characteristics that might be described as neuropsychological syndromes. There are admittedly other ways of describing and classifying neuropsychological deficit, but the syndrome approach has the advantage of providing rather graphic phenomenological descriptions of different kinds of brain-damaged patients. However, it runs the risk of suggesting that every brain-damaged patient can be classified as having some specific, identifiable syndrome—something that is not at all true. Therefore, it is important to understand that the syndromes are classic types of various disorders that are in fact seen in some patients. However, there are many brain-damaged patients who do not have classic-type syndromes; their symptomatology reflects an often complex combination of portions of several syndromes. Heilman and Valenstein (1993), in the way in which they outlined their clinical neuropsychology text, suggested a useful and workable classification of syndromes. First of all, there are the communicative disorders that may be subdivided into aphasia and the specialized language or language-related disorders, including reading impairment (alexia), writing disorders (agraphia), and calculation disorders (acalculia). Second, there are the syndromes associated with some aspect of perception or motility. These include the perception of one's body (the body schema disturbances), the various visual-spatial disorders (which may involve perception, constructional abilities, or both); the gnostic disorders (impairment of visual, auditory, and tactile recognition); the neglect syndromes; and the disorders of skilled and purposeful movement, called apraxias. Third, there are the syndromes that involve primarily general intelligence and memory-dementia and the amnesic disorders. Associated with this latter type are the relatively unique syndromes associated with damage to the frontal lobes. These three general categories account for most of the syndromes in adults. The DSM-IV based categorization can perhaps be most productively viewed as supplemental to the type of neuropsychological system used by Heilman and Valenstein (1985), rather than as an alternative to it. It plays a major role in describing the noncognitive kinds of symptomatology that are often associated with structural brain damage, particularly for those cases in which these personality and affective changes are the predominant symptoms. These considerations are of the upmost clinical importance because the failure to recognize the organic basis for some apparently functional symptom, such as a personality change, may lead to initiating totally inappropriate treatment or the failure to recognize a life-threatening physical illness.

Alterations in brain function can give rise to symptoms that look like functional personality changes, but the reverse can also occur. A nonorganic personality change, notably the acquisition of a depression, can produce symptoms that look like they have been produced by alterations in brain function. The term generally applied to this situation is "pseudodementia," and it is most frequently seen in elderly people who become depressed. The concept of pseudodementia or depressive pseudodementia is not universally accepted, but it is not uncommon to find elderly patients who are diagnosed as demented when in fact the symptoms of dementia are actually produced by depression. The point is proven when the symptoms disappear or diminish substantially after the depression has run its course or the patient is treated with antidepressant medication. Wells (1979, 1980) pointed out that this differential diagnosis is difficult, and cannot be accomplished satisfactorily with the usual examinational, laboratory, and psychometric methods. He suggests that perhaps the most useful diagnostic criteria are clinical features. For example, patients who have pseudodementia tend to complain about their cognitive losses, whereas patients who have dementia tend not to complain. In a later formulation, Caine (1986) pointed to the many complexities of differential diagnosis in the elderly and referred in particular to the abundant evidence for neuropsychological deficits in younger depressed patients and to the not uncommon coexistence of neurological and psychiatric impairments in the elderly. Based on extensive review, Nussbaum (1994) concluded that pseudodementia may have anatomical substrates and may be a real dementia caused by pathology of the subcortical portion of the brain.

EPIDEMIOLOGY

The epidemiology of the organic mental disorders varies with the underlying disorder, and so is unlike what is the case for most of the other diagnostic categories in DSM-IV. Here, we will sample only from those disorders in which epidemiological considerations are of particular interest. There are some exceptionally interesting and well-documented findings for multiple sclerosis, in which prevalence is directly related to the latitude in which one resides; the farther from the equator, the higher the prevalence. Further study of this phenomenon has tended to implicate an environmental rather than an ethnic factor.

The epidemiology of head trauma has been extensively studied, and gender, age, and social class turn out to be important considerations. Head trauma has a higher incidence in males than in females (274 per 100,000 in males and 116 per 100,000 in females in one study) (Levin, Benton, & Grossman, 1982). It is related to age; risk peaks between ages 15 and 24 and occurs more frequently in individuals from lower social classes. Alcohol is a major risk factor, but marital status, a preexisting psychiatric disorder, and a previous history of head injury have also been implicated. The major causes of head injury are motor vehicle accidents, falls, assaults, and recreational or work activities; motor vehicle accidents are clearly the major cause (50–60%) (Smith, Barth, Diamond, & Giuliano, 1998).

The epidemiology of Huntington's disease has also been extensively studied. The disease is transmitted as an autosomal dominant trait, and the marker for the gene has been located on the short arm of chromosome 4 (Gusella et al., 1983). Prevalence estimates vary between 5 and 7 per 100,000. There are no known risk factors for acquiring the disorder; the only consideration is having a parent who has the disease. If that is the case, the risk of acquiring the disorder is 50%. A test is available now to detect carriers of the defective gene, and its availability and usage may eventually reduce the prevalence of Huntington's disease.

There is a great interest in the epidemiology of Alzheimer's disease because the specific cause of the disease is not fully understood and preventing exposure to risk factors for this disease and related disorders remains a possibility. General health status considerations do not constitute risk factors, but some time ago there were beliefs that a transmissible infective agent existed and that exposure to aluminum might be a risk factor. The aluminum hypothesis has largely been discarded. Now, it seems well established that an infective agent is responsible in the case of a rare form of dementia called Creutzfeldt–Jakob disease, but Alzheimer's disease is apparently not associated with infection. Recently, it has been reported that Creutzfeldt–Jakob disease resembles "mad cow disease," and it is thought that a risk factor may be eating beef from cattle possibly exposed to "mad cow disease." Recently, episodes of head trauma have been implicated as a possible risk factor for Alzheimer's disease. A reasonably solid genetic association involving chromosome 21 trisomy has been formed between what appears to be an inherited form of Alzheimer's disease and Down's syndrome.

Much of the epidemiology of the organic mental disorders merges with general considerations regarding health status. Cardiovascular risk factors such as obesity and hypertension put one at greater than usual risk for stroke. Smoking is apparently a direct or indirect risk factor for several disorders that eventuate in brain dysfunction. The diagnosis of dementia associated with alcoholism is now relatively widely accepted, although it was controversial at one time. Alcohol, most clearly, and perhaps several other abused substances, are significant risk factors. In some cases, the crucial risk factor is provided not by the individual, but by the mother of the individual during pregnancy. Existence of fetal alcohol syndrome is well established, and evidence for an association between birth defects and other forms of substance abuse during pregnancy is increasing. Until recently, the risk of acquiring brain disease by infection had diminished substantially, but that situation has changed markedly due to the appearance of human immunodeficiency virus, or HIV-1 infection, or acquired immunodeficiency syndrome (AIDS) dementia (Grant et al., 1987; Van Gorp et al., 1989). Since the last edition of this book appeared, it has become increasingly clear that AIDS is frequently transmitted to children during pregnancy or from breast feeding. At this time, a new anti-infection medication is going through extensive clinical trials and shows great promise.

In summary, the prevalence and incidence of organic mental disorders vary substantially, ranging from very rare to common diseases. The number of risk factors also varies, ranging from complete absence to a substantial number. The genetic and degenerative diseases, notably Huntington's and Alzheimer's disease, possess little in the way of risk factors, and there is not much that can be done to prevent their occurrence. The development of a test for the risk of transmitting Huntington's disease has opened up the admittedly controversial and complex matter of genetic counseling. On the other hand, such disorders as dementia associated with alcoholism, and perhaps stroke, are preventable by good health maintenance. Indeed, the incidence of major stroke has declined in recent years.

Clinical Picture

The variability among organic mental disorders is attributable to a number of factors, including the following considerations: (1) the location of the damage in the brain, (2) the neuropathological process that produced the damage, (3) the length of time the brain damage has been present, (4) the age and health status of the individual at the time the damage is sustained, and (5) the individual's premorbid personality and level of function. Thus, there is no prototypical clinical picture that characterizes all of these disorders. Rather, a neuropsychological approach to the conceptualization of these disorders has been taken that identifies a number of behavioral parameters along which the manifestations of brain dysfunction can be described and classified. The most frequently considered dimensions are intellectual function, language, memory, visual-spatial skills, perceptual skills, and motor function. Studies of brain-damaged patients have shown that particular structures in the brain mediate relatively discrete behaviors. Of particular importance is the consideration that the left and right hemispheres mediate different functions: the left hemisphere is important for language, and the right for spatial abilities. Neurologists and neuropsychologists have identified a number of syndromes in such areas as language dysfunction, memory disorder, and general intellectual impairment. It was pointed out that there are also major variations in the courses of organic mental disorders. Some are transient and leave little or no residual; some are permanent but not progressive; others are either slowly or rapidly progressive. These disorders most profoundly and commonly involve impairment of cognitive, perceptual, and motor skills, but sometimes personality changes of various types are the most prominent symptoms. More often than not, personality and affective changes appear in brain-damaged patients along with their cognitive, perceptual, and motor disorders. Thus, an affective disorder or such symptoms as delusions and hallucinations may be sequelae of brain damage for various reasons. In this section we will concentrate on dementia because it provides the most common picture clinicians are likely to see. Dementia appears most frequently in the elderly, and it is now thought that the most common form of dementia is Alzheimer's disease. A recent estimate indicates that about half a million people in this country have Alzheimer's disease. This figure will increase markedly in the future because of continued increasing longevity.

Because Alzheimer's disease is a progressive disorder, the clinical presentation changes as times passes. It is a disease of insidious onset, and its earliest signs may not be recognized, or recognized only retrospectively. Most typically, the first sign is forgetfulness, which then merges into increasingly blatant impairment of memory. It is felt by some investigators that the first indication of the disorder is onset of a depression, followed by progressive loss of memory, but that view has not yet been extensively documented. It has been noted that as the disorder progresses, the severity of depression becomes milder, ostensibly because patients becomes increasingly less capable of assessing their status. As the disorder progresses, other cognitive functions become impaired, notably abstract reasoning and language abilities. The language deficit may begin with word finding difficulties and develop into impoverished, sometimes incomprehensible speech. Eventually all mental abilities deteriorate to a greater or lesser extent, although basic perceptual and motor skills remain relatively preserved. Alzheimer's disease, unlike other progressive disorders, such as Huntington's disease or multiple sclerosis, does not produce severe difficulties in ambulation or loss of sensory functions. The representative, middle-stage Alzheimer patient may be ambulatory but will demonstrate obvious failure to recollect recent events, and may either speak incoherently, or coherently but with limited content. Names of objects and people may be forgotten, and spatial orientation may be significantly impaired. Gradually, the names of very familiar people, such as family members, may become increasingly less likely to be recalled, and familiar locations will be forgotten. The progression of the disorder has functional and psychopathological, as well as cognitive aspects. Functionally, there is gradual dilapidation of self-care skills, and though social skills may remain relatively preserved, numerous problems with activities of daily living emerge and increasingly compromise independent living. As time passes, the need for assistance in performing self-care activities increases, and placement in a nursing home is often required during the end stage of the disorder. Alzheimer's disease patients who live with their families become increasingly difficult to manage, and the tragedy of the disorder for family members may become a significant clinical condition. With regard to psychopathology, Alzheimer patients may sometimes develop delusions, often characterized by suspiciousness.

Agitation may also become problematic, and the patient may occasionally have angry verbal outbursts. Sometimes there is physical aggressiveness without apparent stimulation. Possible environmental stimuli for these behaviors have been suggested, but it is unclear in any general way that agitation seen in the elderly is either completely endogenous or is provoked by perhaps subtle environmental triggers.

It is generally reported that the course of the disorder from the appearance of first symptoms until death is 5 years. However, with good family and nursing care, patients with Alzheimer's disease often survive longer than that. There is no effective treatment for the disorder itself, but adequate health maintenance and support can increase longevity, as well as the quality of life, through the duration of the disorder.

COURSE AND PROGNOSIS

The course and prognosis for organic mental disorders also vary with the underlying disorder. We will review the basic considerations here by first introducing some stages of acceleration and development. Then we will provide examples of disorders that have courses and prognoses consistent with various accelerative and developmental combinations. The accelerative stages are steady state, slow, moderate, and rapid. The developmental stages are the perinatal period, early childhood, late childhood and adolescence, early adulthood, middle age, and old age. The accelerative stages have to do with the rate of progression of the disorder, and the developmental stages characterize the age of onset of symptoms.

Mental retardation is a disorder whose course involves onset during the perinatal period and steady-state acceleration. Mental retardation is one of those disorders in which there is little if any progression of neuropathology, but there may be a slowly progressive disability because of increasing environmental demands for cognitive abilities that the individual does not possess. Other developmental disorders, such as specific learning disability, do not have their onsets during the perinatal period but rather during early childhood when it is first expected that academic skills will be acquired.

In contrast to these disorders, stroke is typically characterized by onset during middle age. The acceleration of the disorder is first extremely rapid, then slows down, and gradually reaches a steady state. Thus, at the time of the stroke, the stroke patient becomes seriously ill very rapidly, and this is followed by additional destructive processes in the brain. Assuming a good outcome, a gradual recovery period follows, and the brain is restored to a relatively normal steady state. On the other hand, malignant brain tumors, which also tend to appear during middle age, progress rapidly and do not decelerate unless they are successfully surgically removed.

Progressive dementias generally appear during middle or old age and accelerate slowly or moderately. Huntington's disease generally progresses less rapidly than Alzheimer's disease, and so Huntington's patients may live long lives with their symptoms. Head trauma is a disorder that may occur at any age, but once the acute phase of the disorder is over, the brain typically returns to a steady state. Thus, if recovery from the acute condition is satisfactory, the head trauma patient may have a normal life expectancy with an often dramatic picture of deterioration immediately following the trauma until the resolution of the acute phase is completed and is followed by substantial recovery. However, the degree of residual disability may vary widely.

Briefly summarizing these considerations from a developmental standpoint, the most common organic mental disorder associated with the perinatal period is mental retardation and its variants. During early childhood, the specific and pervasive developmental disorders begin to appear. Head trauma typically begins to appear during late childhood and adolescence, and incidence peaks during young adulthood. Systemic illnesses, notably cardiovascular, cardiopulmonary, and neoplastic disease, most commonly impact negatively on brain functions during middle age. Dementia associated with alcoholism also begins to appear during early middle age. The progressive degenerative dementias are largely associated with old age. With regard to acceleration, developmental, vascular, and traumatic disorders tend to be relatively stable after the period surrounding the acquisition of the disorder. Malignant tumors and certain infectious disorders may be rapidly progressive, but the degenerative disorders progress at a slow to moderate pace.

The connotation of the term progressive is progressively worse, but not all organic mental disorders remain stable or get worse. There is recovery from certain disorders as a natural process or with the aid of treatment. In the case of head trauma, there is a rather typical history of initial unconsciousness that lapses into coma for a varying length of time, awakening, a period of memory loss and incomplete orientation called posttraumatic amnesia, and resolution of the amnesia. Rehabilitation is often initiated at some point in this progression, sometimes while the patient is still in a coma. The outcome of this combination of spontaneous recovery and rehabilitation is rarely, if ever, complete return to preinjury status, but often allows for a return to productive living in the community. Recovery from stroke is also common, and many poststroke patients can return to community living. Among the most important prognostic indicators for head trauma are the length of time in a coma and the length of posttraumatic amnesia. General health status is a good predictor for stroke outcome and potential for recurrence. Patients who maintain poor cardiac status, hypertension, inappropriate dietary habits, or substance abuse are poorer candidates for recovery than poststroke patients who do not have these difficulties. Some patients, particularly those who have chronic, severe hypertension, may have multiple strokes that resolves into a condition called multi-infarct dementia.

The efficacy of rehabilitation for head trauma and stroke patients remains a controversial area, but there is increasing evidence that rehabilitation may often have beneficial effects over and above spontaneous recovery. With regard to the developmental disorders, enormous efforts have been made in institutional and school settings to provide appropriate educational remediation for developmentally disabled children, often with some success. Effective treatment at the time of onset of acute disorder also has obvious implications for prognosis. The use of appropriate medications and management following trauma or stroke and the feasibility and availability of neurosurgery are major considerations. Tumors can be removed, aneurysms can be repaired, and increased pressure can be relieved by neurosurgeons. These interventions during the acute phase of a disorder are often mainly directed toward preserving life but also have important implications for the outcomes of surviving patients.

FAMILIAL AND GENETIC PATTERNS

Organic mental disorders are based on some diseases of known genetic origin, some diseases in which a genetic or familial component is suspected, and some that are clearly acquired disorders. It is well established that Huntington's disease and certain forms of mental retardation, notably Down's syndrome, are genetic disorders. There is evidence of a hereditary form of Alzheimer's disease, although the genetic contribution to Alzheimer's disease in general is not fully understood. Recently, a relative rare genetic subtype has been identified.

The great majority of individuals who have this subtype have a gene on chromosome 14, called Apolipoprotein E, that promotes development of the amyloid plaques that constitute the major brain pathology associated with the disease. Whether or not multiple sclerosis has a genetic component remains under investigation, although it is clearly not a hereditary disorder like Huntington's disease.

Of great recent interest is the role of genetics in the acquisition of alcoholism and subsequently dementia associated with alcoholism or alcohol amnestic disorder. Briefly, evidence suggests that having an alcoholic parent places one at higher than average risk for developing alcoholism. The specific genetic factors are far from understood, but the association in families is present. Whether having a family history of alcoholism increases the risk of acquiring dementia associated with alcoholism is not clear, but it has been shown that nonalcoholic sons of alcoholic fathers do more poorly on some cognitive tests than matched controls. The matter is substantially clearer in the case of the alcohol amnestic disorder of Korsakoff's syndrome. A widely cited study by Blass and Gibson (1977) showed that acquisition of Korsakoff's syndrome depends on the existence of a genetic defect in a liver enzyme called transketolase in combination with a thiamine deficiency.

Other genetic and familial factors associated with organic mental disorders relate largely to the genetics of underlying systemic disorders. Thus, the genetics of cancer might have some bearing on the likelihood of acquiring a brain tumor, and the genetics of the cardiovascular system might have some bearing on the risk of stroke. Disorders such as hypertension and diabetes run in families and have varying incidences in different ethnic groups. Ethnic specificity is sometimes quite precise (but this is rare), as in the case of Tay–Sachs disease, a degenerative disorder of early childhood, that is found almost exclusively in eastern European Jews.

Diagnostic Considerations

Neuropsychological assessment has become the state-of-the-art method for diagnosing organic mental disorders. Patients who have these disorders are often not amenable to structured diagnostic interviews, nor would an interview be an optimal methodology for determining the presence or absence of the various DSM-IV criteria for the organic mental disorders. Before describing the various assessment methods, however, something should be said about the purposes of diagnosing organic mental disorders because they differ in some respects from those of diagnosing the other mental disorders described in DSM-IV.

In the case of all disorders, the diagnostic process is concerned with whether a patient meets the criteria for a particular disorder or for more than one disorder. In the case of organic disorders, however, it seems that there may be particular concern with whether the patient's condition is treatable and reversible. In view of the dismal prognosis for many organic disorders and the aura of pessimism that surrounds them, it seems particularly incumbent upon the diagnostician to consider treatment possibilities. Common examples in the literature are the use of shunting to reverse dementia associated with normal-pressure hydrocephalus and appropriate medical treatment to reverse or reduce dementias associated with various metabolic or endocrinological disorders.

Beyond the issue of treatment and reversibility, establishing the presence of an organic mental disorder often does not have the same heuristic value as for other disorders. For example, establishing the diagnosis of attention-deficit hyperactivity disorder may immediately suggest a course of effective pharmacological intervention. Establishing the diagnosis of dementia makes no such suggestion. Generally, one needs a great deal more information to make a reasonable attempt at management and treatment planning. One usually wants to know something about the kinds of deficits present, their severity, and about the presence or absence of potentially compensatory preserved abilities. The task of gaining this knowledge is generally accomplished by a neuropsychological assessment. If the diagnosis of an organic mental disorder has not been established because of a difficult differential diagnostic problem, neuropsychological assessment may be helpful in answering the diagnostic question. In other words, it can help in determining whether the patient's symptoms are based on structural brain damage. Recent developments in neuroimaging have allowed diagnosticians to view the brain far more directly than was possible in the past, and so the role of neuropsychological tests has diminished somewhat in regard to answering the presence or absence question. A computed axial tomography (CT) or magnetic resonance imaging (MRI) scan has become a routine part of the diagnostic workup for an organic mental disorder.

In recent years, neuropsychological assessment has become increasingly involved in determining the extent of deficit in various cognitive functions and describing the patterns of impaired and preserved abilities. There are many neuropsychological tests and many theoretical approaches to neuropsychological assessment. We will provide a general outline of what a comprehensive neuropsychological assessment should contain, regardless of the particular tests used or theoretical approach taken.

General Orientation

A neuropsychological assessment generally consists of administering a series of individual tests or a group of tests incorporated into a battery. Typically, the tests are the performance type with rare use of rating scales or self-report questionnaires. To be characterized as a neuropsychological test, a procedure has to have demonstrated sensitivity to brain dysfunction. In a screening or comprehensive assessment, tests are selected to evaluate a number of functions and abilities. There are also specialized neuropsychological assessments that concentrate on one or a limited number of abilities. Many of the tests commonly used, such as the Wechsler intelligence scales, have been borrowed from the general collection of available tests, but their use in neuropsychology is based primarily on research using these tests with brain-damaged patients. There is a general consensus that the tests included in a comprehensive assessment should tap the areas of abstract reasoning and problem-solving ability, attention, memory, language, visual-spatial skills, and perceptual and motor skills. It is also often useful to obtain academic achievement scores, a general measure of intelligence (IQ), and a global index of the severity of impairment.

Abstract Reasoning and Problem Solving

These abilities are often significantly impaired in dementia, and such impairment constitutes perhaps the major obstacle to engaging in adaptive behavior. Brain-damaged patients typically have difficulty in organizing varying items of information so that inferences can be drawn in the form of concepts or abstractions. They are described as concrete, meaning that they react to the specific characteristics of environmental events with limited capability to generalize from experience. Tests of abstraction and problem solving consist mainly of sorting tests in which the subject has the task of organizing varying stimuli according to a concept that has to be learned by exposure to the stimuli. For example, in a procedure called the Wisconsin Card Sorting Test, the subject has to learn that cards containing colored geometric forms can be sorted by form, color, or the number of forms on the card.

Attention

Attentional dysfunction is the most prominent symptom of delirium, but attentional deficits, albeit of lesser severity, are common in other organic mental disorders. Brain-damaged patients may be distractible, disinhibited, or unable to maintain concentration. There is a form of attention dysfunction seen only in brain-damaged patients called unilateral neglect, and it is seen mainly in stroke patients or patients who have other forms of unilateral brain damage. The phenomenon is the inability to attend to either the right or left side of space. Neglect is most apparent in vision but may occur in the tactile or auditory modalities. Neuropsychologists generally test for neglect, as well as for other aspects of attention, with such tasks as repeating digits, discriminating between sound patterns, and performing psycho-motor tasks that require sustained concentration.

Memory

Some degree of memory impairment is seen in all organic mental disorders but is most clearly evident in pure amnesias or organic amnestic disorders. For purposes of neuropsychological assessment, it is important to distinguish among several forms of memory because the specific form of memory disorder found is often diagnostic. Thus, tests of short-term and long-term memory are usually administered, as are tests for recalling verbal and nonverbal material. Delayed recall, in which material presented about 20–30 minutes previously must be recalled, is a particularly sensitive neuropsychological measure. The Wechsler Memory Scale or some other short battery of memory tests is often included in a neuropsychological assessment.

Language

Impairment of language is less ubiquitous than impairment of abstraction and memory in organic mental disorders but is commonly seen. It is seen in its most dramatic forms in aphasia and in the impoverished language of the advanced Alzheimer's disease patient. Aspects of language generally evaluated by neuropsychologists are verbal intelligence and basic language functions. Verbal intelligence in general is evaluated with the verbal subtests of the Wechsler intelligence scales. Basic language functions are evaluated with one of many available aphasia tests. As part of a comprehensive evaluation, a full aphasia test is typically not administered, but one of several aphasia screening tests is used. The basic skills usually examined are word finding; repetition of spoken language; comprehension of spoken and written language; ability to read letters, words, and sentences; ability to perform simple calculations; and ability to produce extemporaneous speech. Sometimes the language evaluation also includes educational achievement tests.

Visual-Spatial Skills

Brain-damaged patients may become spatially disoriented, and may have difficulty finding locations without verbal cues. More often, however, they have difficulty in forming or analyzing spatial representations such that they become impaired in nonverbal problem solving. They cannot construct objects in two- or three-dimensional space and may have difficulty recognizing spatial complex patterns. They often have difficulty copying even relatively simple geometric forms. Neuropsychological assessment makes extensive use of complex perceptual, copying and other drawing, and constructional tasks to assess visual-spatial abilities.

Perceptual and Motor Skills

Patients who have organic mental disorders frequently have accompanying significant physical disabilities. On the sensory side they may be completely or partially blind, they may be completely or partially deaf, or they may suffer from significant losses of the senses of touch, smell, or taste. The stroke patient, for example, may have some degree of dementia, aphasia, and paralysis of the right side of the body. Multiple sclerosis sometimes produces progressive blindness. Neuropsychologists may do limited evaluations of basic sensory and motor status but typically are more concerned with these functions at a skill level. Thus, in the case of vision, the interest would be less in visual acuity than in the capacity to identify objects or recognize faces. The important point here is that these skill-level deficits can exist in the presence of completely normal sensory or motor function. In the case of motor function, the patient may not be paralyzed but may be unable to pantomime or make pretended movements and gestures when asked to do so. Thus, a comprehensive neuropsychological assessment contains tests of a variety of perceptual and motor abilities such as the ability to recognize objects by touch, motor speed, and dexterity and the ability to identify or analyze simple and more complex visual stimuli, such as overlapping or ambiguous geometric forms.

Academic Achievement and IQ

For various reasons, academic achievement tests are used as components of neuro-psychological assessment of children and adults. Some neuropsychological tests require some degree of reading ability, and therefore it is important to know whether the patient has a sufficient reading level to produce valid performance on these tests. A second reason is that these tests conveniently provide material for extended examination of those disorders that impair academic skills. There are conditions called acquired alexia, agraphia, and acalculia in which the ability to read, write, or calculate is impaired by structural brain damage, usually stroke or head trauma. Finally, neuropsychologists typically assess individuals who have either developmental or acquired brain disorders. The distinction made in DSM-IV between "Disorders Usually First Diagnosed in Infancy, Childhood, or Adolescence" and "Delirium, Dementia, and Amnestic and Other Cognitive Disorders" does not work well for neuro-psychology because both developmental and acquired conditions are viewed by neuropsychol-ogists as neurobehavioral disorders. Indeed, there is extensive neuropsychological research and practice in the areas of learning disability and other pervasive and specific developmental disorders. Some time ago, it was documented that learning disability, once considered a disorder of children, may persist into adulthood (Spreen, 1987).

The use of intelligence tests in neuropsychological assessment is not generally to obtain an IQ for classification or selection purposes but is more typically used to supplement procedures that are more specifically defined as neuropsychological tests. The Wechsler Verbal IQ is often used as an indicator of premorbid level, but it is not an unequivocal indicator, particularly in the case of aphasic patients. Several of the performance subtests, particularly Block Design and Digit Symbol, are highly sensitive to many forms of brain dysfunction. Large discrepancies between verbal and performance IQs sometimes suggest specific damage to one or the other cerebral hemisphere.

Extent of Impairment

It is useful as part of a neuropsychological assessment to provide a global index of the extent of impairment, in addition to a profile of specific impaired and preserved abilities. Such indexes of impairment are useful in estimating the overall degree of disability and capacity for independent function. There are several ways of obtaining these indexes, including converting all individual test scores to standard scores and calculating the mean standard score or counting the number of tests that fall above or below cutoff scores for impairment that are empirically established for each test. The latter method is more useful and is the most commonly used.

SUMMARY

Delirium, Dementia, and Amnestic and Other Cognitive Disorders, formerly known as Organic Mental Disorders, are a variety of conditions that adversely affect behavior by structural damage to the central nervous system. At the most general level, they are classified into the categories of delirium, dementia, amnesia, and other syndromes that primarily affect personality, mood, or anxiety level. The etiology of this set of disorders is extremely heterogeneous because the central nervous system may suffer most of the disorders and diseases that affect other systems and organs of the body and also has its own diseases, such as multiple sclerosis and Huntington's disease. The age of onset, course, and the outcome of these disorders depend on the specifics of the various pathologies.

Clinically, it is important to note that structural brain damage has major implications for cognitive function. It can impair reasoning ability, attention, memory, language, spatial abilities, and a variety of perceptual and motor skills, such as visual recognition or manual dexterity. Therefore, the disorders associated with structural brain damage are often severely and permanently disabling conditions. These cognitive impairments are sometimes associated with physical disability, such as blindness or paralysis, and with personality changes, such as the development of impulse control difficulties. It is critically important to know the expected course of the disorder because it is essentially impossible to do rational treatment planning without such knowledge. Some of these disorders, such as Alzheimer's disease, are unremitting, progressive illnesses. Others, once acquired, do not change much beyond the acute period, and the patient may live a normal life span with varying amounts of residual disability.

Appropriate diagnosis involves an interdisciplinary neurobehavioral evaluation, which should include a preliminary mental status and physical neurological examination, appropriate neuroimaging studies, additional laboratory tests as indicated, such as an EEG, and a neuropsychological assessment. Traditionally, diagnosis has been emphasized for good reasons. First, there is a need to determine whether the disorder is directly treatable or reversible to a greater or lesser extent. Second, these disorders are often quite complex, and detailed neuropsychological assessment is required to identify the specific nature of the syndrome or the pattern of impaired and preserved abilities that the patient has. Knowledge of these patterns is of obvious import for treatment planning, management, and rehabilitation.

ACKNOWLEDGMENT.   Indebtedness is expressed to the Medical Research Service, Department of Veterans Affairs for support of this work.

REFERENCES

American Psychiatric Association. (1987). *Diagnostic and statistical manual of mental disorders*, 3rd ed., rev. (DSM-III-R). Washington, DC: Author.

Blass, J. P., & Gibson, G. E. (1977). Abnormality of a thiamine-requiring enzyme in patients with Wernicke–Korsakoff syndrome. *The New England Journal of Medicine, 297,* 1367–1370.

Butters, N., & Cermak, L. S. (1980). *Alcoholic Korsakoff's syndrome.* New York: Academic Press.

Caine, E. D. (1986). The neuropsychology of depression: The pseudodementia syndrome. In I. Grant & K. M. Adams (Eds.), *Neuropsychological assessment of neuropsychiatric disorders* (pp. 221–243). New York: Oxford University Press.

Grant, I., Atkinson, J. H., Hesselink, J. R., Kennedy, C. J., Richman, D. D., Spector, S. A., & McCutchan, J. A. (1987). Evidence for early central nervous system involvement in the acquired immunodeficiency syndrome (AIDS) and other human immunodeficiency virus (HIV) infections. *Annals of Internal Medicine, 107,* 828–836.

Gusella, J. F., Wexler, N. S., Conneallly, P. M., Naylor, S. L., Anderson, M. A., Tanzi, R. E., Watkins, P. C., Ottina, K., Wallace, M. R., Sakaguchi, A. Y., Young, A. B., Shoulson, I., Bonilla, E., & Martin, J. B. (1983). A polymorphic DNA marker genetically linked to Huntington's disease. *Nature, 306,* 234–238.

Heilman, K. M., & Valenstein, E. (Eds.). (1993). *Clinical neuropsychology*, 3rd ed. New York: Oxford University Press.

Levin, H. S., Benton, A. L., & Grossman, R. G. (1982). *Neurobehavioral consequences of closed head injury.* New York: Oxford University Press.

Levin, H. S., Eisenberg, H. M., & Benton, A. L. (1989). *Mild head injury.* New York: Oxford University Press.

McCue, M., & Goldstein, G. (1991). Neuropsychological aspects of learning disability in adults. In B. P. Rourke (Ed.), *Neuropsychological validation of learning disability subtypes* (pp. 311–329). New York: Guilford.

Neils, J., Boller, F., Gerdeman, B., & Cole, M. (1989). Descriptive writing abilities in Alzheimer's disease. *Journal of Clinical and Experimental Neuropsychology, 11,* 692–698.

Nussbaum, P. D. (1994). Pseudodementia: A slow death. *Neuropsychology Review, 4,* 71–90.

Smith, R. J., Barth, J. T., Diamond, R., & Giuliamo, A. J. (1998). Evaluation of head trauma. In G. Goldstein, P. D. Nussbaum, & S. R. Beers (Eds.), *Neuropsychology* (pp. 135–170). New York: Plenum.

Spreen, O. (1987). *Learning disabled children growing up: A follow-up into adulthood.* Lisse, The Netherlands: Swets & Zeitlinger.

Van Gorp, W. G., Miller, E. N., Satz, P., & Visscher, B. (1989). Neuropsychological performance in HIV-1 immunocompromised patients: A preliminary report. *Journal of Clinical and Experimental Neuropsychology, 11,* 763–773.

Wells, C. E. (1979). Pseudodementia. *American Journal of Psychiatry, 136,* 895–900.

Wells, C. E. (1980). The differential diagnosis of psychiatric disorders in the elderly. In J. O. Cole & J. E. Barrett (Eds.), *Psychopathology in the aged.* New York: Raven Press.

IV

Child Treatment:
Introductory Comments

The growing awareness of etiological factors in childhood disorders, combined with the burgeoning body of research attesting to their short- and long-term deleterious consequences, has led to a dramatic upsurge in clinical and investigative interest in remediation strategies for youth. Findings that attest to the magnitude and complexity of many childhood disorders have led to an increase in interdisciplinary approaches in this area. In particular, work in the fields of psychiatry, developmental psychology, and special education has had a substantial impact on the directions of child treatment in recent years. The chapters in this part of the book reflect the expanded and widened scope of endeavors directed toward ameliorating childhood disorders.

In Chapter 22, Kevin O'Connor, Karyn Ewart, and Ilizabeth Wollheim present an overview of psychoanalytical interventions for children. They provide a variety of strategies under this rubric (e.g., free association, play therapy, and transference) and discuss the similarities and differences between child and adult psychoanalytic therapy. The range of behavioral interventions is discussed by Lisa W. Coyne and Alan M. Gross (Chapter 23). These authors examine treatment techniques derived from classical and operant conditioning, observational learning, and cognitive therapy. They also underscore the importance of integrating approaches from other disciplines (e.g., developmental psychology) and emphasize the empirical evaluation of treatment effects. Pharmacological interventions are presented by Keith Cheng and Kathleen Myers (Chapter 24). Here, the use of medications to treat psychiatric disorders, emotional problems, and behavioral symptoms in children and adolescents is comprehensively covered. Special considerations (e.g., choice of drug, regulation of dose, and monitoring of beneficial and adverse effects) in using pharmacological approaches are discussed.

22

Psychodynamic Psychotherapy with Children

Kevin J. O'Connor, Karyn Ewart, and Ilizabeth Wollheim

Introduction

The term psychodynamic is used in this chapter to refer to all forms of psychotherapy that derive from classical psychoanalysis developed by Sigmund Freud (1938). Briefly stated,

> In classical psychoanalysis, a client presents with a *neurotic symptom* that is the result of *internal conflict* operating out of the client's conscious awareness due to the use of *defense mechanisms*. In the therapy sessions the client divulges material related to the areas of conflict, usually in the form of *free associations*. It is the therapist's task to organize this material in a manner consistent with psychoanalytic personality theory, and to offer understanding of the client's personality dynamics to the client in the form of *interpretations*. Once the client gains *insight*, and then works *through* the material interpreted by the therapist, alleviation of the neurotic symptom occurs. The client is then free to choose to make behavioral changes on the basis of greater self-understanding.

As can be seen from this brief summary, psychoanalytic theory and practice tend to be bogged down by a language all of its own, which can seem intriguing at its best and undecipherable at its worst. The details of the model, including definitions of the italicized terminology, are presented in this chapter. The reader should be aware that the definition and use of many psychoanalytic terms vary from one psychoanalytic writer to another. What this chapter attempts to provide is an integrated, consensual view of the range of psychoanalytic and psychodynamic psychotherapies for children. In so doing, some liberties have been taken in simplifying the material presented.

Most of the psychodynamic therapies developed for use with adults are derived from classical Freudian analysis, but psychodynamic therapies for children generally derive from the child analytic models of either Anna Freud or Melanie Klein. These two fundamental

Kevin J. O'Connor, Karyn Ewart, and Ilizabeth Wollheim • California School of Professional Psychology, Fresno, California 93727.

Advanced Abnormal Psychology, Second Edition, edited by Hersen and Van Hasselt. Kluwer Academic/Plenum Publishers, New York, 2001.

models of child analysis differ with respect to the very nature of psychopathology, the age at which children are considered suitable candidates for analysis, the role of the child's play in the analysis, and the way in which interpretations are delivered to the child client. Out of their work came two specific psychodynamic models, Object Relations Theory and Ego Psychology. Both expand on the basic concepts of Freud's psychoanalytic model. In recognition of these differences, psychodynamic variations of basic psychoanalytic theory and practice are highlighted throughout the chapter.

The chapter begins with a discussion of the psychoanalytic theory of personality development and structure as well as the Object Relations Theory and Ego Psychology modifications of that model that underlie the practice of child psychodynamic psychotherapy. An extensive discussion of the therapy process follows.

PERSONALITY THEORY

Sigmund Freud's contribution to psychological knowledge and treatment is remarkably comprehensive in that he developed the psychoanalytic theory of personality development and functioning and also the treatment model that follows from the theory. Important components of his theory include models of psychosexual development, the structure and topography of personality, and psychopathology. In conceptualizing the relationship between psychoanalytic personality theory and child psychodynamic therapy, it is most important to recognize the developmental aspects of the model. Freud conceptualized two parallel lines of development. One line involves the child's progression through five psychosexual stages, and the other consists of the development of a balanced personality structure.

Psychosexual Stages

Psychoanalytic theory proposes that children progress through five psychosexual stages between birth and adolescence (Freud, 1905). Each stage is grounded on the anatomical or bodily focus of the child's instinctual sexual energies. Note that Freud used the term sexual rather loosely to include all bodily functions that give an individual pleasure. All such sexual energy, it was thought, drives individuals toward survival. This drive to survive was labeled *libido* and the underlying sexual energy is called *libidinal* energy. Libidinal energy, it was thought, propels the individual through the process of development. Each stage also includes developmental tasks that must be negotiated for development to proceed optimally.

Object Relations Theory added to the developmental model in two ways. One addition was the notion that development was driven and structured by libidinal energy and also by a person's early interactions. Winnicott (1964, 1965) suggested that environmental influences, specifically parental figures, strongly influence a child's development. Bowlby (1958, 1988) and Ainsworth et al. (1978) elaborated on the idea of "good enough mothering." Specifically, this is the notion that infants need a period of early adequate parenting to develop into mentally healthy children and adults. They contended that the existence and nature of the children's bonds or attachments to their primary caregivers were essential to healthy development (Shirk & Russell, 1996). This increased focus on early relationships led to a greater focus on Freud's description of the oral stage and to the proposal of significant substages.

The first stage of Freud's (1905) model is called the *oral stage*. It lasts from birth until approximately age 2. The focus of libidinal energy during this first phase is the mouth, which is biologically adaptive in that it focuses the infant on receiving nourishment. The most significant developmental task of the oral stage is the formation of a secure attachment to a primary caretaker(s). To the extent that this is achieved, trust is also developed, and the stage is set for successfully negotiating the process of separation and individuation from the caretaker as the child transitions out of the oral stage.

For the purposes of this chapter, Margaret Mahler's (1979) theory will be used to describe the oral substages that are a key element of Object Relations Theory. Mahler believes that at birth, the infant is unable to differentiate between self and other. (The concept of self versus other/object is further discussed in the section on Personality Structures.) In other words, the infant does not have a concept of self distinct from anything else. Object Relations calls this first substage the autistic stage. In this undifferentiated stage, the infant is unable to distinguish between internal and external reality and thus cannot differentiate self from others. However, there is some controversy between Object Relations theorists as to whether there really is a normal autistic stage. Mahler contends that there is but Bettelheim (1967), Klein (1932), and others disagree. The second substage is the symbiotic stage. In this stage, infants start to become aware that their needs are being met by some outside entity. However, the object and self are still fused. The third substage, separation-individuation, is composed of three phases: differentiation, practicing, and rapprochement. During these phases, the infant further recognizes the relationship between self and others. In other words, a healthy split develops between self and other. In the course of making this split, the infant also develops an awareness of good and bad feelings. Early on, children tend to see objects and their own feelings as either all good or all bad. They do not perceive shades of gray in feelings. The ability to feel ambivalent develops somewhat later when children should be able to tolerate more ambiguity within themselves and within the caretaker. Objects can now be seen as both rewarding and frustrating. From the perspective of Object Relations, the health of future relationships depends on the patterns that are established in these early interactions (Mahler, 1979; Roser, 1996).

From approximately ages 2 to 4, children are expected to negotiate tasks associated with what Freud called the *anal stage*, when libidinal energy is focused on the process of elimination. The major tasks of this period include developing both internal and external control, as well as *self-* and *object-constancy*. These last two terms refer to the child's ability to view itself and those around it as separate individuals whose stable characteristics endure over time. If development proceeds as expected, the child emerges from the anal stage with a rudimentary sense of autonomy.

During the *phallic stage*, libidinal energy is concentrated on the penis, its presence in the case of boys and its absence in the case of girls. It is during this time that the *oedipal conflict* occurs. The oedipal conflict refers to the period of a child's development when, it is theorized, boys hope to eliminate their fathers and keep their mothers for themselves and girls hope to eliminate their mothers in hopes of obtaining a penis or its substitute, a child, from their fathers. Boys successfully negotiate the oedipal conflict by defensively identifying with their fathers and relinquishing their mothers as objects of sexual desire. Girls must abandon their fantasy of impregnation by their fathers and identify with their mothers to resolve the conflict. It should be noted that the female child's experience of the oedipal conflict remains one of the most controversial aspects of psychoanalytic theory.

From the resolution of the oedipal conflict until the onset of adolescence, the child is in the *latency stage*. During this long period, cognitive and social development are more prominent than psychosexual development. The tasks of this period include forming peer relationships, adjusting to major changes in body development and body image, and developing new cognitive skills and interests.

Finally, at adolescence, children enter the *genital stage*, where they remain throughout adulthood. During this phase, libidinal energy is focused on the genitals. The primary task of the stage is the development of a stable, one-to-one, intimate relationship with another adult.

Personality Structures

Simultaneous with the child's progress through the psychosexual stages just described, Freud (1933) postulated that human behavior can be understood in terms of three psychological configurations or structures which account for all human experience and behavior.

The first of these, the *id*, is the original structure, present at birth. Driven by biological forces, including libido, the id acts on impulse and operates according to the *pleasure principle*, in that it is solely interested in gratifying basic needs, irrespective of external constraints. It is the domain of instincts, wishes, needs, and fantasies. Id-dominated thought is referred to as *primary process*. Primary-process thought is magical, grounded in imagery, based on internal rather than external stimulation, and unconcerned with the limitations of reality.

Next to develop is the *ego*, which compels the id to work within the constraints of reality. The word ego, as originally intended by Freud, means "self," and is a shorthand way of speaking about the entire range of conscious mental functioning. The ego operates according to the reality principle. It is dominated by secondary process (goal-directed, logical, reality-oriented) thinking. It is assumed that the ego begins to develop as the child separates from its primary caretaker because at this point external reality begins to have meaning for the child. Infants do not concern themselves with reality so long as their id impulses are satisfied. As children separate, they recognize that some of the sources of their satisfaction are external to themselves and that they must delay gratification in some circumstances. These realizations are the beginnings of ego functioning.

Again, Object Relations Theory expanded on the notion of the ego. Winnicott proposed an entity beyond the ego called the self. Although Winnicott saw the ego as a regulatory mechanism, he viewed the self as the development of the core person who perceives feelings and relatedness to others. The self is comprised of those conscious and unconscious mental representations that the individual constitutes as "me." In counterpoint to the development of the self, individuals develop a sense of the *other* or *object*. The object is the person, fantasy, or place that is the focus of emotional energy. It is not necessarily a reality-based tangible object.

Last to develop is the *superego*. It is the internal representation of the traditional values and ideals of a society reflected and imposed by the parents through rewards, punishment, and overt, as well as unconscious communication. This structure is colloquially referred to as the "conscience." Sigmund Freud and Anna Freud (1936) hypothesized that the superego forms as the child resolves the oedipal conflict at approximately age 5. On the other hand, Melanie Klein (1932) hypothesized that the successful negotiation of separation and individuation, which occurs at about age 2, resulted in the child's development of a primitive superego. This superego is the result of the child's virtual absorption of an image of the primary caretaker, including all of the caretaker's rules and expectations, to make separations tolerable. In other words, the child's mental representation of the parent consoles the child and controls its behavior in the parent's absence. The relevance of this theoretical debate to the treatment of young children is discussed later.

Personality Topography

In addition to conceptualizing the structure of the human psyche according to the tripartite model discussed earlier, Freud (1900, 1915) also developed a *topographical* or depth model. This paradigm divides the mind into the *conscious*, the *preconscious*, and the *unconscious*. The conscious, which includes everything in awareness at any given time, accounts for a very small portion of that which is contained in the mind or psyche. It has often been called the "tip of the iceberg." The dominant portion of the psyche is the unconscious, which includes most id and superego elements. Thus, most behavior is driven and/or contained by forces outside of a person's awareness. According to Freudian theory, unconscious thoughts enter consciousness only in veiled or symbolic form. Finally, the preconscious, which is topographically located "between" the conscious and the unconscious, includes thoughts that, although not part of one's continuous awareness, can be easily brought to consciousness.

Normality and Pathology

Optimal functioning is evidenced when the id, ego, and superego interact in a delicate balance (Freud, 1923). The id pushes the child to seek gratification of basic needs and drives, whereas the superego strives to direct the child to satisfy the id within the constraints imposed by its parents and society. When a conflict arises between the two structures, the ego mediates and attempts to find a realistic way to gratify the id within the constraints imposed by the superego. When a compromise is not possible in reality, the ego uses *defense mechanisms* to circumvent the conflict to allow the child to continue functioning. The term *defense mechanisms* refers to characteristic ways the ego has of distorting reality so as to diffuse a conflict. As the child progresses through its psychosexual stages, it learns more complex and adaptive defense mechanisms. The ego of a young child is likely to use the defense of *denial*, where the ego simply refuses to recognize that a conflict or conflict-producing situation exists. For example, a young child may simply act as if its mother has not died even when faced with evidence that the event is real. The ego of an older child might respond to the same event with the defense of *projection*, which the child attributes its own pain to someone else, perhaps by talking about how sad its dolls are about mom's death while stating that it is not suffering. When older children use more primitive defenses, it is considered diagnostic of serious problems.

Within a psychoanalytic framework, psychopathology generally, it is thought, ensues from one of two underlying phenomena. *Neurotic* pathology is seen as resulting from conflict between the id and superego, which the ego is unable to resolve either in reality or by using defense mechanisms (A. Freud, 1926). Then, the child becomes overwhelmed by anxiety or uses defense mechanisms excessively and reflexively, resulting in the development of a neurotic symptom.

When the child begins to experience a neurotic symptom, *regression* or *fixation* becomes a possibility. This is the tendency during times of psychological tension or distress to revert to developmentally earlier patterns of responding. The particular developmental phase to which the child regresses is determined by the extent to which it successfully negotiated the tasks associated with each of the psychosexual stages. If the child was overly frustrated or gratified at a particular stage, it will continue to proceed through the subsequent stages, but responds to stress in a manner consistent with the stage at which the frustration occurred. If the frustration was so severe or the gratification so overwhelming that further development becomes impossible, then fixation is said to have occurred.

When working with children, both Anna Freud and Melanie Klein discovered that some clients did not respond to their interpretive, insight-oriented interventions. Thus, both theorists began to hypothesize the existence of a second, nonneurotic type of pathology. They proposed that some children exhibited ego deficits. In other words, instead of the problem being a conflict between existing structures, these children lacked fully formed structures—their egos were not fully developed. Additionally, these structural deficits in the ego, it was hypothesized, resulted from environmental as opposed to intrapsychic causes (Shirk & Russell, 1996).

According to Object Relations Theory, nonneurotic pathology resulted when there were problems with one's early interactions with the caregiver and is associated with distorted Object Relations (Blanck & Blanck, 1979, 1994). Object Relations conceptualizes three types of pathology that correspond to whatever stage of development or individuation was disrupted. Again, individual Object Relations theorists conceptualize pathology somewhat differently, but the overall structure each describes is similar. For the purpose of this discussion, Masterson's model adapted from Masterson and Klein's 1995 text is used.

According to Masterson, there are three types of personality disorders: schizoid, borderline, and narcissistic. Technically, none of these disorders manifest in children whose personalities are still in a state of flux and thus much more amenable to treatment. However, it is children's very amenability to treatment that makes it so important to recognize and treat the precursors of these severe personality disorders early.

In schizoid personalities, individuals are distrustful of relationships and thus isolate themselves. Schizoid personality is seen as resulting from attachment-related problems. For these individuals, the model on which they base relationships parallels the master–servant dyad. These individuals feel that they must present themselves as dependent slaves to objects who will serve as masters. Schizoid individuals often feel that any attempts toward individuation will lead to being ignored, devalued, criticized, punished, and rejected. Thus, these individuals feel that assertion is dangerous and results in exile and abandonment. As a consequence, schizoid individuals feel safe only if they are either not connected to others or if they completely become what the other person wants them to be. They often exhibit patterns of getting close and then distancing as they attempt to balance their need for closeness with their fear of rejection. Some characteristics of schizoid individuals include paranoia, sensitivity, and problems with attunement, self-reflection, and self-evaluation. Schizoid individuals are often difficult to treat in therapy because they expect the therapist to reenact the master–slave dyad.

Borderline pathology results from disruptions during the practicing and rapprochement phases of the oral stage. These individuals display a pull for dependency, helplessness, and regression. Borderline children learn that they get their needs met by being inadequate. For them, the maternal object offers approval for regressive and clingy behaviors. Individuals who have borderline personalities fear taking initiative or being competent because they believe that if they assert these behaviors, they will no longer get their needs met. Borderline individuals have an inadequate and negative sense of self. Some characteristics of borderline individuals include poor perception of reality, frustration tolerance, ego boundaries, and impulse control. One of the defining characteristics of borderline personalities is the tendency to exhibit *splitting*. Individuals who split see objects as all good or all bad. They believe that someone who meets their needs is all good, but should that person deny even the most trivial need, the borderline individual becomes enraged and forgets everything good ever received. Suddenly, the person is all bad. This characteristic makes borderline individuals particularly challenging clients as they vacillate between adoring and hating the therapist (Kernberg, 1975).

A narcissistic personality is the consequence of fusion between the object and self and is seen as arising from development postrapprochement disruptions and individuation. Narcissistic individuals believe that the only way to maintain a successful attachment relationship is to fuse with the object. The problem occurs when parents derive their ego strength from the child by aggrandizing the infant. The parents increase their own sense of self-worth by seeing the child as a perfect extension of themselves. On the one hand the infant feels that it can do no wrong, yet at the same time the child is forced to disregard its own aspirations in favor of mirroring the parent's needs and desires. People see themselves as valuable only so long as they are perceived as valuable by parents. Later in life, they obsessively seek out those who will adore them and value them the way their parents did. To get this adoration, they will attempt to mirror those around them just as they mirrored the parent. They fail to develop a real sense of either the other person or themselves. Like a reflection in a mirror, they are transient and one dimensional. They develop a defensive or false self that covers up feelings of inadequacy. Characteristics of narcissistic individuals include grandiosity, lack of empathy, and an exaggeration of achievements or talents.

Ego psychology distinguishes itself by focusing on the adaptive function of the ego (Blanck & Blanck, 1994). Ego psychology introduced the notion of a continuum of function from unstructured clients, those individuals who have schizoid, borderline, or narcissistic conditions who have experienced arrested development resulting in incomplete separation-individuation, to structured clients, who have more neurotic conditions. Structured individuals were able to go through separation-individuation in their development that resulted in the emergence of a distinct identity. They exhibit a relatively intact ego that can tolerate frustration and endure conflict. This continuum integrates the psychoanalytic and Object Relations models of psychopathology.

CLIENTS

Inclusion Criteria

Neurotic symptoms and related regression is the type of pathology that is considered most responsive to psychoanalytic intervention. Anna Freud (1945) believed that children under age 5, who have not yet resolved the oedipal conflict or developed a superego, cannot experience internalized conflict and subsequent neurosis. Therefore, preoedipal children are considered unsuitable candidates for psychoanalysis, as are those who suffer from personality level pathology. In addition to the presence of internalized conflict, Neubauer (1978) suggests that a child is suitable for analysis if the child has some verbal abilities and the parents are both willing to participate in the child's treatment and able to tolerate therapeutic gains that lead to an improvement in the child's development. An additional criterion is the ability to establish a relationship with the therapist, which may preclude treating children younger than age 3. This is due to the fact that, under normal circumstances, relationship skills begin to develop during the oral stage and become solidified through separation and individuation during the anal stage of development.

Melanie Klein's (1932) contention that children develop a primitive type of superego by age 2 led her to believe that very young children can experience internalized conflict and thus are suitable candidates for psychoanalysis. Additionally, dynamic modifications of psycho-analysis, most notably Ego Psychology and Object Relations Theory, allow for *creation* and *strengthening*, as well as modifying, personality structures in therapy. This opens up the possibility of treating children who have more severe forms of psychopathology, which are thought to have their roots in earlier, that is, preoedipal experience, and may be manifest by apparent insufficient ego or superego development.

Indications for Treatment

With children at different developmental levels, there are likely to be particular symp-toms and manifestations of psychopathology, which we briefly discuss here. Some behavior or symptoms should be considered pathological regardless of the age of the child in which they appear. For example, homicidal thinking would be considered pathological in all children. Alternatively, some behavior or symptoms are only viewed as pathological when they are not consistent with the child's current developmental level. For example, extreme fear of strangers is very common and developmentally appropriate in 9-month-old children, but it is considered unhealthy in a 4-year-old. The same principle applies when one looks at the types of ego defense mechanisms used by children of different ages.

CHILDREN UNDER 6

Children in this age range are most likely to present in therapy as a result of failure to meet developmental milestones. Examples of such departures may include a 2-year-old child who is evidencing extreme separation anxiety, a 3-year-old who is not speaking, or a 5-year-old who is not toilet trained. As opposed to the older child or adult who regresses to earlier ways of functioning in the face of stress, these types of presenting problems represent current fixations.

CHILDREN 6–11

When children enter the school system, parents are likely to bring them for therapy to address what they perceive as peer-related difficulties. At the lower end of this age range, children make the sometimes difficult transition from functioning only within their families to functioning in a large peer group. Because this is a new step in the process of separation and individuation, children who have been able to function previously may begin to manifest symptoms at this time. Depression is also a somewhat common presenting problem among school-age children, and because a complete personality structure should have developed by now, early signs of defects in that structure are sometimes observed.

ADOLESCENTS

Major developmental tasks for adolescents include achieving independence and responsibility and developing their own identities within the context of family and peer group. Parents of adolescents are often concerned that these tasks are not being negotiated adequately and are particularly worried about their adolescents' peer group identification. Adolescents often enter treatment secondary to these concerns and fears. Most adolescents present with symptoms of either behavioral or affective disturbances, particularly oppositional behavior and depression.

THERAPISTS

The theory of personality, psychopathology, and treatment underlying child analysis is remarkably complex, and a thorough grasp of all of this is necessary to competently and ethically engage in its practice. Therefore, advanced postdoctoral training at an analytic institute is required (O'Connor, 1991). This level of training is not required of all therapists who adhere to one or another of the psychodynamic modifications because these treatment modalities are often less complex and intensive. However, regardless of the therapeutic modality one practices, it is still of great importance to operate from a strong theoretical base.

THEORY OF TREATMENT

Strategy/Cure

Theoretically, the task of psychoanalytic work with children consists of two parts and is much the same as work with adults, as described in the opening paragraph of this chapter. Initially, the neurotic conflict is brought to consciousness by interpretation. Once this is accomplished, the work of analysis involves reorganizing the personality structures to allow addressing the conflict in reality rather than through excessive use of defense mechanisms (O'Connor, Lee, & Schaefer, 1983). If this work is successful, the optimal result is behavioral change and a subjective experience of no longer being "stuck."

Because reorganizing of the personality structures that the child spent years developing is viewed as such a labor-intensive task, analytic work has always consisted of frequent sessions conducted over a long period of time. The frequency of therapy sessions is one of the things that distinguishes analysis from its psychodynamic modifications. Traditionally, both child and adult analysis have, by definition, occurred daily, either five or six times per week. Some analysts, including Anna Freud (Sandler, Kennedy, & Tyson, 1980), maintain that the reasons for modifying this practice are extratherapeutic (e.g., financial or a matter of convenience for parents) rather than in the best interest of the child, and thus are not justifiable. Most psychodynamic therapists do not see their clients more than one or two times per week, which is considered adequate contact to do the work indicated. Similarly, analysts tend to continue their client's therapy for a period of years, whereas many psychodynamic therapists terminate therapy in a matter of months. This difference is largely due to the fact that psychodynamic therapies do not attempt to accomplish the same degree or depth of reorganization that analysis attempts.

Psychodynamic therapy modifies psychoanalytic work in that the model views the child as a work in progress—one whose development is ongoing and whose personality structures are in the process of being formed. The therapist must, therefore, address any existing conflicts or arrests plus ever changing developmental factors (Chethik, 1989). Accordingly, therapy focuses on fostering the development of personality structures and strengthening existing elements. As such, it is considered a more supportive therapy that promotes building ego strength. Specifically, Anna Freud recommends two options when working with children who have ego deficits. One method involves therapists using their interactions with the child to provide a corrective emotional experience for the child. In other words, the therapist models a healthy relationship with the child, and this interaction fosters ego development. The second method involves working directly with the parents to make the child's environment more adaptive and thus more likely to promote healthy ego development (Shirk & Russell, 1996). Both ego-building strategies and collateral work with parents are addressed later in this chapter.

Object Relations Theory also proposes that the early treatment of more disturbed clients moves in three stages. In the first stage, the therapist confronts the client's defenses so that these can be recognized. In the second stage, the therapist looks at the individual's style of interpersonal interaction. For example, the therapist seeks to determine whether an individual's relationships are most characterized by avoiding (indicative of a schizoid personality), by helplessness (indicative of a borderline personality), or by deferring or devaluing (indicative of narcissism). In the third stage, the therapist looks at the way the client typically portrays or perceives objects. For example, therapists would determine whether the clients perceive themselves as damaged, brilliant, perfect, in exile, abandoned, or lonely. Once these early stages are completed, the therapist may go on to pursue more traditional psychoanalytic work. Several technical modifications are considered necessary, depending on the specific nature of the client's psychopathology. When working with schizoid clients, Object Relations therapists avoid confrontation but attempt to be up-front and clear because schizoid clients tend to be paranoid. Therapists use confrontation with borderline clients, to make these individuals responsible for their own behavior. Finally, with narcissistic clients, therapists focus on helping the clients accept who they are, including their inadequacies, while attempting to avoid sensitivity of these clients to criticism. Again, it should be noted that these disorders do not typically manifest full blown in children; rather it is the precursors that are assessed and treated.

Regardless of the frequency and duration of therapy and whether the treatment is analytic or dynamic, the client's *free association* and *transference* provide the primary sources of material to be interpreted by the therapist.

Free Association and Play

Briefly, free association is a "talking-out" technique that involves having patients articulate everything that enters their minds without allowing their internal censors to screen out thoughts, feelings, or fantasies that their conscious minds consider inappropriate. Although the succession of articulations are likely to appear random or even bizarre to an outside observer, the assumption is that there are extremely relevant unconscious connections among the sequential thoughts in the free associations. It is the therapist's role to recognize, make sense of, and ultimately to interpret the repetitive patterns (O'Connor, 1991).

Not surprisingly, children often have cognitive and emotional difficulty in trying to associate freely. In response to this, Melanie Klein (1955) viewed the child's play as the virtual equivalent of free association, and thus directly interpretable. From a psychodynamic perspective, Miller (1996) modified this view by noting that the therapist must attune to and even join the child's inner world to understand the child's play. Anna Freud (1926) viewed play primarily as a tool analysts use to develop relationships with their clients. Hence, she saw the function of play as a preparation for the "real," that is, verbal work of therapy rather than as the substance of treatment itself. Consistent with current practice in the United States, the model presented here tends to take an integrative position on this issue. Play may be used both for relationship building and as a source of symbolic content to be interpreted. Therapeutic play is not recreational, and although sometimes skills are attained, the purpose of therapeutic play is not primarily educational. Finally, play is not conducted for its abreactive value, although in cases of acute traumatic neurosis, there is a place for abreaction (O'Connor, 1991).

Because play is such a significant part of therapy with children, the use of toys becomes important. Two important questions to consider are "Which toys should be made available to the child?" and "How should the toys be used?" A discussion of therapy rooms and the materials used in child therapy provides an excellent opportunity to represent the wide range of approaches legitimately called psychodynamic.

Within the context of traditional analysis, there is a split regarding which toys should be made available to children when they enter treatment and which ones in subsequent sessions. Anna Freud (Sandler et al., 1980) discusses how, historically, a large number of very realistic looking miniature toys were made available to all children; the thinking was that children would use them to recreate the issues most pressing in their own lives, as well as to express their fantasies. Similarly, in treatment settings that employ a very child-centered, nondirective approach, all materials are available, and very few restrictions, if any, are placed on what the children may use or the manner in which they use them (Axline, 1947).

Alternatively, other analysts disagree with the notion of making all toys available to all children; they believe instead that a few toys should be chosen for each child. Often the toys selected are those that are most likely to elicit material relevant to the issues addressed in therapy; "in order to provide the most suitable way for the child to display what he cannot express in words" (Sandler et al., 1980, p. 127). In addition, the therapist almost always has information about what is occurring in the child's life outside of therapy. If a client is hesitant or resistant to bringing that material to sessions, the therapist might provide toys related to that event. For example, knowing that the client responded strongly to having witnessed a fight between its parents, a therapist might provide obvious "Mommy" and "Daddy" figures for that session. This is very different from Anna Freud's view that the analytic situation itself pulls for enough regression, which should not be encouraged by using toys that elicit even greater regression.

Transference/Relationship

The importance of the therapeutic relationship or *transference* is twofold. First, a strong relationship sustains the child through the inevitable stress of analysis. Second, the transferential aspects of the relationship, to be defined later, provide a vital source of material for interpretation. Because she did not believe in the appropriateness of directly interpreting children's play, this was the focus of Anna Freud's (1926) work.

The term transference refers to a central component of the psychoanalytic therapist–client relationship. Sandler et al. (1980) define transference as *"the ways in which the patient's view of and relations with his childhood objects are expressed in his current perceptions thoughts, fantasies, feelings, attitudes, and behavior in regard to the analyst"* (p. 78). In other words, when the therapeutic relationship evokes feelings for an important person in the client's life and the client responds to the therapist as he or she would to that person, the client is responding transferentially. By definition, anything that is evoked by the "real" relationship between patient and therapist is not transferential. However, in most dynamic therapies today, the term transference is used more loosely to refer to any strong feelings or responses the patient has to the therapist.

Transference is considered an extremely useful phenomenon by all psychodynamic theorists primarily because it is usually more beneficial to observe a client's characteristic ways of responding than it is to hear the client tell you about experiences retrospectively and in an inevitably subjective manner. However, even in the case of adult analysis, determining what is real and what is transference-based is difficult. In working with children, the issue of transference is both more complicated and, not surprisingly, more controversial (O'Connor & Lee, 1991). By definition, as we have discussed, transference responses are related to events and relationships in the patient's past, usually connected to the parents and the psychological environment of the family of origin. When adult clients respond to their therapists in a manner similar to the way they respond to their mothers, it is not difficult to point out and/or interpret the "unreality" of such a response. However, for a child, whose relationship with primary caretakers is immediate and currently developing rather than entrenched in characteristic patterns, it is illogical to talk about the "re-creation" of early, that is, parental, relationships within the analytic setting (O'Connor, 1991). Further, with young children in particular, all relationships with adults are characterized, *in reality*, by dependency needs and a hierarchical structure. It is unrealistic to expect a child to see the "unreality" of treating the therapist in a parentified manner, particularly when the child's parents have participated in creating a care-taking role for the analyst. In fact, the child client's perception of the therapist as a caretaker or authority figure is accurate.

In working with a child client, a therapist is likely to engage in developmentally appropriate activities that would rarely, if ever, occur in the context of a therapeutic relationship with an adult. Some of these activities may be maternal and will elicit or provoke both transferential and reality-based responses in the child. That there is a response at all is *not* transferential, but rather based on something very real that the therapist did. Conversely, the idiosyncratic nature of the response may indeed contain transferential elements. For example, it would be unusual for a child to fail to respond to being hugged or touched. However, assuming the touch is relatively neutral and in reality neither seductive nor threatening, it can be assumed that the child who responds by refusing to let go of the embrace, as well as the child who shirks away in terror, is responding to something beyond the physical action of the therapist. There is clearly an element of transference in both of these responses.

The possibilities for manifesting transference reactions are limitless. However, certain types of responses are encountered more frequently than others in children. At various ages children are likely to respond to their therapists as primary love objects, as a parent, as a mirror image of the parent, or as a powerful and magical being. Any and all of these manifestations would provide suitable content for interpretation and therapeutic work.

Countertransference

The counterpoint to the client's transference is the therapist's countertransference. Perhaps no psychoanalytic concept is more controversial or anxiety-provoking, particularly for novice therapists, than the thought that their own intrapsychic issues may be unconsciously interfering with the course of their patients' treatment. The definition of countertransference offered by Chethik (1989) is closely aligned with the above statement, as well as with the traditional psychoanalytic meaning of the term: "… special feelings a child may elicit in a therapist that stem from a therapist's unique childhood experiences and his own neurotic tendencies" (p. 23). Generally, it is assumed that countertransference is a phenomenon to guard against and that strong feelings elicited by a client signal that something is amiss or inappropriately occurring.

Most psychodynamic therapists, those who work with adults as well as those who work with children, adopt a much broader and more balanced view of countertransference and of the phenomenon of affective responses to clients in general. In fact, the emotions reported by child therapists need not signal the therapist's "latent neurotic tendencies," but rather can be thought of as predictable, natural, and in many cases quite useful in terms of the therapeutic work. Some of the more common feelings that emerge with clients are overattachment, detachment, or anger toward the child, its parents, or others in its environment. Such counter-transferential feelings can be useful in that they are, in most cases, reality-based and, as such, a good indication of the way a particular child is responded to by others in its extratherapeutic life. That is not to say that child as well as adult therapists and analysts do not have to be aware of the ways in which they bring their own individual, particularly childhood, issues into the treatment relationship with their clients. It is the rare adult who does not carry some unresolved feelings about early life into *all* interpersonal relationships, and it is reasonable to expect therapists to strive to become and remain as conscious of the impact of such feelings on their work as possible.

Ego Building

For structured or neurotic clients, psychoanalysis is the preferred treatment modality. As previously stated, in psychoanalysis the interventions focus on bringing unconscious feelings and conflicts into consciousness to resolve conflicts between personality structures. Interpretation of transference and countertransference is viewed as an essential element of analysis. Relatedly, interpreting resistance before content is usually the rule (Blanck & Blanck, 1994).

Traditional analysis is not seen as an appropriate or effective intervention for less structured, nonneurotic clients. These clients are not thought to have the ego strength to tolerate the ambiguity and depth of interpretive work. They cannot tolerate bringing their unconscious conflicts to consciousness. For unstructured clients or nonneurotic clients, therapy first focuses on structure building. Therapy is viewed as a corrective experience that will promote higher levels of object relations. Many psychodynamic therapists see supportive therapy as strengthening the client's defenses by focusing on promoting ego strength, thereby serving to get clients to a place where they can tolerate psychoanalysis (Blanck & Blanck, 1994).

Ego psychologists ally themselves with the client's ego to promote ego strength as a catalyst for psychological growth (Blanck & Blanck, 1994). Ego-building techniques vary, depending on the client's level of structural organization (Blanck & Blanck, 1979). When treating an unstructured client, therapists provide a benign climate where they focus on the client and not the procedure. Therapists do not dictate how clients should conduct their lives but allow clients to find their own way in a supportive environment that offers guidance not ultimatums. Relatedly, when therapists use confrontations, they attack the behavior and not the individual. Therapists verbalize their thoughts only to the extent that they promote the growth process and they take care not to attempt to gratify clients' infantile wishes. Specifically, therapists promote growth in the context of the client–therapist relationship. Therapists do this by connecting with clients at their current level of functioning and then strive to promote higher levels of functioning. The therapist tries to maintain a position of neutrality by attempting to stay evenly suspended between the client's id, ego, and superego. The therapist listens to the client with evenly suspended attention or a "third ear" that is attuned to the client's unconscious, affect, pattern of object relations, transference manifestations, and resistances. The therapist connects to the client by becoming attuned to the client's affective state. Relatedly, the therapist encourages the client to develop and display a range of affect. The therapist is seen as the new object with which the client can pursue higher levels of object relations. This reenactment allows clients to reorganize their personality structures so that they are more adaptive. Through these new patterns of object relations, the therapist promotes the client's self-esteem.

Interpretation

Interpretation is the most powerful intervention used by psychoanalysts to help their patients bring unconscious conflicts to consciousness (O'Connor, 1991). Although this is the primary function of interpretation for both child and adult clients, interpretation serves an additional, preliminary function in work with children. To the extent that their verbal capacities are limited, much of what children experience and store in memory occurs in the absence of linguistic labels. It is thus difficult if not impossible for memories of these experiences to be retrieved by using language (O'Connor, 1991). Interpretation can be a powerful way of providing verbal meaning to children's experiences.

Anna Freud (1928) and Melanie Klein (1955) differed in the way they proposed to use interpretation in child analysis. Anna Freud believed that a child's ego structure was too fragile to tolerate deep interpretation. In fact, because the child's experience and conflict were all viewed as relatively recent and available, deep interpretation was seen as unnecessary. Alternatively, Melanie Klein favored the use of primary process interpretation, often directly labeling the child's primitive, sexualized fantasies from the outset of the treatment. This is considered one of the most controversial aspects of Kleinian analysis because it tends to offend the sensibilities of most parents and even therapists in the United States. Beyond these two views there are various models of interpretation, as well as numerous systems for classifying them (Lewis, 1974; Lowenstein, 1957). The model presented here (O'Connor, 1991) integrates important aspects of various other classification systems.

LEVELS OF INTERPRETATION

The first level of interpretation in this system is called *reflection*. This differs somewhat from the use of the term by Carl Rogers (1951). Rogerian reflections are generally simple restatements of the client's verbalizations or behavior. In the present model, a reflection includes an emotional component that is added to the observation or paraphrase of the child's words or actions. Reflections serve three purposes. They help the child to label its internal experience, expand its affective vocabulary, and have an educative function by teaching children that feelings are an integral part of therapy.

The second level is *present-pattern* interpretation, in which current and observable patterns of behavior are identified and labeled. Initially, only the patterns within session are interpreted. Later, when the therapist has gathered sufficient data, patterns of behavior observed across sessions are interpreted. Present pattern interpretations teach the child that its behavior is consistent and meaningful rather than random and arbitrary.

Simple dynamic interpretations move beyond the interpretation of behavior to making the explicit connections between affect and patterns of behavior, thus combining and expanding the two previous levels of interpretation. Simple dynamic interpretations are still limited to the content of the child's sessions.

Generalized dynamic interpretations "identify for children the operation of their personal dynamics both in- and out-of-session behaviors" (O'Connor, 1991, p. 249). In addition to preparing children for the final level of interpretation, generalized dynamic interpretations assist children in applying the therapy process outside the sessions.

Genetic interpretations draw connections between the child's current behavior and personal history and are the types of interpretations considered most useful by psychoanalysts. These interpretations are generally made after the therapy has been underway for some time and the child has been suitably prepared.

REGULATING THE IMPACT

Just as the therapist should gradually build up to genetic interpretations to maximize the child's receptiveness and diminish the possibility that it will become overwhelmed, Miller (1996) also warns against making premature interpretations and notes the value of following the child's lead. The impact of interpretations can be modulated in various other ways. First, interpreting *within the play* by focusing on the dolls or figures the child is using can be significantly less disruptive or threatening than directly interpreting the child's behavior or feelings. Second, using *as if* interpretations, which suggest that the client's experience is common to many children, provides distance from the content and allows the child to feel less isolated from others. Finally, the impact can be limited by focusing the interpretations primarily on the content of the therapeutic relationship. In addition to reducing anxiety, this can be helpful in building therapeutic rapport.

Interpretations must be conceived and offered according to the child's developmental level. The cognitive and particularly the linguistic abilities of the child will be the most important determinant of how much interpretive work can be accomplished in session. For children under age 6, interpretation needs to be concrete and conducted primarily within play. Much of the therapeutic work may have to be done through activity and experience rather than discussion and interpretation. For children between ages 6 and 11, a balance can be struck between language and action, depending on the particular characteristics and needs of the child. With most adolescents, interpretation will load heavily on language with a minimal emphasis on play.

WORKING THROUGH

In psychoanalysis, interpretation is followed by the principal work of treatment, a process known as *working through*. Anna Freud defined this process as the "constant reiteration of the interpretation ... the elaboration and the extension of the interpretation in different contexts" (Sandler et al., 1980, pp. 182–183). If one thinks about how easily things slip out of the minds of adults, let alone children, it becomes obvious that a single interpretation, though potentially effective and even powerful, is insufficient to create any kind of lasting effect or change. Rather, change occurs as "patient's behavior and mental life gradually take in and integrate new knowledge and patterns of behavior as the process of working through proceeds" (Sandler et al., 1980, p. 182). Working through can be observed when the course of development is reestablished along expected lines.

If this description of working through sounds elusive and difficult to grasp, it is probably because many practitioners of psychoanalysis have difficulty defining the process and speak of knowing in very intuitive terms, that working through is in process or has been sufficiently completed. However, some psychodynamic modifications view working through as a process of *ego-based problem solving* (O'Connor, 1991) or of finding an affectively satisfactory way of "being in the world." Again, developmental considerations are of paramount importance in structuring the experience for the child client.

The burden of helping the very young child work through its conflicts falls primarily on the therapist, who is often quite involved in working to change the client's real, that is, extratherapeutic, environment. There may still be some environmental manipulation needed in work with 6- to 11-year-old clients, but working through now begins to focus on helping the child to think about its interactions with family and peers. Group psychotherapy may be suggested for the child in this age group as a collateral activity aimed at furthering the working through of peer-related conflicts. With children older than 11, the process of working through resembles adult work, and the goal is fostering as much independent ego-based problem solving as possible.

Collateral Involvement of Parents

In adult treatment, the closer one is to the analytic end of the analytic–dynamic continuum, the greater the emphasis on preventing the contamination of the therapist-client relationship, and the less likely it is that the therapist will involve anyone other than the client in the treatment process. In child treatment, such "purity" is neither possible nor desirable. It is not possible because the continuity of the therapy depends on the parents bringing the child to treatment and paying the bills. It is not desirable because successful child therapy necessitates the support of parents, and in most cases that means some involvement.

Anna Freud (Sandler et al., 1980) believed that the age of the child and the pathology of both the child and parent(s) should be considered in deciding how to involve parents. Contexts in which parents may be seen by their child's therapist range from a true analytic relationship with the parent as client to one in which the therapist provides didactic parenting skills training. Most psychodynamic therapies fall somewhere in between these polar extremes, where parents are not themselves considered clients, yet are more actively involved in their child's treatment than didactic training implies. The more traditionally psychoanalytic the treatment, the less likely it is that collateral involvement will extend beyond the child's parents. However, more systemic therapists may involve other significant persons in the child's life, including members of family and medical, educational, and legal systems in which a particular child may be embedded (O'Connor, 1991).

Confidentiality also affects the decision as to how to involve the parents because information from both parties is received by the therapist at various points during treatment. It is vitally important that an explicit agreement be made among therapist, child, and parents at the outset of treatment regarding sharing such information and that the boundaries around this issue be clear and protected.

Termination

Given the central importance of the analytic relationship, the question of when to end analysis is obviously of great significance. Theoretically, the answer is quite simple: When there is evidence that the child understands and is better able to mediate the conflicts that brought it to therapy, it is appropriate to consider termination. Such evidence includes recognition by the therapist that the child has returned to an appropriate developmental level and has maintained the concomitant behavioral changes (O'Connor, 1991).

Unfortunately, in practice, the question of when to terminate is much more complex than this simple guideline implies. First, it is not always clear when the treatment goals have been accomplished, largely because treatment goals are often modified during the course of therapy. In addition, there are unfortunate circumstances in which a particular client and therapist cannot work together, in which case all efforts should be made to transfer the child smoothly to another therapist. Finally, there are often external (i.e., extratherapeutic) circumstances that dictate the timing of termination, such as the therapist's or client's departure from the area, financial restraints, or parental unwillingness to continue to support treatment.

SUMMARY

This chapter presented an overview of psychoanalytic or psychoanalytically derived psychodynamic interventions with children. It is noted that psychoanalytic and psychodynamic models have many points in common. For example, they both view symptoms as dynamic, constantly growing, changing, and diverse. In addition, both theories believe in psychic determinism, meaning that individuals are influenced by both internal and external experience and that nothing is accidental. Also, both theories are developmental. Psychoanalytic thought emphasizes the drives underlying developmental processes, whereas Object

Relations emphasizes the importance of external, relationship factors. Finally, both theories contend that individuals' current behavior relates strongly to their pasts.

The two central differences between psychoanalytic and psychodynamic theories involve (1) their conceptualization of the relationship between personality structures and psychopathology and (2) the early goals of treatment. Psychoanalysis is seen as best suited for clients who have developed all three personality structures (id, ego, superego) and whose difficulties arise from conflicts among those structures. Psychodynamic theorists expanded the psychoanalytic model to address more severely disturbed clients whose personality structures are not fully developed. Object Relations Theory and Ego Psychology both emphasize the importance of the ego in both client's development and the therapy process. In psychoanalytic therapy, the focus is on uncovering and resolving major conflicts. In psychodynamic therapy, the focus is on building structures, particularly on strengthening the ego.

Additionally, reference was made on numerous occasions to the ways in which child and adult psychoanalytic treatments converge and differ. With regard to child treatment, a developmental frame was emphasized. Given the advances that have been made in psychoanalytic treatment for children and the expansion of the original model into a wide array of psychodynamic interventions in the last half century, it is certain these will continue to be a dominant force in child psychotherapy well into the future.

REFERENCES

Ainsworth, M., Blehar, M., Waters, E., & Wall, S. (1978). Patterns of attachment. Hillsdale, NJ: Erlbaum.

Axline, V. (1947). *Play therapy*. Cambridge, MA: Houghton Mifflin.

Bettelheim, B. (1967). *The empty fortress: Infantile autism and the birth of the self*. New York: The Free Press.

Blanck, G., & Blanck, R. (1994). *Ego psychology: Theory and practice* (2nd ed.) New York: Columbia University Press.

Blanck, G., & Blanck, R. (1979). *Ego psychology II: Psychoanalytic developmental psychology*. New York: Columbia University Press.

Bowlby, J. (1958). The nature of the child's tie to his mother. *International Journal of Psycho-Analysis, 39*, 350–373.

Bowlby, J. (1988). *A secure base: Parent–child attachment and healthy human development*. New York: Basic Books.

Chetnik, M. (1989). *Techniques of child therapy: Psychodynamic strategies*. New York: Guilford.

Freud, A. (1926). *The psychoanalytic treatment of children*. London: Imago Press, 1946.

Freud, A. (1928). *Introduction to the technique of child analysis* (L. P. Clark, trans). New York: Nervous and Mental Disease Publishing.

Freud, A. (1936). *Ego and the mechanisms of defense*. New York: International Universities Press.

Freud, A. (1945). Indications for child analysis. *Psychoanalytic study of the child, 1*, 127–149.

Freud, A. (1965). *Normality and pathology in childhood: Assessment of development*. New York: International Universities Press.

Freud, S. (1900). *The interpretation of dreams, Standard edition*, Vol. 5. London: Hogarth, 1957.

Freud, S. (1905). Three assays on the theory of sexuality. In J. Stratchey (Ed.), *The complete works of Sigmund Freud*, Vol. 7. London: Hogarth, 1957.

Freud, S. (1915). *The unconscious, Standard edition*, Vol. 14. London: Hogarth, 1957.

Freud, S. (1923). The ego and the id. *Collected papers*. London: Hogarth.

Freud, S. (1933). *Collected papers*, London: Hogarth.

Freud, S. (1938). *An outline of psychoanalysis, Standard edition*, Vol. 23. London: Hogarth, 1961.

Kernberg, O. (1975). *Borderline conditions and pathological narcissism*. New York: Jason Aronson.

Klein, M. (1932). *The psycho-analysis of children*. London: Hogarth.

Klein, M. (1955). The psychoanalytic technique. *American Journal of Orthopsychiatry, 25*, 223–237.

Lewis, M. (1974). Interpretation in child analysis: Developmental considerations. *Journal of the American Academy of Child Psychiatry, 13*, 32–53.

Lowenstein, R. (1957). Some thoughts on interpretation in the theory and practice of psychoanalysis. *The Psychoanalytic Study of the Child, 12*, 127–150.

Mahler, M. (1979). *Infantile psychosis and early contributions.* New York: Jason Aronson.

Masterson, J. F., & Klein, R. (1995). *Disorders of the self: New Therapeutic horizons.* New York: Brunner/Mazel.

Miller, J. P. (1996). *Using self psychology in child psychotherapy.* Northvale, NJ: Jason Aronson.

Neubauer, P. (1978). The opening phase of child analysis. In J. Glenn (Ed.), *Child analysis and therapy* (pp. 263–274). New York: Jason Aronson.

O'Connor, K. (1991). *The play therapy primer: An integration of theories and technique.* New York: Wiley.

O'Connor, K., & Lee, A. (1991). Advances in psychoanalytic psychotherapy with children. In M. Hersen, A. Kazdin, & A. S. Bellack (Eds.), *The clinical psychology handbook*, 2nd ed. (pp. 580–595). New York: Pergamon Press.

O'Connor, K., Lee, A., & Schaefer, C. (1983). Psychoanalytic psychotherapy with children. In M. Hersen, A. Kazdin, & A. S. Bellack (Eds.), *Clinical psychology handbook* (pp. 543–564). Elmsford, NY: Pergamon.

Rogers, C. (1951). *Client-centered therapy.* Boston: Houghton Mifflin.

Roser, K. (1996). A review of psychoanalytic theory and treatment of childhood autism. *The Psychoanalytic Review, 83*(3), 325–341.

Sandler, J., Kennedy, H., & Tyson, R. (1980). *The technique of child analysis: Discussions with Anna Freud.* Cambridge, MA: Harvard University Press.

Shirk, S., & Russell, R. (1996). *Change processes in child psychotherapy.* New York: Guilford.

Winnicott, D. (1964). *The child, the family and the outside world.* London: Penguin.

Winnicott, D. (1965). *The maturational process and the facilitating environment.* New York: International Universities Press.

23

Behavior Therapy

Lisa W. Coyne and Alan M. Gross

Introduction

Behavior therapy is a treatment strategy, guided by learning theory, that emphasizes functional behavior–environment relationships. Its primary goals are to enhance adaptive behaviors and eliminate or reduce maladaptive behaviors in daily life. Maladaptive functioning, whether motor, cognitive, or physiological, is conceptualized as the product of faulty learning. Thus, behavior therapists attempt to treat behavioral problems by functionally assessing and modifying environmental contingencies that foster and maintain them. Since its inception, behavior therapy has been used to address a variety of different issues, including psychological disorders, child maltreatment, behavioral health, and prevention efforts, among others (Hersen & Ammerman, 1989).

In the 1950s, behavior therapy grew in response to what many learning theorists believed was the failure of more traditional treatment paradigms, such as psychoanalysis. Behaviorists criticized psychoanalysts for their zeal in drawing causal inferences about behavior from introspective techniques and their lack of rigorous scientific methods. In contrast, behavior therapy coupled the goal of treating overt behaviors with formulating verifiable hypotheses (Thorpe & Olson, 1996). Its earliest procedures were derived from laboratory research and involved basic classical and operant principles. In 1966, Wolfe and Lazarus published *Behavior Therapy Techniques*, which detailed standard strategies of aversion therapy, the token economy, and systematic desensitization for use with adult populations (Thorpe & Olson, 1996). Despite initial resistance from the proponents of more established therapeutic paradigms, behavior therapy gained popularity due to this adherence to experimentally supported theories of behavioral change.

The earliest behavioral work with children may be traced to Watson and Raynor's investigation of fear acquisition with "little Albert" in 1920 and Mary Cover Jones' examination of counterconditioning (Peterson, 1997). In the 1930s, Mowrer and Mowrer developed the "bell-and-pad" treatment of nighttime enuresis, a classical conditioning technique (Hersen & Ammerman, 1989). Basic studies such as these led to conclusions that children, like adults,

Lisa W. Coyne and Alan M. Gross • Department of Psychology, University of Mississippi, University, Mississippi 38677.

Advanced Abnormal Psychology, Second Edition, edited by Hersen and Van Hasselt. Kluwer Academic/Plenum Publishers, New York, 2001.

are subject to the basic laws of learning. As such, they could also benefit from behavior therapy. In the mid to late 1970s, child behavior therapists began applying behavioral techniques to child problems such as food refusal and noncompliance. Moreover, these procedures gained impetus for use with youngsters who were mentally retarded and autistic—problems deemed untreatable by psychoanalysts (Peterson, 1997; Williams & Gross, 1994). As with early adult behavior therapies, procedures for children were somewhat simplistic, either derived from animal models or based on variants of adult treatments. Many of these closely followed Skinnerian operant principles applied either to children, their parents, or both. As child behavior therapy grew in popularity and perceived applicability, its procedures necessarily became more complex. For example, later treatments began to capitalize on developmental phenomena such as children's desire and capacity to model others (Peterson, 1997).

Currently, the field of child behavior therapy has begun to address, as Peterson (1997) puts it, the "complexity of a child's world." For example, at the forefront of investigation and treatment are emphases on how coercive peer or caretaker relationships maintain inappropriate behavior patterns (Frick, 1998; Hembree-Kigin & McNeil, 1995; Patterson, 1982). Further, behavior therapists have begun to look at unique developmental issues, such as the particulars of adolescence, as well as more specific stressors such as childhood grief after the loss of a caretaker, a divorce, or school transitions (Peterson, 1997). Attention to the history of family, peer, and other contextual influences has provided insight to guide preventive approaches (Chorpita, 1997a). Finally, many recent publications testify to the interchanges between behavior therapy and neuropsychology, psychopharmacology, and psychological testing, which many argue have enriched and informed behavioral treatments (Hersen & Ammerman, 1989).

This chapter reviews a number of issues involved in assessing and treating children and examines current trends in child behavior therapy. An examination of theoretical issues, classic therapeutic techniques, and empirical findings characteristic of a behavioral approach is also provided. Finally, current issues and areas for future growth are addressed.

Behavioral Assessment

The application of behavioral techniques is preceded by the issue of behavioral assessment strategies. To manipulate environmental factors that give rise to problematic behaviors, it is necessary first to elucidate their functional properties. This goal is primary to the functional analytic method, which strives to identify and measure meaningful response units and their controlling variables, whether environmental or organismic, to understand and alter behavior (Nelson & Hayes, 1981). Nelson and Hayes suggest adherence to an S-O-R-C model to guide data collection. "S" indicates the antecedent stimulus purported to set the stage for the target behavior. "O" includes organismic variables, such as past learning history, physiology, or genetics, that may mediate responses, or "R." Finally, "C" denotes environmental consequences that occur contingent on performance of the target behavior. To identify such contingencies, behavior therapists conduct behavioral observations. They isolate highly specific situations in which an antecedent is controlled and a consequence altered (e.g., presentation of a reinforcer or removal of an aversive stimulus) contingent on the occurrence of the target behavior. Should the target response change in a reliable way, behavioral function can be assumed (Lalli & Kates, 1998). In recent years, strict use of behavioral observation has been augmented by a number of alternative but empirically sound assessment devices, such as rating forms.

Though they provide a strong basis for empirically assessing childhood psychopathology, functional analytic methods may not be sufficient for a thorough evaluation (Williams & Gross, 1994) due in part to their lack of attention to normal developmental processes and normative comparisons (Ollendick & Hersen, 1984). Strict focus on observable behavior reduces subjective inference, but it leaves behavioral assessment methods insensitive to the maturational aspects of learning. Thus, a number of behavioral assessment devices that take normative data and developmental information into account have gained precedence in recent years (e.g., Achenbach, 1991; Achenbach & Edelbrock, 1983). In addition, many argue that behavioral assessment methods should be augmented by the concurrent use of both cognitive abilities and neuropsychological tests (e.g., Goldstein, 1979; Horton & Miller, 1985; Nelson, 1980). In particular, a battery of cognitive abilities and achievement tests may be useful in more specific assessment of a child's developmental lags or deficits than strict behavioral observation. Neuropsychological tests may help to rule out organic causes for behavioral deficits. In any case, both types of test may assist in identifying specific problems that merit treatment focus and may be used as dependent measures when evaluating treatment effectiveness (Williams & Gross, 1994).

INTERDISCIPLINARY INFLUENCES

Developmental Influences

Behavioral and developmental psychology developed somewhat independently of one another. Whereas behaviorists stress the study of environmental factors in the development and maintenance of maladaptive behaviors, developmentalists concerned themselves with normal maturational processes. Moreover, the two fields were divided by deep methodological differences. In testing their hypotheses, developmental psychologists often relied on unobservable psychological constructs to infer causality (e.g., Piaget's holistic structures). Behaviorists relied solely on basic conditioning paradigms to explain developmental processes. Nonetheless, behaviorists came to recognize that learning occurs through a progression of changes, influenced by factors such as age and developmental level, in children's interactions with their environment. Rather than viewing children as simply scaled-down versions of adults, behaviorists recognized the importance of developmental issues and milestones in designing and applying behavior therapy and assessment.

In the late 1980s, child behavior therapists began to integrate work accumulating in the field of developmental psychology into both assessment and treatment procedures. Knowledge of developmental norms, sex differences, children's developmental ability to participate in treatment, and developmental phases characterized by extreme stress, as in adolescence, were examined with greater interest (Hersen & Ammerman, 1989). For example, Achenbach and colleagues (Achenbach, 1974, 1991; Achenbach & Edelbrock, 1978, 1979, 1981, 1983) collected extensive normative data on children aged 2–3 and 4–16 using the Child Behavior Checklist (CBCL; Achenbach & Edelbrock, 1983). The CBCL, which may be completed by either parent or teacher, addresses common behavioral problems and difficulties in social interaction. Children's responses are compared against normative data and used to generate a profile of the child's current functioning relative to age-appropriate peers. The CBCL enjoys widespread use as an assessment tool in both clinical and research settings. However, caution in generalization is merited because the norms reflected in the CBCL may not appropriately represent variation in socioeconomic and ethnic groups (Williams & Gross, 1994).

Behavior therapists increasingly acknowledge the impact of developmental factors on both children's ability to participate in and benefit from therapy. For example, young or developmentally delayed children may have difficulty comprehending instructions in imagery or relaxation techniques because these treatments were originally designed for adults (see, for example, Koeppen, 1974; Morris & Kratochwill, 1991). Consequently, child behavior therapists have altered such techniques to fit children's specific developmental needs. Further, children's unique social contexts—such as family, classroom, or peer relationships—have been recognized as important agents of therapeutic change. Treatments that incorporate parents or teachers as cotherapists, as in many parent-training interventions, have become prominent (e.g., Briesmeister & Schaefer, 1998; Forehand & McMahon, 1981).

Developmental factors also may make assessing treatment outcome problematic. For example, many behaviors may change due to development alone rather than as a consequence of intervention. Further, some suggest that symptom substitution may occur as children age. In other words, children's problematic behavior may shift to become more developmentally relevant, as new levels are reached. Thus, it is important to disentangle these factors when designing and applying behavioral treatments. Collection of follow-up data may be helpful in clarifying specific mechanisms that result in behavioral change.

Cognitive-Behavioral Influences

Strict definitions of child behavior therapy have broadened to incorporate cognitive-behavioral techniques and theories (Craighead, Meyers, & Wilcoxon Craighead, 1985; Hart & Morgan, 1993; Kendall & Braswell, 1985; Knell, 1993). Cognitive-behavior modification first appeared in the treatment literature in the late 1960s and early 1970s and drew a great deal of attention. This was in response to the field's growing dissatisfaction with the narrow scope of radical behaviorism and a burgeoning interest in cognitive mediators of behavioral responses and the phenomenon of self-control (Hart & Morgan, 1993; Kendall & Braswell, 1985). As early as the 1930s, Edward C. Tolman posited the existence of cognitive mediators of the learning process. In the 1960s, the work of Albert Ellis (rational-emotive therapy) and Albert Bandura (observational learning theory) gained precedence. These emerging models of cognitive learning theory led to the expansion of the behavioral stimulus–response model to include mediation by the organism's cognitive processes (Hart & Morgan, 1993). In the clinical realm, these treatments acknowledged cognitive components of learning, and they also made these the foci around which behavioral change might occur. Although some behavior analysts viewed this as a major paradigm shift, others recognized it as an extension of behavioral theory (Spence, 1994).

THERAPEUTIC TECHNIQUES BASED ON CLASSICAL AND OPERANT CONDITIONING

Classical conditioning, also known as respondent or Pavlovian conditioning, is a learning paradigm developed from the work of Ivan Pavlov in the early 1900s. It describes the process by which an organism's reflexive behavioral responses are brought under stimulus control. To elaborate, reflexive responses are triggered by particular environmental stimuli. By repeatedly pairing a neutral stimulus with an unconditioned stimulus, one that elicits an unlearned, or unconditioned response, an association is formed between the two. Through this association, the formerly neutral stimulus, now the conditioned stimulus, has gained the power to evoke the conditioned response. Development of this basic and elegant paradigm fostered a wealth of empirical inquiry into the development of clinical treatments. Currently, classical conditioning procedures, such as systematic desensitization, and exposure-based treatments, such as flooding, are commonly used for a variety of fear and avoidance disorders, such as simple phobias (Ollendick & King, 1998; Silverman & Eisen, 1993), test anxiety (Strumpf & Fodor, 1993), separation anxiety (Last, 1989), and obsessive–compulsive disorder (Hagopian & Ollendick, 1997; Laurent & Potter, 1998).

Whereas classical conditioning procedures deal with learning reflexive behavioral responses, operant procedures address more complex, goal-directed behaviors. The operant conditioning paradigm assumes a lawful relationship between behavior and environment. The probability of these complex behaviors, called *operants* by B. F. Skinner, is affected by their consequences. That is, reinforcing consequences increase, and punishing consequences decrease the probability of a behavior's occurrence. It follows that altering the consequences of one's behavior results in behavioral change. When targeting behavior for treatment, it is important to elucidate the environmental contingencies that support those behaviors. During treatment phases, both antecedents and consequences of behaviors may be shifted to effect more adaptive patterns of responding. These basic tenets form the foundation of child behavior therapy. Therapies based on operant conditioning principles, such as reinforcement, punishment, extinction, and contingency management, have been used successfully with conduct problems (Frick, 1998), ADHD (Pelham, Wheeler, & Chronis, 1998), fears and anxieties (Barrios & O'Dell, 1998), and behavioral health issues (Slifer, Cataldo, & Kurtz, 1998).

Systematic Desensitization

Systematic desensitization, pioneered by Joseph Wolpe in the late 1950s, was conceptualized in terms of the classical conditioning process of reciprocal inhibition (Hagopian & Ollendick, 1997). Since then, it has become one of the most commonly used treatments for alleviating anxiety-related complaints such as phobias (Ollendick & King, 1998). Its goal is to reduce subjectively reported fears and other anxiety-related behaviors via three therapeutic components. First, relaxation training is conducted to foster deep muscle relaxation and induce a state incompatible with anxiety responses during the systematic desensitization phase. Next, a hierarchy of anxiety-provoking stimuli is constructed by the client; the least feared items are ranked lowest, and those most feared are ranked highest. Finally, each stimulus on the graduated list is presented to clients while they are engaged in relaxation. This pairing may take place either *in vivo* or imaginally. As each stimulus level is mastered, that is, experienced without anxiety, a higher level stimulus is presented until the highest may be encountered with no difficulty (Laurent & Potter, 1998).

In the relaxation training segment of treatment, the child is first taught to attend to the tension and relaxation of specific muscle groups. During this phase, it is important to modify relaxation training scripts, most often formulated for adults, to approximate the child's developmental level. For example, children's scripts are usually shorter than those used for adults (Laurent & Potter, 1997). Koeppen (1974) has made scripts more relevant to a child's imaginative capacity. When requiring children to focus on facial and jaw muscles, he asks them to pretend to bite down hard on a jawbreaker and then let up. Further, child scripts usually limit the number of muscle groups to be tensed and relaxed to no more than three per session. Finally, one must consider whether the child can in fact learn relaxation techniques (Laurent & Potter, 1997). Relaxation training sessions usually range from 15 to 20 minutes and should not extend beyond that. Children are encouraged to practice these skills until they achieve mastery in quickly achieving a relaxed state. The level of relaxation is typically assessed by behavioral observation during the exercise. Difficulty in relaxing is operationalized by persistent movements, fluttering eyelids, and facial tension. Should these responses be present, the therapist may consider a modeling procedure to assist the child (Morris & Kratochwill, 1991).

In constructing an anxiety hierarchy, both child and parent are requested to make a list of feared stimuli. Then, these stimuli, usually 20 to 25 items, are arranged in a hierarchy of least to most anxiety-provoking based on the child's subjective anxiety state (Hagopian & Ollendick, 1997). For example, for a child who feared the dark, a relatively benign stimulus might be a dimly lit room after dinner. A highly fear-eliciting stimulus might involve a fully darkened room with only an illuminated night light.

During the systematic desensitization procedure, the child is first engaged in a relaxation exercise during which she or he imagines a pleasant image. When an optimal state of relaxation is reached, the therapist encourages the child to encounter or imagine as vividly as possible the least anxiety-producing situations in the hierarchy. It is crucial that the child experience or visualize the scene until mild anxiety is experienced. After indicating fear by a raised finger, the child then refocuses on a pleasant image and returns to a relaxed state. If anxiety becomes excessive, the therapist may back up a step or two in the hierarchy to help the child remain relaxed. When the child learns to visualize the feared stimulus with little or no anxiety, the next step is introduced, and so on. Treatment is complete when the child can imagine all levels in the hierarchy without fear (Hagopian & Ollendick, 1997).

A number of variations in systematic desensitization procedures have been used in child populations. In addition to the classic and *in vivo* techniques, a procedure involving emotive imagery developed by Lazarus and Abramovitz (1962) shows some promise. In this procedure, the use of relaxation training is replaced with instructions for children to visualize an adventure of their favorite superhero. Exposure to items from the anxiety hierarchy takes place in the story's context, and in this way, positive feelings elicited by the story, it is thought, counter fears elicited by those items (Ollendick & King, 1998). For example, one recent study by Cornwall, Spense, and Schotte (1997) investigated the efficacy of emotive imagery with twenty-four darkness-phobic children ranging in age from 7 to 10. Children were randomly assigned either to the experimental condition or to a wait-list control group. On a number of different measures, including trait anxiety, child ratings on a fear thermometer, and behavioral observations during a darkness tolerance task, results indicated significant improvement over the control group. Although these results appear promising, replication is needed (Ollendick & King, 1998).

In a 1998 review of treatments for childhood anxiety disorders, Ollendick and King found that both imaginal and *in vivo* desensitization were "probably efficacious" for treating simple phobias, although they also point out the paucity of existent empirical support as a cautionary note in drawing such a conclusion (Ollendick & King, 1998). Further, systematic desensitization may be inappropriate for children under age 9 because they may have trouble pairing relaxation and imagery. This may be due in part to difficulty in specifying discrete muscle responses during relaxation and clearly imagining the fear-eliciting stimulus (Laurent & Potter, 1998). Nonetheless, this treatment may be implicated in cases where more intense exposure-based interventions, as in flooding, are not acceptable to parent or child (Hagopian & Ollendick, 1997).

Flooding and Response Prevention

Flooding and other variants of exposure-based interventions are based on the classical conditioning principle of extinction. This procedure differs from systematic desensitization in that the most feared stimuli are presented early in treatment. In this technique, repeated exposure, whether *in vivo* or imaginally, to the feared stimulus in the absence of an unconditioned stimulus weakens the power of the feared stimulus to evoke a fear response. Thus, anxiety responses are eventually extinguished. Further, it is crucial to prevent escape from the feared stimulus and keep the stimulus present until the child's level of anxiety decreases. Failure to do so may strengthen avoidant responding because escape provides some immediate relief from the feared situation (Hagopian & Ollendick, 1997). Francis and Beidel (1995) caution that although the best results are achieved when the child is confronted specifically with the anxiety-provoking stimulus, this technique may cause a great deal of distress in younger children. Thus, they recommend that the rationale for treatment be explained to the child in age-appropriate terms (Francis & Beidel, 1995).

Flooding and response prevention techniques are often used in treating child obsessive–compulsive disorder (OCD). Response prevention, based on operant theory, involves prohibiting the child from engaging in the compulsive behavior that occurs subsequent to exposure to the anxiety-eliciting stimulus (Hagopian & Ollendick, 1997). Preventing compulsive responses, as in preventing avoidance behaviors, results in extinction. For example, in a recent multiple-baseline design across subjects, Knox, Albano, and Barlow (1996) investigated the efficacy of a graduated *in vivo* and imaginal exposure and response prevention treatment in which both parents and therapists assisted. Participants were four children aged 8 to 13 who feared monsters, contamination, loss of possessions, and harm by others. In addition, they demonstrated associated compulsions. The durations of these anxieties and compulsions ranged from 6 months to 4 years. After a 4-week treatment program, consisting of three sessions 90 minutes long per week, results indicated reductions in both subjective distress and compulsive rituals. These gains were maintained at 3- and 12-month follow-ups (Knox, Albano, & Barlow, 1996).

Several variations of this procedure have appeared in the literature. These include implosion, imaginal flooding, and reinforced practice. *Implosion* is quite similar to flooding—its only difference lies in its focus on exaggerated anxiety-eliciting cues rather than imagined situational cues (Laurent & Potter, 1998). As in flooding, the child continues to imagine the cues until a state of relative calm is reached. In the *imaginal flooding* technique, a fear hierarchy is constructed, as in systematic desensitization. However, the child is asked to begin imagining an item ranked in the middle of the list and to continue doing so until fear subsides. *Reinforced practice* involves rewards for prolonged periods of exposure to an authentic feared stimulus. The children remain in the presence of the stimulus for as long as they will tolerate it. After this initial threshold has been set, rewards are delivered for lengthening the periods of exposure (Barrios & O'Dell, 1998).

In using flooding and other prolonged exposure techniques, it is important to consider for whom such interventions are appropriate. For example, flooding may be implicated when rapid extinction is crucial (Williams & Gross, 1994) or when other treatments, such as systematic desensitization, have been deemed inappropriate (see for example Screenivasan, Manocha, & Jain, 1979; Yule, Sacks, & Hersov, 1974). Another issue that merits consideration is the distress that younger children experience in exposure treatments. This may warrant the use of caution with younger populations and at the very least, careful, age-appropriate explanations of treatment rationale, as suggested by Francis and Beidel (1995). Finally, flooding and response prevention seem indicated in treating childhood compulsive behaviors, as in OCD (Barrios & O'Dell, 1998; Knox, Albano, & Barlow, 1996).

Positive Reinforcement

Reinforcement procedures are based on operant conditioning theory. Positive reinforcers delivered after the occurrence of a behavior increase the probability that that behavior will occur in the future. For example, if a child is given verbal praise after completing a homework problem correctly, that child may work harder in the future to complete assignments and get the right answers. For positive reinforcement to work, acquisition of the reinforcer is made contingent on the child's completion of a desired response. Reinforcers are determined solely by their effects on a child's behavior, rather than by their assumed values, nature, or appearance (Parrish, 1997). Nonetheless, as a rule of thumb, positive reinforcers are usually inherently pleasing stimuli such as food or verbal praise, but may also be stimuli that have acquired reinforcing properties through association with another pleasant stimulus. A large body of research concerning the application and efficacy of positive reinforcement has accumulated. In fact, it is one of the most effective methods of increasing the frequency of desirable behavior, and although not explicitly stated, is a component in a myriad of behavioral treatment packages (Handen, 1998).

Repp and Karsh (1994) provide an illustrative study in which positive reinforcement was used. Investigators functionally assessed the problem behaviors of two students, who had developmental disabilities, in their classroom environments. Students demonstrated tantrum behaviors, including kicking, crying, falling to the floor, and throwing objects, in addition to finger stereotypies. Previous interventions using time-out and various restraint procedures had failed to produce behavioral change. Behavioral observations of demand situations and teacher interviews suggested that the children's problematic behaviors were maintained by positive reinforcement; specifically, teacher attention. Thus, investigators posited that shifting teacher attention from undesirable to desirable behaviors would lead to a behavioral change. Teachers were instructed to withdraw attention, specifically, verbal pleas, physical struggles, soothing comments, and reprimands, from tantrum behaviors. Instead, they were asked to attend to on-task behaviors with either verbal praise or physical reinforcement, such as pats on the back or high-fives. Initially, teachers provided reinforcement on a fixed-interval, 15-s schedule, which eventually lengthened to 90-s intervals. In addition, teachers reinforced appropriate social behavior with the children's favorite activities, such as music tapes or magazines. For each 2- to 3-minute interval during which the children interacted appropriately with their teachers, a positive reinforcer was delivered. Results indicated that tantrum behaviors decreased significantly immediately following intervention and at a 1-year follow-up (Repp & Karsh, 1994).

How reinforcers are delivered impacts their effectiveness as agents of behavioral change. For example, reinforcers delivered immediately are more powerful than those delivered after a waiting period. In addition, the magnitude of a reinforcer is also important: small, immediately delivered reinforcers work better than larger, delayed ones. To illustrate, consider attempts at improving study skills. It is much easier to watch the Simpsons (small, immediate reinforcer) than to resist and study to acquire a good exam grade (large, distant reinforcer). Finally, reinforcement schedule also plays a role in how quickly and how well behavior may change. Reinforcement may be presented in either continuous, interval, or ratio schedules. On a continuous reinforcement schedule, a reinforcer is presented after every response. In interval and ratio schedules, which may be either fixed or variable, reinforcers are presented after the occurrence of the target response following the elapsed time interval or after a specified number of responses, respectively. For example, if children in a classroom setting are required to initiate verbal interactions with peers on a fixed-ratio schedule, they will receive a reinforcer after the specified number of responses. Research has indicated that intermittent reinforcement is more efficient than continuous reinforcement because it increases a behavior's resistance to extinction. However, when initiating positive reinforcement, it is important for a therapist to reinforce a child continuously (i.e., after each desirable response). After the target behavior has increased to an acceptable level, the therapist may begin reinforcing responses intermittently.

Three basic methods of positive reinforcement are commonly used. These are the use of primary reinforcers, the token economy, and differential reinforcement. *Primary reinforcers* are those stimuli that are inherently reinforcing. In a *token economy*, the child receives "token" reinforcers—such as poker chips or coupons—that are traded later (e.g., at the end of the class period) for desired primary reinforcers. *Differential reinforcement* is often used to increase the probability of a desired response while decreasing an undesirable one. For example, a child might be differentially reinforced for on-task classroom behaviors while off-task behaviors are ignored. Failure to deliver reinforcement after inappropriate behaviors leads, it is thought, to the extinction of those responses.

Two types of differential reinforcement procedures may be used to increase the probability of desirable behaviors while reducing undesirable ones. In the first, *differential reinforcement of incompatible behaviors*, or DRI, a child may be reinforced for acts that preclude completion of an undesirable target response. This technique has been used to treat hand stereotypies in a mentally retarded population: keeping hands still or handling toys were reinforced to reduce stereotyped hand motions (Handen, 1998). The second technique, called *differential reinforcement of other behaviors*, or DRO, involves providing reinforcement during a period in which a specific undesirable behavior has not occurred. Benefits of these two procedures include highly specific recognition of behaviors incompatible with the undesired response. These behaviors should be naturally occurring and should serve the same function as the undesirable behavior (Handen, 1998).

When a child is learning an entirely new behavior, a technique called *shaping* may be appropriate. In this procedure, therapists use a method of "successive approximations" to teach a desired behavior. Simply put, components of a desirable response are taught in increments and are reinforced at each step. Gradually, the criteria for receiving reinforcement change until the goal behavior is added to the child's repertoire. As the child's behavioral skill increases, the involvement of the therapist decreases to encourage the child to demonstrate mastery independently (Parrish, 1997). Although shaping is commonly used, there is a lack of agreement as to the optimal speed at which a behavior should be developed (Williams & Gross, 1994).

Some research has indicated that there may be negative side effects from using reinforcement. For example, it is commonly believed that extrinsic positive reinforcement reduces intrinsic motivation, task interest, and creativity (Eisenberger & Cameron, 1996). However, these detrimental effects may occur only under specific conditions, such as presenting a singular reinforcer noncontingently on task performance, followed by a period of nonreinforcement. Further, decrements in performance in such situations are quite small (Handen, 1998).

Punishment

In contrast to positive reinforcement procedures, punishment is used to decrease the probability of undesirable behaviors. In punishment procedures, either an aversive stimulus is added or a positive stimulus is removed contingent upon completion of an undesired behavior. These methods are called "positive punishment" and "omission," respectively. In a *positive punishment* procedure, if a child hits a sibling, his parents may verbally reprimand him. In *omission*, his parents may withdraw television privileges contingent on the aggressive behavior. As in positive reinforcement, the effect of a particular stimulus on behavior rather than stimulus quality determines its usefulness as a punisher. However, stimuli used in positive punishment, such as physical punishment, are typically inherently aversive. Like positive reinforcement, punishment may be presented in either continuous, interval, or ratio schedules.

Punishment procedures are rarely used on their own. Rather, they are often paired with positive reinforcement. The decrease of an undesirable behavior's frequency is an improvement, but children often may need to build their repertoires of desirable behaviors by increasing desirable responses. Further, such a strategy may aid children in understanding differential consequences for their appropriate and inappropriate behaviors.

Several types of punishment procedure are commonly used. One variety of positive punishment if *overcorrection*. In this technique, a child overcorrects the environmental effects resulting from an inappropriate act. This component of overcorrection, called *restitution*, involves restoration of the environment to a better state than it was before the undesirable act. For example, a child who dumped the dishes in the drying rack on the floor would be required to sweep the kitchen floor, as well as all the floors in the rest of the house. In addition to the correction of environmental effects, the child is required to practice "overly correct" forms of appropriate behavior. This is called *positive practice* and involves repeating behaviors that are incompatible with the undesired behavior. For example, when dealing with self-stimulatory behaviors, such as head-weaving in an autistic population, one might require children engaging in these behaviors to hold their heads in a stationary position and engage in very prescribed head movements for a short duration (see Foxx & Azrin, 1973).

There are also two varieties of omission. In a *time-out* procedure, positive reinforcers are taken away from the child by removing that child from a reinforcing environment. For example, when a child hits a peer in a classroom, that child may be placed in a chair away from the class activity. The general recommendation for duration of time-out is one minute per year in age. However, time may be added for inappropriate behaviors, such as tantrumming or kicking, while in time-out. For this technique to work, it is important that the child have limited access to positive reinforcers—even those verbalizations provided by the teacher or therapist to enforce the time-out may inadvertently reinforce undesirable behaviors. To reduce verbal contact with a child in time-out, Reitman and Drabman (1996) have presented a technique in which children are informed that they receive additional minutes of time-out for speaking. Rather than verbally telling a child about the added time, a therapist counts words spoken on fingers, each finger signifying an additional minute in time-out.

Response cost, another form of omission, involves removing a positive reinforcer after an undesired behavior. Although frequently used for aggressive behavior and behavioral non-compliance, response cost is often included with other interventions in a comprehensive treatment package. To ensure its effectiveness, the "cost" to the child contingent upon performing an undesired behavior must be salient. In other words, the stimulus removed from the child must have some value to that particular child.

Although time-out is often used to treat childhood aggression in the classroom, one of its drawbacks is the need to withdraw the child from the academic environment for a short period of time, which may interfere with learning. In addition, time-out procedures may lack acceptability to parents or teachers due to difficulty in implementation or the belief that "they won't work." In contrast, a response cost procedure in which positive reinforcers such as tokens or points are removed allows teachers to provide consequences for undesirable behavior and at the same time allow the child to remain in the classroom. Further, response cost may have a higher acceptability to parents and educators than time-out.

In a multiple baseline design across subjects, Reynolds and Kelley (1997) evaluated the efficacy of a response cost-based treatment package for managing aggressive behaviors in preschool children. Target behaviors that led to loss of positive reinforcers included hitting, kicking, taking a toy from a peer, destroying class materials, throwing objects, name-calling, and excluding peers from an activity. At the beginning of each observation interval, the children were provided with a "GOOD BEHAVIOR CHART" that included five smiley faces. For each instance of inappropriate behavior, a smiley face was removed while the teacher repeated the contingency. If children retained one or more smiley face after a 40-minute period, they were allowed to choose a small prize, such as play in a desired center, a special snack, or helping the teacher. If at the end of the week children had retained at least one smiley face each for 4 or 5 days, they were permitted to choose a toy from a grab bag. The intervention resulted in substantial decreases in aggressiveness.

Due to ethical considerations, positive punishers are used only when less aversive methods fail or when children's behaviors place them at risk of serious medical, physical, or educational consequences (Parrish, 1997). For a number of reasons, many researchers suggest that any use of punishment should follow consideration and application of positive reinforcement methods. First, positive reinforcement strategies are usually at least as or more effective than punishment. Second, punishment may lead to problematic relationship-based side effects. For example, if a child associates a particular person (parent, teacher, or therapist) with punishment, that person may become less socially reinforcing to the child. Finally, misapplied punishment techniques may cause harm (Parrish, 1997). In the light of these considerations, a treatment hierarchy in which nonaversive methods are first considered and evaluated may be appropriate. However, if situations arise in which rapid suppression of a behavior is warranted, as in cases of harm to self or others, punishment may be the treatment of choice (Williams & Gross, 1994). Whatever the case, therapists should make decisions concerning the use of punishment carefully based on the information obtained thorough idiographic analysis.

Extinction

Extinction, yet another operate technique, also decreases the frequency of an undesired behavior. To extinguish undesirable responding, one must withhold reinforcement following a behavior that was previously maintained by that reinforcement. For example, if a child's disruptive behavior is maintained by positive adult attention, withdrawal of attention, or *planned ignoring*, will decrease that behavior. If an aberrant behavior, such as tantrumming, is reinforced negatively by terminating demands made on the child, then extinction would involve maintaining those demands to prevent "escape." In any case, it is crucial to identify specific reinforcers responsible for maintaining a behavior. Planned ignoring works only if attention is in fact the reinforcer responsible for the occurrence of a behavior. To accurately identify maintaining reinforcers, observation of the rate of undesirable behavior following the systematic removal of likely reinforcers is suggested. This may prove difficult, however, if behaviors are maintained by "thin," intermittent schedules of reinforcement, or if more than one reinforcer maintains a behavior across a variety of settings (Williams & Gross, 1994).

Several considerations are involved in ensuring the effectiveness of an extinction paradigm. As mentioned previously, reinforcers that maintain an undesirable behavior must be clearly identified. After identification, these reinforcers must be withheld consistently. The danger of not doing so would be the inadvertent institution of an intermittent reinforcement schedule, which makes behavior *resistant* to extinction. Controlling reinforcers may prove extremely difficult, especially when a child is in a classroom where inadvertent social reinforcers are abundant. Further, children who experience an extinction procedure may engage in pouting, crying, or tantrum behaviors that are difficult to ignore. *Extinction bursts*, or increases in the frequency or intensity of a behavior following an extinction procedure, may also prove hard to handle. In a classroom setting, these types of disruptions may cause teachers to stop using extinction procedures. However, when coupled with positive reinforcement for desirable behaviors, extinction side effects may be diminished (Handen, 1998). It is also important to educate treatment mediators about such bursts. Finally, extinguished behaviors may recur. This *spontaneous recovery* may diminish if reinforcement remains withheld (Parrish, 1997).

Francis (1988) provides an illustrative case example of extinction of compulsive reassurance-seeking in an 11-year-old obsessive–compulsive child. In addition to persistent fears of death or handicap from diseases, the child presented with a number of compulsions, such as persistently asking his parents for reassurance regarding his health or mortality. The child's parents were instructed to ignore all reassurance-seeking behaviors for a phase of eight consecutive days. Following a return to baseline in which parents resumed attention to reassurance-seeking, they were again instructed to return to the extinction phase for 20 days. Once treatment was initiated, the child experienced an extinction burst during which he was extremely tearful, panicky, and demanding. However, his rate of reassurance-seeking dropped to zero after 6 days. During the return to baseline, his behavior worsened, but dropped again in the subsequent extinction phase. At a 1-month follow-up, his rate of reassurance-seeking remained at zero (Francis, 1988).

Extinction is a gradual but effective process because extinguished behavior tends to remain so for long periods of time (Handen, 1998). Typically, extinction procedures are provided in comprehensive treatment packages and often work best when coupled with positive reinforcement. It is perhaps most useful in situations in which maintaining reinforcers are clearly identifiable and easily controlled. Because the effects of extinction are delayed, this technique may not be indicated for use when risk of harm to self or others is evident, as in self-injurious or aggressive behavior.

Contingency Management

Contingency management programs use a variety of operant techniques to change children's behavior. Specifically, they incorporate positive reinforcement, punishment, and extinction paradigms, among others. Parents, peers, and teachers are often trained to implement these programs. A basic component of contingency management programs involves specifying clear behavioral goals. These goals, as well as the consequences of failure to meet them, are typically communicated to a child by using *contingency contracting*. In this procedure, a behavioral contract that specifies a number of criteria is established jointly by the therapist and the child. First and foremost, both appropriate and inappropriate behaviors, as well as the consequences of each, must be clearly specified. Rules that detail the use of contingencies must also be clearly stated, in addition to any "bonus clauses" for appropriate behavior above and beyond the contract. Last, the contract should include an explicit statement of terms under which the contract is abandoned or terminated (Williams & Gross, 1994). Contingency management has been used with success for a diversity of childhood problems including school refusal (Kearney & Tillotson, 1998), anxiety (Barrios & O'Dell, 1998), and for parents who maltreat their children (Donohue, Ammerman, & Zelis, 1998).

An interesting case study in which contingency management was coupled with a response prevention component to treat nocturnal enuresis of a 9-year-old male is provided by Luciano, Molina, Gomez, and Herruzo (1993). After 2 weeks of baseline data were collected, Salvadore, who wet the bed nightly, was placed on a contingency management protocol. In this procedure, Salvadore was taught a number of retention (response prevention) exercises. Positive social reinforcers were provided for such behaviors as correct completion of retention exercises and awakening to an alarm clock with a dry bed in the morning. Natural aversive consequences, such as experiencing a wet diaper or bedsheets and cleaning up both himself and his bedsheets, were contingencies for failure to retain his urine. Records of his progress were kept by Salvadore himself, while the therapist wrote praising comments in the same journal. After 40 weeks, his nocturnal enuresis had been reduced significantly (Luciano et al., 1993).

MODELING

Modeling therapies are derived from Albert Bandura's principles of observational learning. Bandura believed that individuals acquired much of their adaptive repertoires via observation of others (Bandura, 1977). Modeling provides an opportunity for children to learn by observing a "model" engage in a target behavior and experience its consequences. The functions of modeling are threefold (Thorpe & Olson, 1996). First, children may acquire new behavior patterns by combining responses in novel ways. Second, modeling may have either inhibitory or disinhibitory effects on behavior. For example, a child who learns through modeling that consequences for biting another result in time-out may *inhibit* aggressive behavior in the future. On the other hand, a child who fears snakes may handle one after observing peers or teachers do the same in the absence of aversive consequences. Thus, the child's behavior becomes *disinhibited*. Finally, modeling may facilitate appropriate social responses. In the case of a socially phobic child, watching a peer or therapist initiate social interactions may encourage that child to do the same. Modeling has been used successfully for a variety of childhood disorders, including anxiety and phobias (Barrios & O'Dell, 1998), parent treatment in child abuse and neglect (Azar & Wolfe, 1998), and externalizing behavior disorders (Kendall & Braswell, 1985).

Several factors influence how well and how efficiently children learn behaviors through modeling procedures. The extent to which children recognize vicarious consequences, as well as experience direct consequences resulting from their own attempts to perform a given behavior, determines how well that behavior is learned. Further, modeling may be more efficient if incentives to learn a behavior are provided. The more salient the consequences, the better attention children will pay, and the more motivation they will demonstrate (Thorpe & Olson, 1996). Modeling efficiency may also be enhanced through verbal coding of observed responses. This may facilitate a child's retention of a given behavioral sequence. Finally, practice makes perfect: the more opportunities children have to perform a modeled behavior, the higher the likelihood that learning will occur (Thorpe & Olson, 1996).

In a basic modeling procedure, a child is exposed to a live model who performs target behaviors. Modeling may take place in a "graduated" fashion, in which the model engages in progressively more difficult behaviors. This approach proves especially useful when treating childhood phobias. Further, children may be "guided" by models, in other words, given feedback on their own performance from the model. In addition to these techniques, a few other common variants exist. These include symbolic modeling, covert modeling, and participant modeling. In a *symbolic modeling* procedure, children may view a film in which a model performs desired target responses. *Covert modeling* requires children to imagine either themselves or a model with similar characteristics performing a target behavior appropriately. Finally, *participant modeling*, involves the child's direct or indirect observation of a model and subsequent practice of the target behaviors. This practice is usually augmented with guided instruction and support from the model.

Matson (1983) provides an illustrative study in which participant modeling was used to treat fear of small animals in a multiple-baseline design. Jane, age 3, was referred for her debilitating fear of small animals, which manifested as freezing, going into a fetal position, and shaking as soon as she saw the feared animal. Treatment was implemented by the child's mother. First, procedures were explained to Jane in a manner appropriate to her developmental level. During subsequent training sessions, her mother first presented a stuffed dog and cat, with which they played for 5-minute intervals. The mother would repeat that these were nice animals and model affectionate behavior. After Jane could hold the stuffed animals for a period of 1 minute, live animals were introduced. During this phase, her mother repeated that these were nice animals and patted them for 3- to 4-minute periods. This procedure was repeated until Jane's fearful behaviors diminished significantly. Improvements were maintained at a 1-year follow-up (Matson, 1983).

When utilizing modeling techniques, it is important to distinguish between mastery models and coping models. *Mastery models* demonstrate perfect performance of target behaviors. For example, while engaging in a behavior, the model demonstrates no frustration, anxiety, or need for practice. In contrast, a *coping model* demonstrates requisite coping strategies for dealing with difficult tasks, or even failures. Thus, coping models make errors and may demonstrate skills of persistence and practice. In so doing, the coping model may be more like the child and perhaps more salient (Kendall & Braswell, 1985). Research has indicated that coping models may be superior to mastery models in effectiveness (e.g., Kazdin, 1974; Meichenbaum, 1972).

BEHAVIORAL PARENT TRAINING

Behavioral parent training refers to interventions based on behavior modification principles and grounded in learning theory. Although varied in the extent to which they adhere to behavioral methods, these treatments are bound by a few common themes. Proponents of these approaches posit that children's maladaptive behaviors are developed and maintained through reciprocal coercive familial interactions (see Hembree-Kigin & McNeil, 1995; Patterson, 1982). As such, emphasis is placed on identifying the functional nature of such interactive patterns and making them therapeutic targets for change. Because parents play a primary role in constructing and managing their child's environment, the behavior therapist trains them to become agents of behavioral change. Parents learn more effective ways of communicating and applying contingencies to their children. Specifically, they learn to recognize and modify both the antecedents and consequences of their children's problematic behavior. Each intervention is tailored to the child's target behavior, as well as to idiosyncratic family needs. Behavioral parent training has been used for a variety of childhood problems in a range of settings, including conduct and oppositional-defiant disorders (Brestan & Eyberg, 1998; Frick, 1998; Hembree-Kigin & McNeil, 1995; Serketich & Dumas, 1996), ADHD (Pelham, Wheeler, & Chronis, 1998), disruptive classroom behavior (Funderburk, Eyberg, Newcomb, McNeil, Hembree-Kigin, & Capage, 1998), and a number of others.

Behavior therapists may provide parents with either didactic instruction (Lutzker, Huynen, & Bigelow, 1998), via instructional materials, videotapes, or even on-the-spot coaching (Hembree-Kigin & McNeil, 1995). In addition, therapists may use more active training methods such as modeling, rehearsal, feedback, and homework assignments. Techniques commonly imparted to parents involve differential reinforcement, contingency management, response cost, and extinction (Briesmeister & Schaefer, 1998). For example, training in using contingency schedules may help parents ascertain whether to deliver reinforcers continuously or intermittently. The appropriate use of time-out procedures may also assist parents in providing consistent and effective consequences for their children's undesirable behaviors.

Lutzker et al. (1998) outlined three major approaches to parent training. *Contingency management training* teaches parents to issue simple, direct commands and apply consistent consequences to their children's target behaviors. This procedure is often used for noncompliance and difficulty following instructions. *Planned activities training* assists parents in structuring antecedents to increase appropriate behaviors and minimize opportunities for inappropriate behaviors. Finally, *behavioral momentum* or *errorless compliance training* involves first teaching parents to issue requests with a high probability of child compliance. Gradually, instructions for more complex and less probable behaviors are phased in (Ducharme & Popynick, 1993; Ducharme & Worling, 1994).

The influence from developmental psychology is a strong guiding force in parent training interventions. For example, Hembree-Kigin and McNeil's (e.g., 1995) parent–child interaction therapy (PCIT) is a behavioral treatment that has a strong developmental thrust (Vernberg, 1998). PCIT conceptualizes early-onset behavior disturbances such as noncompliance, as frequent, repetitious, negative, affective interchanges with parents (Hembree-Kigin & McNeil, 1995). In addition to using parents as cotherapists and teaching parenting skills through on-the-spot coaching techniques, this intervention emphasizes early recognition of psychopathology and its precursors, as well as vulnerability or risk factors. The importance of understanding why a particular child has entered a deviant developmental pathway is stressed, as well as the biological, social, and psychological factors involved in determining it (Vernberg, 1998). A common problem in many behavior therapies that do not take developmental factors into consideration is the failure to address age-specific interpersonal information-processing deficits and to develop "age appropriate language pragmatics" (Vernberg, 1998). PCIT utilizes bug-in-ear technology to help parents match their language usage to their child's developmental level and facilitate positive reinforcement for appropriate child play. Finally, PCIT conducts follow-ups to determine the length of treatment effects because children may struggle with similar issues when new developmental stages have been reached (Funderburk et al., 1998; Hembree-Kigin & McNeil, 1995).

Recent work by Schuhmann, Foote, Eyberg, Boggs, and Algina (1998) provides interim results of a study investigating the effectiveness of PCIT with preschool-age children who have oppositional-defiant disorder. Sixty-four families were assigned randomly to either a treatment or a wait-list control condition. Participants in the treatment condition were taught both child-directed interaction (CDI), in which they learned nondirective play therapy skills and parent-directed interaction (PDI). In the PDI phase, parents learned to direct their children's behavior with clear, direct, age-appropriate instructions and to deliver consistent consequences. Further, parents were directed to give praise for compliance and time-out for noncompliance. Treatment was terminated when parents demonstrated mastery of skills. Results indicated that parents in the treatment condition interacted more positively with their children than those in the wait-list control. Further, parents in the treatment group reported significant improvements in their children's behavior.

Many behavior therapists view behavioral parent training as one of the field's outstanding achievements. A number of publications have appeared in the recent literature detailing the efficacy of these techniques (e.g., Briesmeister & Schaefer, 1998; Pelham, Wheeler, & Chronis, 1998; Serketich & Dumas, 1996). Initial results have been promising, but additional research and follow-up studies will enhance further development of assessment strategies and address relapse prevention (Briesmeister & Schaefer, 1998). Moreover, there is still room for expanding and refining parent training procedures. For example, more attention must be paid to the reciprocal nature of parent–child interactions regarding how children's behavior affects their parents' capacity to function. Another future direction of this research involves the identifying risk factors and assessing preventive efforts.

Cognitive-Behavioral Approaches

Cognitive-behavioral therapy (CBT) stresses the role of covert behaviors—specifically, cognitive variables—in the learning process. Specifically, it focuses on the way children respond to their cognitive interpretations of experience (Kendall & Panichelli-Mindel, 1995). As does behavior therapy, cognitive-behavioral theory posits that environmental contingencies play a central role in the psychological development of children. However, CBT underscores the primacy of information-processing capacity in acquiring, maintaining, and remediating maladaptive functioning (Kendall, 1993). Central to cognitive-behavioral theory and technique is the concept of reciprocal determinism. *Reciprocal determinism* posits that cognitive factors interact with environmental contingencies bidirectionally to produce an organism's response repertoire (Craighead, Meyers, & Wilcoxon Craighead, 1985). It follows that changes in cognition produce changes in behavior, and vice versa. Thus, cognitive-behavioral therapies focus on both modalities to produce therapeutic change.

In treating children, cognitive-behavioral interventions emphasize the instruction of adaptive thinking processes (Kendall & Braswell, 1985). It is believed that deficiencies in cognitive processing play a role in developing and maintaining some childhood psychopathology (Hart & Morgan, 1993). Consequently, cognitive-behavioral therapists attempt to teach children new strategies for modifying their thought processes to control behavior. This type of intervention tends to focus on three different areas of children's maladaptive functioning, each of which has given rise to a different therapeutic procedure. First, children may demonstrate difficulty in verbal control of behaviors. Luria (1959, 1961) suggested that when children initially learn behaviors, they are under the verbal control of adults. Through self-talk, however, children eventually learn to control their own behavior, first by talking to themselves out loud and subsequently by internalizing self-instructions. Emphasis on this area of cognitive functioning led to the formulation of "self-instructional training" by Meichenbaum (Meichenbaum & Goodman, 1971). Children's cognitive-behavioral therapy also focuses on developing self-control (or self-regulation) in children, which is defined as the ability to choose a previously low-probability behavior when a higher probability behavior is available. This has given rise to therapies geared toward helping children self-reward with the goal of developing and maintaining new cognitive or behavioral responses. Finally, cognitive therapies also focus on children's ability to solve problems. A number of creative interventions exist to enhance skills deficits in this area.

Self-Instructional Training and Problem-Solving Skills Training

Self-instructional training involves teaching children to use "self-talk" to negotiate difficult tasks or situations. This technique is often used with impulsive children (Frick, 1998; Kendall & Braswell, 1985; Lochman, 1992). First, the therapist models appropriate behaviors for children while verbalizing self-instructions aloud. The child is required to imitate this behavior while the therapist again repeats self-instructions that correspond to the child's behavior. Finally, the child also learns, via prompting by the therapist, to verbalize the self-instructional statements while performing the behavior. After much practice, therapist prompts are faded as the child develops increasing ability to covertly produce self-instructions while engaging in the desired responses.

Problem-solving skills training (PSST) posits the existence of interpersonal skills deficits in behaviorally disordered children. In fact, many empirical studies have investigated the relationship between behavioral adjustment and interpersonal problem-solving skills. In most cases, children who exhibit adjustment difficulties generate fewer appropriate alternative solutions to interpersonal problems. Further, they are less able to identify consequences of their behaviors than their well-adjusted counterparts. Finally, they have difficulty correctly identifying goal-directed behavior in others (Frick, 1998). As a result, many problem-solving skills training programs have been developed to remedy these deficits. Treatment may incorporate the use of scripts, role plays, or games initiated by the therapist to expose children to a variety of interpersonal conflict situations in a safe environment. Then, children are asked to offer possible solutions, and they receive feedback and verbal praise from the therapist when they come up with appropriate answers.

One program that emphasizes both self-instructional and problem-solving training was developed by Lochman (1992) for aggressive children. This approach focuses on the deficits in social cognition characteristic of aggressive children and adolescents. In the first phase of the program, children are taught to use self-instructional statements, such as "Stop and think!" when they become aware of physiological arousal. These statements are used to inhibit impulsive aggressive responses. The program's second phase guides children through a variety of perspective-taking tasks. For example, children are asked to view photographs of ambiguous social situations and to label and discuss the intention of the persons in the photos. Further, children role-play the situations to demonstrate how individuals may misjudge the intentions of others. Finally, the third portion of the program addresses anger control. During this phase, children are taught to recognize the physiological signs of anger and use these signals as discriminative cues to begin a problem-solving process (Frick, 1998). The results of a 3-year follow-up study of this approach indicate that children who participated demonstrated lower rates of drug and alcohol use, as well as higher self-esteem and problem-solving skills (Lochman, 1992).

A number of studies point to the efficacy of cognitive-behavioral treatments for adolescent depression (Kaslow & Thompson, 1998; Lewinsohn, Clarke, Hops, & Andrews, 1990), anxiety disorders (Kendall & Southam-Gerow, 1996; Ollendick & King, 1998; Ollendick, 1995; March, 1995), impulsive children (Kendall & Braswell, 1985), antisocial behavior (Brestan & Eyberg, 1998; Kazdin, Bass, Siegel, & Thomas, 1989), and enuresis (Ronen & Wozner, 1995). Frick (1998) outlined a number of treatment packages that incorporate both approaches for conduct-disordered children (e.g., Bierman & Greenberg, 1996; Lochman & Wells, 1996). However, one shortcoming of this treatment for conduct-disordered youth is that behavioral gains made often do not generalize well outside the clinical environment. Effectiveness may be enhanced if parents are incorporated into the treatment as cotherapists (Frick, 1998). More research is needed in clinical populations to evaluate the efficacy of this treatment for other types of childhood disorder, such as ADHD and anxiety (Kendall, 1993).

ETHICAL ISSUES IN TREATING CHILDREN

The extent to which children should be involved in treatment decisions is no simple matter in any psychological intervention, but especially in behavior therapy. Because behavior therapies are heavily educational and directive, it is of utmost importance that participants be as well-informed as possible. For example, in exposure-based treatments, it would be unethical to present highly fear-inducing stimuli to a client without first explaining the treatment rationale. However, children are often viewed as incapable of comprehending treatment, much less of participating in treatment decisions. Further, because they are most often other-referred, they may be disenfranchised from the decision to participate in therapy at its outset. It is common for therapists to enlist significant others involved in the child's life as treatment mediators without consulting the child. Yet children merit the same ethical considerations in psychological treatment as adults. To what extent should children and adolescents be involved in their own treatment?

Even though children are often referred for treatment by teachers or parents, this does not necessarily preclude them from being active participants in therapeutic choices. As with adults, children at risk of harming themselves or others are not capable of making significant contributions. Similarly, very young children or those who have limited cognitive abilities may be incapable of participating in such decisions. The distinction between child and adult blurs, however, when one considers adolescents. For example, in a study by Weithorn (1980), 14-year-olds rivaled adults in comprehending treatment issues. Further, even 9-year-olds demonstrated basic, although simplistic, agreement with treatment decisions made by older groups. Belter and Grisso (1984) found that by age 15, adolescents presented with their rights in a therapy analog exhibited the same degree of understanding as 21-year-old participants. Further, minors who have learning and behavioral problems are capable of identifying the risks and benefits of treatment (Kaser-Boyd, Adelman, & Taylor, 1985). This suggests that therapists should remain open to including adolescents and even children who demonstrate suitable competence in making treatment choices.

Other ethical issues arise in the consideration of child confidentiality. Often, when children are seen in therapy, they are not alone. Many behavioral interventions stress the necessity of involving parents, teachers, and peers in the treatment process. For example, consider parent training programs, in which both child and parents are considered clients. In such situations, the child's confidentiality is often at risk. Further, it seems increasingly the case that children are legally allowed to participate in therapy without parental consent. These situations may arise in cases of alleged sexual or physical abuse, pregnancy, or substance abuse (Gustafson & McNamara, 1995). In such cases, it is important for the therapist to consider a number of issues when making decisions about handling confidentiality agreements. These include considering the child's age, needs and desires, the parent's concerns, the presenting problem, and relevant state statutes. It may also be helpful to make at least an informal assessment of cognitive abilities and developmental level (Gustafson & McNamara, 1995). When these issues are dealt with, an agreement needs to be clarified between therapist, child, and parents about how confidentiality will be approached.

CURRENT ISSUES AND FUTURE DIRECTIONS IN BEHAVIOR THERAPY

Regardless of gains made in technical complexity and efficacy, as well as the increasing acceptance from both the clinical community and managed care, behavior therapy is still a fledgling science. As such, there is much room for improvement. Two major practical goals for the beginning of the next century will be survival in an age of managed care and increased effectiveness and palatability for the consumer (Chorpita, 1997b). Chorpita details a number of ways to advance the field, including more reliance on actuarial decision making, better computerized assessment, abandonment of a "cure" model, and development of a more appropriate nosological system (Chorpita, 1997b). Issues apropos to such advancement include the empirical validation of behavior therapy, how the field will negotiate the issue of psychiatric diagnosis, and efforts to increase generalization of treatment effects.

Empirical Validation

Behaviorists stress the necessity of dimensional, behavior-based views of psychopathology, but the move toward empirical validation of treatment has gained momentum. Such an impetus could allow the field greater mobility and acceptance in the emerging realm of managed care. Thus, the American Psychological Association Division 12 Task Force on the Promotion and Dissemination of Psychological Procedures was convened in 1995. The purpose of this task force was to standardize the search for empirically valid treatments and to isolate what treatment works for whom across a number of categorical, high-frequency childhood psychopathologies. Thus, a number of inclusion criteria were detailed, and the results were published in a recent review issue of the *Journal of Clinical Child Psychology*. These criteria stressed the methodological rigor of study design, as well as strength of empirical support (see Lonigan, Elbert, & Johnson, 1998). For example, "well-established" interventions were those in which at least two group-design studies or more than nine single-case design studies were conducted and results indicated that treatment was superior to a placebo or alternative treatment. Further, in these studies, treatment manuals were used, and sample characteristics were clearly specified. Criteria for "probably efficacious" interventions were somewhat less stringent (Lonigan, Elbert, & Johnson, 1998).

Behavioral and cognitive-behavioral interventions fared well across a range of childhood disorders such as ADHD (Pelham, Wheeler, & Chronis, 1998), depression (Kaslow & Thompson, 1998), anxiety (Ollendick & King, 1998), autism (Rogers, 1998), and conduct disorders (Brestan & Eyberg, 1998). It is clear that many behavioral therapies are efficacious and merit a long and continuing history of research and application (Lonigan, Elbert, & Johnson, 1998). However, these strategies are most effective when used in prescribed research versus clinical settings and for highly discrete and well-defined psychopathologies. For example, further research is still needed in treating disorders where the incidence of comorbidity is high. More work may also be necessary to address the dimensional components of psychological dysfunction within current categories of disorder. For example, the range of behaviors from mild to severe or overt to covert aggression may warrant different types or intensities of treatment. Issues such as these are not addressed adequately in the existing literature. Kazdin and Kendall (1998) detailed a number of steps to guide future treatment development and research. They emphasize the need to assess etiological factors, the necessity of manuals to guide treatment delivery and replication, and stress the importance of both process and outcome measures. Factors such as treatment focus, duration, and intensity with regard to psychological or behavioral disturbances also merit further investigation (Kazdin & Kendall, 1998).

Behavioral Assessment and Psychiatric Diagnosis

Chorpita (1997a) noted that although much of child psychopathology is defined in terms of behaviors rather than categories of diagnosis, the assessment process is broadening. This seems evident in the movement toward matching treatments to disorders. Some behavior analysts fear that behavior therapy will become unmoored from its theoretical roots via subsumption into a medical model that holds that treatment "cures" and that psychopathology is categorical (Chorpita, 1997b). Others, however, believe that the use of a common diagnostic system fosters better communication within the field. The current DSM-IV (American Psychiatric Association, 1994) has expanded its focus on childhood disorders and may prove useful when coupled with behavioral assessment strategies.

It must be noted that a serious limitation of the DSM-IV is its emphasis on the topography of problematic behavior while ignoring its function in a specific context (Watson & Gresham, 1998). However, not all behaviors lend themselves to direct experimental manipulation to assess their function—take, for example, behaviors that occur during sleep, covert acts, or rarely occurring behaviors. Such behaviors may be more suited to a descriptive assessment (Watson & Gresham, 1998). Hersen and Van Hasselt (1987) argued that strict adherence to "narrow band" behavioral assessment strategies precludes considering such issues as etiology, precipitating stressors and onset, chronicity, and severity. Further, such an approach may cloud the issue of the way target behaviors and symptoms may interrelate within a particular diagnostic category (Williams & Gross, 1994). Yet the field seems to be moving away from an "either ... or" dilemma and toward better integration of the two systems. Chorpita (1997b) reiterates that more empirical investigation is needed to examine the interrelationship between diagnostic categories and functional assessment. The end result of such an endeavor may be the establishment of "a more complex and representative nosology" (Chorpita, 1997b, p. 581).

Generalization of Treatment Effects

Generalization of treatment effects is a problem for all current psychotherapies, including behavior therapy. Behavioral gains made in treatment may fail to demonstrate stability across four generalization domains—specifically, setting, time, behaviors, or participants (Allen, Tarnowski, Simonian, Elliot, & Drabman, 1991). Treatment generalization across time, or *response maintenance* studies, evaluate whether gains made in therapy remain stable when treatment is discontinued. Those studies that investigate across settings look at how well behavior gains are maintained across different situations. *Response generalization* indicates the extent to which behaviors not specifically targeted toward treatment may also change. Studies that assess generalization across nontreated individuals examine whether these individuals exhibit behavioral changes similar to those receiving treatment. One recent review by Allen et al. (1991) found that 46.9% of studies presented generalization data. However, of these, most did not meet specified criteria—maintenance of treatment gains at 6-month follow-up (Allen et al., 1991).

Kazdin (1989) proposed a number of strategies to help ensure generalization of treatment effects. First, therapists should strive to teach behaviors that will eventually come under the control of natural environmental contingencies. He also stresses the importance of training teachers, parents, and peers in using behavioral programs. If extrinsic reinforcers or punishers are used, they should be gradually faded to resemble natural contingencies. In addition to more strict behavioral strategies, it may also prove useful to teach children to self-monitor, self-evaluate, and self-reward. Finally, therapists should incorporate the use of cognitive-behavioral procedures, such as problem-solving skills training, to enhance awareness of cognitive mediators of behavior (Kazdin, 1989).

Although behavior and cognitive-behavioral therapies have a wealth of empirical support for their treatment efficacy in clinical trials, there is some question as to how well they generalize to more ecologically valid clinical settings. Happily, some have proposed models for "bridging the gap" between outcome researchers and practitioners. These methods may include clinicians in private practice or managed care settings, identification of factors in research settings which may influence positive outcomes, and exporting laboratory-tested procedures to clinics (Weisz, Donenberg, Han, & Weiss, 1995). Further, the conceptualization of treatment as "cure" may mislead consumers to believe that behavior therapy works across all imaginable situations. This view may also preclude understanding the necessity of research that addresses generalization. Clearly, the use of reversal designs suggests that behavior therapy predicts the possibility of its own failure. This does not mean that it is designed to fail, but that it recognizes its own limitations, especially in the area of generalization. Thus, revising the "cure" model of treatment may be necessary (Chorpita, 1997b).

SUMMARY

Behavior therapies focus on environmental determinants of behavior and posit that behavioral change occurs by manipulating behavioral contingencies. Because of their emphasis on studying overt behavior and their strong foundation on experimentally evaluated procedures, behavior therapies have gained widespread acceptance in the scientific community. These types of treatment have been used for a variety of disorders, first in adult populations, and later, with children.

As behavioral approaches to assessment and treatment have matured during the past three or four decades, they have integrated influences from a number of different areas. In the area of assessment, many argue for using cognitive abilities and achievement tests, as well as neuropsychological tests, in addition to functional analytic and observational methods. In the area of treatment, influences from cognitive-behavioral treatments, developmental psychology, psychological testing, and pharmacology may often augment pure behavioral techniques.

Behavior therapies are based on principles of both classical and operant conditioning. Systematic desensitization and flooding derived from classical principles are commonly used for treating childhood fears and anxieties. Operant procedures such as response prevention, reinforcement, punishment, extinction, and contingency management, have been successfully used for a myriad of childhood behavior problems. Modeling techniques derived from Bandura's social learning theory also fall under the rubric of behavior therapies. The field of behavioral interventions has broadened to include cognitive-behavioral approaches such as self-instruction and problem-solving skills training programs. Finally, ethical issues that surround the treatment of children have helped to elucidate appropriate roles of both children and adolescents in the treatment process.

A number of current issues delineate areas for future growth in both treatment application and outcome research in the field of behavior therapy. In recent years, psychologists have sought to validate therapeutic interventions empirically across the spectrum of clinically diagnosed childhood disorders. Both behavioral and cognitive-behavioral treatments demonstrated certain levels of efficacy. Debate about the current nosological system continues to trouble the field, yet there has been some recent movement toward integration. In addition, treatment generalization has gained the interest of many researchers, and several guidelines exist for enhancing the ecological validity of behavioral procedures.

REFERENCES

Achenbach, T. M. (1974). *Developmental psychopathology*. New York: Ronald Press.
Achenbach, T. M. (1991). *Manual for the Child Behavior Checklist*. Burlington, VT: Author.
Achenbach, T. M., & Edelbrock, C. S. (1978). The classification of child psychopathology: A review and analysis of empirical effects. *Psychological Bulletin, 85*, 1275–1301.

Achenbach, T. M., & Edelbrock, C. S. (1979). The Child Behavior Profile II. Boys aged 12, 16, and girls aged 6–11 and 12–16. *Journal of Consulting and Clinical Psychology, 47,* 223–233.

Achenbach, T. M., & Edelbrock, C. S. (1981). Behavioral problems and competencies reported by parents of normal and disturbed children aged four through sixteen. *Monographs of the society for research in child development, 461* (no. 188).

Achenbach, T. M., & Edelbrock, C. S. (1983). *Manual for the child behavior checklist and revised child behavior profile.* Burlington: University of Vermont Press.

Allen, J. S., Jr., Tarnowski, K. J., Simonian, S. J., Elliott, D., & Drabman, R. S. (1991). The generalization map revisited: Assessment of generalized treatment effects in child and adolescent behavior therapy. *Behavior Therapy, 22,* 393–405.

American Psychiatric Association. (1994). *Diagnostic and statistical manual of mental disorders,* 4th ed. Washington, DC: Author.

Azar, S. T., & Wolfe, D. A. (1998). Child physical abuse and neglect. In E. J. Mash and R. A. Barkley (Eds.), *Treatment of childhood disorders,* 2nd ed. (pp. 501–544). New York: Guilford.

Bandura, A. (1977). *Social learning theory.* Englewood Cliffs, NJ: Prentice-Hall.

Barrios, B. A., & O'Dell, S. L. (1998). Fears and anxieties. In E. J. Mash and R. A. Barkley (Eds.), *Treatment of childhood disorders,* 2nd ed. (pp. 249–337). New York: Guilford.

Belter, R. W., & Grisso, T. (1984). Children's recognition of rights violations in counseling. *Professional Psychology: Research and Practice, 15,* 899–910.

Bierman, K. L., & Greenberg, M. T. (1996). Social skills training in the FAST Track program. In R. D. Peters and R. J. McMahon (Eds.), *Preventing childhood disorders, substance abuse, and delinquency* (pp. 65–89). Thousand Oaks, CA: Sage.

Brestan, E. v., & Eyberg, S. M. (1998). Effective psychosocial treatments of conduct-disordered children and adolescents: 29 years, 82 studies, and 5,272 kids. *Journal of Clinical Child Psychology, 27,* 180–189.

Briesmeister, J. M., & Schaefer, C. E. (1998). *Handbook of parent training: Parents as co-therapists for children's behavior problems.* New York: Wiley.

Chorpita, B. F. (1997a). Children, promises, and behavior therapy: Commentary on "behavior therapy's promise for child treatment: Where we've been, where we may be going." *Behavior Therapy, 28,* 543–546.

Chorpita, B. F. (1997b). Since the operant chamber: Is behavior therapy still thinking in boxes? *Behavior Therapy, 28,* 577–583.

Craighead, W. E., Meyers, A. W., & Wilcoxon Craighead, L. (1985). A conceptual model for cognitive-behavior therapy with children. *Journal of Abnormal Child Psychology, 13,* 331–342.

Cornwall, E., Spence, S. H., & Schotte, D. (1997). The effectiveness of emotive imagery in the treatment of darkness phobia in children. *Behaviour Change, 13,* 223–229.

Donohue, B., Ammerman, R. T., & Zelis, K. (1998). Child physical abuse and neglect. In T. S. Watson and F. M. Gresham (Eds.), *Handbook of child behavior therapy* (pp. 183–202). New York: Plenum.

Ducharme, J. M., & Popynick, M. (1993). Errorless compliance to parental requests: Treatment effects and generalization. *Behavior Therapy, 24,* 209–226.

Ducharme, J. M., & Worling, D. E. (1994). Behavioral momentum and stimulus fading in the acquisition and maintenance of child compliance in the home. *Journal of Applied Behavior Analysis, 27,* 639–647.

Eisenberger, R., & Cameron, J. (1996). Detrimental effects of reward: Reality or myth? *American Psychologist, 51,* 1153–1166.

Forehand, R., & McMahon, R. J. (1981). *Helping the noncompliant child: A clinician's guide to parent training.* New York: Guilford.

Foxx, R. M. & Azrin, N. H. (1973). The elimination of autistic self-stimulatory behavior by overcorrection. *Journal of Applied Behavior Analysis, 6*(1), 1–14.

Francis, G. (1988). Childhood obsessive–compulsive disorder: Extinction of compulsive reassurance-seeking. *Journal of Anxiety Disorders, 2,* 361–366.

Francis, G., & Beidel, D. C. (1995). Cognitive-behavioral psychotherapy. In J. S. March (Ed.), *Anxiety disorders in children and adolescents* (pp. 321–340). New York: Guilford.

Frick, P. J. (1998). *Conduct disorders and severe antisocial behavior.* New York: Plenum.

Funderburk, B. W., Eyberg, S. M., Newcomb, K., McNeil, C. B., Hembree-Kigin, T., & Capage, L. (1998). Parent-child interaction therapy with behavior problem children: Maintenance of treatment effects in the school setting. *Child and Family Behavior Therapy, 20*(2), 17–38.

Goldstein, G. (1979). Methodological and theoretical issues in neuropsychological assessment. *Journal of Behavioral Assessment, 1,* 23–41.

Gustafson, K. E., & McNamara, R. (1995). Confidentiality with minor clients: Issues and guidelines with therapists. In

D. N. Bersoff (Ed.), *Ethical conflicts in psychology* (pp. 193–197). Washington, DC: American Psychological Association.

Hagopian, L. P., & Ollendick, T. H. (1997). Anxiety disorders. In R. T. Ammerman & M. Hersen (Eds.), *Handbook of prevention and treatment with children and adolescents: Interventions in the real world context* (pp. 431–454). New York: Wiley.

Handen, B. L. (1998). Mental retardation. In E. J. Mash & R. A. Barkley (Eds.), *Treatment of childhood disorders*, 2nd ed. (pp. 369–415). New York: Guilford.

Hart, K. J., & Morgan, J. R. (1993). Cognitive-behavioral procedures with children: Historical context and current status. In A. J. Finch, W. M. Nelson, III, & F. S. Ott (Eds.), *Cognitive-behavioral procedures with children and adolescents: A practical guide* (pp. 1–24). Boston: Allyn & Bacon.

Hembree-Kigin, T. L., & McNeil, C. B. (1995). *Parent-child interaction therapy*. New York: Plenum.

Hersen, M., & Ammerman, R. T. (1989). Overview of new developments in child behavior therapy. In M. Hersen (Ed.), *Innovations in child behavior therapy* (pp. 3–31). New York: Springer.

Hersen, M., & Last, C. G. (1988). How the field has moved on. In M. Hersen & C. G. Last (Eds.), *Child behavior therapy casebook* (pp. 1–10). New York: Plenum.

Hersen, M., & Van Hasselt, V. B. (1987). Developments and emerging trends. In M. Hersen & V. B. Van Hasselt (Eds.), *Behavior therapy with children and adolescents. A clinical approach* (pp. 3–28). New York: Wiley.

Horton, A. M., & Miller, W. G. (1985). Neuropsychology and behavior therapy. In M. Hersen, R. M. Eisler, & P. M. Miller (Eds.), *Progress in behavior modification*, Vol. 19 (pp. 1–55). New York: Academic Press.

Kaser-Boyd, N., Adelman, H., & Taylor, L. (1985). Minors' ability to identify risks and benefits of therapy. *Professional Psychology: Research and Practice, 16*, 411–417.

Kaslow, N. J., & Thompson, M. P. (1998). Applying the criteria for empirically supported treatments to studies of psychosocial interventions for child and adolescent depression. *Journal of Clinical Child Psychology, 27*, 146–155.

Kazdin, A. E. (1974). Covert modeling, model similarity, and reduction of avoidance behavior. *Behavior Therapy, 5*, 325–340.

Kazdin, A. E. (1989). *Behavior modification in applied settings*, 3rd ed. Homewood, IL: Dorsey.

Kazdin, A. E., Bass, D., Siegel, T., & Thomas, C. (1989). Cognitive-behavioral therapy and relationship therapy in the treatment of children referred for antisocial behavior. *Journal of Consulting and Clinical Psychology, 57*, 522–535.

Kazdin, A. E., & Kendall, P. C. (1998). Current progress and future plans for developing effective treatments: Comments and perspectives. *Journal of Clinical Child Psychology, 27*(2), 217–226.

Kearney, C. A., & Tillotson, C. A. (1998). School attendance. In T. S. Watson & F. M. Gresham (Eds.), *Handbook of child behavior therapy* (pp. 143–162). New York: Plenum.

Kendall, P. C. (1993). Cognitive-behavior therapies with youth: Guiding theory, current status, and emerging developments. *Journal of Consulting and Clinical Psychology, 61*, 235–247.

Kendall, P. C., & Braswell, L. (1985). *Cognitive-behavior therapy for impulsive children*. New York: Guilford.

Kendall, P. C., & Panichelli-Mindel, S. M. (1995). Cognitive-behavioral treatments. *Journal of Abnormal Child Psychology, 23*(1), 107–124.

Kendall, P. C., & Southam-Gerow, M. A. (1996). Long-term follow-up of a cognitive-behavioral therapy for anxiety-disordered youth. *Journal of Consulting and Clinical Psychology, 64*, 724–730.

Knell, S. M. (1993). *Cognitive-behavioral play therapy*. Northvale, NJ: Jason Aronson.

Knox, L. S., Albano, A. M., & Barlow, D. H. (1996). Parental involvement in the treatment of childhood obsessive compulsive disorder: A multiple baseline examination incorporating parents. *Behavior Therapy, 27*, 93–115.

Koeppen, A. S. (1974). Relaxation training for children. *Elementary School Guidance and Counseling, 9*, 14–21.

Lalli, J. S., & Kates, K. (1998). The effect of reinforcer preference on functional analysis outcomes. *Journal of Applied Behavior Analysis, 31*(1), 79–90.

Last, C. G. (1989). Anxiety disorders. In T. H. Ollendick & M. Hersen (Eds.), *Handbook of child psychopathology*, 2nd ed. (pp. 219–228). New York: Plenum.

Laurent, J., & Potter, K. L. (1998). Anxiety-related difficulties. In T. S. Watson & F. M. Gresham (Eds.), *Handbook of child behavior therapy* (pp. 371–392). New York: Plenum.

Lazarus, A. A., & Abramovitz, A. (1962). The use of emotive imagery in the treatment of children's phobias. *Journal of Mental Science, 108*, 191–195.

Lewinsohn, P. M., Clarke, G. N., Hops, H., & Andrews, J. (1990). Cognitive-behavioral treatment for depressed adolescents. *Behavior Therapy, 21*, 385–401.

Lochman, J. E. (1992). Cognitive-behavior intervention with aggressive boys: Three-year follow-up and preventive effects. *Journal of Consulting and Clinical Psychology, 60*, 426–432.

Lochman, J. E., & Wells, K. C. (1996). A social-cognitive intervention with aggressive children: Prevention effects and contextual implementation issues. In R. D. Peters & R. J. McMahon (Eds.), *Preventing childhood disorders, substance abuse, and delinquency* (pp. 111–143). Thousand Oaks, CA: Sage.

Lonigan, C. J., Elbert, J. C., & Johnson, S. B. (1998). Empirically-supported psychosocial interventions for children: An overview. *Journal of Clinical Child Psychology, 27,* 138–145.

Luciano, M. C., Molina, F. J., Gomez, I., & Herruzo, J. (1993). Response prevention and contingency management in the treatment of nocturnal enuresis: A report of two cases. *Child and Family Behavior Therapy, 15*(1), 37–51.

Luria, A. R. (1959). The directive function of speech development and dissolution. *Word, 15,* 341–352.

Luria, A. R. (1961). *The role of speech in the regulation of normal and abnormal behaviors.* New York: Liveright.

Lutzker, J. R., Huynen, K. B., & Bigelow, K. M. (1998). Parent training. In V. B. Van Hasselt and M. Hersen (Eds.), *Handbook of psychological treatment protocols for children and adolescents* (pp. 467–500). Mahwah, NJ: Erlbaum.

March, J. S. (1995). Cognitive-behavioral psychotherapy for children and adolescents with OCD: A review and recommendations for treatment. *Journal of the American Academy of Child and Adolescent Psychiatry, 34*(1), 7–18.

Matson, J. L. (1983). Exploration of phobic behavior in a small child. *Journal of Behavior Therapy and Experimental Psychiatry, 14,* 257–260.

Meichenbaum, D. H. (1972). Examination of model characteristics in reducing avoidance behavior. *Journal of Behavior Therapy and Experimental Psychiatry, 3,* 225–227.

Meichenbaum, D. H., & Goodman, J. (1971). Training impulsive children to talk to themselves: A means of developing self-control. *Journal of Abnormal Psychology, 77,* 115–126.

Morris, R. J., & Kratochwill, T. R. (1991). Childhood fears and phobias. In T. R. Kratochwill & R. J. Morris (Eds.), *The practice of child therapy,* 2nd ed. (pp. 76–114). New York: Pergamon.

Nelson, R. O. (1980). The use of intelligence tests within behavioral assessment. *Behavioral Assessment, 2,* 417–423.

Nelson, R. O., & Hayes, S. C. (1981). The nature of behavioral assessment. In M. Hersen & A. S. Bellack (Eds.), *Behavioral assessment,* 2nd ed. (pp. 3–33). New York: Pergamon.

Ollendick, T. H. (1995). Cognitive-behavioral treatment of panic disorder with agoraphobia in adolescents: A multiple baseline design analysis. *Behavior Therapy, 26,* 517–531.

Ollendick, T. H., & Hersen, M. (1984). *Child behavioral assessment: Principles and procedures.* New York: Pergamon Press.

Ollendick, T. H., & King, N. J. (1998). Empirically supported treatments for children with phobic and anxiety disorders: Current status. *Journal of Clinical Child Psychology, 27,* 156–167.

Parrish, J. M. (1997). Behavior management: Promoting adaptive behavior. In M. L. Batshaw (Ed.), *Children with disabilities,* 4th ed. (pp. 657–686). Baltimore: Paul H. Brookes.

Patterson, G. R. (1982). *Coercive family process.* Eugene, OR: Castalia.

Pelham, W. E., Jr., Wheeler, T., & Chronis, A. (1998). Empirically supported psychosocial treatments for attention deficit hyperactivity disorder. *Journal of Clinical Child Psychology, 27,* 190–205.

Peterson, L. (1997). Behavior therapy's promise for child treatment: Where we've been, where we may be going. *Behavior Therapy, 28,* 531–541.

Reitman, D., & Drabman, R. S. (1996). Read my fingertips: A procedure for enhancing effectiveness of time-out with argumentative children. *Child and Family Behavior Therapy, 18*(2), 35–40.

Repp, A. C., & Karsh, K. G. (1994). Hypothesis-based intervention for tantrum behaviors of persons with developmental disabilities in school settings. *Journal of Applied Behavior Analysis, 27*(1), 21–31.

Reynolds, L. K., & Kelley, M. L. (1997). The efficacy of a response cost-based treatment package for managing aggressive behavior in preschoolers. *Behavior Modification, 21*(2), 216–230.

Rogers, S. J. (1998). Empirically supported comprehensive treatments for young children with autism. *Journal of Clinical Child Psychology, 27,* 168–179.

Ronen, T., & Wozner, Y. (1995). A self-control intervention package for the treatment of primary nocturnal enuresis. *Child and Family Behavior Therapy, 17*(1), 1–20.

Schuhmann, E. M., Foote, R. C., Eyberg, S. M., Boggs, S. R., & Algina, J. (1998). Efficacy of parent-child interaction therapy: Interim report of a randomized trial with short-term maintenance. *Journal of Clinical Child Psychology, 27,* 34–45.

Screenivasan, U., Manocha, S. N., & Jain, V. K. (1979). Treatment of severe dog phobia in childhood by flooding: A case report. *Journal of Child Psychology and Psychiatry, 20,* 255–260.

Serketich, W. J., & Dumas, J. E. (1996). The effectiveness of behavioral parent training to modify antisocial behavior in children: A meta-analysis. *Behavior Therapist, 27,* 171–186.

Silverman, W. K., & Eisen, A. R. (1993). Phobic disorders. In R. T. Ammerman, C. G. Last, & M. Hersen (Eds.), *Handbook of prescriptive treatments of children and adolescents* (pp. 178–197). Boston: Allyn & Bacon.

Slifer, K. J., Cataldo, M. D., & Kurtz, P. F. (1998). Behavioural training during acute brain trauma rehabilitation: An empirical case study. *Brain Injury, 9,* 585–593.

Spence, S. H. (1994). Practitioner review: Cognitive therapy with children and adolescents: From theory to practice. *Journal of Child Psychology and Psychiatry, 35,* 1191–1228.

Strumpf, J. A., & Fodor, I. (1993). The treatment of test anxiety in elementary school-age children: Review and recommendations. *Journal of Child and Family Behavior Therapy, 15*(4), 19–42.

Thorpe, G. L., & Olson, S. L. (1997). Behavior therapy and its origins. *Behavior therapy: Concepts, procedures, and applications,* 2nd ed. (pp. 5–30) Boston: Allyn & Bacon.

Vernberg, E. M. (1998). Developmentally-based psychotherapies: Comments and observations. *Journal of Clinical Child Psychology, 27,* 46–48.

Watson, T. S., & Gresham, F. M. (1998). Current issues in child behavior therapy. In T. S. Watson & F. M. Gresham (Eds.), *Handbook of child behavior therapy* (pp. 499–504). New York: Plenum.

Weisz, J. R., Donenberg, G. R., Han, S. S., & Weiss, B. (1995). Bridging the gap between laboratory and clinic in child and adolescent psychotherapy. *Journal of Consulting and Clinical Psychology, 63*(5), 688–701.

Weithorn, L. A. (1980). Competency to render informed treatment decisions: A comparison of certain minors and adults. *Dissertation Abstracts International, 42,* 3449B–3450B.

Williams, M. A., & Gross, A. M. (1994). Behavior therapy. In V. B. Hasselt & M. Hersen (Eds.), *Advanced abnormal psychology* (pp. 419–441). New York: Guilford.

Yule, W., Sacks, B., and Hersov, L. (1974). Successful flooding treatment of a noise phobia in an 11-year-old. *Journal of Behavior Therapy and Experimental Psychiatry, 5,* 209–211.

24

Pharmacological Interventions

Keith Cheng and Kathleen Myers

Introduction

The use of psychotropic medications has increasingly become part of comprehensive treatment plans for children and adolescents. Due to the paucity of research, however, pediatric psychopharmacology is more an art than a science. Most rigorous pharmacological studies have focused on attention-deficit hyperactivity disorder (ADHD), and there are clear indications for stimulants as the primary therapy. However, there are fewer and less rigorous well controlled studies of antidepressants in children and adolescents, and even fewer in number and less well designed studies of antianxiety or anxiolytic medications. Thus, recommendations for using them in treatment are not as clear as for ADHD. Despite the lack of rigorous data, psychotropics are increasingly used. Factors contributing to this trend are diverse, including increasing severity of juvenile psychopathology, school mandates to educate youths who have serious psychiatric disorders, parents, and the inability of communities to manage their children's problems sufficiently, lack of appropriate alternative services, the availability of more effective medications that have relatively benign side effects, and pressure to contain costs from managed care.

Classification

Psychotropic medications used in juvenile populations are classified in five major groups: (1) stimulants, (2) antidepressants, (3) mood stabilizers, (4) anxiolytics, and (5) antipsychotics. A medication's classification does not limit its use to one type of psychopathology. For example, antidepressants are more commonly prescribed for anxiety than anxiolytics. Antipsychotics are used to treat schizophrenia and also mania, tic disorders, and severe ADHD. Most psychotropics do not have Food and Drug Administration (FDA) approval for pediatric use, and their use is based on "off-label," or non-FDA approved, indications. FDA approval is

Keith Cheng • Child and Adolescent Treatment Program, Emanuel Hospital, Portland, Oregon 97227.   **Kathleen Myers** • Outpatient Child and Adolescent Psychiatry, Department of Psychiatry, Oregon Health Sciences University, Portland, Oregon 97201.

Advanced Abnormal Psychology, Second Edition, edited by Hersen and Van Hasselt. Kluwer Academic/Plenum Publishers, New York, 2001.

given to medications after rigorous stage testing by the pharmaceutical company. Because the testing for use by children and adolescents is more demanding and costly than for adults, many companies do not seek FDA approval for pediatric indications. Clinical experience has formed the basis for most pediatric psychopharmacology. However, NIMH has recently called for more systematic study of psychotropic medication in youth. Several multisite studies started earlier this decade are still in progress.

Generic versus Brand Name Drugs

Medications are designated by two names. The generic name is the chemical name of a medication. Brand names represent the pharmaceutical companies' patented trade names which are important to initial marketing. Generic medications are usually less expensive, but they may also vary significantly in potency and therapeutic action. This is partially explained by the bioavailability of a medication, the amount that enters cardiovascular circulation. The FDA allows generics to vary up to 20% from standards set for brand medications. Because of this variability, clinicians may specify that generics not be substituted for brand name psychotropics. In this chapter, psychotropic medications will usually be referred to by their generic names because this is the practice in medical sciences and is used in peer-reviewed journals.

Mechanism of Action

Therapeutic actions of psychotropic medications are not known. However, preclinical studies and human experimental imaging studies have elucidated actions that are associated with, if not partially responsible for, the therapeutic actions of various psychotropic medications. Many psychotropics act at one or more of three sites in the central nervous system (CNS): at pre-synaptic receptors to stimulate or block neurotransmission; at the re-uptake pump to block the recycling of neurotransmitters from the synaptic cleft back into the presynaptic receptor; or at the postsynaptic receptor to block, or antagonize, their ability to bind neurotransmitters. In most mechanisms, the end result is "down-regulation," a decrease in either the functional number of postsynaptic receptor sites or a decrease in their binding strength. Other psychotropics facilitate the transmission of peptides or hormones in the CNS. Some stabilize cell membranes. Most psychotropics probably act by more than one mechanism. The neurotransmitters involved with the basic psychotropic groups presented in this chapter will be described.

Pharmacokinetics and Pharmacodynamics

Pharmacokinetics is the way individuals handle drugs and is determined by physiological processes that influence the concentration of a drug in body tissues. These processes depend on four physiological factors: absorption, distribution, metabolism, and excretion. The pharmacokinetics of a drug changes at developmental stages and with physiological changes. Thus, the pharmacokinetics of children differs from that of adolescents, and both differ from that of adults. Children's stomachs are less acidic, and thus acidic medications, such as stimulants, may be absorbed more slowly at younger ages. Then, the absorbed drug is diluted in the bloodstream. Children tend to have a higher volume of distribution throughout the bloodstream and thus lower concentrations of water-soluble medications, such as lithium. Children and adolescents usually display faster drug metabolic rates due to more active hepatic metabolism. In general, they need higher doses of medications per kilogram of weight and multiple daily doses. Excretion of a drug is partially determined by its half-life, the time required for the drug's concentration in circulation to decrease by one-half. Half-life values are helpful in determining dosing intervals. Medications whose half-lives are longer than 24 hours can be dosed once daily, whereas those whose half-lives are shorter require dosing two to four times per day to avoid wide swings in concentrations and thus a variable therapeutic effect. Approximately four half-life periods are needed for a medication to reach a steady-state concentration. If a medication is stopped abruptly, about six half-lives are needed to eliminate the drug completely. These factors are crucial for optimal titration for a single medication and multiagent pharmacotherapy.

Pharmacodynamics is an individual's response to medication. Multiple mechanisms may be involved, including interactions between agonists and antagonists at drug receptor sites. Pharmacodynamics may lead to unexpected outcomes of therapy and adverse effects that are difficult to predict.

Polypharmacy is becoming more common to treat a serious single disorder or comorbid disorders. The result may be enhanced or diminished effects of one or both drugs or the appearance of new effects. The resulting interactions may be therapeutic or adverse. The most important adverse drug interactions occur with drugs that have serious toxicity and a low therapeutic index, so that relatively small changes in drug level can have significant adverse consequences. Lithium is an example. These drug interactions can result from many mechanisms, such as competition at receptor sites, alteration of enzymatic pathways active in metabolism, the displacement of a drug from the protein to which it is bound, and inhibition of drug transport systems. The physician's task is to determine the potential for such interactions and to assess such potential interaction when a patient's response to treatment changes.

Medication Consultation

Many ill children may not need psychotropic medications, but some disorders such as psychotic and bipolar disorders mandate pharmacological intervention as the primary therapy. Other definite indications for a medication consultation include severe depressive and anxiety disorders and failure of behavioral and psychotherapeutic interventions to fully ameliorate aggressive and self-injurious behaviors. More elective indications are failure of nonmedical interventions to resolve depressive and anxiety disorders, attention deficit hyperactivity disorders, and augmentation of psychotherapeutic interventions.

Evaluating any pharmacotherapy includes a comprehensive genetic, perinatal, developmental, family, medical, behavioral, and emotional history in combination with physical, neurological, mental status, and laboratory examinations. Specific disorders may require additional evaluation and monitoring that is discussed in the following sections. Psychological testing is often requested to help clarify diagnostic ambiguities, support clinical impressions, or aid with treatment planning. Close collaboration with pediatricians and schools is needed for baseline assessment, as well as determining treatment response.

Consent and Assent

Consent for pharmacotherapy with youth differs from adults in that a guardian, not the patient, is responsible for consent. The consent process is the physician's education of the patient's parents or guardians as to indications, goals, alternatives, and risks of specific medical treatments. After an appropriate discussion, guardians explicitly grant permission for treatment. Some states allow verbal consent, and others require signed consent. Children cannot consent to treatment with psychotropic medications because they cannot adequately understand treatment issues and risks. Competency for informed consent is generally achieved at age 18. However, individual states may grant this right as early as age 14. This approach is supported by a study which found that 14-year-olds demonstrated the same capabilities as 21-year-olds in understanding complicated medical issues (Weithorn & Campbell, 1982). Nevertheless, the cognitive capacity to understand consent issues does not automatically imply the ability to make mature decisions (Cauffman & Steinberg, 1995). The physician must make individualized determinations regarding teens' ability to consent.

Children may not be capable of consent, but they are generally requested to assent to treatment. The American Academy of Pediatrics (AAP, 1995) provides the following guidelines: (1) helping the child achieve a developmentally appropriate awareness of the nature of its condition, (2) telling the child what to expect from treatment, (3) making a clinical assessment of the child's understanding of the situation and what factors are influencing its response, and (4) solicitation of a statement of the child's willingness to accept the proposed treatment. Though assent is optimal, initiation of treatment requires only the guardian's consent.

Psychodynamics

Taking psychotropic medications raises several psychodynamic issues. Self-image may be affected. Heckling peers may use derogatory terms to tease children who receive medication at school. Side effects, such as tremors, sedation, or drooling may stigmatize youth. Medication can be a daily reminder that something is wrong with them. Children may refuse medications because a relative is being treated with the same or similar drug. The psychopathology itself may influence a youth's attitude. A manic adolescent may refuse lithium because it dulls the mania. A psychotic patient may refuse medications because of paranoid delusions. Finally, one of the most common psychodynamics is opposition to authority figures. When the physician is sensitive to youths' perceptions about medications for psychiatric problems, compliance usually improves.

Clinical Collaboration

Collaboration with other caregivers is the rule, rather than the exception, in treating juvenile disorders. Medication and psychotherapy are often provided by different clinicians. This multimodal arrangement has both advantages and disadvantages. Patients can benefit from the combined expertise of more than one clinician. But coordination may lapse, clinicians may not agree on treatment issues, and the patient may present different agendas to different team members that may disrupt treatment planning. Clinicians often disagree about medicating children (Schowalter, 1989). To avoid these difficulties, caregivers must communicate openly, agree on the goals and methods of treatment, and engage the patient and guardians in consent for communication among team members. Treatment team members should prospectively plan for compromises in treatment in cases of suicidality, medication noncompliance, relapses, and major life stresses. Treatment team members should have distinct and well-defined responsibilities (Kingsbury & Tekell, 1999).

Treatment is ideally provided by clinicians who have expertise in psychiatric disorders. However, there is a shortage of child and adolescent psychiatrists (Thomas & Holzer, 1999). Thus, many pediatricians, family physicians, and nurse practitioners prescribe psychotropic medications. These clinicians' skills may vary from expert to limited. The recent approval of specialty board certification in developmental and behavioral pediatrics should increase the available expertise in pediatric psychopharmacology. Regardless of who prescribes these medications, pharmacotherapy should not comprise the sole treatment. Childhood and adolescent disorders require multimodal and individualized interventions. Too often, the treatment of juvenile psychopathology is left to the prescription pad.

The remainder of this chapter surveys the psychotropic medications used for children and adolescents, including basic indications, contraindications, mechanism of action, pharmacokinetics, medical workup, adverse reactions, and course of treatment. Further details may be obtained from the additional reading list at the end of the chapter.

STIMULANTS

Background

Stimulants are the most commonly prescribed psychotropic medications for child and adolescent psychiatric disorders. Charles Bradley's (1937) paper, "The Behavior of Children Receiving Benzedrine," described the academic and social benefits that children who have "Minimal Brain Dysfunction" derived when amphetamines were prescribed. In the past three decades, little has changed in the medical treatment of such children who have primary deficits in cognitive and motor control. Stimulants have continued to be the drugs of choice for ADHD. Since the 1970s, commonly prescribed stimulants include methylphenidate (Ritalin), dextroamphetamine (Dexedrine, Dextrostat), methamphetamine (Desoxyn), pemoline (Cylert), and a combination of four amphetamine salts, dextroamphetamine saccharate, dextroamphetamine sulfate, amphetamine aspartate, and amphetamine sulfate (Adderall). All of the stimulants, except Cylert, are classified by the FDA as schedule II drugs, the most restrictive classification for clinically used drugs. The majority of Schedule II medications have great potential for abuse and dependence and are highly regulated through restrictive prescription regulations. Cylert is classified as a Schedule IV medication because it does not have high abuse potential. Cylert is the least euphorigenic of the stimulants and has failed to show self-administration properties in animal models. Stimulants are prescribed annually for more than 1.5 million children, approximately 2.8% of the school-age population (Safer, Zito, & Fine, 1996). Methylphenidate is the most commonly prescribed stimulant and accounts for more than 90% of the prescriptions. Its popularity may arise from fewer side effects on growth than the other stimulants. Although little has changed pharmacologically, research during the past six decades has elucidated the psychopathology of these young people, focusing first on their cognitive deficits, later on their motor dyscontrol, and most recently on their inattention. Currently, the term Attention-Deficit Hyperactivity Disorder (ADHD) is used to describe youths who have primary deficits of inattention, hyperactivity, and/or impulsivity. Initially, it was thought that the stimulants had a "paradoxical effect" in "calming" these children. It is now known that the stimulants' mechanisms of actions are not paradoxical and are the same in both adults and children.

Mechanism of Action

The stimulants are called such because they increase alertness, arousal, and activity levels in the central nervous system (CNS). They are structurally similar to the catecholamine neurotransmitters, norepinephrine and dopamine, that act directly on the sympathetic nervous system. Because the stimulants act primarily to enhance these catecholamines, the term "sympathomimetic" is often used to describe their actions. The precise mechanisms of action are still poorly understood. Recent studies suggest that the stimulants may enhance neuronal connections and neurotransmission of the catecholamines between the orbital-frontal and limbic regions of the CNS. Stimulants, it is thought, act by inhibiting dopamine re-uptake transporters and increasing the time that dopamine has to bind to its receptors on other neurons. This ultimately leads to a greater capacity to inhibit and regulate impulsive behaviors, have more internalized speech, and better self-control.

Indications

The FDA-approved indications for stimulant use by children are ADHD and narcolepsy. The core target symptoms in ADHD are inattentiveness, hyperactivity, and impulsivity. Secondary improvements in adjunctive symptoms such as disorganization, forgetfulness, intrusiveness, and noisiness also occur. The core symptoms of at least 70–80% of youngsters will respond positively to one of the stimulants in the first trial. If three stimulants are tried, the response rate to at least one of the stimulants increases to 85–90% (Cantwell, 1996). Some children respond better to one stimulant than to another, but such response is idiosyncratic and cannot be predicted. The medications target symptoms relevant to classroom behavior, academic achievement, and productivity. They enhance performance in measures of vigilance, reaction time, fine motor coordination, impulse control, short-term memory, and specific types of verbal and nonverbal learning. Nevertheless, improved functioning in more traditional measures of cognitive abilities, such as intelligence tests, have not been found. Thus, these medications help children to demonstrate their innate intelligence and knowledge, but do not increase their intelligence. However, effects on overall academic achievement appear more complicated. Productivity and accuracy may improve, but overall ability with grade level material may not. Short term gains in performance have also been repeatedly documented, but longer term scholastic success has not. This may reflect methodological problems in longitudinal studies, especially the failure to discriminate pure ADHD youths from those who have serious comorbid disorders. These findings have produced lively discussions of the pros and cons of stimulants.

Irritability, which may be mistaken for a comorbid mood disorder, may resolve with stimulant treatment. The intensity and quality of interactions with parents, teachers, and peers often improves from stimulant administration and makes these youths more socially appealing. Even more intriguing, comorbid symptoms, such as opposition, defiance, aggression, and conduct disturbances, may also improve. These changes allow children to participate better in group activities, such as sports, Scouts, and church.

Apart from their indication for and effectiveness in ADHD, stimulants often improve cognitive and motor performance in other CNS-related behavioral disturbances, such as mental retardation, autism, organic brain dysfunction, or genetic syndromes with behavioral dysregulation. However, stimulants do not improve learning disabilities in the absence of ADHD.

Several factors affect the effectiveness of the stimulants. Age is surprisingly important. Younger children, especially preschoolers, do not respond as well as older children and may have more frequent and odd side effects. The older literature indicated that children "outgrew" ADHD during adolescence, and/or that teens did not respond to stimulants. This may occur because their hyperactivity is less evident. However, other symptoms, especially inattention, persist in more than 50% of ADHD children into adolescence and are responsive to stimulants. Gender is not well studied, although girls respond similarly to boys. Comorbid disorders decrease the effectiveness of the stimulants, especially in anxiety disorders, which may be exacerbated by the stimulants.

Dextroamphetamine and Adderall are FDA approved for treating ADHD for age 3 and older. Methamphetamine, methylphenidate, and pemoline are FDA-approved for age 6 and older.

Pharmacokinetics and Administration

Stimulants are readily absorbed from the gastrointestinal tract into the circulatory system and then easily cross the blood brain barrier into the CNS. They are metabolized in the liver and then excreted in the urine. The onset of action for methylphenidate and dextroamphetamine is usually within 30–60 minutes. Peak plasma concentration for methylphenidate is reached within 1 to 3 hours, and for dextroamphetamine in 3 to 4 hours. Behavioral benefits last approximately 3 to 4 hours for both stimulants, thus requiring twice daily administration. Both are available in extended release forms, which may allow once daily administration, thereby avoiding dosing at school. However, many children do not respond as well to longer acting preparations as to equivalent doses of the regular preparation. Pemoline, Adderall, and methamphetamine have longer elimination half-lives which often allow once daily dosing. Typically, the longer acting medications have a delayed onset of action which may make the morning and early classes more difficult than later classes. Therefore, some clinicians prescribe a combination of the regular preparation and the longer acting preparation in the morning to derive the benefits of quick onset, as well as sustained action. When pemoline is used, 3 to 4 weeks are usually required for improvement in ADHD symptoms.

Contraindications and Adverse Effects

Relative contraindications to stimulants include current psychosis, pregnancy, growth retardation, cardiovascular abnormalities, and substance abuse. Patients whose liver function is impaired should not receive pemoline because of potential liver failure. Abbott Pharmaceutical Company, the makers of pemoline (Cylert), recently reported that 17 deaths occurred during the last two decades due to liver failure attributed to pemoline. They recommend pemoline only as a second- or third-line treatment for ADHD, accompanied by monitoring of liver function (Pizzuti, 1999). Recent treatment with monoamine oxidase inhibitors (MAOIs) also precludes the use of stimulants because of potential hypertensive crises.

The use of stimulants with preexisting tic disorders is controversial. Stimulants can exacerbate tics, but recent evidence suggests that many children who have preexisting tic disorders may be treated with stimulants without exacerbation (Gadow, Sverd, Sprafkin, Nolan, & Grossman, 1999). When tics are associated with stimulants treatment, alternative medications are generally sought.

ADHD children treated with stimulants are not at greater risk than untreated ADHD children for substance abuse later in life (Weiss, Hechtman, Milroy, & Perlman, 1985). However, youths who have a history of drug and alcohol abuse are generally treated with other psychotropics for their ADHD symptoms. Some substance abusing adolescents misuse or sell their stimulants. For example, they may crush their stimulant and snort the powder for a euphoric effect (Garland, 1998). Because of their potential for abuse and their side effects, various special interest groups periodically demand a ban on the use of stimulants by children. Ironically, of all the psychotropic medications used by children, stimulants are considered among the safest, as documented in several longitudinal studies.

All stimulants have similar side effects, although an individual child may experience side effects from one stimulant and not from another. Stimulants may cause many uncomfortable, but not serious, side effects. Nervousness and insomnia are the most common side effects, followed by headache, anorexia, nausea, dizziness, rapid pulse, and increased blood pressure. These side effects often resolve spontaneously within 2 weeks. They may also be managed by decreasing the dose or stopping dosages late in the day. Rare, but serious, complications which mandate stopping medication include psychosis and seizures. Dysphoria is common in young children. Although stimulants may decrease the seizure threshold stimulants are successfully and safely prescribed for many youths who have comorbid seizures and ADHD (Feldman, Crumrine, Handen, Alvin, & Teodori, 1989).

Some children experience a syndrome of worsened hyperactivity, irritability, and moodiness when the medication wears off at the end of the day. This phenomenon is called "rebound." Frequently, a late afternoon dose can resolve rebound reactions without causing sleep disturbance. Generally, stimulants can be abruptly discontinued. However, withdrawal reactions occasionally occur; these include irritability, insomnia, or marked hyperactivity, especially when children have been taking stimulants for long periods at higher doses. Withdrawal reactions can be minimized by gradually tapering the stimulant during seven to ten days. Parents frequently worry about growth retardation associated with decreased appetite. However, longitudinal research indicates that although growth may fall off initially, chronic stimulant use does not affect final adult stature.

Medical Workup

In addition to completing the usual medical history and physical evaluation before any medication trial, the initiation of a stimulant trial requires several additional considerations. Special attention should be given to assessing illnesses that may mimic ADHD, including petit mal epilepsy, hyperthyroidism, lead poisoning, anemias, and postconcussive syndromes. Other behavioral disorders can also be mistaken for ADHD, including learning, depressive, bipolar, psychotic, anxiety, and conduct disorders. Stimulant medication could exacerbate these illnesses. Clinicians also need to be alert to comorbid disorders that may decrease the effectiveness of stimulant treatment. The presence of comorbid disorders may greatly influence what stimulant, if any, should be started. Finally, certain medical illnesses, including cardiac problems, liver dysfunction, epilepsy, tics, and growth abnormalities may preclude a stimulant trial. It is also helpful to know whether any relatives have been treated with stimulants and to know of their responses and any untoward effects.

Baseline weight and height are needed to monitor growth because many youths will experience appetite suppression. Similarly, baseline pulse and blood pressure need to be monitored because stimulants could cause hypertension and tachycardia. If a child's physical exam is normal or if pemoline is used, laboratory tests are usually not mandatory unless the history leads to suspicions about the aforementioned medical problems. Patients for whom pemoline is prescribed require baseline and then follow-up liver function tests.

It is also helpful to obtain baseline behavior rating scales from parents, teachers, and/or other relevant adults such as day care providers. Some clinicians obtain a baseline continuous performance test (CPT). Comparing baseline and follow-up scores from rating scales and CPTs assists clinicians with stimulant dose titration.

The use of baseline electroencephalograms (EEG) and single photon emission computed tomography (SPECT) is controversial. The American Academy of Child and Adolescent Psychiatry does not advocate the use of these tests in routinely assessing ADHD (Dulcan, 1996).

Course of Treatment

A low dose of methylphenidate or dextroamphetamine is usually started once or twice daily with meals. The dose is adjusted by small increments weekly, according to clinical response or significant side effects. Occasionally, some children may require dosages higher than usually recommended. In some of these cases, treatment with other medications or augmentation with other psychotropics should be considered. Children who are early risers or fast metabolizers of stimulants will sometimes need dosing three to four times daily. Side effects, vital signs, and rating scales should be followed regularly during the initial months. The liver function of patients on pemoline should be assessed at least every six months.

Because one of the main purposes of stimulants is to help improve academic performance, these medications are sometimes not administered on weekends or during the summer months. There are no specific guidelines for discontinuing stimulant medications. The decision to stop treatment is usually based on school and parent reports. Up to 20% of children may be able to discontinue medication after 12 months of treatment (Werry, 1999). A medication holiday of 1 to 2 weeks once a year is usually recommended to determine how a child functions without medication.

Noticeable improvements occur in 60–85% of studied populations. If a youth does not respond to an initial stimulant medication, a second or even third trial of a different stimulant is recommended before alternative medications, such as bupropion, guanfacine, or tricyclic antidepressants are considered.

The role of psychotherapy or behavioral therapy in conjunction with stimulants requires comment. Despite current opinion that medications are the primary treatment for ADHD and that other interventions have not demonstrated synergistic effects, most clinicians recommend that all youths should be evaluated for other therapeutic interventions and services. These children need to learn social skills, parents need behavior management training, and teachers need specific educational strategies. Multimodal interventions are still recommended. Research continues into their roles in the overall treatment of ADHD youths.

ANTIDEPRESSANTS

Background

The first antidepressants, the monoamine oxidase inhibitors (MAOIs) and tricyclic antidepressants (TCAs), were developed in the 1960s, and remained the only antidepressants available for clinical use for two decades. Their chemical structures and predominant effects on the neurotransmission of norepinephrine led to the "catecholamine theory of depression." Commonly used TCAs include imipramine (Tofranil), amitriptyline (Elavil), desipramine (Norpramin), doxepin (Sinequan), and clomipramine (Anafranil). MAOIs include tranylcypromine (Parnate), phenelzine (Nardil), and isocarboxazid (Marplan). In the 1980s, the effectiveness of selective serotonin re-uptake inhibitors (SSRIs) led to the "serotonin theory of depression." Now five SSRIs are available in the United States: fluoxetine (Prozac), paroxetine (Paxil), sertraline (Zoloft), fluvoxamine (Luvox), and citalopram (Celexa). Newer antidepressants introduced in the 1990s, however, have more varied chemical structures, neurotransmitter effects, and mechanisms of action. They underscore the complex pathophysiology of depression and drug mechanisms. The newer antidepressants are nefazodone (Serzone), venlafaxine (Effexor), mirtazapine (Remeron), and bupropion (Wellbutrin).

Despite their diverse chemical structures and mechanisms, all antidepressants are equally effective at therapeutic dosages in adults. Although individuals may experience differential responses to different antidepressants, large controlled studies have shown that approximately 75% of depressed adults achieve remission in 4 to 12 weeks of treatment regardless which type of antidepressant is administered. Thus, the popularity of the newer antidepressants reflects their more benign side effects, not their greater effectiveness.

Antidepressants have been prescribed for children and adolescents for three decades. However, there has been a tremendous antidepressant prescription increase during the 1990s. This trend reflects the increasing recognition of depression in youths, a cohort effect for increasing rates of depression among young people (Ryan, Williamson, Iyengar, Orvaschel, Reich, Dahl, & Puig-Antich, 1992), earlier age of onset (Kovacs & Gastonis, 1994), the development of safer antidepressants, the limitations of psychotherapy for severe depressions, and financial pressure from managed care. Increasingly, psychologists are collaborating with physicians to treat depressed children and adolescents.

Indications and Efficacy

Although case studies suggested that the TCAs are efficacious in child and adolescent depression, multiple, well-designed, single-site studies have failed to demonstrate the superiority of TCAs over a placebo (Birmaher, Ryan, Williamson, Brent, Kaufman, 1996b; Myers & McCauley, 1997). Recently, a large multisite study confirmed these earlier results (Wagner, 1999). Many explanations for the lack of efficacy have been offered. Phenomenological explanations focused on the high rate of comorbidity of juvenile depression, a known factor in decreasing response among depressed adults. Pathophysiological explanations focus on immature neurotransmitter systems. In particular, the development of monoaminergic storage capacity and synthesis continues throughout childhood and may not be capable of responding to antidepressant stimulation (Goldman-Rakic, Brown, 1982). Neuroendocrine theories have noted that the hypothalamic–pituitary–adrenal axis, which is dysregulated in depressed adults, is highly resilient in children (Dahl, Ryan, Puig-Antich, Nguyen, al-Shabbout, Meyer, & Perel, 1991).

SSRIs appear more promising. Three double-blind, placebo-controlled studies have suggested that SSRIs are efficacious in both children and adolescents during 6 to 12 weeks of treatment. The first was a single-site study with a small sample (Simeon, Dinicola, Ferguson, & Copping, 1990). Two-thirds of the patients in each group demonstrated mild to moderate improvement, and there was a trend to higher scores in the fluoxetine-treated groups. In another study based in a larger sample and more careful screening for early placebo responders, fluoxetine was superior to a placebo, and the response rate was 56% versus a 33% nonresponse rate (Emslie, Rush, Weinberg, Kowatch, Hughes, Carmody, & Rintelmann, 1997). In the only multisite study of paroxetine, it was similarly superior to both imipramine and a placebo (Wagner, 1999). Interestingly, SSRI-treated youths in all three studies improved at approximately the same rate as in previous TCA studies: 55–65%. The lower placebo response in the latter two studies led to statistically significant differences between the two treatment conditions. However, even these studies showed rather high placebo response rates, a feature of all juvenile antidepressant studies. Not all outcome measures also detected improvements in certain depressive symptoms. Finally, the fluoxetine-treated youths tended to relapse during a year of naturalistic follow-up. Similar results from the multisite study have not yet been published. Thus, available studies do suggest that the SSRIs are efficacious in juvenile depression, but many questions remain. Clearly, further work is needed to clarify the role of SSRIs in juvenile depression (Ryan, 1992). The newer antidepressants have not been systematically studied in youths. However, case studies suggest that they may be safely used by youth. None of the antidepressants has FDA approval for treating depression. Their use in children and adolescents is based on an off-label indication.

The TCAs have a long history as a second-line medication for ADHD, for youths who cannot take a stimulant, do not respond to stimulants, or have comorbid depression. Many studies have documented that TCAs, particularly desipramine, are efficacious in improving attention and hyperactivity, although less so than stimulants (Cantwell, 1996). More recently it has been shown that bupropion is comparable to TCAs in treating ADHD (Conners, Casat, Gualtieri, Weller, Reader, Reiss, Weller, Khayrallah, & Ascher, 1996) and has replaced TCAs as a stimulant alternative. It is particularly preferred for ADHD youths who have comorbid substance abuse because bupropion reduces cravings for addictive substances. Both TCAs and bupropion are off-label indications for ADHD.

Both TCAs and SSRIs have been widely used to treat juvenile anxiety disorders, just as in adults (Bernstein, Borchardt, & Perwein, 1996). For two decades, controversy has centered on whether TCAs are effective in treating separation anxiety. However, SSRIs have now replaced TCAs as the preferential treatment for anxiety, despite limited study with youths (Birmaher, Waterman, Ryan, Cully, Balach, Ingram & Brodsky, 1994).

The best pharmacological studies of anxiety disorders have been conducted for obsessive-compulsive disorder (OCD). Both clomipramine (DeVeaugh-Geiss, Moroz, Biederman, Cantwell, Fontaine, Greist, Reichler, Katz, & Landau, 1992) and fluvoxamine (Riddle, Claghorn, Gaffney, et al., 1996; March, Kobak, Jefferson, Mazza, & Greist, 1990) have been FDA-approved for children more than 10-years old, and sertraline for children more than 6-years old (March, Biederman, Wolkow, Safferman, 1998). Paroxetine has been efficacious in open label studies (Rosenberg, Stewart, Fitzgerald, Tawile, & Carroll, 1999), and is likely to be approved soon because a multisite study has just been completed. Fluoxetine has shown promise in small single-site studies (Riddle, Scahill, King, Hardin, Anderson, Ort, Smith, Leckman, Cohen, 1992). Most SSRI studies have resulted in approximately a 50% improvement during 8 to 20 weeks of study. Trichotillomania may also respond to clomipramine.

Finally, TCAs are prescribed for migraine headaches and enuresis. TCAs may prevent the migrainous cycle of vascular constriction and dilation. Imipramine is still a commonly prescribed TCA for enuresis. Its effectiveness may be due to its anticholinergic side effects. Although more than 75% of youths will reduce the frequency of bed wetting, only 25% will achieve total dryness. Enuresis is the only FDA-approved indication for a TCA. The dosages for migraine and enuresis are lower than for depressive and anxiety disorders.

Mechanisms of Action

As with other psychotropics, the mechanisms of action of antidepressants are not known. Their acute effects have been most studied. TCAs stimulate norepinephrine stimulation from presynaptic receptors. SSRIs block the serotonin re-uptake pump. Burpopion blocks the re-uptake pump for dopamine, and its metabolite blocks the pump for norepinephrine. Mirtazapine antagonizes postsynaptic serotonin-2 receptors. The other antidepressants have more complex mechanisms. For example, venlafaxine acts on both serotonin and norepinephrine re-uptake inhibition (SNRIs). Trazodone and nefazodone block, or antagonize, serotonin receptor sites both pre- and postsynaptically (SARIs).

These mechanisms of action are evident during acute treatment. Long-term mechanisms are not as clear, but, it is hypothesized, involve neuroadaptive changes of a specific receptor subtype, perhaps the delayed desensitization of neurotransmitter autoreceptors, and other adaptive changes (Hyman & Nestler, 1996). Furthermore, these therapeutic mechanisms have not been investigated in the developing CNS. Immature hormonal effects may interfere with receptor binding and down-regulation, thereby decreasing antidepressants' efficacy. Overall, the diversity of neurotransmitters and their mechanisms of action suggest greater complexity in the etiology and treatment of depression than current theories explain.

Pharmacokinetics and Administration

All of the antidepressants are metabolized in the liver. Several factors contribute to the pharmacokinetics of antidepressants, such as whether the drug has an active metabolite and its degree of protein binding. TCAs have been fairly well studied (Myers & McCauley, 1997), particularly imipramine (Preskorn, Bupp, Weller, & Weller, 1989; Wilens, Biederman, Baldessarini, Puopolo, & Flood, 1992) and nortriptyline (Geller, Cooper, Chestnut, Abel, & Anker, 1984; Geller, Cooper, & Chestnut, 1985). Steady-state levels are achieved by the seventh day, consistent with those for adults. The half-lives of specific TCAs vary widely and are partially determined by age. For example, the half-life of nortriptyline ranges from 11 to 42 hours in 5- to 12-year-olds, from 14 to 74 hours in 13- to 16-year-olds, and 15 to 93 hours in adults. Similarly, clomipramine's half-life ranges from 5–17 hours in 5- to 19-year-olds compared to 19 to 37 hours in adults. These differences mean that the younger the youth, the more variable may be the serum levels, and thus mood and behavior, during a 24-hour period. Therefore, TCAs are usually administered multiple times daily (Wilens et al., 1992).

The pharmacokinetics of SSRIs in children and adolescents has not been systematically studied, but some extrapolation may be drawn from adult studies (Leonard, March, Rickler, & Allen, 1997). Several issues affect the pharmacokinetics of the SSRIs, including potency, half-life, the presence of active metabolites, dose-plasma concentrations, and protein binding. The potencies of SSRIs vary greatly, but potency does not correlate with efficacy. SSRIs also vary in their selectivity. For example, although SSRIs are very selective for serotonin, at higher dosages they all inhibit the re-uptake of norepinephrine and to a smaller degree dopamine, possibly producing more adverse reactions. Paroxetine, fluvoxamine, and sertraline are the most potent and most selective, and fluoxetine and clomipramine are the least potent and least selective.

Metabolism during prepuberty is approximately twice that of adults for all SSRIs and reaches the adult rate by age 15. Therefore, children may require higher milligram per kilogram dosages and twice daily dosing. However, metabolism of individual SSRIs varies, reflecting the different half-lives of parent drugs and their metabolites. Fluoxetine has the longest half-life, as well as the most potent primary metabolite. Therefore, it takes several weeks to reach steady-state concentration, and the SSRI remains active for several weeks after discontinuation. This could complicate recovery from an adverse effect and initiation of another medication. By contrast, paroxetine has the shortest half-life, and its metabolite is inactive. Thus, it clears the system more quickly, eases recovery from adverse effects, and facilitates a switch to another medication. There is, however, an increased risk for a withdrawal syndrome.

The degree of protein binding of SSRIs relates to their potential for drug interactions. Fluvoxamine has the least protein binding, and thus drug interactions are less likely. By contrast, fluoxetine, sertraline, and paroxetine are all highly protein bound and can displace other bound drugs from protein sites, causing drug interactions.

Contraindications and Adverse Effects

TCAs have many minor side effects that are variably tolerated, such as blurred vision, dry mouth, rashes, photosensitivity, jitteriness, and gastrointestinal symptoms. Weight gain is one of the main reasons for their unpopularity. More serious complications have led to replacing them by newer medications. Hematologic impairments may produce lethal infection. Neurological effects may range from mild sedation to cognitive dulling, interference with learning, agitation, and seizures. Neurobehavioral effects may include nightmares, agitation, and the precipitation of psychosis or mania. Abrupt discontinuation of TCAs may produce a flu-like syndrome due to withdrawal of the anticholinergic side effects of TCAs. This may even occur within a day of discontinuation for younger children who metabolize TCAs rapidly. Thus, cessation of TCAs should be tapered during 1–2 weeks.

Of greatest concern are cardiac complications. All TCAs slow the conduction of electrical signals in the heart, generally a benign effect unless there is preexisting cardiac disease (Leonard, Meyer, Swedo, Hamburger, Allen, Rapoport, & Tucker, 1995; Walsh, Greenhill, Giardina, Bigger, Waslick, Sloan, Bilich, Wold, & Bagiella, 1999; Wilens, Biederman, Baldessarini, Geller, Schleifer, Spencer, Birmaher, & Goldblatt, 1996). Many youths experience changes in heart rate and blood pressure, generally without clinical effects. These usually benign side effects have been of greater concern during the past decade when several children who took TCAs, particularly desipramine, died suddenly (Riddle, Nelson, Kleinman, Rasmusson, Leckman, King, & Cohen, 1991; Varley & McClellan, 1997). These deaths were never causally associated with desipramine (Biederman, Thisted, Greenhill, & Ryan, 1995; Riddle et al., 1991). Nevertheless, most physicians now avoid TCAs for children and adolescents.

In general, SSRIs have fewer and less serious side effects than TCAs. Generally benign side effects that may limit using SSRIs include gastrointestinal distress, appetite changes, motor effects, tremors, neurobehavioral effects, sleep disturbances, anxiety, agitation, and headaches. The most serious potential complication is the precipitation of mania or psychosis, similar to other antidepressants, and the emergence of self-destructive ideation (King, Riddle, Chappell, Hardin, Anderson, Lombroso, & Scahill, 1991). Due to their increased metabolism, children may experience withdrawal symptoms daily. Thus, SSRIs, especially those whose half-lives are shorter, may have to be administered twice to thrice daily. The most serious complication of any SSRI is "serotonin syndrome," which is uncommon, but potentially lethal. Serotonin syndrome results when there is an overactivity of serotonergic receptor sites. The syndrome is commonly accompanied by a cluster of overstimulation symptoms, including jitteriness, insomnia, diarrhea, and a sensation of jumping out of one's skin. A serious overdose of SSRIs causes short-term illness, but no long-term sequelae (Riddle, Brown, Dzubinski, Jetmalani, Law, & Woolston, 1989).

The newer SNRIs and SARIs have not been sufficiently examined in children and adolescents to describe their side effects or dosing schedules systematically. However, low dosages of trazodone are widely prescribed for sleep disturbances, often in combination with SSRIs, without major adverse effects. Bupropion is widely used in clinical practice without major morbidity. The greatest concern is an increased risk for seizures, particularly in bulimia.

Medical Evaluation and Monitoring

Before starting any antidepressant, children and adolescents should receive the usual initial evaluation and physical examination. Initiating a TCA requires additional assessment.

An electrocardiogram (EKG) is indicated to rule out preexisting cardiac disease and to establish a baseline for comparison during treatment. An electroencephalogram (EEG) may be indicated for potential seizure/disorder or other central nervous system disorders because TCAs may decrease the seizure threshold. The EKG, blood pressure, and pulse should be repeated as dosages are increased and should be monitored periodically thereafter. The use of TCA blood levels has been controversial. Some authors advise blood levels after any dosage increase; others eschew blood levels if EKGs remain normal. However, when additional medications are prescribed that affect hepatic metabolism, TCA blood levels should be rechecked because TCA levels may rise to toxic levels or drop to subtherapeutic levels.

SSRIs, SNRIs, SARIs, and bupropion do not require routine monitoring. Neither therapeutic benefits nor adverse effects have been correlated with blood levels.

Course of Treatment

Results of naturalistic outcome studies suggest that antidepressant treatment of youth should last 6 to 18 months (Birmaher, Ryan, Williamson, Brent, Kaufman, Dahl, Perel, & Nelson, 1996a; Birmaher et al., 1996b; Myers & McCauley, 1997). However, many depressed youths do not fully remit during treatment (Emslie et al., 1997), and up to 70% will experience another depressive episode within 5 years (Myers & McCauley, 1997; Birmaher et al., 1996b). Thus, treatment decisions must be individualized according to the youth's degree of morbidity and complications with depression. If depression recurs, the antidepressant is usually reinstituted for another 6 months. Some youths may appear to become resistant to an antidepressant during the course of treatment. In these cases, higher dosages, lower dosages, or change to another antidepressant may be tried. Occasionally, youths who have severe, recurrent depressions that respond poorly to pharmacotherapy receive augmentation. This may be with a low dose of another class of antidepressant, with thyroxine, or with a mood stabilizer, most often lithium. However, empirical evidence to support this approach with youths is limited (Strober, Freeman, Rigali, Schmidt, & Diamond, 1992).

Up to 25% of early-onset depressed youths develop manic "switching" during treatment (Geller, Fox, & Clark, 1994; Strober, Lampert, Schmidt, & Morrel, 1993). This "switch" could represent antidepressant activation or unmasking of an underlying bipolar disorder. Subsequent treatment with a mood stabilizer is common.

The onset of depression in young people has significant morbidity in multiple domains of functioning. Thus, no depressed youth should receive antidepressants as the sole therapy. Ongoing or intermittent psychotherapy is always indicated. In fact, in most cases, psychotherapy should comprise the initial therapy.

MOOD STABILIZERS

Background

Mood stabilizers are a class of medication used to stabilize mood swings, particularly of Bipolar Disorder (BPD). The three most commonly used mood stabilizers for both adults and children are lithium, divalproex (Depakote), and carbamazepine (Tegretol). Lithium, a naturally occurring element, has been the primary treatment for BPD since its discovery by Australian William Cade in the 1950s. At that time it was hailed as a "miracle drug" that allowed severely ill BPD patients to live in the community, instead of institutions. Lithium was also the first psychotropic that prevented relapses of mania and depression. The FDA approved lithium for treating BPD in 1970. In the past two decades, newer mood stabilizers have emerged. Selected anticonvulsants have shown the ability to control the mood cycles of BPD. Divalproex and carbamazepine have been the most intensely studied and are generally accepted as a first- or second-line treatment for BPD. They are used in place of, or in conjunction with, lithium.

BPD has always been, but is increasingly becoming, a difficult disorder to control. BPD is a mood disorder with alternating episodes of mania and major depression (MDD), generally separated by days to months of relatively normal mood. There are several forms of BPD. Bipolar I Disorder (BPDI) is the classic form in which patients experience alternating, distinct episodes of both mania and depression. Bipolar II Disorder (BPDII) patients experience recurrent MDD episodes and days to weeks of low grade hypomania which may not produce major impairment. When four or more cycles of BPDI or BPDII occur in a year, it is termed Rapid Cycling Bipolar Disorder. Individuals may experience multiple episodes of rapid cycling within weeks, days, or even hours. Some individuals experience "mixed episodes" of mania and MDD concurrently. The subtype of BPD relates to treatment response and prognosis. BPDI and BPDII have been better studied, and respond best to available pharmacotherapies. Rapid cycling and mixed episodes respond more poorly.

Historically, it was thought that BPD begins in late adolescence or young adulthood when the traditional subtype, BPDI, could be observed. However, research during the past 5 years has identified BPD in early adolescence and even in prepuberty (Geller & Luby, 1997; Wozniak, Biederman, Kiely, Ablon, Faraone, Mundy, & Mennin, 1995). No epidemiological studies exist to estimate the prevalence of BPD in children and adolescents. However, studies of BPD adults and their relatives indicate that 20 to 40% of BPD presents during adolescence (Akiskal, Downs, Jordan, Watson, Daugherty, & Pruitt, 1985; Strober, Morrell, Burroughs, Lampert, Danforth, & Freeman, 1988); and prospective juvenile studies show that more than 31% of MDD children (Kovacs & Pollock, 1995; Geller, Fox, & Fletcher, 1993; Geller, Fox, & Clark, 1994b), and 28% of MDD adolescents develop mania within 5 years (Strober, 1992; Strober et al., 1993). When the onset of BPD is in prepuberty and early adolescence, it is the rapid-cycling or mixed-episode type (Geller, Sun, Zimmerman, Luby, Frazier, & Williams, 1995; Geller & Luby, 1997). Due to the difficulty in differentiating the distinct manic and depressive episodes in these subtypes and the high rate of comorbidity, BPD is often misdiagnosed in young people (Carlson & Weintraub, 1993; Faraone, Biederman, Wozniak, Mundy, Mennin, & O'Donnell, 1997; Weller, Weller, & Fristad, 1995; West, McElroy, Strkowski, Keck, & McConville, 1995). Children and adolescents may be expected to be less responsive to treatment than adults. However, longitudinal outcome studies and controlled treatment studies remain to be completed. Thus, guidelines for treating juvenile BPD are based on adaptations of adult treatment and limited available studies (Geller, 1997).

Indications and Efficacy

Lithium is a highly effective treatment for acute mania. It is most effective for classic, uncomplicated mania, in patients who have good interepisode functioning, a limited number of episodes, and BPD cycles in which the index or initial episode is manic. It stabilizes mood; reduces psychomotor agitation, irritability, and insomnia; and may even resolve psychotic symptoms. In the one controlled study of adolescents, lithium was significantly more effective than a placebo (Geller, 1997). In a naturalistic treatment study, adolescents who discontinued lithium experienced a significantly higher relapse rate than those who continued lithium long term (Strober, Morrell, Lampert, Burroughs, 1990). These results are consistent with adult studies, which show that intermittent lithium therapy may produce a worse outcome than continuous therapy and that it is difficult to restabilize patients with lithium after interruptions of treatment. This may be especially true for patients who have multiple episodes of BPD and a remitting and relapsing course. Because adolescents have a remitting and recurring course, they may be advised to maintain lithium throughout their teenage years. However, longer term treatment of acute episodes remains controversial for adults and is likely to be so for youths until longitudinal studies are available. Because of these complex developmental issues, lithium's use and effectiveness in children is more complicated (Geller, Cooper, Zimmerman, Sun, Williams, & Frazier, 1994a). However, it is the only FDA-approved medication for maintenance treatment of BPD in youths more than 12-years-old.

BPD marked by complicated manic and depressive episodes, repeated episodes, rapid cycling, mixed episodes, and impaired interepisode functioning is not as responsive to lithium. Additionally, recurrent episodes of BPD escalate the course of the disorder, similar to the course of recurrent epilepsy, a phenomenon called "kindling." These observations led to trials of anticonvulsants in patients who had complicated BPD and responded suboptimally to lithium. Adult studies showed that carbamazepine (Tegretol) and divalproex sodium (Depakote) may provide better control of BPD episodes as adjuncts to lithium or as primary medications.

Recognition of early onset BPD as predominantly of the rapid-cycling or mixed-episode subtypes and acceptance of divalproex sodium as a first-line medication for rapid cycling in adults led to successful trials with adolescents (Papatheodorou & Kutcher, 1993). Additionally, divalproex sodium's better tolerated side effects and its greater safety in overdose have led to its preferential use in youths, often as the first-line treatment, even though its effectiveness has not been systematically investigated. Carbamazepine and divalproex sodium are both FDA-approved for treating seizure disorders in children. Divalproex sodium recently received FDA approval for treating mania in adults, but not in children and adolescents. Other anticonvulsants, particularly lamotrigine (Lamictal) and gabapentin (Neurontin), which are increasingly used for adult BPD, have not been well studied in youths. However, many child and adolescent psychiatrists empirically use them as third-line medications, especially for treatment-refractive youths.

Decisions about longer term maintenance therapy must be individualized. The World Health Organization recommends maintenance treatment after two episodes of BPD. However, many patients will not readily accept long-term treatment, and many clinicians want to avoid long-term exposure to medications that have potential serious complications. The risks and benefits must be clearly reviewed with youths and their parents. BPD episodes are likely to recur in youths (Strober, Schmidt-Lackner, Freeman, Bower, Lampert, & DeAntonio, 1995). When episodes recur, they may not respond to previously successful pharmacotherapy. Thus, prognosis may worsen, and polypharmacy may be required. Both lithium and divalproex sodium are off-label indications for the maintenance treatment of juvenile BPD. Maintenance therapy may prevent recurrence and also allow for other interventions. As with adults, many youths will have residual symptoms that are impairing or even incapacitating. They will require other therapies to facilitate acceptance of illness, treatment compliance, and psychosocial adaptation.

Other off-label indications for lithium include the augmentation of antidepressants in treatment-resistant MDD and the prevention of future MDD episodes in patients who have recurrent unipolar MDD. Lithium has also been recommended for the children of parents who have BPD, when the children have behavior problems with affective instability, but not clear mood disorders. Lithium and the other mood stabilizers may also ameliorate severe aggression and explosive behaviors in youths who have various disorders, including ADHD, autism, and mental retardation.

Divalproex sodium and carbamazepine are increasingly used for the same off-label indications as lithium. Additionally, they are often used concurrently with psychotropics for youths who have comorbid psychiatric disorders and seizure disorders. They may also be helpful in treating behavior disturbances in youths who have underling organicity, such as brain damage or fetal alcohol effects. Preliminary evidence indicates that carbamazepine may be an alternative to stimulants for ADHD (Silva, Munoz, & Alpert, 1996).

Mechanism of Action

Like other psychotropics, lithium's mechanism of action is uncertain. Preclinical studies suggest two mechanisms. Lithium inhibits phosphatidyl inositol monophosphatase, an enzyme that is involved in neurotransmitter metabolism. Lithium also alters neuronal G-proteins which changes neuronal transmission. It is not clear how these mechanisms relate to clinical effects.

The mechanisms of action of carbamazepine and sodium divalproex in BPD are not known. It is well known that they interact with γ-amino-butyric acid (GABA). However, correlation with clinical effects remains to be elucidated.

Pharmacokinetics and Administration

Lithium occurs as a simple salt that has no metabolites and is excreted exclusively in the urine. Its half-life ranges from 20 to 24 hours in adults. In children and adolescents, the half-life is lower because of the higher volume of distribution and more efficient renal clearance (Geller & Luby, 1997). This shorter half-life requires dosing lithium at least twice daily. Because lithium has a narrow therapeutic window and high potential for toxicity, its use is complicated for patients who have renal disease. However, the lack of active metabolites and protein binding reduce the risks for interactions with other medications. Therapeutic effects usually occur in one week.

Divalproex and carbamazepine are both metabolized in the liver. They both have relatively short half-lives, so they are usually administered two to three times a day. At therapeutic doses, it may take 1 to 3 weeks before therapeutic effects become clinically apparent.

Contraindications and Adverse Effects

Relative contraindications to lithium include pregnancy, renal disease, cardiovascular disease, thyroid disease, and dehydration. There are many medications that can increase lithium levels into toxic ranges, including carbamazepine, selected antibiotics, diuretics, and nonsteroidal anti-inflammatory agents like ibuprofen. Alcohol, antihypertensives, and antipsychotics may interact with lithium to produce confusional states. Lithium taken in overdose may be lethal or result in permanent neurological damage. Because of lithium's narrow therapeutic window and potential for toxicity when levels exceed this window, any factor that increases lithium's serum level could cause toxic reactions. For example, patients who take lithium must be careful to prevent dehydration during sports or gastrointestinal illnesses. Caution is warranted when prescribing lithium for suicidal patients.

Lithium has many annoying side effects: nausea, vomiting, diarrhea, malaise, sedation, tremor, and weight gain. More rare, but also more serious side effects include renal dysfunction and hypothyroidism. In children there are special concerns that lithium can affect bone development by mobilizing calcium from immature bones. In general, lithium can be safely used by children (Geller & Fetner, 1989), but they may experience more side effects (Campbell, Silva, Kafantaris, Locascio, Gonzalez, Lee, & Lynch, 1991), particularly very young children (Hagino, Weller, Weller, Washing, Fristad, & Kontras, 1995). Most clinicians eschew the use of lithium by very young children.

The side effects of the anticonvulsants have been well described in medical publications. Of most recent concern, divalproex sodium is associated with polycystic ovary disease in women who have seizure disorders (Isojarvi, Laatikainen, Pakarinen, Juntunen, & Myllyla, 1993). Caution is warranted in prescribing divalproex sodium as a mood stabilizer for female psychiatric patients who have comorbid seizure disorders.

Medical Workup

In addition to the usual initial evaluation, there is a protocol for initiating lithium. Required laboratory evaluation includes complete blood count, thyroid function tests, electrolytes, renal function tests, urinalysis, and an EKG. Abnormalities in these tests do not always preclude treatment with lithium, but more caution and monitoring may be necessary. Decisions must be individualized, depending on the severity of BPD episodes and patients' other medical and social needs. In children, regular monitoring of physical growth is needed, especially height. Lithium levels need to be checked shortly after initiating lithium and regularly as the dosage is increased. After stabilization, lithium levels are monitored annually or when the youth experiences psychiatric or medical complications.

Divalproex sodium and carbamazepine also have an evaluative protocol. Required laboratory evaluations include complete blood count and liver function tests. Serum levels are checked shortly after initiating treatment, regularly with dosage increases, and then annually. These anticonvulsants may induce their own metabolism, and thus serum levels may fall in the few months after apparent stabilization. Rechecks are needed, especially if the youth experiences an exacerbation of symptoms. Because these anticonvulsants are so highly protein bound, they can also be displaced when other medications such as antidepressants are added, leading to increased serum levels. Thus, serum levels should be monitored when selected medications are added.

Course of Treatment

Most early-onset BPD results in recurrent episodes. No guidelines are yet available for the length of treatment. Current experience suggests that treatment will be very long term, especially when the onset of BPD is earlier. The clinician is guided by the individual youth's degree of illness and complications. Polypharmacy is common. This may include more than one mood stabilizer and/or the addition of an antipsychotic medication. In general, antidepressants are avoided in BPD due to the risk of escalating manic episodes. However, although mood stabilizers may prevent future cycles of mania and depression, they are not good antidepressants once a youth becomes depressed. Thus, an antidepressant must often be tried.

Finally, youths who have BPD occasionally have comorbid ADHD. Although early experience suggested that the stimulants are contraindicated in BPD, many of these youths will benefit from the addition of a stimulant if ADHD symptoms persist after the control of mania. Other youths may experience exacerbation of their mania. When conduct disorders develop, more vigorous pharmacotherapy may reduce the acting out. Alternatively, it is help-ful to enlist the aid of the juvenile justice system or residential treatment programs.

Early-onset BPD is a difficult disorder to treat. Pharmacotherapy is the primary interven-tion. Some youths may be able to profit from psychotherapy; others may benefit from their parents' learning behavior management techniques. School interventions will almost always be needed. Thus, the role of the treatment team will be varied and challenging, especially because there will be times when these youths will not be able to participate easily in treatment. Child and adolescent psychiatrists are still learning the basic methods for treating these youths.

ANXIOLYTICS

Background

Anxiolytic medications are among the medications most commonly prescribed for adults. The use of benzodiazepines to treat anxiety symptoms in children and adolescents, however, is relatively uncommon. In the past, anxiolytics have been known as "sedative-hypnotics," or "minor tranquilizers." Traditionally, benzodiazepines and barbiturates were the two major types of psychotropics in the anxiolytic class of drugs. In the 1960s and 1970s, barbiturates were commonly prescribed for anxiety symptoms, but because of serious addiction problems, barbiturates are not used by adults or children for anxiety problems. The usual medications used in treating anxiety symptoms in children, in addition to benzodiazepines, are anti-histamines and buspirone. Buspirone is a relatively new anxiolytic that is FDA-approved for use by adults, but not by children.

The benzodiazepines can be classified according to the length of their half-life and po-tency. Clonazepam is a benzodiazepine that has a long half-life and high potency. Low-potency benzodiazepines that have long half-lives are chlordiazepoxide (Librium), diazepam (Valium), clorazepate (Tranxene), flurazepam (Dalmane), nitrazepam (Mogadon). High-potency benzodiazepines that have short half-lives are lorazepam (Ativan), alprazolam (Xanax), and triazolam (Halcion). The low-potency, short half-life benzodiazepines group consists of oxazepam (Serax) and temazepam (Restoril). Ironically, the medications most commonly used in treating childhood anxiety disorders are serotonin re-uptake inhibitors and tricyclic antidepressants, not anxiolytics. Concerns about tolerance and chemical dependency keep benzodiazepines from being more widely prescribed for children and adolescents. Some clinicians feel this has led to an underutilization of benzodiazepines by children and adoles-cents. Other medications used in treating anxiety are beta-blockers and antihistamines. MAOIs are also known for anxiolytic effect, but are virtually never used for children because of side-effect risks.

Mechanism of Action

Three neurotransmitter systems are implicated in the biological basis of anxiety. They are the norepinephrine, serotonin, and GABA systems. Benzodiazepine relieves anxiety symptoms via the GABA system. Antidepressants decrease anxiety symptoms through their influence on norepinephrine and serotonin systems. Buspirone's most prominent action is on serotonin receptor sites, though it also binds weakly to dopamine receptor sites. Theoretically, buspirone decreases anxiety through its effect on serotonin. Antihistamines, it is thought, ease anxiety symptoms by inducing sedation. The sedating qualities of antihistamines is through their blockade of histamine receptors.

Indications

There are FDA-approved indications for using some benzodiazepines in treating childhood anxiety. Lorazepam and chlorazepoxide are FDA-approved for use by children 12 years and older for anxiety symptoms. Oxazepam (Serax) is FDA-approved for managing anxiety disorders and short-term relief of symptoms of anxiety in children, though its safety and effectiveness in children age 6 and less has not been established. Clonazepam is FDA-approved for treating seizure disorders in infants, children, and adults. It is also FDA-approved for treating panic disorders only in adults. Lorazepam is frequently used in hospital settings for treating acute agitation. This off-label use is common in both adult and adolescent populations. Other pediatric off-label indications for the using benzodiazepines include panic disorder, mania, and sleep disturbances. In general, the use of benzodiazepines by children and adolescents is usually considered a second-line treatment. None of the benzodiazepines (flurazepam, triazolam, and temazepam) used primarily as sleeping pills is FDA-approved for use by children.

The safety and effectiveness of buspirone have not been determined in pediatric populations. Therefore its use as an anxiolytic by children and adolescents would be considered an off-label indication. There are some case studies that show that buspirone has promise for treating childhood anxiety disorders (Pfeffer, Jiang, & Domeshek, 1997; Carrey, Wiggins, & Milin, 1996; Hanna, Feibusch, & Albright, 1997). But at this time there are no well-controlled studies that show the efficacy of buspirone in treating childhood anxiety disorders.

The antihistamine hydroxyzine (Vistaril) is FDA-approved for use by children. Hydroxyzine is indicated in treating anxiety states in both adults and children. It is commonly used to augment pain medication pre- and postoperatively. Recent studies of adults confirm that hydroxyzine is more effective than a placebo in treating generalized anxiety disorders (Ferreri & Hantouche, 1998).

Contraindications

Relative contraindications for using benzodiazepines include youth who have histories of disinhibitory reactions, substance abuse, liver dysfunction, and take the anti-AIDS medication zidovudine. Benzodiazepines should also be avoided in cases of comorbid sleep apnea. For buspirone, the relative contraindications are liver or kidney dysfunction. In addition, benzodiazepines should not be given concurrently with MAOIs. Antihistamines should be avoided in a number of medical conditions, including narrow angle glaucoma and urinary or gastrointestinal obstruction. Caution should also be used when antihistamines are combined with pain medications. Antihistamines tend to potentiate the effects of analgesics such as sedation.

Pharmacokinetics

All of the benzodiazepines are available for oral administration. The half-life values for benzodiazepines can vary widely from 1 to 200 hours. The onset of action, however, for anxiolytic effect or sleep induction is usually within the first 30 to 60 minutes of administration. Of all the benzodiazepines, only lorazepam is well absorbed intramuscularly (im). This makes lorazepam ideal for treating acute agitation in children who refuse to take medications orally. For insomnia, the use of short half-live benzodiazepines is recommended. Benzodiazepines that have longer half-lives are more prone to cause "hangovers" and daytime sedation. As with most medications, preadolescent children generally require more frequent doses than adolescents and adults because of their rates of liver metabolism.

Buspirone is available only orally. Its onset of action is slower than benzodiazepines in treating anxiety. In contrast to anxiety relief in minutes for benzodiazepines, buspirone may take several weeks before symptom relief is achieved.

Hydroxyzine is available in both oral and injectable forms. In low doses, hydroxyzine acts as an anxiolytic. In high doses, it can induce sleep. Its onset of action is usually within 30 minutes.

Adverse Reactions

The most common side effects of benzodiazepines are sedation, dizziness, and fatigue. Sometimes there are significant problems with disinhibition. This can make children more agitated and out of control than their clinical status before benzodiazepine treatment. Decreased coordination and cognitive performance are also occasional adverse reactions that plague children and adolescents. Benzodiazepines are known to have a high risk of addiction. Therefore, clinicians are reticent to prescribe them for adolescents who have histories of substance abuse. In rare instances, the long-term use of benzodiazepines can result in liver dysfunction or low white blood cell counts.

In contrast to benzodiazepines, buspirone does not cause dependency problems, and there are rarely problems of sedation. Common side effects include dizziness, insomnia, gastrointestinal upset, headache, fatigue, and irritability.

Medical Workup

Aside from a physical examination, there are no other special or unique medical baseline tests for the use of antihistamines, buspirone, or the short-term use of benzodiazepines. If benzodiazepines are used on a long-term basis, regular follow-up blood tests to check liver function and white blood cell counts should be obtained.

Course of Treatment

Because problems of addiction are strongly associated with the length of anxiolytic administration, it should be limited. Uncomplicated insomnia is often transient and intermittent, but short-term use is usually sufficient. The prolonged use of benzodiazepines for insomnia is usually not indicated. The daily use of benzodiazepines for insomnia for more than 14–28 days is not recommended. If sleep problems persist, an evaluation for other psychopathology should be undertaken to clarify the etiology of insomnia. There are no clinical guidelines available to determine the length of treatment for anxiety symptoms. Most clinicians attempt to keep treatment as brief as possible.

Buspirone is not known for any withdrawal reactions from abrupt cessation. Therefore, discontinuing it does not usually require a tapering schedule.

Antihistamines are not known for problems of addiction, but brief treatment periods are the usual guideline for using them in childhood anxiety and sleep disorders. If anxiety or insomnia persists for more than 2 to 4 weeks, other psychopathology should be considered.

ANTIPSYCHOTICS

Background

The positive psychotic symptoms of hallucinations and delusions are hallmarks of both adult and childhood onset schizophrenia. Currently, antipsychotic medications are the cornerstone of treatment for psychotic symptoms. Chlorpromazine, the first antipsychotic medication, was administered to schizophrenic patients in the early 1950s. When first introduced, antipsychotic medications were referred to as major tranquilizers. Later the term "neuroleptics" was used when it was discovered that the neurotransmision of dopamine was affected because these medications blockade postsynaptic dopamine in the central nervous system. Currently, these dopamine blocking medications are referred to as typical or traditional antipsychotics. This is in contrast to the new "atypical" antipsychotics which are known for their better-side-effect profiles. Examples of traditional antipsychotics in order of low to high potency are chlorpromazine (Thorazine), thioridazine (Mellaril), perphenazine (Trilafon), trifluoperazine (Stelazine), thiothixene (Navene), fluphenazine (Prolixin), haloperidol (Haldol), and droperidol (Inapsine). Examples of atypical antipsychotics include clozapine (Clozaril), risperidone (Risperdal), olanzapine (Zyprexa), and quetiapine (Seroquel). Atypical antipsychotics are now considered first-line treatments for psychotic adults. There is no FDA approval for their use by children, but atypical antipsychotics are also considered first-line medications for children and adolescents who have psychotic symptoms. Atypical antipsychotics have several advantages over the traditional ones. They have fewer problems with side effects and they are more effective in reducing the negative symptoms of schizophrenia. Because atypical antipsychotics have more favorable side-effect profiles, patients are more compliant with their medications and are ultimately hospitalized less frequently due to medication noncompliance (Neumann, 1999; Rosenheck, Cramer, Allan, Erdos, Frisman, Xu, Thomas, Henderson, & Charney, 1999; Addington, Jones, Bloom, Chouinard, Remington, & Albright, 1993).

Mechanism of Action

For the past several decades, it has been observed that drugs that increase dopamine activity can sometimes produce positive psychotic symptoms. For example, amphetamines, which cause dopamine release, can cause paranoid delusions that are indistinguishable from paranoid schizophrenia. This is known as the "dopamine hypothesis" of schizophrenia. It is also known that drugs that decrease dopaminergic activity will decrease or stop positive psychotic symptoms. The traditional antipsychotics such as chlorpromazine and haloperidol mainly block postsynaptic dopamine receptors. This dopamine receptor blockade in the mesolimbic parts of the brain is, in theory, the way these medications ameliorate positive psychotic symptoms. Atypical antipsychotics block dopamine receptors relatively more weakly compared to traditional antipsychotics, but they also block some specific serotonin receptor sites. It is believed that the blockade of both dopamine and serotonin receptors makes atypicals effective because no antipsychotic effect is present in experimental drugs that block serotonin receptors alone. Therapeutic doses of risperidone in adults block about 60% of "5HT2a" serotonin receptors and 50% of postsynaptic dopamine receptors simultaneously. These results were shown in positron emission tomography (PET) studies. Future PET scanning data may help determine the optimal dopamine to serotonin receptor blockade ratio for antipsychotic medications.

Indications

As noted earlier, psychotic disorders such as schizophrenia are the main indication for using antipsychotic medications. However, antipsychotics are also indicated for a variety of childhood psychopathologies. For example, haloperidol is also indicated in treating tic disorders and Tourette's syndrome, attention deficit hyperactivity disorder, and episodes of severe combative and explosive behavior in children. Chlorpromazine, thioridazine, and trifluoperazine are also indicated in this short-term treatment of severe disruptive behaviors. These traditional antipsychotics are FDA-approved for use by children. Chlorpromazine is FDA-approved for use by children as young as 6 months (as a preanesthetic), thioridazine is approved for children 2 years and older, haloperidol is approved for children 3 years and older, and trifluoperazine is approved for children age 6 and older. Droperidol is commonly used for acute combative behavior in hospital settings (Joshi, Hamel, Joshi, & Capozzoli, 1998). It is also interesting to note that many of the traditional antipsychotics such as fluphenazine, haloperidol, and prochlorperazine (Compazine) are indicated for treating nausea.

At this time, none of the atypical antipsychotics has FDA approval for use by children or adolescents. However, they all have off-label indications for treating childhood psychotic disorders. Risperidone has also been identified as a useful treatment for tic disorders (Lombroso et al., 1995), as an effective augmentation agent for SSRIs in treating obsessive–compulsive disorder (Stein, Bouwer, Hawkridge, & Emsley, 1997), and for aggressive and disruptive disorder symptoms (Schreier, 1998).

Contraindications

Strong contraindications to treatment with traditional antipsychotics include bone marrow suppression and liver dysfunction. Other relative contraindications include a history of neuroleptic malignant syndrome, pregnancy, obtundation, and concomitant use of strong CNS depressants. There is a relative contraindication to using traditional antipsychotics with lithium because of reported drug-induced delirium-like states.

In general, except for clozapine, atypical antipsychotics have no major contraindications. Any blood disease is an absolute contraindication for using clozapine because of its bone marrow suppression tendencies. Other contraindications include uncontrolled epilepsy, severe hypotension, and cardiorespiratory disease. The major contraindication to the use of risperidone, olanzapine, and quetiapine is a known allergic response from previous use.

Pharmacokinetics

In general, children require higher doses of antipsychotic medication per kilogram than adults because they have a higher rate of hepatic metabolism and because children as a whole have a lower percentage of body fat in which these lipophilic medications are stored. Oral doses of neuroleptics usually reach peak concentrations 2 to 3 hours after ingestion. Intramuscular doses reach peak concentrations in 30 to 60 minutes. Haloperidol and fluphenzine have an added advantage for treating noncompliant patients. They come in a long-acting "depot" form. A deep intramuscular injection can provide enough medication so that a patient may not need another injection for 2 to 4 weeks. Thus, reliance on patients to take their pills every day is eliminated.

Traditional antipsychotics range in half-life from several hours to several days. Most are metabolized by the liver and have active metabolites. Their onset of action ranges from a few days to a few weeks. They sometimes stabilize psychotic symptoms faster than atypical antipsychotics, but this is probably due to their stronger sedating qualities, rather than an actual antipsychotic effect. Psychotic individuals who are more sedated and groggy appear less symptomatic than those who are still wide awake and verbalizing incoherently. Most traditional antipsychotics are available in both oral and injectable forms. This allows more flexibility in delivering medication in acute psychotic states when medication refusal is common.

Atypicals are available only in oral preparations. Risperidone is available in liquid form, which can be helpful for children who resist swallowing pills. No depot form of atypicals exists at this time. The serum half-lives of atypical antipsychotics range from 4 to 10 hours for quetiapine, to 6 to 12 hours for risperidone, and 20–70 hours for olanzapine. Based on these half-life values, it is recommended that quetiapine be dosed three to four times a day and risperidone two times a day. Olanzapine can usually be dosed once a day. Onset of action for atypicals is usually 1 to 3 weeks.

Adverse Reactions

Traditional antipsychotics are known for extrapyramidal side effects (EPS). The more potent the traditional antipsychotic, the greater the risk of EPS. EPS manifests commonly as akathisia or generalized restlessness, Parkinson's disease-like tremor, and dystonic reactions such as acute muscle spasms or dyskinetic muscular reactions. In general, there is a higher rate of dystonic reactions in children and adolescents than in adults. In particular, adolescent males are known for having severe dystonic reactions or unrelenting muscle spasms. The most serious adverse reaction is neuroleptic malignant syndrome (NMS). NMS is potentially lethal if not recognized early and treated emergently. It usually presents with acute "board-like" rigidity of abdominal muscles, high fever, and delirium. Tardive dyskinesia (TD) develops from chronic or long-term treatment with antipsychotic medications. TD is a hypersensitive reaction to dopamine in the substantia nigra portion of the midbrain and manifests as involuntary movements, usually in the tongue, lips, jaw, face, and less frequently in the trunk. Other common adverse reactions to antipsychotic medication include sedation, low blood pressure, dizziness, dry mouth, constipation, and headache. Antipsychotics lower seizure threshold and should be used with caution by children and adolescents who have epilepsy. In rare cases, liver dysfunction and bone marrow suppression may result from antipsychotic treatment. Galactorrhea or milk-like secretion from the nipples in females can be a very troubling side effect for teenage girls. Weight gain is also a common problem for youth on antipsychotic medications. On a average, a 3–5% weight gain is associated with traditional antipsychotic treatment.

In general, except for clozapine, atypical antipsychotics have a much lower rate of side effects than typical antipsychotics. However, there are some caveats to keep in mind. In adults the rate of EPS for individuals who receive risperidone is considered no greater than a placebo in therapeutic doses. However, a recent report showed higher rates of EPS in risperidone-treated adolescents than in adults (Grcevich, 1996). Risperdal and olanzapine are known for problems with weight gain. In one study, the average patient gained 16 pounds on risperidone (Kelly, Conley, Love, Horn, & Ushchak, 1998). Compared with all of the atypicals, olanzapine causes an even greater problem of weight gain than risperidone (Wirshing, Wirshing, Kysar, Berisford, Goldstein, Pashdag, Mintz, & Marder, 1999). It is not uncommon for adolescents to gain 10 to 20 pounds on olanzapine. Seroquel tends to be the most sedating of the atypical antipsychotics currently available. This may be an advantage over the other atypicals for psychotic youth who have insomnia. Clozapine is known for a high rate of bone marrow suppression. One out of a hundred patients treated during a year's time with clozapine will develop bone marrow suppression. Because of this, the pharmaceutical company requires that anyone who takes clozapine get a complete blood count once a week. Blood test refusal results in pharmacies refusing to supply the medication.

Medical Workup

Important parts of the medical workup before starting antipsychotic medication, in addition to a physical exam, include measuring height and weight and neurological examination for tics, stereotypies, extrapyramidal disorders, and tardive dyskinesia. Baseline laboratory tests that are recommended include a complete blood count, liver function tests, and electrocardiogram. The "Abnormal Involuntary Movements Scale" (AIMS) or similar instrument should be used to assess for involuntary movements before antipsychotic treatment. For children, follow-up AIMS administration is recommended at least once every 6 months to detect developing TD.

In general, the medical workup for atypical antipsychotics is much less rigorous than for typical antipsychotics. Electrocardiograms are not recommended for baseline measurement. Seroquel has one special baseline exam recommended by its manufacturer. Baseline and follow-up eye exams are recommended to identify problems of cataract formation. Baseline complete blood counts are mandatory for clozapine.

Course of Treatment

Because of the risk of TD, antipsychotic treatment must be started with caution. Treatment for acute psychosis is commonly initiated in the hospital. In this controlled setting, the doses of medication are usually higher than for patients who are being treated for less severe psychotic symptoms and disruptive behaviors. Psychotic youth are typically treated for several months to a year before considering a medication holiday. If these medications are stopped abruptly, a withdrawal syndrome could develop. Problems with nausea, vomiting, loss of appetite, sweating, insomnia, agitation, and irritability are common withdrawal symptoms. In children who have tic disorders, abrupt cessation of antipsychotic medications can result in severe withdrawal dyskinesias. These involuntary twitches can be more pronounced than the tics that existed before initiating treatment. Tapering medications over 1 to 2 weeks usually can ameliorate withdrawal symptoms. There are no clear guidelines for the length of antipsychotic treatment of pediatric populations. Research is needed to help guide clinicians in this area.

MISCELLANEOUS MEDICATIONS

Medications that are not classified among the psychotropics are often useful in treating emotional and behavioral problems in children and adolescents. Among these are guanfacine, clonidine, propranolol, naltrexone, and diphenhydramine. These medications are used in pediatric populations for various off-label indications which are described following.

Clonidine and Guanfacine

Clonidine (Catapres) and guanfacine (Tenex) are both classified as antihypertensive agents and effectively lower blood pressure in hypertensive individuals. Chemically, they stimulate selective adrenergic (norepinephrine) receptors in the CNS and are called alpha-2 adrenergic agonists. Both medications bind to postsynaptic alpha-2a adrenergic receptors in the prefrontal cortical regions, which are implicated in attentional and organizational functions. Clinical benefits include improved working memory and attention regulation (Chappell, Riddle, Scahill, Lynch, Schultz, Arnsten, Leckman, & Cohen, 1995). The half-lives of guanfacine and clonidine are approximately 12 hours in children. However, the duration of action of guanfacine is longer at about 24 hours compared to 8 hours for clonidine. Both medications have shown therapeutic benefits in childhood disorders characterized by hyperaroused cognitive or motor states.

Both clonidine and guanfacine are used as second- or third-line medications in the primary treatment of ADHD. They are also used in conjunction with stimulants when hyperactivity and impulsivity persist, despite good stimulant control of inattention and other cognitive symptoms. Because of its greater sedating qualities, clonidine is more effective in controlling hyperactivity, but guanfacine is better in improving attention span (Jakala, Riekkinen, Sirvio, Koivisto, Kejonen, Vanhanen, & Riekkinen, 1999).

Clonidine and guanfacine have also been effective in decreasing tics in Tourette's disorder (Chappell et al., 1995). Improvement in both tics and disruptiveness have been reported. Their ability to control tics is less well investigated and understood than their effect on disruptiveness and attention. Theoretically, guanfacine and clonidine may ameliorate tic and disruptive symptoms by regulating the activity of central norepinephrine.

Clinical experience is also increasing the understanding of alpha-2 agonist effects in treating PTSD, usually as a second-line treatment. In a small case series, clonidine has shown effects in improving anxiety, hyperactivity, and social behaviors in preschool children who have PTSD (Harmon & Riggs, 1996), and guanfacine ameliorates PTSD nightmares (Horrigan, 1996).

The most common side effects for both alpha-2 agonists are sedation, followed by headache, dizziness, and lowered blood pressure. Clonidine presents with more adverse effects than guanfacine. Most children experience some decrease in blood pressure and pulse while remaining asymptomatic. Practically speaking, open trials of guanfacine have shown few side effects.

The use of clonidine became controversial when methylphenidate and clonidine were concurrently prescribed for several children who died. No direct association was ever identified (Wilens, Spencer, Conners, & Cantwell, 1999), but considerable controversy persists. Some clinicians feel that more caution should be used when prescribing clonidine because of possible cardiac side effects (Cantwell, Swanson, & Conners, 1997), whereas others observe that there is not enough evidence to link clonidine to potentially lethal reactions. Interestingly, the American Heart Association does not recommend baseline and follow-up EKGs for clonidine or guanfacine in pediatric populations (Gutsgesell, Atkins, Barst, Buck, Franklin, Humes, Ringel, Shaddy, & Taubert, 1999). Because of the controversy, many clinicians prefer an initial trial of guanfacine, rather than clonidine, due to its more selective profile for alpha-2a agonism and thus lessened risk for cardiac complications. However, guanfacine is much more expensive, and some managed care companies will not approve its preferential use.

Reflex hypertension may occur if administration of clonidine or guanfacine is stopped abruptly. This can be potentially life-threatening. Thus, these medications are always tapered down when a decision is made to discontinue treatment.

Naltrexone

Naltrexone (Trexan) has traditionally been used to reverse the effects of narcotic-induced respiratory depression in opiate overdose. It is classified as an opiate blocker. Naltrexone has been used to treat developmentally disabled children who have self-injurious behaviors. It has been hypothesized that children who bite themselves, bang their heads, or otherwise self-mutilate are not sufficiently sensitive to painful stimuli. Naltrexone may decrease their pain threshold, thereby making self-inflicted injury more aversive. Some initial case studies showed some positive outcomes in this difficult to treat population. However, larger, more recent studies have not consistently demonstrated that naltrexone decreases self-injurious behaviors.

There have been some reports that naltrexone may reduce hyperactivity in autistic children (Kolmen, Feldman, Handen, & Janosky, 1995). However, there are no controlled studies comparing naltrexone to other psychotropics, like stimulants.

The most common side effects from naltrexone are insomnia, nervousness, stomach-aches, nausea, and headaches. In rare instances, there can be liver dysfunction. So it is recommended that children who receive long-term naltrexone treatment be provided with routine monitoring of liver function tests.

Diphenhydramine

There is a long history of using antihistamines in dealing with childhood sleep problems and fussy behavior in infants. However, a Medline search of the literature of the past ten years reveals no controlled studies to support this popular off-label indication. Sleep disorders in infants and young children can be very exhausting to parents. Behavioral methods are preferred, but there is some evidence that short use of diphenhydramine (Benadryl) might be effective. Similar use may be helpful for insomnia connected with a minor illness or psycho-social stress, or when parents are overwhelmed (Richman, 1985).

The sedating effects of diphenhydramine, it is thought, are mediated through its blockade of histamine receptors in the CNS. Its long term use for allergic reactions, rashes, and upper respiratory infection symptoms has shown that diphenhydramine is safe for youths. However, there are some bothersome side effects, including dilated pupils and dry mouth and skin. The most serious adverse reaction is delirium usually secondary to overdosage, particularly in young children who may hallucinate during the delirum. If supportive measures are not taken in this condition, it is potentially lethal. Note that some children experience an idiosyncratic reaction to antihistamines. They become agitated or hyperactive in response to this medica-tion. Diphenhydramine is available over-the-counter and does not require a prescription.

Propranolol

Propranolol (Inderal) is classified as a beta-blocker medication. Beta-blockers were initially used to treat high blood pressure and other cardiovascular conditions in adults. In adults, off-label indications include performance anxiety, lithium tremor, akathisia, hyperven-tilation attacks, PTSD, alcohol withdrawal, and generalized anxiety symptoms. There are no FDA approved behavioral indications for using propranolol in pediatric populations, but beta-blockers have shown some promise in treating aggression in children who have brain damage, PTSD, and generalized anxiety symptoms. In a study of sexually and physically abused children, propranolol was used to treat the symptoms of PTSD. Scores on an inventory of PTSD symptoms indicated that the children exhibited significantly fewer symptoms while receiving propranolol than before or after they received this medication (Famularo, Kin-scherff, & Fenton, 1988). The studies that examined the effectiveness of propranolol in treating aggression in brain-damaged children were uncontrolled and used small numbers of subjects

(Williams, Mehl, Yudofsky, Adams, & Roseman, 1982; Yudofsky, Williams, & Gorman, 1981; Kuperman & Stewart, 1987). These small studies did show that there were fewer aggressive outbursts and physical assaults with propranolol treatment. As noted, these studies were uncontrolled, and a number of the subjects were taking other medications that targeted their aggressive behavior. Side effects from propranolol are considerable. Bradycardia, bronchoconstriction, depression, hallucinations, hypotension, nausea and vomiting, dizziness and hypoglycemia make the use of propranolol rather unpopular in any population.

Summary

The use of psychotropic medications to treat childhood psychopathology is taking on a more primary role in comprehensive treatment planning. Aided by recently mandated federal grants, pediatric psychopharmacological research during the 1990s made great progress. With this increase in available study data, more indications for using psychotropics in children and adolescents have been found, but the knowledge base of childhood psychopharmacology is still well behind adult levels. Future research is still needed to delineate safe, appropriate, and effective uses for psychotropic agents in pediatric populations. Medication helps keep many children, who have debilitating psychopathology, developmentally on track and able to live relatively normal lives. But despite the sometimes dramatic effects of psychotropics, it should be remembered that medication is part of a treatment plan, not the whole plan. The most important aspect of working with children and adolescents is providing parental support, education, guidance, and counseling.

Additional Readings

Stahl, S. M. (1996). *Essential psychopharmacology: Neuroscientific basis and clinical applications.* Cambridge, England: Cambridge University Press.

Werry, J. S., & Aman, M. G. (1999). *Practitioner's guide to psychoactive drugs for children and adolescents.* 2nd ed. New York: Plenum Medical Book.

References

Addington, D. E., Jones, B., Bloom, D., Chouinard, G., Remington, G., & Albright, P. (1993). Reduction of hospital days in chronic schizophrenic patients treated with risperidone: A retrospective study. *Clinical Therapy, 15,* 917–926.

Akiskal, H. S., Downs, J., Jordan, P., Watson, S., Daugherty, D., & Pruitt, D. B. (1985). Affective disorders in referred children and younger siblings of manic depressives. *Archives of General Psychiatry, 42,* 996–1003.

American Academy of Pediatrics, Committee on Bioethics (1995). Informed consent, parental permission, and assent in pediatric practice. *Pediatrics, 95,* 314–317.

Bernstein, G., Borchard, C., & Perwein, A. (1996). Anxiety disorders in children and adolescents: A review of the past ten years. *Journal of the American Academy of Child and Adolescent Psychiatry, 35,* 1110–1119.

Biederman, J., Thisted, R. A., Greenhill, L. L., & Ryan, N. D. (1995). Estimation of the association between desipramine and the risk for sudden death in 5- to 14-year-old children. *Journal of Clinical Psychiatry, 56,* 87–93.

Birmaher, B., Ryan, N. D., Williamson, D. E., Brent, D. A., Kaufman, J., Dahl, R. E., Perel, J., & Nelson, B. (1996a). Childhood and adolescent depression: A review of the past 10 years. Part I. *Journal of the American Academy of Child and Adolescent Psychiatry, 35,* 1427–1439.

Birmaher, B., Ryan, N. D., Williamson, D. E., Brent, D. A., & Kaufman, J. (1996b). Childhood and adolescent depression: A review of the past 10 years. Part II. *Journal of the American Academy of Child and Adolescent Psychiatry, 35,* 1575–1583.

Birmaher, B., Waterman, G. S., Ryan, N., Cully, M., Balach, L., Ingram, J., & Brodsky, M. (1994). Fluoxetine for childhood anxiety disorders. *Journal of the American Academy of Child and Adolescent Psychiatry, 33,* 993–999.

Bradley, C. (1937). Behavior of children receiving benzedrine. *American Journal of Psychiatry, 94,* 577–585.

Campbell, M., Silva, R. R., Kafantaris, V., Locascio, J. J., Gonzalez, N. M., Lee, D., & Lynch, N. S. (1991). Predictors of side effects associated with lithium administration in children. *Psychopharmacology Bulletin, 27,* 373–380.

Cantwell, D. P. (1996). Attention deficit disorder: A review of the past 10 years. *Journal of the American Academy of Child and Adolescent Psychiatry, 35,* 978–987.

Cantwell, D. P., Swanson, J., & Conners, D. F. (1997). Case study: Adverse response to clonidine. *Journal of the American Academy of Child and Adolescent Psychiatry, 36*(4), 539–544.

Carlson, G. A., & Weintraub, S. (1993). Childhood behavior problems and bipolar disorder: Relationship or coincidence? *Journal of Affective Disorders, 28,* 143–153.

Carrey, N. J., Wiggins, D. M., & Milin, R. P. (1996). Pharmacological treatment of psychiatric disorders in children and adolescents: Focus on guidelines for the primary care practitioner. *Drugs, 51,* 750–759.

Cauffman, E., & Steinberg, L. (1995). The cognitive and affective influences on adolescent decision making. *Temple Law Review, 68,* 1763–1789.

Chappell, P. B., Riddle, M. A., Scahill, L., Lynch, K. A., Schultz, R., Arnsten, A., Leckman, J. F., & Cohen, D. J. (1995). Guanfacine treatment of comorbid attention-deficit hyperactivity disorder and Tourette's syndrome: Preliminary clinical experience. *Journal of the American Academy of Child and Adolescent Psychiatry, 34,* 1140–1146.

Committee on Bioethics (1995). Informed consent, parental permission, and assent in pediatric practice. *The American Academy of Pediatrics, 95,* 314–317.

Conners, C. K., Casat, C. D., Gualtieri, C. T., Weller, E., Reader, M., Reiss, A., Weller, R. A., Khayrallah, M., & Ascher, J. (1996). Bupropion hydrochloride in attention deficit disorder with hyperactivity. *Journal of the American Academy of Child and Adolescent Psychiatry, 35,* 1314–1321.

Dahl, R. E., Ryan, N. D., Puig-Antich, J., Nguyen, N. A., al-Shabbout, M., Meyer, V. A., & Perel, J. (1991). 24-hour cortisol measures in adolescents with major depression: A controlled study. *Biological Psychiatry, 30*(1), 25–36.

DeVaugh-Geiss, J., Moroz, G., Biederman, J., Cantwell, D., Fontaine, R., Greist, J. H., Reichler, R., Katz, R., & Landau, P. (1992). Clomipramine hydrochloride in childhood and adolescent obsessive–compulsive disorder: A multicenter trial. *Journal of the American Academy of Child and Adolescent Psychiatry, 31,* 45–49.

Dulcan, M. (1997). Practice parameters for the assessment and treatment of children, adolescents, and adults with attention-deficit/hyperactivity disorder. *Journal of the American Academy of Child and Adolescent Psychiatry, 36*(10 Supplement), 85S–121S.

Emslie, G. J., Rush, A. J., Weinberg, W. A., Kowatch, R. A., Hughes, C. W., Carmody, T., & Rintelmann, J. (1997). A double-blind, randomized, placebo-controlled trial of fluoxetine in children and adolescents with depression. *Archives of General Psychiatry, 54,* 1031–1307.

Famularo, R., Kinscherff, R., & Fenton, T. (1988). Propranolol treatment for childhood posttraumatic stress disorder, acute type. A pilot study. *American Journal of Diseases of Children, 142,* 1244–1247.

Faraone, S. V., Biederman, J., Wozniak, J., Mundy, E., Mennin, D., & O'Donnell, D. (1997). Is comorbidity with ADHD a marker for juvenile-onset mania? *Journal of the American Academy of Child and Adolescent Psychiatry, 36,* 1046–1055.

Feldman, H., Crumrine, P., Handen, B. L., Alvin, R., & Teodori, J. (1989). Methylphenidate in children with seizures and attention-deficit disorder. *American Journal of Diseases of Children, 143,* 1081–1086.

Ferreri, M., & Hantouche, E. G. (1998). Recent trials of hydroxyzine in generalized anxiety disorder. *Acta Psychiatrica Scandinavica, Supplementum, 393,* 102–108.

Gadow, K. D., Sverd, J., Sprafkin, J., Nolan, E. E., & Grossman, S. (1999). Long-term methylphenidate therapy in children with comorbid attention-deficit hyperactivity disorder and chronic multiple tic disorder. *Archives of General Psychiatry, 56,* 330–336.

Garland, E. J. (1998). Intranasal abuse of prescribed methylphenidate. *Journal of the American Academy of Child and Adolescent Psychiatry, 37,* 1242–1243.

Geller, B. (1997). Double-blind placebo-controlled study of lithium for adolescents with comorbid bipolar and substance dependency disorders. Presented at the *Annual Midyear Institute of the American Academy of Child and Adolescent Psychiatry,* March 19–21, Hamilton, Bermuda.

Geller, B., Cooper, T. B., Chestnut, E. C., Abel, A. S., & Anker, J. A. (1984). Nortriptyline pharmacokinetic parameters in depressed children and adolescents: Preliminary data. *Journal of Clinical Psychopharmacology, 4,* 265–269.

Geller, B., Cooper, T. B., & Chestnut, E. C. (1985). Serial monitoring and achievement of steady state nortriptyline plasma levels in depressed children and adolescents: Preliminary data. *Journal of Clinical Psychopharmacology, 5,* 213–216.

Geller, B., Cooper, T. B., Zimerman, B., Sun, K., Williams, M., & Frazier, J. (1994a). Double-blind placebo-controlled study of lithium for depressed children with bipolar family histories. *Neuropsychopharmacology, 10*(S-122), 541S.

Geller, B., & Fetner, H. H. (1989). Children's 24-hour serum lithium level after a single dose predicts initial dose and steady-state plasma level. *Journal of Clinical Psychopharmacology, 9,* 155.

Geller, B., Fox, L. W., & Clark, K. A. (1994b). Rate and predictors of prepubertal bipolarity during follow-up of 6- to 12-year-old depressed children. *Journal of the American Academy of Child and Adolescent Psychiatry, 33,* 461–468.

Geller, B., Fox, L. W., & Fletcher, M. (1993). Effect of tricyclic antidepressants on switching to mania and on the onset of bipolarity in depressed 6- to 12-year-olds. *Journal of the American Academy of Child and Adolescent Psychiatry, 32,* 43–50.

Geller, B., & Luby, J. (1997). Child and adolescent bipolar disorder: A review of the past 10 years. *Journal of the American Academy of Child and Adolescent Psychiatry, 36,* 1168–1176.

Geller, B., Sun, K., Zimmerman, B., Luby, J., Frazier, J., & Williams, M. (1995). Complex and rapid-cycling in bipolar children and adolescents: A preliminary study. *Journal of Affective Disorders, 34,* 259–268.

Goldman-Rakic, C. P., & Brown, R. M. (1982). Postnatal development of monoamine content and synthesis in the cerebral cortex of rhesus monkeys. *Developmental Brain Research, 4,* 339–349.

Grcevich, S. J., Findling, R. L., Rowane, W. A., Friedman, L., & Schulz, S. C. (1996). Risperidone in the treatment of children and adolescents with schizophrenia: A retrospective study. *Journal of Child and Adolescent Psychopharmacology, 6,* 251–257.

Gutgesell, H., Atkins, D., Barst, R., Buck, M., Franklin, W., Humes, R., Ringel, R., Shaddy, R., & Taubert, K. A. (1999). Cardiovascular monitoring of children and adolescents receiving psychotropic drugs. *Circulation, 99,* 979–982.

Hagino, O. R., Weller, E. B., Weller, R. A., Washing, D., Fristad, M. A., & Kontras, S. B. (1995). Untoward effects of lithium treatment in children aged four through six years. *Journal of the American Academy of Child and Adolescent Psychiatry, 34,* 1584–1590.

Hanna, G. L., Feibusch, E. L., & Albright, K. J. (1997). Buspirone treatment of anxiety associated with pharyngeal dysphasia in a four-year-old. *Journal of the American Academy of Child and Adolescent Psychiatry, 7* 137–143.

Harmon, R. J., & Riggs, P. D. (1996). Clonidine for posttraumatic stress disorder in preschool children. *Journal of the American Academy of Child and Adolescent Psychiatry, 35,* 1247–1249.

Horrigan, J. P. (1996). Guanfacine for PTSD nightmares. *Journal of the American Academy of Child and Adolescent Psychiatry, 35,* 975–976.

Hyman, S. E., & Nestler, E. J. (1996). Initiation and adaptation: A paradigm for understanding psychotropic drug action. *American Journal of Psychiatry, 153,* 151–162.

Isojarvi, J. I., Laatikainen, T. J., Pakarinen, A. J., Juntunen, K. T., & Myllyla, V. V. (1993). Polycystic ovaries and hyperandrogenism in women taking valproate for epilepsy. *New England Journal of Medicine, 329,* 1383–1388.

Jakala, P., Riekkinen, M., Sirvio, J., Koivisto, E., Kejonen, K., Vanhanen, M., & Riekkinen, P., Jr. (1999). Guanfacine, but not clonidine, improves planning and working memory performance in humans. *Neuropsychopharmacology, 20,* 460–470.

Joshi, P. T., Hamel, L., Joshi, A. R., & Capozzoli, J. A. (1998). Use of droperidol in hospitalized children. *Journal of the American Academy of Child and Adolescent Psychiatry, 37,* 228–230.

Kelly, D. L., Conley, R. R., Love, R. C., Horn, D. S., & Ushchak, C. M. (1998). Weight gain in adolescents treated with risperidone and conventional antipsychotics over six months. *Journal of Child and Adolescent Psychopharmacology, 8,* 151–159.

King, R. A., Riddle, M. S., Chappell, P. B., Hardin, M. T., Anderson, G. M., Lombroso, P., & Scahill, L. (1991). Emergence of self-destructive phenomena in children and adolescents during fluoxetine treatment. *Journal of the American Academy of Child and Adolescent Psychiatry, 30,* 179–186.

Kingsbury, S. J., & Tekell, J. L. (1999). What are the advantages and disadvantages of using different providers for psychotherapy and drug treatment? *Harvard Mental Health Letter, 15*(11), 8.

Kolmen, B. K., Feldman, H. M., Handen, B. L., & Janosky, J. E. (1995). Naltrexone in young autistic children: A double-blind, placebo-controlled crossover study. *Journal of the American Academy of Child and Adolescent Psychiatry, 34,* 223–231.

Kovacs, M., & Gatsonis, C. (1994). Secular trends in age at onset of major depressive disorder in a clinical sample of children. *Journal of Psychiatric Research, 28*, 319–329.

Kovacs, M., & Pollock, M. (1995). Bipolar disorder and comorbid conduct disorder in childhood and adolescence. *Journal of the American Academy of Child and Adolescent Psychiatry, 34*, 715–723.

Kuperman, S., & Stewart, M. A. (1987). Use of propranolol to decrease aggressive outbursts in younger patients. Open study reveals potentially favorable outcome. *Psychosomatics, 28*, 315–319.

Leonard, H. L., March, J., Rickler, K. C., & Allen, A. J. (1997). Pharmacology of the selective serotonin reuptake inhibitors in children and adolescents. *Journal of the American Academy of Child and Adolescent Psychiatry, 36*, 725–736.

Leonard, H. L., Meyer, M. C., Swedo, S. E., Richter, D., Hamburger, S. D., Allen, A. J., Rapoport, J. L., & Tucker, E. (1995). Electrocardiographic changes during desipramine and clomipramine treatment in children and adolescents. *Journal of the American Academy of Child and Adolescent Psychiatry, 34*, 1460–1468.

Lombroso, P. J., Scahill, L., King, R. A., Lynch, K. A., Chappell, P. B., Peterson, B. S., McDougle, C. J., & Leckman, J. F. (1995). Risperidone treatment of children and adolescents with chronic tic disorders: A preliminary report. *Journal of the American Academy of Child and Adolescent Psychiatry, 34*, 1147–1152.

March, J., Biederman, J., Wolkow, R., & Safferman, A. (1998). Sertraline in children and adolescents with obsessive compulsive disorder: A multicenter double-blind placebo-controlled study. *Journal of the American Medical Association, 280*, 1752–1756.

March, J. S., Kobak, K. A., Jefferson, J. W., Mazza, J., & Greist, J. H. (1990). A double-blind, placebo-controlled trial of fluroxamine versus imipramine in outpatients with major depression. *Journal of Clinical Psychiatry, 51*, 200–202.

Myers, K., & McCauley, E. (1997). Treatment of depressive disorders during adolescence. In D. L. Dunner (Ed.), *Current psychiatric therapy II*, 2nd ed. (pp. 458–467). Philadelphia: W.B. Saunders.

Neumann, P. J. (1999). Methods of cost-effectiveness analysis in the evaluation of new antipsychotics: Implications for schizophrenia treatment. *Journal of Clinical Psychology, 60*(Suppl 3), 9–14, discussion 15.

Papatheodorou, G., & Kutcher, S. P. (1993). Divalproex sodium treatment in late adolescent and young adult acute mania. *Psychopharmacology, 29*, 213–219.

Pfeffer, C. R., Jiang, H., & Domeshek, L. J. (1997). Buspirone treatment of psychiatrically hospitalized prepubertal children with symptoms of anxiety and moderately severe aggression. *Journal of Child and Adolescent Psychopharmacology, 7*, 145–155.

Pizzuti, D. (1999, June). Cylert (pemoline) patient information/consent form. *Abbott Pharmaceutical Products Division*, 99F-110-6993A.

Preskorn, S. H., Bupp, S. J., Weller, E. B., & Weller, R. A. (1989). Plasma levels of imipramine and metabolites in 68 hospitalized children. *Journal of the American Academy of Child and Adolescent Psychiatry, 28*, 373–375.

Richman, N. (1985). A double-blind drug trial of treatment in young children with waking problems. *Journal of Child Psychology and Psychiatry and Allied Disciplines, 26*, 591–598.

Riddle, M. A., Brown, N., Dzubinski, D., Jetmalani, A. N., Law, Y.,& Woolston, J. L. (1989). Fluoxetine overdose in an adolescent. *Journal of the American Academy of Child and Adolescent Psychiatry, 23*, 587–588.

Riddle, M. A., Claghorn, J., Gaffney, G., et al. (1996). Fluvoxamine for children and adolescents with OCD: A controlled multicenter trial. Presented at the *43rd Annual Meeting of the American Academy of Child and Adolescent Psychiatry*, October 25, Philadelphia.

Riddle, M. A., Nelson, J. C., Kleinman, C. S., Rasmusson, A., Leckman, J. F., King, R. A., & Cohen, D. J. (1991). Sudden death in children receiving Norpramin: A review of three reported cases and commentary. *Journal of the American Academy of Child and Adolescent Psychiatry, 30*, 104–108.

Riddle, M. A., Scahill, L., King, R. A., Hardin, M. T., Anderson, G. M., Ort, S. I., Smith, J. C., Leckman, J. F., & Cohen, D. J. (1992). Double-blind, crossover trial of fluoxetine and placebo in children and adolescents with obsessive–compulsive disorder. *Journal of the American Academy of Child and Adolescent Psychiatry, 31*, 1062–1069.

Rosenberg, D. R., Stewart, C. M., Fitzgerald, K. D., Tawile, V., & Carroll, E. (1999). Paroxetine open-label treatment of pediatric outpatients with obsessive–compulsive disorder. *Journal of the American Academy of Child and Adolescent Psychiatry, 38*, 1180–1185.

Rosenheck, R., Cramer, J., Allan, E., Erdos, J., Frisman, L. K., Xu, W., Thomas, J., Henderson, W., & Charney, D. (1999). Cost-effectiveness of clozapine in patients with high and low levels of hospital use. Department of Veterans Affairs Cooperative Study Group on clozapine in refractory schizophrenia. *Archives of General Psychiatry, 56*, 565–572.

Ryan, N. D. (1992). The pharmacologic treatment of child and adolescent depression. *Psychiatric Clinics of North America, 15*, 29–40.

Ryan, N. D., Williamson, D. E., Iyengar, S., Orvaschel, H., Reich, T., Dahl, R. E., & Puig-Antich, J. (1992). A secular increase in child and adolescent onset affective disorder. *Journal of the American Academy of Child and Adolescent Psychiatry, 31*, 600–605.

Safer, D. J., Zito, J. M., & Fine, E. M. (1996). Increased methylphenidate usage for attention deficit disorder in the 1990s. *Pediatrics, 98*, 1084–1088.

Schowalter, J. E. (1989). Psychodynamics and medication. *Journal of the American Academy of Child and Adolescent Psychiatry, 28*, 681–684.

Schreier, H. A. (1998). Risperidone for young children with mood disorders and aggressive behavior. *Journal of Child and Adolescent Psychopharmacology, 8*(1), 49–59.

Silva, R. R., Munoz, D. M., & Alpert, M. (1996). Carbamazepine use in children and adolescents with features of attention-deficit hyperactivity disorder: A meta-analysis. *Journal of the American Academy of Child and Adolescent Psychiatry, 35*, 352–358.

Simeon, J., Dinicola, V. B., Ferguson, H. B., & Copping, W. (1990). Adolescent depression: A placebo controlled fluoxetine treatment study and follow-up. *Progress in Neuropsychopharmacology and Biological Psychiatry, 14*, 791–795.

Stein, D. J., Bouwer, C., Hawkridge, S., & Emsley, R. A. (1997). Risperidone augmentation of SSRIs in obsessive compulsive and related disorders. *Journal of Clinical Psychiatry, 58*(3), 119–122.

Strober, M. (1992). Relevance of early age-of-onset in genetic studies of bipolar affective disorder. *Journal of the American Academy of Child and Adolescent Psychiatry, 31*, 606–610.

Strober, M., Freeman, R., Rigali, J., Schmidt, S., & Diamond, R. (1992). The pharmacotherapy of depressive illness in adolescence: II. Effects of lithium augmentation in nonresponders to imipramine. *Journal of the American Academy of Child and Adolescent Psychiatry, 31*, 16–20.

Strober, M., Lampert, C., Schmidt, S., & Morrell, W. (1993). The course of major depressive disorder in adolescents: I. Recovery and risk of manic switching in a follow-up of psychotic and nonpsychotic subtypes. *Journal of the American Academy of Child and Adolescent Psychiatry, 32*, 34–42.

Strober, M., Morrell, W., Burroughs, J., Lampert, C., Danforth, H., & Freeman, R. (1988). A family study of bipolar I disorder in adolescence: Early onset of symptoms linked to increased familial loading and lithium resistance. *Journal of Affective Disorders, 15*, 255–268.

Strober, M., Morrell, W., Lampert, C., & Burroughs, J. (1990). Relapse following discontinuation of lithium maintenance therapy in adolescents with bipolar I illness: A naturalistic study. *American Journal of Psychiatry, 147*, 457–461.

Strober, M., Schmidt-Lackner, S., Freeman, R., Bower, S., Lampert, C., & DeAntonio, M. (1995). Recovery and relapse in adolescents with bipolar affective illness: A five-year naturalistic prospective follow-up. *Journal of the American Academy of Child and Adolescent Psychiatry, 34*, 724–731.

Thomas, C. R., & Holzer, C. E. (1999). National distribution of child adolescent psychiatrists. *Journal of the American Academy of Child and Adolescent Psychiatry, 38*, 9–15.

Varley, C. K., & McClellan, J. (1997). Case study: Two additional sudden deaths with tricyclic antidepressants. *Journal of the American Academy of Child and Adolescent Psychiatry, 36*, 390–394.

Wagner, K. D. (1999). Multisite study of paroxetine versus imipramine and placebo in the treatment of children and adolescents with major depression. Paper presented at Oregon Health Sciences University, June 18.

Walsh, B. T., Greenhill, L. L., Giardina, E. V., Bigger, J. T., Waslick, B. D., Sloan, R. P., Bilich, K., Wolk, S., & Bagiella, E. (1999). Effects of desipramine on autonomic input to the heart. *Journal of the American Academy of Child and Adolescent Psychiatry, 38*, 1186–1192.

Weiss, G., Hechtman, L., Milroy, T., & Perlman, T. (1985). Psychiatric status of hyperactives as adults: A controlled prospective 15-year follow-up of 63 hyperactive children. *Journal of the American Academy of Child and Adolescent Psychiatry, 24*, 211–220.

Weithorn, L. A., & Campbell, S. B. (1982). The competency of children and adolescents to make informed treatment decisions. *Child Development, 53*, 1597–1598.

Weller, E. B., Weller, R. A., & Fristad, M. A. (1995). Bipolar disorder in children: Misdiagnosis, underdiagnosis, and future directions. *Journal of the American Academy of Child and Adolescent Psychiatry, 34*, 709–714.

Werry, J. S., & Aman, M. G. (1999). *Practitioner's guide to psychoactive drugs for children and adolescents*, 2nd ed. New York: Plenum Medical Book.

West, S. A., McElroy, S. L., Strkowski, S. M., Keck, P. E., Jr., & McConville, B. J. (1995). Attention deficit hyperactivity disorder in adolescent mania. *American Journal of Psychiatry, 152*, 271–273.

Wilens, T. E., Spencer, T. J., Swanson, J. M., Connor, D. F., & Cantwell, D. (1999). Combining methylphenidate and clonidine: A clinically sound medication option. *Journal of the American Academy of Child and Adolescent Psychiatry, 38*, 614–619, discussion 619–622.

Wilens, T. E., Biederman, J., Baldessarini, R. J., Geller, B., Schleifer, D., Spencer, T. J., Birmaher, B., & Goldblatt, A.

(1996). Cardiovascular effects of therapeutic doses of tricyclic antidepressants in children and adolescents. *Journal of the American Academy of Child and Adolescent Psychiatry, 35*, 1491–1501.

Wilens, T. E., Biederman, J., Baldessarini, R. J., Puopolo, P. R., & Flood, J. G. (1992). Developmental changes in serum concentrations of desipramine and 2-hydroxydesipramine during treatment with desipramine. *Journal of the American Academy of Child and Adolescent Psychiatry, 31*, 691–698.

Williams, D. T., Mehl, R., Yudofsky, S., Adams, D., & Roseman, B. (1982). The effect of propranolol on uncontrolled rage outbursts in children and adolescents with organic brain dysfunction. *Journal of the American Academy of Child and Adolescent Psychiatry, 21*, 129–135.

Wirshing, D. A., Wirshing, W. C., Kysar, L., Berisford, M. A., Goldstein, D., Pashdag, J., Mintz, J., & Marder, S. R. (1999). Novel antipsychotics: Comparison of weight gain liabilities. *Journal of Clinical Psychiatry, 60*, 358–363.

Wozniak, J., Biederman, J., Kiely, K., Ablon, J. S., Faraone, S. V., Mundy, E., & Mennin, D. (1995). Mania-like symptoms suggestive of childhood-onset bipolar disorder in clinically referred children. *Journal of the American Academy of Child and Adolescent Psychiatry, 34*, 867–876.

Yudofsky, S., Williams, D., & Gorman, J. (1981). Propranolol in the treatment of rage and violent behavior in patients with chronic brain syndromes. *American Journal of Psychiatry, 138*, 218–220.

V

Adult Treatment: Introductory Comments

Of the three modalities implemented for treating adult psychological disorders, the pharmacological approach has the longest history and can be traced back to antiquity. Dynamic psychotherapy, with its roots in Freudian psychoanalysis, had its inception at the turn of the twentieth century. Behavior therapy, on the other hand, is primarily a creature of the second part of the twentieth century and now the twenty-first century, but it too can be traced to ancient times with some very specific and interesting historical examples. Although the philosophical underpinnings of the three approaches are vastly different, each is basically devoted to the relief of psychological suffering. With respect to empirical documentation of efficacy, the behavioral and pharmacological strategies have been the most open to scientific scrutiny. However, as the reader will see in Chapter 25, there is a movement among dynamic psychotherapists to subject their treatments to the empirical test as well.

In Chapter 25, David L. Wolitzky, Morris Eagle, and Lester Luborsky discuss the use of dynamic psychotherapy. Specifically, they review several main observations about psychodynamic psychotherapy and psychoanalysis. In particular, they distinguish two main types of therapy: the more traditional, and the more contemporary. Further, research that has led to great strides in the field of psychodynamics, psychotherapy, and psychoanalysis is presented, and illustrations of representative treatment techniques are provided. In Chapter 26, which is on behavior therapy, Kevin T. Larkin and Michael J. Zvolensky outline anxiety-reduction strategies, operant approaches, and those that combine elements of the aforementioned. Impressive improvements in behavior therapy are documented, and behavior therapy strategies are now considered treatments of choice for simple phobia, obsessive–compulsive disorder, posttraumatic stress disorder, and sexual dysfunction. Many unanswered questions remain, however, particularly with regard to identifying mechanisms of change.

In Chapter 27, Daniel M. Harris, William Wilson, and Ann Marie Hamer examine the contemporary use of pharmacological interventions for a variety of disorders. As they cogently point out, pharmacological interventions now play an essential role in treatment and are best viewed as one element of a comprehensive, individualized treatment plan. They indicate that integration of biological, psychological, and social modalities offers the best hope for efficacious intervention and positive treatment outcome.

25

Dynamic Psychotherapy

DAVID L. WOLITZKY, MORRIS EAGLE,
AND LESTER LUBORSKY

THE DYNAMIC THEORY OF THE MIND

The terms "dynamic psychotherapy" and "psychodynamic psychotherapy" have been used interchangeably with "psychoanalytic psychotherapy" or "psychoanalytically oriented psychotherapy." Freud borrowed the term "psychodynamic" from physics, where "dynamic" refers to the interaction of forces as in thermodynamics or aerodynamics and conveys the idea of an interplay of forces in the mind, particularly conflicting forces.[1] In fact, Kris (1947), an influential psychoanalytic theorist, defined psychoanalysis as that discipline that views behavior from the perspective of inner conflict. Thus, one of the basic questions a traditional psychodynamic therapist would consider in clinical situations would be, With which inner core conflict is this patient struggling?

What is the nature of inner conflict? According to traditional psychoanalytic theory, our basic conflicts express the opposition between unconscious wishes and the defenses against these wishes so that they are blocked from conscious awareness and from being implemented in action. Based on both clinical experience with his early cases and his understanding of

---

[1]Since Freud's time, psychodynamic has come to be a broad term that subsumes Freudian treatment approaches, as well as other theories and intervention methods. It also stresses intrapsychic conflict but does so in the context of basic assumptions concerning human motivation that are at variance with Freud's. We should also point out that some clinicians (whether Freudian in orientation or not) make a sharp distinction between "psychoanalysis" as a particular form of psychodynamic psychotherapy; others tend to blur the distinction and see it on a continuum with psychoanalysis. Those who stress the distinction emphasize that in psychoanalysis there is a more systematic focus on transference and resistance (concepts we shall define later), a greater reliance on dreams and free associations, and the exploration and interpretation of the patient's past history as well as current realities. These differences are said to be facilitated by the use of the couch and the frequency of sessions (usually three to five sessions per week in psychoanalysis, as opposed to one or two times per week in psychoanalytic psychotherapy).

DAVID L. WOLITZKY • Department of Psychology, New York University, New York, New York 10003-6634. **MORRIS EAGLE** • Derner Institute, Adelphi University, Garden City, New York 11530. **LESTER LUBORSKY** • Department of Psychiatry, University of Pennsylvania, Philadelphia, Pennsylvania 19104.

Advanced Abnormal Psychology, Second Edition, edited by Hersen and Van Hasselt. Kluwer Academic/Plenum Publishers, New York, 2001.

Darwinian evolutionary theory, Freud believed at first that it is primarily sexual wishes and desires that are implicated in conflict and defense.[2]

How did Freud come to emphasize the centrality of unconscious conflict in psychic life and the therapeutic goal of making these conflicts conscious? When Freud first came on the scene, the available methods of therapeutic intervention were rest, massage, hydrotherapy, and faradic stimulation (the application of low-voltage electrical stimulation to symptomatic parts of the body). These methods did not address causes of the patient's tensions and suffering. Instead, they were aimed at providing symptomatic relief. They were relatively ineffective and rarely produced stable benefits.

Freud studied with two famous hypnotists of his era: Charcot and Bernheim. He came away impressed with the power of hypnosis to induce and remove symptoms. He began to use these methods in his own work. At first, he would put the patient in a hypnotic trance and suggest that the symptoms disappear and that the patient have a posthypnotic amnesia for his suggestion. This approach met with limited success. Freud then experimented with variations of this approach. In one instance, he was called in to treat a woman who had just given birth, but was morose, agitated, and unable to nurse (there was no breast milk coming despite her conscious desire to feed her infant). His direct hypnotic suggestions that the milk start flowing had only a temporary effect. Freud then suggested, again with the directive for posthypnotic amnesia for his suggestion, that when she awoke from the hypnotic trance the patient would become angry at her family and complain that they were giving her insufficient care and attention, demand food, and insist that under the conditions that existed they could not expect her to feed her baby adequately. She awoke, carried out the suggestions, and very quickly became symptom-free (Freud, 1892–1893).

What was the underlying basis of this patient's symptoms and what was the insight that led Freud to this successful therapeutic maneuver with this patient who apparently was suffering from a postpartum depression? We can assume that the patient did and did not want to feed her infant—she was in a state of psychological conflict. Further, we can assume that part of this conflict was unconscious; as far as the patient consciously knew, she wanted to nurse her baby. To consciously wish not to feed and in that way to harm her infant would produce painful feelings of guilt. Freud discerned that she was angry at having to assume the role of the nurturant one, particularly if it meant that she would not have her own wishes satisfied and that she would not be cared for. The inability to nurse was implicitly seen as a psychological symptom based on this conflict. Being given permission by an authority figure to express one side of her feelings apparently was necessary to shift the dynamic balance of the conflict. (Actually, this example also illustrates that a psychodynamic understanding was used as the basis for a behavioral manipulation, a kind of assertiveness training through hypnotic suggestion.)

Cases such as these formed the basis for Freud's psychodynamic approach and for the key concepts of psychic determinism and unconscious motivation. By psychic determinism, Freud meant to emphasize that mental activity can be shown to have lawful regularities. By unconscious motivation, he meant to imply that a great deal of psychological activity goes on outside of awareness, that it is actively kept out of awareness, and that, nonetheless, it exerts a continuing, powerful impact on conscious experience and behavior.

[2]It should be noted that for Freud, the term "sexual" includes *infantile sexuality*, such as oral and anal wishes and impulses. "Sexual" should be understood in the sense of *sensual*. The term "infantile" means early in development and should have no pejorative connotations. Freud's point was that from an early age certain bodily zones (mouth, anus, genitals) were special sources of bodily pleasure.

Although Freud certainly was not the first major psychologist to state that there are unconscious influences on conscious thought, he was the first to develop a systematized, comprehensive theory of the dynamic unconscious as the underpinning of the development of normal as well as pathological behavior. It is in this sense that repression (the automatic exclusion of conflict-laden ideas from awareness) was regarded as the "cornerstone" of psychoanalytic theory.

Defense, Anxiety, and Symptom Formation

At first, Freud used the terms repression and defense as synonymous. Later, repression came to be seen as only one of the defenses. Other common defenses include reaction formation, projection, and denial, to name just a few. Any mental activity or behavior, in which a person engages to avoid anxiety, may be said to have a defensive function. Thus, an idea that one might think would generate considerable anxiety could be fully in awareness if its emotional significance is not consciously experienced. For instance, because of the defense of isolation of affect, one might consciously contemplate murderous ideas, but cut off from their normal emotional accompaniments. Freud believed that it was the disavowal of unacceptable wishes that was the critical factor that makes the person vulnerable to a neurosis. Defense required the expenditure of mental (psychic) energy. If the unconscious wishes were sufficiently strong and/or the defenses could not adequately conceal the wishes, the result would be an outbreak of neurotic symptoms.

In Freud's original locational theory, the mind was divided into an unconscious, a preconscious, and a conscious portion. Freud thought that the moral prohibitions directed against sexual wishes were consciously opposing the unconscious wishes. Conflict was initially conceptualized as opposition between conscious (or preconscious) psychic elements and unconscious ones. By 1923, Freud had realized that moral prohibitions and defenses against instinctual wishes could and often were unconscious and that repression was not the only way of defending against unacceptable wishes. Thus, Freud maintained the centrality of conflict but came to realize that its essential nature was not just the opposition between unconscious and conscious forces.

These are some of the main reasons that Freud then developed the three-part structural theory of the id, ego, and superego that reflected the major sources of mental conflict. Freud also came to recognize that aggression is coequal with sex; the two are the major instinctual drives. Finally, Freud realized that conflict was not an abnormal condition, but an inevitable, ubiquitous feature of mental life. Emotional disturbance occurred not because of conflict *per se*, but because of the maladaptive solutions to which it could give rise in the person's effort to avoid the outbreak of serious anxiety and/or symptoms.

In its final form, Freud's theory of anxiety focused on key danger situations that could lead to traumatic anxiety in which people feel totally helpless, overwhelmed, and unable to satisfy their essential needs. These danger situations, in order of their appearance in the course of development, are the loss of the object, loss of the object's love, castration anxiety, and superego anxiety (guilt). Each of these potential anxieties persists throughout life and small-scale signals of the full-blown experience of any of them is an automatic trigger for initiating defenses. Hence, this theory is referred to as the signal theory of anxiety. A fuller statement of these concepts and the theory of symptom formation can be found in Waelder (1960), Brenner (1982), Eagle and Wolitzky (1992), and Luborsky (1996).

THE GOALS OF TREATMENT AND OF ACHIEVING GOOD HEALTH: AWARENESS AND CONFLICT RESOLUTION

Two basic assumptions in the traditional psychoanalytic theory of pathology and of treatment—that have their roots in the prepsychoanalytic thinking of Charcot and Janet—are (1) that isolation of mental contents from the rest of the personality is pathogenic, and (2) that bringing to consciousness and assimilating such contents are therapeutic. These basic prepsychoanalytic ideas have remained central. In fact, a good part of the early history of psychoanalytic treatment can be understood as a continuing evolution of conceptions about those mental contents that are to be made conscious and the techniques for achieving this goal. For example, in Freud's earliest writings, it was primarily traumatic memories that were to be made conscious, and it was originally through hypnosis that this goal was to be achieved.

Freud believed that if we could restore to conscious awareness what was banished from it, we would free the patient of disabling symptoms. Early on, Freud believed that so-called pathogenic or traumatic, unconscious memories were the cause of the symptoms. The affect connected to these memories, it was thought, exists in a "strangulated" state. If the memory could be retrieved into consciousness, the feelings associated with it could be "abreacted" (expressed and reexperienced), lose their intensity, and be "associatively reabsorbed" into consciousness (that is, take their place in the patient's mass of conscious ideas and memories). At first, hypnosis was the way to achieve these ends. However, matters were quickly seen as more complex. Hypnotic "cures" were often short-lived, and some patients were resistant to hypnosis, leading Freud to try related methods. He would let patients talk (to achieve catharsis) in the context of which he would urge them to recall traumatic events. Sometimes he would use the so-called pressure technique of placing his hand on the patient's forehead and insisting that a forgotten memory would be retrieved. As one can see, these methods, including the use of reclining on a couch while talking, were remnants of the hypnotic procedure and were still based on the idea that the recovery of specific memories would lead to symptom removal.

Eventually, Freud came to the famous "fundamental rule" of free association. Now, the directive was to speak freely without inhibiting or editing the thoughts and feelings that came into one's mind. Over time, Freud came to several realizations that increased the complexity of his task of designing an effective treatment: (1) patients experienced not only the pain of ego-alien, discrete symptoms, but also had disturbed patterns of adaptations for which they sought help; the aim of treatment expanded to deal with specific symptoms and also with the person's total character; (2) accordingly, it was not only that a few key repressed memories were the source of the patient's suffering, but rather the maladaptive patterns of thought, feeling, and behavior that developed over many years; now the reduction of the symptoms as well as the amelioration of the maladaptive patterns were approached more indirectly through a more general, open-ended exploration of the patient's personality; (3) whereas Freud originally thought that memories of sexual seduction played a major role in the patient's emotional disturbances, he came to believe that for many patients what he had taken as memories of actual seduction turned out to be *fantasies*.

The abandonment of the "seduction theory" was a decisive turning point in the history of psychoanalysis for it put the issue of the patient's "psychic reality" in the primary position as a major determinant of psychopathology. This should not be taken to mean that what happens to one is unimportant or that seductions and other traumatic events very rarely take place. Rather, it broadens one's focus to include not only the events themselves, but the *personal meanings*, both conscious and unconscious, of the events. The task of treatment is uncovering these personal meanings as expressed in the context of the patient's relationship with the therapist.

And treatment should aim to increase the *awareness* of who one is, how and why one got to be that way, and what unacceptable needs and wishes one has been hiding from one's self.

RESISTANCE

One important factor that interferes with achieving the goal of awareness and resolution of inner conflict is the operation of defenses in the treatment. Thus, just as outside of therapy one generally defends against becoming aware of certain wishes because of the anxiety that such awareness would entail, so in the therapy situation one continues to resist awareness for the same basic reason. There is no reason to expect that such anxiety would disappear because one is in treatment. Indeed, under certain circumstances in treatment, anxiety may be intensified. Therefore, resistance has been defined as defense operating in the interpersonal context of treatment. The term resistance has had a pejorative connotation because it suggests opposition to the aims of treatment. But, when we recognize that its primary motive is the avoidance of anxiety, then this connotation should be removed. Resistance may take many forms, both blatant and subtle. For example, refusing to talk is an overt opposition to self-exploration, whereas forgetting one's dreams may be a more indirect form of avoidance.

Another basic way to conceptualize resistance is in terms of the patient's reluctance to give up infantile wishes (e.g., that one will be loved or nurtured unconditionally) and the fantasy that such wishes can be and will be gratified. Although patients consciously want to change and be rid of their neurotic symptoms and distress, they do not necessarily link (except perhaps in a highly intellectual way) their distress to the compulsive pursuit of infantile wishes. And for many patients, the prospect of giving up central infantile wishes and fantasies is experienced at some deep unconscious level as rendering life empty or meaningless. Clearly, patients need to feel emotionally convinced that more realistic meanings, pleasures, and gratifications are possible to be able to yield essentially unattainable gratifications or fantasies.

One of the concrete implications of the role of resistance in treatment is the practical rule of thumb that analysis of the patient's defenses (including resistances) should precede analysis of wishes and impulses. Unless defenses are dealt with, awareness of wishes and impulses will be hindered. In the development of psychoanalysis, the analysis of defenses increasingly became an important part of treatment.

TRANSFERENCE

One of the most central concepts in the psychoanalytic theory of treatment is the concept of transference. Freud even stated that if the concepts of transference and resistance were central in a theory, then whatever the approach might be called, it was psychoanalytic. It is interesting that Freud singled out both transference and resistance, for in the psychoanalytic theory of psychotherapy, transference functions both as a kind of resistance and as the most important tool for therapeutic change.

In what way is transference a form of resistance? If transference is understood as transferring onto the therapist one's infantile wishes and fantasies and the conflicts and defenses in which they are embedded, then one can see that at an unconscious level the patient hopes that the therapist will gratify his or her infantile wishes. Indeed, from a traditional psychoanalytic perspective, the essence of transference can be understood as an expression of a persistent fantasy that one's basic wishes and needs will be gratified—this time by the therapist. But as noted earlier, the fantasy that one's infantile wishes will be gratified is a core aspect of resistance. Hence, the conclusion that transference is a primary expression of resistance.

In what way(s) is transference a tool for therapeutic change? Generally speaking, as Freud (1912a) recognized, a positive transference is often a precondition for therapeutic change and for interpretations to "take hold." A more specific function of transference is that it provides experiences that have a here-and-now emotional immediacy. It is one thing to talk about wishes, conflicts, and reactions to persons from one's distant past; it is another matter to relive in an emotionally vivid way new editions of these past experiences in relation to the therapist, who is present. And, as Freud (1912a) observed, it is difficult to slay a dragon in effigy.

In fact, most analysts would agree that a good part of psychoanalytic psychotherapy consists in analyzing the transference—that is, making interpretations that help bring the patient's transference reactions to awareness and that help patients understand these reactions as mirrors of their neurotic patterns. Malan (1963, 1976) describes the ideal transference interpretation as one that facilitates a "triangle of insight," by which he means interpretations that help the patient make insightful connections among patterns of reactions to the therapist, to other important current figures (e.g., wife, husband, lover, boss, friend, etc.), and to parental figures in the patient's past. According to classical psychoanalytic theory, therapeutic changes consist essentially in bringing awareness by analyzing or mastering the "transference neurosis," that is, a version of the neurotic pattern, but now in relation to the therapist.

One final set of comments about the concept of transference needs to be made. In recent years, the traditional view of transference as a *distortion* (that is, patients distort their perception of therapists and react to them as if they were parental figures) has been severely criticized by Gill (1982). He argues for a relativistic position in which the therapist attempts to understand the patient's perceptions and behaviors not as complete distortions, but as plausible reactions to cues emitted by the therapist and to aspects of the therapist's real behavior. As an example (Luborsky, 1996), a patient in analysis who was very prone to highly conflictual reactions to feeling rejected, "heard a scratching noise" which she interpreted as a sign that her analyst had become distracted and was scratching" a spot off of his sleeve. She went even further in interpreting the noise when she inferred that the behavior she "perceived" was a sign that the analyst was uninterested in her. The whole experience was momentarily forgotten until the next session when she recovered it and explained to the therapist what had happened. For Gill, such transference experiences are broadly conceived and seem to be virtually synonymous with the patient's experience of the therapeutic relationship. For many, including the authors of this chapter, Gill's views are a welcome corrective to the classical position that analysts are "blank screens" onto which patients projects their wishes, fantasies, conflicts, and defenses. Having endorsed Gill's corrective, we still find it useful to regard transference as a selective and biased reading of the present in terms of the past, even though that reading also tends to be based on current "reality hooks."

COUNTERTRANSFERENCE

The concept of countertransference is complementary to the concept of transference, but now the focus is on the therapist rather than the patient. In its early meaning (Freud, 1910), countertransference referred to the therapist's reactions to the patient, particularly to the patient's transference, that were strongly influenced by the therapist's unresolved unconscious conflicts, wishes, and fantasies. Thus, it was of primary importance that therapists should try to become aware of and attempt to deal with countertransference reactions, lest they seriously interfere with their understanding of the patient and the progress of treatment. Indeed, Freud (1910) maintained that the progress of therapy was limited by the therapists' unresolved countertransference reactions. If the therapist could not deal with interfering counter-transference reactions through introspection and self-analysis or consultation with a colleague, then further psychoanalytic treatment for the therapist was in order.

It can be seen that in this traditional account of countertransference, it is essentially an impediment, an obstacle to treatment, that must be resolved. In more recent years, however, the concept of countertransference has been extended so that for some it includes virtually every aspect of the therapist's reactions to the patient. Note the parallel between the broadening of the concept of countertransference so that it includes the totality of therapists' reactions to their patients and the earlier noted extension of the meaning of transference so that it includes the totality of the patient's reactions to the therapist.

Instead of viewing countertransference reactions as unwanted intrusions, the more recent view emphasizes their potential usefulness in treatment, particularly as possible clues to what the patient might be "pulling for" in the therapist and to subtle features of the patient–therapist interaction. It seems to us that the key words in this account are "potential" and "possible." The therapist's emotional reactions to the patient are *potentially* useful and represent *possible* clues to what the patient is "pulling for" and to important aspects of the patient–therapist interaction. However, as a therapist, one cannot automatically assume—as seems to be the case in some of the recent literature—that one's emotional reactions to the patient are always those that the patient is "pulling for" and are *necessarily* clues to what is going on in the patient. Therapists must reflect upon their emotional reactions to patients and attempt to understand their origin and their nature. They are likely to be the complex product of many different sources and factors. For example, there can be many different reasons for feeling angry (or bored or anxious or sexually aroused or pitying or many other feelings) with a patient. One cannot automatically assume that the anger (or boredom or anxiety or sexual arousal or pity) can be accounted for entirely on the basis that this emotion is what the patient was unconsciously eliciting from the therapist.

FREE ASSOCIATION

As noted earlier, Freud moved from reliance on hypnosis to the eventual use of free association, which continues to be a basic psychoanalytic technique. In classical psycho-analysis, the patient lies on the couch; the analyst sits behind and out of view, and the patient is expected to follow the "fundamental rule of psychoanalysis" (Freud, 1912a) of saying whatever comes to mind regardless of how trivial, irrational, irrelevant, or embarrassing it may seem. This is the patient's primary task in psychoanalysis. Based on an association model of the mind, Freud believed—as do most contemporary analysts—that free association, in contrast to more directed and socially conventional thought, would facilitate the emergence of unconscious material that would at least partly escape defense and censorship. Of course, because defenses and censorship continue to operate during free association (just as they continue to operate during dreams), the material that emerges continues to be disguised and hence requires deciphering and interpretation (a topic we cover in the next section). Although the "basic rule" is simple—merely saying what comes to mind—it is not simple to follow.

The difficulties patients encounter are not unlike those people experience when they attempt to practice meditation—habitual modes of thought keep intruding and taking over.

A basic theoretical assumption that underlies the use of free association is that unconscious ideas and wishes influence and direct the course and content of the patient's associations. Thus, contiguous ideas, though of very different manifest content are assumed to possess an underlying thematic connection. For example, a patient begins an early analytic session by saying she finds it difficult to express her thoughts, but fears that once she begins, she may not be able to stop. Her next thought is to ask the therapist where the ladies room is located. On the face of it, these two ideas have no apparent connection. The therapist, however, may begin to form the tentative hypothesis that the patient is making an unconscious connection between control of thought and speech and control of bowel and bladder functions.

Although free association is the "fundamental rule" in long-term psychoanalysis, its use is modulated and modified in psychodynamic psychotherapy, particularly when the therapy is carried out with the patient sitting up and facing the therapist. In that situation, patients would normally be encouraged to speak about what is on their minds and of immediate concern rather than to free associate. Indeed, in many forms of time-limited psychodynamic psychotherapy, there is an agreement between patient and therapist that primarily certain therapeutic goals will be dealt with in the treatment.

INTERPRETATION AS A BASIC TECHNIQUE

As noted before, the patient's free associations (as well as dreams) are subject to defense and disguise and hence require interpretation to make their meaning clear. Interpretation is the main psychoanalytic tool for achieving the therapeutic goals of "making the unconscious conscious" and facilitating the patients' resolutions of their underlying conflicts. We noted earlier that in contemporary conceptions of psychoanalytic treatment, analysis of resistance and defense takes up a major part of therapeutic work. This means that many interpretations made in treatment are likely to deal with the patient's defenses and resistances to change. They attempt to clarify not only that patients are resisting, but why, what, and how they are resisting.

There is widespread agreement among analysts and psychodynamic therapists that the most effective interpretations are accurate ones that are presented tactfully and with proper timing, when patients are almost able to reach the same understanding themselves. It should be apparent that there are many interventions, other than interpretations, that the therapists makes in the course of treatment. Examples of these are questions, confrontations, clarifications, explanations about the rationale of treatment, and occasional suggestions and advice (though there is general agreement that this last type of intervention should be used quite sparingly or not at all because a basic value that undergirds the entire process is that the patient benefits from moving in a more autonomous direction). There is also general agreement that interpretations that focus on the transference and its links to the patient's current and past unconscious conflicts, wishes, and fantasies are the most effective interventions. As note earlier, Malan (1963, 1976) presented some evidence that such interpretations, which presumably facilitate a "triangle of insight," are related to positive therapeutic outcome.

As we shall see, in some of the recent psychoanalytic literature, interpretation and insight have been pitted against each other as therapeutic factors, in particular, the therapeutic relationship. Thus, some have argued that the therapeutic relationship, rather than the interpretation and insight, is the primary therapeutic agent. It seems to us, however, that it is not especially fruitful to dichotomize these two therapeutic factors because they operate together.

Thus, the therapeutic impact of an interpretation, including how it is heard and received, is likely to reflect the nature of the patient–therapist relationship, and conversely, an empathic, well-times, tactful, and insightful interpretation is likely to strengthen the relationship.

Finally, we will comment briefly on the issue of the validity of interpretations. There is a rather large literature, both psychoanalytic and philosophical, on the question of how one validates an interpretation. For example, what kind of evidence would validate (or invalidate) for a patient an interpretation involving the attribution of an unconscious wish? The answers that have been given to this question include the impact of the interpretations on the patients' subsequent associations (e.g., Schmidl, 1955) and the patient's ultimate conscious acknowledgment of the wish attributed to them (Mischel, 1963, 1966). Consider another question: What kind of evidence would validate (or invalidate) an interpretation pertaining to the patient's early experiences? The difficulties inherent in answering this kind of question have led some theorists to argue that in making interpretations and reconstructions of the patient's past, the analyst cannot claim "historical truth," but only "narrative truth," that is only a plausible and convincing account (Spence, 1982).

Some recent work (e.g., in Luborsky & Crits-Christoph, 1990) suggests possible means of determining the validity of at least some interpretations. It is a method by which clinical raters can assess patients' "Core Conflictual Relationship Themes" (CCRTs) from transcription of psychotherapy sessions. Based on the patient's account of relationship episodes, clinical raters can reliably assess the dominant *wishes* (W) expressed, the *experienced and expressed reactions from others* (RO), and consequent *reactions of the self* (RS). Luborsky and his colleagues find that patients, like people in general, tend to have a limited number of stable CCRTs. The heart of the method is this principle: For a given patient, the accuracy of a therapist's interpretations can be operationally measured by determining degree of agreement with independently assessed ratings of the patient's predominant CCRTs (Crits-Christoph, Cooper, & Luborsky, 1988). Such a measure of accuracy of interpretation defined in the manner described is positively correlated with positive therapeutic outcome. This discovery is the first systematic demonstration that accuracy of interpretation is related to positive therapeutic outcome.

Therapists' ability to offer "accurate," well-timed, tactfully expressed interpretations is facilitated by their capacity to recognize patients' central relationship patterns and the awareness and proper management of counertransference reactions and by a capacity for empathy. By empathy, we mean that the therapist is able to experience partial, transient identification with the patient in which there is a cognitive/affective "knowing" of the patient's inner world of experience. In this sense, empathy is a process of data gathering and forms the basis for whatever interpretation the therapist ultimately offers. In some theories, which we shall refer to later, empathy is seen as essential to understanding, and also the act of empathic communication of one's understanding is regarded as a vital therapeutic factor in itself.

ANALYTIC NEUTRALITY AND ABSTINENCE AS A BASIC TECHNIQUE

Most analysis agrees that the therapist should assume a neutral role in the treatment. How neutrality is defined, however, is of great importance. Freud (1912b) recommended that analysts remain "opaque" or "blank screens" onto which the patients would project their wishes, conflicts, fantasies, so on. According to this view, the "blank screen" role of the therapist would ensure that the patient's projections were "pure," uncontaminated by real characteristics of the therapist. A similar rationale was provided for the "principle of abstinence"—the withholding of transference gratification. It was assumed that frustration of transference wishes would most efficaciously stimulate the patient's wishes, conflicts, and fantasies, and center them on the person of the analyst.

As discussed earlier, the idea that the therapist could remain a "blank screen" is really not tenable. We are always emitting cues to others, whether we intend to or not. Furthermore, such an unrealistic conception of analytic neutrality led to its caricatured implementation—some analysts mistakenly equated neutrality with coldness, aloofness, stodginess, and excessive and unresponsive silence.

Given the untenability of the "blank screen" idea, what remains of the concept of analytic neutrality? It seems clear to us that a very useful and defensible aspect of analytic neutrality requires the therapist not to take sides in the patient's inner conflicts. If the conflict is truly an intrapsychic one, the therapist's advocacy or alignment with one or another side will not be very useful in achieving the goal of inner resolution. A clinical anecdote illustrates this point.

Some years ago one of us was supervising a novice therapist who presented a case in which an undergraduate female student from a very traditional immigrant family had been considering moving to her own apartment. The patient's father was outraged at this possibility and communicated his opposition in no uncertain terms. The patient was very upset by the situation in which she found herself and came to treatment (at a university clinic) for help. As the case was reported, it became apparent that the therapist, a young graduate student herself, identified with the patient and sided with the latter's desire to acquire her own apartment. Indeed, she largely conceived of her therapeutic role as one in which she would support the patient's move toward "autonomy." The supervisor noted that what was being represented solely as a conflict between the patient and her father might well also include and mask an inner conflict (e.g., between the desire to move, on the one hand, and anxieties regarding separation and independence on the other) in which one side of the conflict (separation anxiety) was externalized and represented by father's opposition and hence, need not be confronted and experienced. The supervisor also cautioned that the therapist's role in supporting the patient's desire to move could also contribute to a shutting out and denial of conflicted feelings about moving. As it turned out, under the impact of the patient's mother's peacemaking and mediating efforts, the father relented somewhat in his opposition and took a "do what you want" attitude. He was now ready to negotiate about such matters as how frequently the patient would return home for meals, etc. At this point, external opposition softened, and the patient's own conflictual and ambivalent feelings about moving away from home fully surfaced. But because the therapist had taken the role of supporter of "autonomy," the patient found it difficult to work on her conflictual feelings and instead left treatment.

THE THERAPEUTIC OR THE HELPING ALLIANCE

Although some analysts (e.g., Brenner, 1979) have not found it useful to distinguish between transference and the therapeutic alliance, most have found the distinction useful. The concept of therapeutic alliance is generally intended to emphasize the importance of establishing and maintaining a safe, therapeutic atmosphere in which the therapist's compassion, humanness, and respect for the patient are evident (Greenson, 1965) and in which the patient feels a bond with and is supported by the therapist as they cooperatively engage in pursuing a common goal. Some analysts (e.g., Zetzel, 1966) believe that the therapeutic alliance constitutes a precondition for fostering the analytic process and also is therapeutic in its own right—

for example, it facilitates a "new ego identification" (Zetzel, 1966, p. 92) with the analyst and thereby permits and facilitates the patient's growth.

Much systematic empirical work has been carried out in this area by Luborsky and his colleagues (e.g., Luborsky, 1976; Luborsky, Crits-Christoph, Alexander, Margolis, & Cohen, 1983; Morgan, Luborsky, Crits-Christoph, Curtis, & Solomon, 1982). Luborsky (1984, 2000a,b) has used the term "helping alliance" to refer to the "degree to which the patient experiences the relationship with their therapist as helpful or potentially helpful in achieving the patient's goals in psychotherapy" (p. 79). He and his colleagues have been able to define this construct operationally. He found that one could obtain reliable judgments about the helping alliance, that scores on this measure were reasonably consistent from earlier and later stages of treatment, and that early indications of a positive helping alliance predicted therapeutic improvement. Progressively during the last three decades, this area of research and clinical applications has rapidly grown and its predictive validity has become better established (Horvath & Symonds, 1991; Luborsky, 1984).

SOME RECENT CONCEPTIONS OF DYNAMIC PSYCHOTHERAPY

Although many of the concepts we have discussed—transference, counter-transference, resistance, and interpretation—play a central role in all "schools" of dynamic psychotherapy, in the preceding account we have presented mainly a traditional or broadly Freudian view. The history of psychoanalysis has also been marked by dissent and pluralism. Thus, a complete discussion of psychoanalytic theories of treatment would include the work of Freud and of ego psychologists and also the approaches of neo-Freudians, the work of Melanie Klein, the British school of object relations theorists, and the work of Kohut (e.g., 1984). Obviously, we cannot cover all of these approaches in a brief, introductory chapter. (Those who want to read further in these areas can refer to Eagle, 1984; Eagle & Wolitzky, 1992; Greenberg & Mitchell, 1983; Luborsky, 2000b). What we will do is present some ideas and conceptualizations of psychotherapy that have been especially influential during the past three decades, particularly in North America. These ideas and conceptualizations have been mainly derived from the work of Kohut (1971, 1977, 1984) and other self-psychologists, from the writings of Fairbairn (1952) and Winnicott (1958, 1965) on object relations theory, and from the work of Weiss, Sampson, and their colleagues (1986) on control-mastery theory. Although these theoretical approaches differ in important ways on many issues, there are some central features that are common to all of them.

THE THERAPEUTIC RELATIONSHIP

In many contemporary psychoanalytic approaches to psychotherapy, there is a reduced emphasis on the therapeutic role of insight and an increased emphasis on the patient–therapist relationship as a *direct* therapeutic agent. Although the importance of the patient–therapist relationship is recognized in traditional psychoanalytic theory, it has largely an *indirect* role. The therapeutic relationship serves as a precondition for treatment and makes it possible for the insight and analysis of the transference to operate. By contrast, in some contemporary views, the relationship itself is directly therapeutic. The factors and processes that are invoked to account for the supposed therapeutic efficacy of the relationship include identification with the therapist and a resumption of arrested development facilitated by the experience of a benevolent, understanding, and constructive relationship. This relationship partially compensates for what was traumatically missing in early development. Thus, Fairburn (1952) maintains that in successful psychotherapy, an earlier "bad" object situation is replaced by a "good" object situation. In ordinary language, this means that earlier experiences of deprivation, frustration, neglect, rejection, and nonunderstanding are replaced by understanding and acceptance.

In a similar vein, Kohut (1977, 1984) directly and explicitly conceptualizes the therapeutic process in terms of resuming developmental growth. In particular, Kohut believes that the patient's self-defects are engendered by early traumatic experiences with a basic drive to repair these self-defects and to complete the development of the self. What makes the achievement of these goals possible is a therapeutic relationship in which early experiences of traumatic empathic failures are replaced by experiences of the therapist's empathic understanding and by "optimal failures." Even when therapists fail to fully understand patients (and one's understanding of another can never be perfect), their failures are not of traumatic proportions. They are "optimal" in the sense that they can be assimilated by the patient and can strengthen their ability to cope and to benefit from "good enough" understanding.

One way of contrasting the traditional Freudian view of psychotherapy with that of self-psychology is to note that from the Freudian perspective, it is the *patient's* insight and understanding that are held to be therapeutic; in the self-psychology view, it is the *therapist's* understanding and the communication of such understanding to the patient that are held to be therapeutic—in the traditional view, *understanding* (one's wishes, conflicts, etc.) is therapeutic, whereas in the self-psychology view, *being understood* is therapeutic.

The degree to which the contemporary psychoanalytic conceptions of treatment are similar to the concepts of Rogers (e.g., 1951) should be noted, particularly because these valuable similarities often go unobserved and unacknowledged. According to Rogers, the experience of a relationship in which the other is nonjudgmentally caring, empathetic, genuine, and accepting will in itself automatically facilitate innate actualizing tendencies and hence bring about change and growth. For Rogers, the growth that is brought about in successful therapy is not so much a resumption of early arrested development, but rather an expression of a life-long actualizing tendency that needs proper interpersonal conditions to find expression.

In the contemporary "control-mastery" theory of Weiss, Sampson, and their colleagues (1986), the therapeutic relationship also plays a critical role but has a somewhat different emphasis than that given by object relations theory or self-psychology. According to Weiss and Sampson, "*unconscious pathogenic beliefs*" acquired in childhood interactions with parental figures are responsible for much neurotic distress and suffering. According to them, patients come to treatment, not to gratify infantile wishes—as claimed in traditional Freudian theory—but to be rid of their pathogenic beliefs. Furthermore, it is assumed that they have an *unconscious plan* for achieving this goal. In general, patients attempt to find conditions in which it is safe to bring forth repressed material; to attempt to master the associated conflicts, anxieties, and traumas; and to attempt to disconfirm their pathogenic beliefs. To determine whether *conditions of safety* are present in treatment and whether or not the therapist will react to them in the same way as parental figures did, patients unconsciously present *tests* to the therapist. If tests are *passed*, the patient is more likely, among other things, to bring out repressed material, to experience less anxiety, and to show evidence of greater depth of experiencing. These patient responses are *not* associated with *test failures*. Much of the clinical richness of Weiss and Sampson's work is expressed in the accounts of what constitutes test-passing and test-failing for each patient. From a research and methodological viewpoint, one of the important contributions of Weiss and Sampson's work is the demonstration that one can obtain reliable ratings and measures of such factors as a patient's unconscious plan, whether a therapeutic intervention constitutes test-passing or test-failing, and the behavioral consequences of test-passing and test-failing.

At this point, we will provide some concrete examples of what Weiss and Sampson mean by pathogenic beliefs and what constitutes test-passing and test-failing. The essence of pathogenic beliefs is that, based on early interactions and implicit parental communications, developmentally normal goals, such as striving toward separation—individuation, are experienced as endangering oneself and others and as threatening vital ties to parents, and hence they increase anxiety and guilt. These pathogenic beliefs can be understood as having an implicit if-then form such as *if* I pursue a goal so as to separate and become more independent, *then* I will be punished, or I will endanger a vital relationship, or I will be hurting someone important to me.

One person might have the pathogenic belief that *"if I pursue the goal of leading an independent life, it can only be at the expense of my parent(s),"* thus engendering intense guilt. Another person may suffer from the pathogenic belief that *"if I pursue my ambition and desire to be successful, I will be severely punished for surpassing my parent(s),"* thus resulting in the experience of "survivor guilt" (Modell, 1983) and the inhibition of ambition striving.

As to what kind of therapist interventions and behaviors constitute test-passing and test-failing, one can state as a general rule of thumb that interventions that tend to *disconfirm* the patient's pathogenic beliefs represent test-passing, whereas those that tend to *confirm* the patient's pathogenic beliefs are experienced as *retraumatizations* and constitute test-failing. A simple clinical example is taken from a recent paper by Weiss (1990). "A woman who feared she would hurt her parents and her male therapist by becoming independent might experiment with independent behavior in her sessions by disagreeing with the therapist's opinions and then unconsciously monitoring him to see if he feels hurt" (pp. 107–108). Obviously, the therapist's tolerance and acceptance of disagreement would constitute test-passing, while the therapist's anger or attempts to direct or control the patient would constitute test-failing.

It will be noted that implicit in Weiss and Sampson's concept of psychotherapy is the idea that test-passing and consequent positive therapeutic changes can occur without interpretations and without explicit insight. And indeed, they have empirically demonstrated that therapeutic changes do occur without interpretation. One can understand these changes largely as a product of the "corrective emotional experiences" (Alexander & French, 1946) provided by the therapeutic relationship. Many contemporary approaches, including those of Rogers and of the object relations theorists, Kohut's self-psychology, and the control-mastery theory of Weiss and Sampson, all of which view the patient-therapist relationship as the primary therapeutic agent, can be understood as different ways of formulating the primary importance of "corrective emotional experiences" in leading to a positive therapeutic outcome.

Another common feature shared by the therapeutic approaches that we have been considering is the assumption of a basic drive toward health. This is especially clear and explicit in Rogers's (1951) concept of an inborn and universal actualizing tendency. It is also expressed in (1) Kohut's (1977, 1984) idea that patients strive to complete developmental growth and will do so under appropriate therapeutic conditions, (2) Winnicott's (1965) idea that a "facilitating environment" (which includes the therapeutic situation) will automatically facilitate maturational growth, and (3) Weiss and Sampson's (1986) claim that patients are motivated to be rid of their unconscious pathogenic beliefs and have an unconscious plan for accomplishing that goal.

All theories of treatment accept the view that the therapist's empathy is a desirable, and even indispensable, aspect of therapy and of the therapeutic relationship. However, for some approaches (e.g., Freudian, cognitive-behavioral), empathy, like patient–therapist rapport, is a *precondition* for the operation of the presumably active therapeutic ingredients (e.g., interpretation and insight, capturing automatic thoughts and relinquishing irrational beliefs). By contrast, in other approaches (e.g., client-centered), empathy is itself an important active therapeutic agent. Indeed, in self-psychology it is the most critical curative agent.

ALTERED CONCEPTION OF TRANSFERENCE

We have been discussing a revised understanding of the nature of transference that is common to all of the more contemporary psychoanalytic approaches to psychotherapy. As discussed earlier, according to traditional theory, an essential aspect of transference is the patients' push for therapists to gratify their infantile wishes. Common to the more contemporary views we have been discussing the rejection of this assumption and replacing it by the basic idea that patients come to treatment with the hope for a *new* set of experiences radically different from the traumatic, pathology-generating experiences of the past. Thus, in Weiss and Sampson's control-mastery theory, patients hope to have their pathogenic beliefs disconfirmed by the therapists' responses. In Kohut's self-psychology, patients hope to receive the empathic mirroring necessary to resume developmental growth, and in object relations theory, patients hope to experience the therapist as a "good object," in contrast to the traumatic "bad objects" of their past. In this new conception of transference, therapeutic change is as likely to occur through such "silent" and implicit processes as disconfirmation of pathogenic beliefs, empathic understanding, and transference–countertransference enactments as through explicit interpretation and insight. Of course, ideally, these implicit and explicit factors will operate together. The traditional view also continues on into the present. It is that the patient comes to treatment with a partly maladaptive transference pattern; one of the desirable benefits of successful dynamic psychotherapy is that patients become more aware of their relationship patterns and can alter the parts of the pattern that are maladaptive. Such a theory is emphasized in many updated and modernized views of the process of dynamic psychotherapy, including Luborsky (1984) and Weiss and Sampson (1986).

SELECTED RESEARCH ON DYNAMIC PSYCHOTHERAPY

This chapter will end with a brief sample of some recent research on dynamic psychotherapy because this is a necessary support for its theory of personality and its treatment techniques.

Weiss, Sampson, and Their Colleagues with the Control-Mastery Theory

Many of the formulations of Weiss and Sampson's (1986) control-mastery theory are buttressed by systematic empirical research. Using detailed process notes and transcripts of tape-recorded psychoanalytic sessions in a single-case design, they showed that independent judges can reliably agree about the nature of the patient's unconscious plan, the contents that been warded off, when the patient has presented a test to the analyst, and whether the analyst has passed or failed the test. They have also shown that test-passing is reliably followed by the patient becoming less anxious, more relaxed, more flexible and spontaneous; bolder in tackling issues in treatment; and friendlier toward others. Finally, in the course of treatment, the patient showed a steady decline in the number of statements in which she complained that she felt compelled to do something she did not consciously want to do or felt unable to do something she consciously wanted to do. (It should be noted that the issue of feeling driven rather than feeling a sense of control was a central complaint of the patient.) Silberschatz, Fretter, and Curtis (1986) reported that for two cases showing, respectively, very good and moderately good outcome, 89 and 80%, respectively, of the therapists' interventions were independently rated as "pro-plan" (that is, they furthered the patient's unconscious plan), whereas 2 and 0%, respectively, of the interventions were "anti-plan." Contrastingly, in a case showing poor outcome, 50% of the therapist's interventions were rated as "pro-plan," 6% as "anti-plan," and 44% as "ambiguous." In a more recent paper, Silberschatz, Curtis, and Nathans (1989) found that when the therapist was rated low on test-passing, the result was a poor outcome "as defined by conventional therapeutic outcome measures" (p. 44) and conversely, when the therapist was rated high on test-passing, the result was a good outcome.

Luborsky and His Colleagues with Supportive–Expressive Psychotherapy and the CCRT

Much of this investigation into the process of psychodynamic psychotherapy has been summarized in a manual for short- and long-term supportive–expressive psychotherapy by Luborsky (1984), Luborsky and his colleagues (1988), and Luborsky and Crits-Christoph (1998), which presents many complex findings. As noted earlier, according to Luborsky, patients' relationship episodes narrated in treatment can be reliably broken down into the wish or need the patient expresses (W), the response from the other (RO), and the subsequent reaction of the self (RS). Further, one can reliably find for each patient the predominant core conflictual relationship themes (CCRT). In Luborsky et al., one finds the following pattern in successful treatment from early to late treatment sessions:

1. a relative stability in the main wish or need expressed
2. a decrease in the percentage of negative responses from the other
3. a decrease in the percentage of negative responses of the self
4. an increase in the percentage of positive responses of the other
5. an increase in the percentage of positive responses of the self

As one can see from this, even in successful treatment, the main wish or need expressed by the patient does not tend to change. What does change is the experienced reaction of the other to one's expressed need or wish and one's own subsequent reaction to the response of the other. That the experienced response of the other changes in the course of treatment provides a clue as to what factors bring about change. The treatment factor that Luborsky most emphasizes as effecting change is the patient's experience of a helping alliance with the therapist. This general factor includes a "Type 1" helping alliance, which is the patient's experience of the therapist as helpful and supportive and a "Type 2" helping alliance, which is the patient's experience of working together with the therapist in a joint effort.

One can link the importance of the helping alliance to the previously noted CCRT changes in experienced responses from others and from the self. According to traditional psychoanalytic theory, the neurotic individual's wishes are linked to conflict and anxiety and set off "expected or remembered helplessness" (Freud, 1926). If patients have been able to express these wishes in the therapy and experience the therapists' responses as helpful and supportive, then they will come to modify their experience and expectation of a negative response from the other and the consequent negative response of the self. According to Luborsky, these changes indicate that patients have developed an increased sense of mastery and a decreased sense of helplessness in dealing with their core relationship problems. Patients are now better able to express their wishes and needs (as well as thoughts and feelings) with reduced anxiety and a greater sense of mastery, as shown in their experience and expectation of a positive response from the other (and of the self). (Note that from the perspective of Weiss and Sampson's [1986] control–mastery theory, this whole sequence can also be understood in terms of the therapist's test-passing and disconfirmation of the patient's pathogenic beliefs.)

Strupp and His Colleagues with the Patient–Therapist Interaction

We come, finally, in our brief sampling of psychotherapy research, to the work of Strupp and his colleagues. Like Luborsky, Strupp has been a pioneer in psychotherapy research. Also like Luborsky, Strupp's work has been too variegated to be subject to a brief summary. However, we can provide a sampling and some highlights.

Strupp understands psychotherapy as, above all, a human relationship and as a process of learning (and unlearning) in the context of that relationship (Strupp, 1986). Along with others, then, psychotherapy for Strupp is more a kind of *education* than a form of treatment. (Interestingly enough, Freud referred to psychoanalysis as "after-education"—that is, so to speak, a second round of postchildhood socialization and education.) In accord with that conception of psychotherapy, much of the research and writing of Strupp and his colleagues has focused on aspects of the *interaction* between patient and therapist in the therapeutic relationship. Thus, like Luborsky, Strupp and his colleagues have stressed the importance of the *therapeutic alliance* between patient and therapist. For example, they have developed the 44-item Vanderbilt University Therapeutic Alliance Scale, which clinical judges can reliably use to rate tape-recorded psychotherapy sessions for the degree of therapeutic alliance (Hartley & Strupp, 1983).

Employing the Vanderbilt scale, Strupp and his colleagues found that there was a strong suggestion that for positive outcome patients, the therapeutic alliance was highest during the first quarter of sessions, in contrast to poor outcome patients whose therapeutic alliance scores *fell* by the end of the first quarter of sessions (Hartley & Strupp, 1983). This pattern, suggesting the importance of the *early* therapeutic alliance for outcome, was reported by Luborsky (1976). In general, Hartley and Strupp (1983) conclude that the therapeutic alliance may be a necessary but not sufficient condition for determining therapy outcome. They concur with Morgan et al.'s (1982) observation that, whereas a poor therapeutic alliance almost always predicted a poor outcome, good outcome occurred in cases with many as well as with few signs of a therapeutic alliance.

In another study on the interaction between patient and therapist, Henry, Schacht, and Strupp (1986) found that positive and total *complementarity* between patient and therapist (complementarity refers to "a given interaction sequence in which the communication of one participant is thought to 'pull for' a complementary communication from the other" [Strupp et al., 1988, p. 693]) was related to good therapeutic outcome, whereas *multiple communications* "which simultaneously communicate more than one interpersonal message (e.g., acceptance and rejection) ... were almost exclusively associated with therapies having poor outcome" (Strupp et al., 1988, p. 693).

Henry, Schacht, and Strupp (1986) found that in poor outcomes, therapists' communications tended to be more hostile and negative. However, what is also quite fascinating is that the therapists' own self-rated introject "at worst" was significantly related to the number of hostile statements made to the patient. And, consistent with this finding, Christensen, Lane, and Strupp (1987) found that the degree of hostility in the therapists' reports of past relationships with their parents predicted similarly poor interpersonal process in the therapy interaction.

There is much else one can discuss regarding the work of Strupp and his colleagues, for example, the relationship between psychotherapy research and practice (e.g., Strupp, 1986), psychotherapy research and practice and public policy (e.g., Strupp, 1986), a manual for short-term psychodynamic psychotherapy (Strupp & Binder, 1986), a manual for short-term psychodynamic psychotherapy (Strupp & Binder, 1984), and the nature of training in psychodynamic psychotherapy (e.g., Strupp et al., 1988). However, we trust that the sampling of psychotherapy research that we presented will provide the reader with an idea of the range and vitality of research, theory, and practice in psychodynamic psychotherapy; additional range is also provided in another overview by Luborsky (2000b).

SUMMARY

Several main observations about psychodynamic psychotherapy and psychoanalysis have been reviewed:

- Two main types of theories have been distinguished: the more traditional and the more contemporary. The more traditional theories focus more on the therapist identifying the main transference pattern and through interpretation guided by assessment of the pattern, helping the patient achieve insight, and thus freeing the patient to master the resultant symptoms (as summarized in the treatment manual by Luborsky, 1984).
- This traditional theory and related techniques still exist alongside of what have been called contemporary theories in this review. They are those that have been given as examples here, including the theory and technique of Carl Rogers, the self-psychology and technique of Heintz Kohut, and the control-mastery theory of Weiss and Sampson (1986).
- The research studies given here as samples have helped the field of psychodynamics, psychotherapy, and psychoanalysis make great steps in understanding the process of the therapies. The examples given include the works of Luborsky and associates, as well as Strupp and associates and the manuals for the treatment techniques that they have developed.
- The next major steps in current research are taking the field toward more specific applications of the theory and techniques for use with different kinds of patients. Eventually, the field will know more about the kind of treatment that each kind of patient should get, so that it will be possible to specify the treatment needed for different kinds of patients.

REFERENCES

Alexander, F., & French, T. M. (1946). *Psychoanalytic therapy: Principles and applications.* New York: Ronald Press.

Brenner, C. (1979). Working alliance, therapeutic alliance and transference. *Journal of the American Psychoanalytic Association, 27*(Suppl.), 137–157.

Brenner, C. (1982). *The mind in conflict.* New York: International Universities Press.

Christensen, J. C., Lane, T. W., & Strupp, H. J. (1987). Pre-therapy interpersonal relations and introject as reflected in the therapeutic process. Paper presented at the *Meeting of the Society for Psychotherapy Research* (SPR), Ulm, West Germany.

Crits-Christoph, L. P., Cooper, A., & Luborsky, L. (1988). The accuracy of therapists' interpretations and the outcome of dynamic psychotherapy. *Journal of Consulting and Clinical Psychology, 56*, 490–495.

Eagle, M. (1984). *Recent developments in psychoanalysis: A critical evaluation.* Cambridge, MA: Harvard University Press.

Eagle, M., & Wolitzky, D. L. (1992). Psychoanalytic theories of psychotherapy. In D. K. Freedheim (Ed.), *History of psychotherapy: A century of change* (pp. 109–158). Washington, DC: American Psychological Association.

Fairbairn, W. R. D. (1952). *Psychoanalytic studies of the personality.* London: Tavistock Publications & Routledge & Kegan Paul.

Freud, S. (1892–1893). A case of successful treatment by hypnotism. *Standard edition*, Vol. 2 (pp. 115–128). London: Hogarth Press, 1966.

Freud, S. (1910). The future prospects of psychoanalytic therapy. *Standard edition*, Vol. 11 (pp. 139–151). London: Hogarth Press, 1957.

Freud, S. (1912a/1958). The dynamics of transference. *Standard edition*, Vol. 12 (pp. 97–108). London: Hogarth Press.

Freud, S. (1912b/1958). Recommendations to physicians practicing psychoanalysis. *Standard edition*, Vol. 12 (pp. 109–120). London: Hogarth Press.

Freud, S. (1914). On the history of the psychoanalytic movement. *Standard Edition*, Vol. 14 (pp. 7–66). London: Hogarth Press, 1957.

Freud, S. (1923). The ego and the id. *Standard edition*, Vol. 19 (pp. 3–59). London: Hogarth Press, 1961.

Freud, S. (1926). Inhibitions, symptoms, and anxiety. *Standard edition*, Vol. 10 (pp. 87–174). London: Hogarth Press, 1959.

Freud, S. (1933). The dissection of the psychical personality. *Standard edition*, Vol. 17 (pp. 57–81). London: Hogarth Press, 1964.

Gill, M. M. (1982). *Analysis of transference.* New York: International Universities Press.

Greenberg, J. R., & Mitchell, S. A. (1983). *Object relations in psychoanalytic theory.* Cambridge, MA: Harvard University Press.

Greenson, R. R. (1965). The working alliance and the transference neurosis. *Psychoanalytic Quarterly, 34*, 155–181.

Hartley, D., & Strupp, H. (1983). The therapeutic alliance: Its relationship to outcome in brief psychotherapy. In J. Masling (Ed.), *Empirical studies of psychoanalytic theory*, Vol. 1 (pp. 1–27). Hillsdale, NJ: Erlbaum.

Henry, W. P., Schacht, T. E., & Strupp, H. H. (1986). Structural analysis of social behavior: Application to a study of interpersonal process in differential psychotherapeutic outcome. *Journal of Consulting and Clinical Psychology, 54*, 27–31.

Horvath, A. O., & Symonds, B. D. (1991). Relation between working alliance and outcome in psychotherapy: A meta-analysis. *Journal of Counseling Psychology, 38*(2), 139–149.

Kohut, H. (1971). *The analysis of the self.* New York: International Universities Press.

Kohut, H. (1977). *The restoration of the self.* New York: International Universities Press.

Kohut, H. (1984). *How does analysis cure?.* New York: International Universities Press.

Kris, E. (1947). The nature of psychoanalytic propositions and their validation. In S. Hook & M. R. Korwitz (Eds.), *Freedom and experience: Essays presented to Horace Kalle* (pp. 239–259). New York: Cornell University Press.

Luborsky, L. (1976). Helping alliances in psychotherapy: The groundwork for a study of their relationship to its outcome. In J. Claghorn (Ed.), *Successful psychotherapy* (pp. 92–116). New York: Brunner/Mazel.

Luborsky, L. (1984). *Principles of psychoanalytic psychotherapy: A manual for supportive-expressive treatment.* New York: Basic Books.

Luborsky, L. (1996). *The symptom-context method—Symptoms as opportunities in psychotherapy.* Washington, DC: American Psychological Association.

Luborsky, L. (2000a). A pattern-setting therapeutic alliance study revisited. *Psychotherapy Research, 10*, 17–29.

Luborsky, L. (2000b). Psychodynamic therapies. In A. E. Kazdin (Ed.), *Encyclopedia of psychology.* Washington, DC; New York: American Psychological Association; Oxford University Press.

Luborsky, L., & Crits-Cristoph, P. (1990). *Understanding transference: The CCRT method.* New York: Basic Books.

Luborsky, L., Crits-Cristoph, P., Alexander, L., Margolis, M., & Cohen, M. (1983). Two helping alliance methods for predicting outcomes of psychotherapy. A counting signs versus a global rating method. *Journal of Nervous and Mental Disease, 17*, 480–492.

Luborsky, L., Crits-Cristoph, P., Mintz, J., & Auerbach, A. (1988). *Who will benefit from psychotherapy?: Predicting therapeutic outcome.* New York: Basic Books.

Luborsky, L., & Crits-Christoph, P. (1998). *Understanding transference*, 2nd ed. Washington, DC: American Psychological Association.

Malan, D. (1963). *A study of brief psychotherapy.* New York: Plenum.

Malan, D. (1976). *The frontier of brief psychotherapy.* New York: Plenum.

Mischel, T. (1963). Psychology and explanations of human behavior. *Philosophy and Phenomenological Research, 23*, 578–594.

Mischel, T. (1966). Pragmatic aspects of explanation. *Philosophy of Science, 33*, 40–60.

Modell, A. (1983). Self-preservation and the preservation of the self: An overview of the more recent knowledge of the narcissistic personality. Paper given at *Symposium on Narcissism, Masochism, and the Sense of Guilt in Relation to the Therapeutic Process*, May 14–15, San Francisco, CA.

Morgan, R., Luborsky, L., Crits-Christoph, P., Curtis, H., & Solomon, J. (1982). Predicting outcomes of psychotherapy by the Penn Helping Alliance rating method. *Archives of General Psychiatry, 39*, 397–402.

Rogers, C. R. (1951). *Client-centered therapy*. Boston: Houghton Miffin.

Schmidl, E. (1955). The problem of scientific validation in psychoanalytic interpretation. *International Journal of Psychoanalysis, 36*, 105–113.

Silberschatz, G., Fretter, P. B., & Curtis, J. T. (1986). How do interpretations influence the process of psychotherapy? *Journal of Consulting and Clinical Psychology, 54*, 646–652.

Silberschatz, G., Curtis, J. T., & Nathans, S. (1989). Using the patient's plan to assess progress in psychotherapy. *Psychotherapy, 26*(1), 40–46.

Spence, D. P. (1982). *Narrative truth and historical truth*. New York: W. W. Norton.

Strupp, H. H. (1986). Research, practice, and public policy (How to avoid dead ends). *American Psychologist, 41*, 120–130.

Strupp, H. H. (1989). Can the practitioner learn from the researcher? *American Psychologist, 44*, 717–724.

Strupp, H. H., & Binder, J. L. (1984). *Psychotherapy in a new key: A guide to time-limited dynamic psychotherapy*. New York: Basic Books.

Strupp, H. H., Butler, S. F., & Rosser, C. L. (1988). Training in psychodynamic therapy. *Journal of Consulting and Clinical Psychology, 56*, 689–695.

Waelder, R. (1960). *Basic theory of psychoanalysis*. New York: International Universities Press.

Weiss, J. (1990). Unconscious mental functioning. *Scientific American, 262*(3), 103–109.

Weiss, J., Sampson, H., & the Mount Zion Psychotherapy Research Group. (1986). *The psychoanalytic process: Theory, clinical observation and empirical research*. New York: Guilford.

Winnicott, D. W. (1958). *Collected papers. Through paediatrics to psychoanalysis*. London: Tavistock.

Winnicott, D. W. (1965). *The maturational processes and the facilitating environment*. London: The Hogarth Press and the Institute of Psycho-Analysis, 1987.

Zetzel, E. (1966). The analytic situation. In R. E. Litman (Ed.), *Psychoanalysis in the Americans* (pp. 86–106). New York: International Universities Press.

26

Behavior Therapy

Kevin T. Larkin and Michael J. Zvolensky

Introduction

The term behavior therapy was first introduced in the 1950s to refer to the application of interventions based on an understanding of learning principles. At the time of the inception of behavior therapy, the prevailing paradigm in clinical psychology was psychodynamic, and since that time there has arguably been a major paradigmatic shift from psychoanalytic approaches to behavioral approaches. This transition was based, at least in part, on the observation that psychoanalytic methods for treating mental/behavioral disorders have not been consistently superior to no treatment, placebo, or other treatment conditions. In contrast, investigations of behavior therapy have emphasized empirical scrutiny and quantifiable behavior change, and therefore behavior therapy applications have been widely recognized as very successful for treating a wide variety of mental/behavioral problems, ranging from anxiety disorders to developmental disabilities.

Defining Characteristics

Behavior therapy differs from other forms of psychological therapies in its commitment to basic research and its link with behavior theory (see Chapter 5). Specifically, behavior therapy is aimed at determining environment–behavior relationships that can explain the cause and/or maintenance of maladaptive behaviors typically seen in clinical settings. Elucidation of these environment–behavior relationships has emerged from behavioral research, most notably operant and classical conditioning (see later). Congruent with the laboratory research upon which it is based, behavior therapy typically focuses on the function rather than the structure of behavior. In the most general sense, structural analyses focus on the *way* people behave (e.g., the form of a particular response), whereas functional analyses focus on the *reason* people behave (e.g., the purpose of a particular response). For example, a behavior therapist seeks to understand why a person is depressed rather than to analyze the constellation of depressive symptoms reported. Using the previous example, structural approaches imply

Kevin T. Larkin and Michael J. Zvolensky • Department of Psychology, West Virginia University, Morgantown, West Virginia 26506-6040.

Advanced Abnormal Psychology, Second Edition, edited by Hersen and Van Hasselt. Kluwer Academic/Plenum Publishers, New York, 2001.

that behavior is caused by some sort of underlying and often unobservable structure (e.g., maladaptive schema, unconscious motive). In contrast, a functional approach suggests that environment–behavior relationships cause and maintain particular types of responding (e.g., a person lost a job and cannot financially support her/his family and therefore experiences a dysphoric mood).

In a functional approach, behavior therapists attempt to explicate the relationship between observable behavior and the contextual variables of the environment, particularly focusing on observable antecedents and consequences to behavioral responses. Indeed, there are often short- and long-term consequences that produce and maintain maladaptive behavior, and the behavior therapist's job is to identify the function of maladaptive behaviors and work toward changing the consequences of such behaviors to produce positive outcomes. For example, if a child's recurrent tantrums in a school classroom are routinely followed by attention from the teacher, a behavior therapist might encourage the teacher to praise the child when he or she is not having a tantrum and ignore the child when a tantrum occurs. Thus, tantrum behavior aimed at receiving attention is not reinforced, thereby changing the function of such responding. This process of assessment, called a *functional analysis of behavior*, is the core of behavior therapy approaches. Following from this general scientific framework, it is clear that behavior therapists adhere to the contention that current behavioral problems are typically caused and maintained by maladaptive learning experiences.

Another theoretical component of behavior therapy is its focus on idiographic (i.e., individual) rather than nomothetic (i.e., group) approaches to assessing and changing behavior. Nomothetic approaches, by definition, focus on identifying the commonalities and differences among traits and dispositions that occur within and between groups of people. Idiographic approaches, on the other hand, focus on variability in the behavior of a person over time and across situations. As such, a second aim of the functional analysis of behavior is to identify consistent sources of variance for a particular person presenting to the clinic with a specific behavioral problem.

Despite the uniformity among behavior therapists commonly perceived by the public, it is important to note that not all behavior therapists are alike. Indeed, there are different behavioral approaches, differing in specific aspects of their clinical approach. Such diversity is reflected in the numerous terms that have been employed to describe the general therapeutic approach of behavior therapy (e.g., applied behavior analysis, behavior modification, and cognitive-behavior therapy). Although these various terminologies describe one's specific approach, behaviorally oriented therapists are all committed to changing maladaptive behavior through functional, idiographic assessment of a specified target behavior. By identifying the controlling variables, it is possible to employ treatment strategies that are based on behavioral principles to alter problematic behavior. To achieve these goals, behavior therapists attempt to provide a new set of learning experiences that are in accord with positive behavioral change within the value system of the patient.

Through sound functional analyses of behavior, behavior therapy approaches have evolved over the years based on new empirical information pertaining to common clinical phenomena. For purposes of this chapter, a clinical case presentation of panic disorder will be considered, with reference to first-, second-, and newer generation behavior therapy approaches.

Case Illustration

Steve is a 46-year-old, married, white male who has a 2-month history of recurrent panic attacks. He describes 5–60 minute unpredictable episodes of panic occurring every 3 to 4 days, associated with the following symptoms: muscle tension in the head and accompanying headache pain, racing and pounding heart, increased rate of breathing, increased sweating, lightheadedness, a "fizzy taste in the mouth," some nausea, feeling sensations of warmth inside his body, decreased attention and concentration, feeling worried and nervous, and being terrified of having a heart attack and dying. Thinking he had some physical disease, Steve was evaluated thoroughly before seeking help at an anxiety disorders clinic, which included cardiac monitoring, thyroid function tests, echocardiogram, ultrasound evaluation of blood vessels in his neck, an exercise stress test, MRI of the head, upper GI series, and ultrasound of the pancreas, all with negative results. Due to the frequency of these panic attacks, Steve began to avoid going out for dinner and to decrease travel opportunities needed to advance his career. No previous history of panic attacks was reported, but Steve reported experiencing separation anxiety at a younger age. His medical history was positive for esophageal reflex and spasms, but otherwise not remarkable for cardiac problems, neurological impairment, or any other chronic medical condition. Steve had already eliminated caffeinated beverages from his diet before intervention and used no other psychoactive substances.

BEHAVIOR THERAPY: FIRST-GENERATION APPROACHES TO TREATMENT

For purposes of illustration, let us imagine that our patient, Steve, sought help for his anxiety condition in 1975, a time when he would have been diagnosed with Agoraphobia with Panic Attacks. At that time, the theoretical foundation of behavior therapy was largely influenced by approaches based on principles of operant and classical conditioning. Before providing a functional behavior analysis of Steve's condition, it is important to understand the theoretical foundations of both operant and classical conditioning.

Operant Conditioning

Operant methods may be broadly classified into two categories: those techniques that increase the probability that a specific behavior occurs and those that decease that probability. Many methods are used to achieve both increases and decrements in behavior. Let us first consider methods to increase behavior, those that employ reinforcement. *Positive reinforcement* methods of behavioral change involve presenting a desirable stimulus contingent on emitting a specified (appropriate) behavior, for example, providing an increase in salary to a worker who exceeded an established productivity level. Applying such an approach, high rates of work productivity presumably will be maintained. *Negative reinforcement*, on the other hand, involves response-contingent removal of an unpleasant stimulus. For example, a person may leave a frightening situation to avoid feeling anxiety and fear, like Steve's decision to avoid eating meals out and not take advantage of travel opportunities. In this case, increased rates of avoidance behaviors will be observed.

Reinforcement strategies can effectively increase performance rates for behaviors already present, but the same cannot be said for behaviors that a person does not know how to emit (e.g., skill level). *Shaping* is a behavioral technique that can be used to amend a skill deficit. Shaping refers to the systematic reinforcement of behaviors that successively approximate a specified behavior. Using a shaping procedure, a person is assessed to identify an activity that can be successfully performed and that, although distinct, is similar to the desired behavior. The emission of this distinct behavior is initially reinforced, and the criterion for reinforcement is shifted closer to the desired behavior. For example, in shaping assertive behavioral responses in a passive-dependent patient, reinforcement may be initially provided for a verbal response of any type. Through successive approximations, the specific content and nonverbal style of presentation can be shifted to arrive at the delivery of more desirable, assertive verbal behavior.

Punishment represents one of the most basic techniques for diminishing responses and can be broadly defined as the provision of a negative consequence following undesired behavior. Historically, there have been questions raised concerning the ethical issues surrounding the use of punishment-based techniques because they may serve as a model for aggressive behavior and/or lead to negative psychological outcomes (e.g., fear). There are several punishment techniques that involve the behavior-contingent application of an aversive stimulus to decrease the likelihood of an identified behavioral response, including spanking, yelling, and ingesting of noxious substances (e.g., lemon juice). Other forms of punishment, however, involve removing a stimulus that a person finds rewarding to decrease behavior. *Response cost*, whereby children forfeit watching a favorite TV show for a set period of time because of their previous problematic behavior is an example of this type of punishment procedure.

Extinction procedures are another operant strategy. Extinction techniques involve nonreinforcment of a specified behavior to decrease the probability of future response. For example, a therapist may not acknowledge negative self-verbalizations by a depressive client who regularly emits them during therapy to get attention from the therapist. Extinction techniques work quite well with externally reinforced behaviors but are less effective with behaviors that are largely internally reinforced (e.g., masturbation). Use of extinction strategies is further complicated by what is termed the "extinction burst," in which increased rates of response occur for a short period before response diminishment is observed. Because extinction bursts are commonly observed, these strategies are not appropriate for self-injurious behaviors, where this temporary increase in behavior has harmful and in extreme cases perhaps fatal consequences.

Two additional methods that combine extinction and reinforcement to decrease inappropriate responding are *Differential Reinforcement of Other* (DRO) and *Differential Reinforcement of Incompatible* (DRI) behaviors. DRO procedures involve reinforcing behavior other than the problem behavior. For example, a child who engages in damaging scratching behavior that produces open sores may have its nonscratching behavior reinforced (DRO). Further, the child may be reinforced for playing with a toy because it is assumed that the child cannot play with a toy and scratch at the same time (DRI)(Nemeroff & Karoly, 1991).

Satiation is another behavioral procedure used to diminish inappropriate behaviors. Satiation involves providing an overabundance of responses or stimuli so that the individual no longer finds them reinforcing. Ayllon (1963), in a classic study of towel hoarding in a psychiatric ward, placed an excessive number of towels in the room of a patient who hoarded the towels. After acquiring a large number of towels (e.g., approximately 600), the patient permanently discontinued the hoarding behavior, presumably because having the towels no longer was reinforcing.

Negative practice, defined as the repeated performance of a problem behavior with little opportunity for rest, and *positive practice*, the repeated performance of appropriate behaviors, may also be used to decrease inappropriate responding. Negative practice is typically used with small motor behaviors (e.g., facial tics) which are generally not under voluntary control and not intrinsically reinforcing. From a theoretical viewpoint, negative practice is considered effective through the removal of the negative reinforcing properties of rest that follow the repeated motor behavior. Positive practice involves the repeated performance of adaptive behaviors and is often combined with *overcorrection*, defined as the restoration of a situation to a state better than that before the disturbance, to facilitate positive behavioral change.

For purposes of treating our patient who has panic attacks, it is important to note that it is well established that operant extinction strategies, including *implosive therapy, flooding, response prevention*, and *exposure therapy*, are quite effective in treating patients who have anxiety disorders. All of these approaches aim to reduce anxiety in the long run by exposing the patient to a feared stimulus (e.g., eating dinner out) and prohibiting the escape and avoidance behaviors from occurring, thereby removing the negatively reinforcing properties of anxiety reduction. Although these procedures are anxiety-evoking in the short term, they result in significant improvement of anxiety symptoms with time.

Classical Conditioning

Because it is well known that some behaviors are quite reflexive (e.g., jumping back when unexpectedly frightened), some behavioral researchers suggested that not all responses fit easily within the confines of an operant conditioning framework. Inspired by the work of the Russian physiologist, Ivan Pavlov, it was shown that these "automatic" behavioral responses are learned quite easily using a different type of conditioning, namely respondent, classical, or Pavlovian conditioning; all three names are synonymous and can be used interchangeably. If a problematic stimulus–response association has been acquired via classical conditioning (e.g., sight of a restaurant induces anxiety symptoms), the stimulus–response association can be deconditioned (i.e., unlearned) using some of the principles of classical conditioning outlined by Pavlov.

In one of the first efforts aimed at creating a deconditioning treatment for problems acquired through classical conditioning, Wolpe (1958) developed *systematic desensitization*, which has been successfully applied as a treatment strategy for anxiety, among other types of disorders (e.g., sexual dysfunction, sleep disturbances). The first step in systematic desensitization involves constructing a hierarchy of approximately 15 to 20 items that are related to the feared stimulus. Then, the patient learns a competing behavioral response, such as progressive muscle relaxation, and is instructed to relax all major muscle groups, and then imagine a fear-evoking scene. The client is then instructed to stop imagining the fear-relevant scene, and the level of anxiety is assessed. If the level of anxiety is below a specified criterion, the next scene in the hierarchy is imagined; if the ratings are higher than the specified criterion, the original scene is repeated. This same procedure is followed for all hierarchical scenes.

Research suggests that systematic desensitization alleviates pathological anxiety across a broad range of anxiety-related disorders (see Paul, 1969, for a review). According to Wolpe (1958), systematic desensitization works as a function of a process called counterconditioning. In counterconditioning, a conditioned stimulus (e.g., sight of a restaurant) is presented with an unconditioned stimulus (UCS) (e.g., relaxation) that is different from the original UCS (e.g., extreme physiological arousal). Once learned, the conditioned response to the new UCS "competes" with the conditioned response produced by the old UCS and lessens the connection between the conditioned response and the old UCS. Wolpe termed the process of teaching a competing response *reciprocal inhibition*. To put it simply, this principle states that a person cannot exhibit the physiological state accompanying relaxation and anxiety simultaneously because each state inhibits the expression of the other. Accordingly, the state of relaxation inhibits the experience of anxiety and serves as the basis for the way systematic desensitization works. Others have disagreed with Wolpe, and suggested that other mechanisms of change could account for the observed changes in behavior (e.g., extinction, changing cognitive processes, habituation, nonspecific treatment factors).

Case Illustration

Let us now return to an analysis of Steve's presenting problem and how it might be addressed by using these first-generation behavioral conceptualizations. First, most behavior therapists would not have difficulty recognizing the negative reinforcement component of Steve's anxiety that occurs with avoidance of work-related travel and pleasurable activities. As depicted in Figure 1, such a functional analysis easily leads the behavior therapist to develop an intervention plan based on knowledge of operant conditioning that focuses on increasing exposure to these feared situations. With some effort, Steve will be able to engage in these activities and his anxious condition will dissipate during repeated exposure sessions.

Alternatively, the behavior therapist may focus on the elements of the situation (e.g., the smells and sounds of a restaurant) that have been conditioned to elicit anxious arousal via classical conditioning. From this perspective, the behavior therapist may devise a desensitization treatment based on a classical conditioning conceptualization. In this case, Steve would learn a counterconditioned response, like progressive muscle relaxation, and gradually approach more diverse out-of-home activities. Using an anxiety hierarchy, like that depicted in Table 1, Steve would demonstrate competency in achieving a relaxed state and would be instructed to relax himself during presentation of progressively more anxiety-evoking images from the hierarchy. Typically within eight to twelve sessions, Steve would be able to imagine the most stressful scene in the hierarchy without experiencing anxiety. Successful imaginal presentations without anxiety would typically be followed by instructions to actually practice engaging in that particular task during intervening weeks of therapy (*in vivo* desensitization). Indeed, examination of the literature reveals that both of these approaches, exposure therapy and relaxation training, have been successful in treating Panic Disorder (Michelson, Mavissakalian, & Marchione, 1988). Other psychiatric disorders have been treated successfully using these behavior therapy approaches based upon operant and classical conditioning perspectives as well. For example, for obsessive–compulsive disorder and posttraumatic stress disorder, exposure and response prevention is considered the treatment of choice. In obsessive–compulsive disorder, patients are exposed to the anxiety-evoking stimuli (e.g., doorknob) and are prevented from engaging in the compulsive ritual that reduces anxiety (e.g., hand washing). In posttraumatic stress disorder, patients are exposed to stimuli surrounding the original trauma (e.g., sirens) and are not permitted to avoid or escape them during exposure in safe

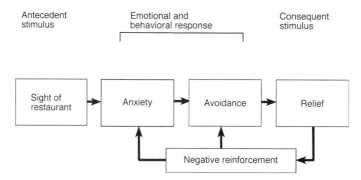

FIGURE 1. A functional analysis of Steve's behavior problem based on a first-generation behavior therapy conceptualization of panic disorder. Note that the negatively reinforcing property of relief from anxiety results in an increase and maintenance of both anxiety symptoms and avoidance behaviors.

TABLE 1. Steve's Hierarchy of Exposure to "Eating Out" Scenes

Step	Scene	SUDS[a]
1	Eating in the backyard at the picnic table	11
2	Driving by favorite restaurant at lunchtime	26
3	Pulling in parking lot of favorite restaurant in midafternoon	33
4	Entering restaurant, ordering soda in midafternoon	42
5	Entering restaurant, eating lunch in midafternoon	55
6	Pulling in parking lot of favorite restaurant at lunchtime	70
7	Pulling in parking lot of favorite restaurant at dinnertime	75
8	Entering restaurant, eating lunch with wife at lunchtime	80
9	Entering restaurant, eating dinner with wife at dinnertime	95
10	Entering restaurant, eating lunch with co-worker at lunchtime	98
11	Entering restaurant, eating lunch alone at lunchtime	100
12	Entering restaurant, eating dinner alone at dinnertime	100

[a]SUDS means subjective units of distress, a 0–100 scale that measures anticipated anxiety/distress associated with engaging in that particular item (adapted from Wolpe, 1958).

settings. In both cases, anxiety responses are extinguished by repeated exposure to the feared stimuli.

BEHAVIOR THERAPY: SECOND-GENERATION APPROACHES TO TREATMENT

Cognitive-Behavior Modification

In the 1970s, behaviorally trained clinicians were often criticized for ignoring what were perceived as important mental events relevant to understanding a patient's presenting symptom picture. Although the validity of these assertions can be immediately called into question upon examining the importance cognitive activity plays in the functional behavioral analysis depicted earlier, these criticisms polarized the field, a state which continued into the 1990s. Some behavior therapists acknowledge the central role of anxiety reduction strategies which evolved from conditioning models of behavioral pathology (Wolpe, 1958), but others have elevated the importance of cognitive or mental events in explaining the etiology of maladaptive behavioral problems (Beck, 1976; Meichenbaum, 1977). This latter group of practitioners, who often are called cognitive-behavioral therapists, have focused on developing new strategies aimed at altering directly the cognitive component of the prevailing problem.

Although advances in cognitive-behavioral strategies have been made with a number of patient populations, there is no more compelling evidence for the efficacy of these procedures than findings from clinical trials of the *cognitive treatment of depression*. Stemming from the belief that people depress themselves by engaging in a variety of negative thinking patterns and perceptual styles in response to environmental events, Aaron Beck (1976) developed and formalized this therapeutic approach. Treatment of depression, according to Beck, involves identifying and challenging common maladaptive thoughts and their deeper cognitive roots (i.e., a belief system referred to as a cognitive schema). Through a collaborative relationship with the therapist, the patient learns to consider alternative thought processes that may be just as valid as the depressing thoughts. For example, upon failing a test, a student might think his poor performance is the result of stupidity or ignorance, which leads to a depressive state. Accordingly, the failure itself does not result in depression, but rather it is the belief that "I failed the test because I am stupid" that results in depressive affect. Alternative conceptualizations discovered through the therapeutic process may include failing the test because it was an extremely difficult test or because the student did not study effectively. In both cases, if evidence exists for the alternative interpretation, the level of the depressive mood can be attenuated. Empirical efforts aimed at examining the efficacy of this approach have provided clear evidence that cognitive therapy for depression results in reduced negative affect (Beck, Rush, Shaw, & Emery, 1979). Further, the magnitude of mood change parallels the effects of commonly accepted therapy with antidepressant medication or electroconvulsive therapy.

Empirically Supported Therapies

In addition to this so-called "cognitive revolution," a number of important developments within the mental/behavioral health care system have shaped the current state of behavior therapy. Foremost among these are the development, evaluation, and dissemination of what have become known as empirically supported treatments. The current movement toward establishing empirically supported therapies for recognized mental/behavioral disorders has been at least partially in response to cost-containment efforts in the health-care system and specific funding-related restrictions for mental/behavioral health services. For example, health-care policy changes have strongly recommended, and in certain cases demanded, that psychological services follow guidelines for relatively brief treatments that have an empirical basis for a positive outcome.

The movement to list categorically empirically supported therapies for target populations was pioneered by the American Psychological Association Division 12 (Clinical Psychology) Task Force on Promotion and Dissemination of Psychological Procedures (Chambless, Baker, Baucom, Beutler, Calhoun, Crits-Christoph, Daiuto, DeRubeis, Detweiler, Haaga, Johnson, McCurry, Mueser, Pope, Sanderson, Shoham, Stickle, Williams, & Woody, 1998). The function of the task force was to review critically the existing empirical psychological treatment literature in an effort to identify those psychosocial interventions that have shown promise in alleviating specific types of psychological distress. Once potential treatments were identified and agreed upon, the task force could then communicate this information to the mental/behavioral health community. The task of charting efficacious treatments is an ongoing process because researchers are continuously examining therapies, refining their components, and assessing their utility across different populations, sites, and time periods.

Briefly, the task force evaluated treatments according to their *efficacy*, that is, the demonstration that an intervention improves psychological status in well-controlled, experimental studies. This research differs slightly from questions of *effectiveness*, defined as the relative degree of utility of a treatment to produce positive outcomes in the context in which treatment most often is sought (Onken, Blain, & Battjes, 1997). Typically, large-scale clinical trials are used to evaluate and demonstrate the efficacy of psychological interventions. Such evaluations are outcome-oriented; they typically involve evaluating a particular type of therapy compared to some type of control group (e.g., placebo, other form of therapy), although a variety of different evaluation formats are also considered (e.g., a series of single-case studies).

The criteria for demonstrating efficacy were next categorized by the task force as either "well-established treatments" or "probably efficacious treatments." Although it is not possible to review here the criteria for each of these domains in their entirety, "well-established therapies" generally have demonstrated superior outcomes compared to a control condition (e.g., placebo) or another treatment on two separate occasions by independent investigators. In contrast, "probably efficacious treatments" generally reflect treatments that have been superior to a waiting-list control group (i.e., persons who desire psychological treatment but are on a waiting list for such treatment). In all cases, the evaluative process involved randomly assigning persons who had a particular type of psychological disorder to specified treatment conditions. For example, patients who had major depression might be randomly assigned to receive an "active" psychological treatment or a separate treatment condition, such as a pill placebo. In these trials, patients were then evaluated in a standardized manner for the same duration using the same types of theoretically relevant dependent measures. Overall, these efforts allowed the task force to evaluate whether a particular therapy reduces psychological distress in a significant and clinically useful way.

Because behavior therapy has always been committed to empirical evaluation and time-efficient strategies, it is not surprising that behavior therapists have been at the forefront of developing empirically supported treatments. As depicted in Table 2, inspection of the titles of the well-established efficacious therapies indicates that behavioral and cognitive-behavioral therapies overwhelmingly top the list of empirically supported therapeutic interventions (Chambless et al., 1998). In fact, of the existing well-established therapies on the treatment list, the vast majority can be considered behavioral. For example, of the "well-established treatments," 93% are listed as behavioral or cognitive-behavioral based on conceptual basis, therapeutic components, and implementation procedures. Likewise, 87% of the "probably efficacious" treatments can also be considered cognitive-behavioral in origin.

In sum, behavior therapy evolved from the 1970s to the 1990s in two primary areas: (1) the growing recognition that internal processes such as thoughts and emotions characterized and affected many important aspects of psychological dysfunctions and (2) the critical value of demonstrating therapeutic efficacy. In contrast to interventions developed during the first generation of behavior therapists, second-generation therapies began to target behavioral change in a number of different response domains (i.e., cognitive, affective, and behavioral). Thus, it is not surprising that second-generation behavioral and cognitive-behavioral interventions can best be described as multicomponent strategies that contain treatment elements based on both basic learning principles from the first-generation approaches and more recent

TABLE 2. Well-Established Empirically Validated Treatments[a]

Cognitive-behavior therapy for panic disorder with/without agoraphobia
Cognitive-behavior therapy for generalized anxiety disorder
Exposure treatment for agoraphobia
Exposure/guided mastery treatment for specific phobia
Exposure and response prevention for obsessive–compulsive disorder
Stress inoculation training for coping with stressors
Behavior therapy for depression
Cognitive-behavior therapy for depression
Interpersonal Therapy for depression
Behavior therapy for headache
Cognitive-behavior therapy for bulimia
Cognitive-behavior therapy for pain associated with rheumatic disease
Cognitive-behavior threapy with relapse prevention for smoking cessation
Behavior modification for enuresis
Parent training programs for parents of children with oppositional disorder
Behavioral marital therapy

[a]Chambliss et al., 1998

developments in cognitive psychology (e.g., memory biases). Although it is not necessarily clear to what extent specific therapy components contribute to treatment outcome and maintenance, there is compelling evidence that each component in these cognitive-behavioral protocols is useful.

Case Illustration

To illustrate how an empirically supported therapy is actually employed in treatment, we now return to Steve, our patient who suffers from panic disorder. How might Steve be treated with a greater focus on integration of cognitive therapeutic strategies and demonstration of efficacy using well-established therapies? If Steve sought help in 1990 for his problem, which would now be diagnosed as Panic Disorder with Agoraphobia, he would most likely participate in a treatment program using Panic Control Therapy (PCT; Barlow, Craske, Cerny, & Klosko, 1989). This multicomponent cognitive-behavioral intervention, listed as a "well-established" treatment (see Table 2), is often guided by using a treatment manual entitled *Mastery of Your Anxiety and Panic-II* (MAP-II; Barlow & Craske, 1994) that articulates the procedures for PCT in a step-by-step fashion. Using this manual-based approach, Steve would first be given educational information about the nature, origin, and course of panic disorder before applying any specific intervention strategies. A model similar to the second-generation functional analysis depicted in Figure 2 would be employed to provide Steve with an effective rationale for the assignments in which he would be engaged during subsequent sessions. Note that the cognitive appraisal of panic sensations possesses a uniquely important role in the functional analysis, in contrast to the first-generation interventions.

The second and ongoing step in Steve's treatment would be to have him monitor both negative emotional experiences and stressful life events to facilitate the recognition and identification of environmental events that contribute to the occurrence of recurrent panic attacks. Identifying such negative life events makes the potential occurrence of panic attacks more predictable and perhaps controllable, thereby lessening their aversiveness. Third, the therapist would train Steve in relaxation and breathing exercises and have him practice these

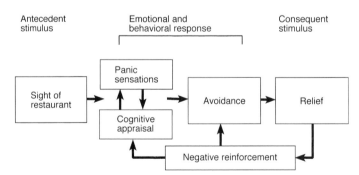

FIGURE 2. A functional analysis of Steve's behavior problem based on a second-generation behavior therapy conceptualization of panic disorder. Although the principle of negative reinforcement is still recognized, note the central role of the cognitive appraisal of the panic sensations in maintaining the disorder. The bidirectional arrows between Panic sensations and Cognitive appraisal reflect that although panic sensations are needed for catastrophic appraisals to occur, catastrophic appraisals contribute further to the problem directly by increasing the intensity of the physiological sensations at that time and indirectly by increasing the patient's general vigilance in detecting what otherwise may have been normal physiological bodily sensations.

exercises until he had acquired the skill of regulating bodily arousal. Breathing retraining is particularly important because it corrects probable imbalances between oxygen and carbon dioxide in the patient's blood by breathing diaphragmatically at a regular rate. Based upon the central importance of cognitive appraisal, Steve would next learn to challenge maladaptive cognitive errors related to worry about the negative consequences of panic attacks. For example, during cognitive restructuring, Steve would be taught to reconceptualize his panic attacks as harmless events that occur in response to particular natural stressors. Cognitive strategies are typically aimed at (1) correcting misappraisals of bodily sensations as threatening, (2) helping patients to predict more accurately the future likelihood of panic attacks, and (3) helping patients to predict more accurately and rationally the likely consequences of panic attacks.

Finally, Steve would participate in repeated trials of interoceptive exposure and if necessary, exteroceptive exposure exercises in both the clinical setting and his natural environment. Briefly, exposure to interoceptive bodily events is achieved through exercises that produce somatic sensations that are similar to panic (e.g., head spinning, hyperventilation induced via breathing through a straw). Situational (or exteroceptive) exposure, on the other hand, involves contacting feared environmental stimuli previously associated with the occurrence of panic attacks. For instance, Steve had already associated certain situations with panic (e.g., travel, eating out), and would be asked to eat a meal out or take a short business trip. Such exercises would be continued until these stimuli no longer elicited significant levels of anxiety.

BEHAVIOR THERAPY: NEW GENERATION APPROACHES TO TREATMENT

Behavior therapy has always been defined by a focus on concrete, quantifiable behavioral change through the application of the principles of behavior modification. In the first generation, the foundations of behavior therapy were based primarily on classical and operant conditioning. In the second generation, the theoretical foundations were extended to include cognitive and social learning principles. Although the evolution of behavior therapy has led toward the development of a wide variety of empirically supported treatment methods for a number of complex behavioral and emotional problems, some behavior therapists have recently suggested that because cognitive-behavioral approaches focus almost exclusively on promoting behavioral change, they may be somewhat limited in nature and scope. Thus, rather than emphasize change-only strategies in behavior therapy, it has been argued that behavioral interventions should also reflect the value of *acceptance* and the relationship between behavioral change and acceptance should be a primary focus of clinical attention (Hayes, Wilson, Gifford, Follette, & Strosahl, 1996). This movement toward applying acceptance-oriented strategies with more traditional cognitive-behavioral strategies represents an emerging new generation of behavior therapy. In fact, acceptance-based behavioral interventions have now been developed for a wide range of behavioral problems, including marital discord, borderline personality disorder, eating disorders, and anxiety and affective dysfunctions.

There have been a number of reasons for the recent emphasis on acceptance-based interventions in behavior therapy. First, despite the great strides made in behavior therapy in developing efficacious treatments for mental/behavioral disorders, therapeutic success does not always occur. For example, behavior therapies, like other psychological and pharmacological interventions, typically produce treatment effects that are specific to particular types of problem behavior (e.g., anxiety levels), rather than more general aspects of life functioning (e.g., job performance). Second, when treatment gains are observed, they often do not generalize to other aspects of behavioral functioning. As one example, although there is growing recognition that anxiety and depressive states are related, empirically supported treatments for depression often do not aim to reduce problematic anxious or fearful responding. Third, most persons who seek professional help for mental/behavioral problems do not neatly "fit" into the DSM-IV syndromal categories. Indeed, persons who seek treatment typically are struggling with behavioral problems across a vast array of life domains (e.g., family, career, personal) in addition to specific types of mental/behavioral problems. Thus, it could be argued that therapies focused on a single disorder are necessarily limited because they do not adequately address these other potentially important aspects of life functioning.

What Is Acceptance?

The majority of behavior therapies to date can be considered change-oriented; that is, they are focused on eliminating problems and producing adaptive, healthy responses to replace maladaptive ones. For example, cognitive-behavioral therapy for depression, as one of the hallmarks of empirically supported treatments, involves teaching patients to consider more positive ways of thinking, rather than the negative manner in which they are accustomed. Although change-oriented approaches have utility, they differ considerably from acceptance-oriented strategies that emphasize "letting go" of the struggle to change and even embracing certain emotional/psychological states that are perceived as problematic. Paradoxically, as patients learn to accept these states, more adaptive behavior emerges because the formerly problematic events no longer serve a maladaptive function. For example, in the case of a woman with depression, once she stops her struggle to make herself "feel better," efforts at engaging in personally adaptive behaviors (e.g., participation in social or work-related activities) tend to increase, and she can thereby attain a more healthy psychological/emotional state.

It is important to note that "change" and "acceptance" should not be considered dichotomous dimensions. In fact, existing acceptance-based therapies share in common a use of both traditional change-oriented *and* acceptance-based strategies. Moreover, both "change" and "acceptance" approaches represent types of behavioral change in themselves and often facilitate other collateral behavioral changes. For example, once a couple gives up the struggle to change each other's behavior in a particular way, previously problematic "change-oriented" behaviors (e.g., blaming, complaining, threatening) typically dissipate. Using an acceptance context, the couple can more easily see that their attempts to solve the problem were in fact part of the problem. Through such efforts, the couple may be in a better position to express their discomfort/dissatisfaction without chastising/blaming one another for being solely responsible for the marital discord. Thus, the problem becomes shared between the couple and now certain change-oriented strategies (e.g., communication skill training) can be applied with greater precision and efficacy.

Behavioral Therapies that Incorporate Acceptance

A variety of behavioral therapies have been developed that focus at least partly on acceptance-based strategies for promoting positive behavioral change, including Dialectical Behavior Therapy for borderline personality disorder, behavioral couples therapy, addiction problems, and more recently behavioral therapy for eating disorders (e.g., Linehan, 1994; Marlatt, 1994). One of the most notable examples of an acceptance-based approach to treatment that represents one intervention in this new generation is *Acceptance and Commitment Therapy* (ACT; Hayes & Wilson, 1994).

ACT is a psychotherapeutic approach that views experiential avoidance, defined as an unwillingness to experience unpleasant thoughts and feelings, as the primary psychological problem and reason for life disruption. There is emerging evidence that experiential avoidance is a common occurrence across various types of psychopathology. As an example, a substantial percentage of persons who have substance abuse and dependence problems use drugs to create positive emotions and/or reduce negative emotions. Similarly, persons who have anxiety disorders such as panic disorder and social phobia often attempt to avoid aversive anxiety experiences by arranging their life to prevent contact with potentially anxiety-provoking situations. In these disorders, as we have described earlier in this chapter, such escape or avoidance behaviors function as a solution for negative emotional experiences and a lack of ability to modulate these internally based negative emotional experiences effectively. Not surprisingly, across disorders, attempts to escape from or avoid emotional events lead to personal problems in the immediate situation and also typically fail as long-term solutions.

Considering the negative consequences of experiential avoidance, in ACT, patients are encouraged to allow aversive feelings to occur without making efforts to control them. For example, a person who has obsessive–compulsive disorder is encouraged to experience intrusive obsessions fully and without defense for what they are (i.e., unpleasant thoughts) and not as what the patient says they are (i.e., signs of impending harm or doom). In this way, patients can learn that anxiety-related emotional events are not the cause of their suffering nor an obstacle to positive psychological well-being. ACT can be contrasted with the first- and second-generation cognitive-behavioral approaches that help the patient learn to control or modify maladaptive thoughts to think and feel differently and presumably behave in more adaptive ways. Another important component of ACT is that it actively teaches patients to distinguish between situations in which direct change efforts are desirable and possible and situations in which emotional acceptance is a more viable, adaptive strategy. For example, patients are encouraged to give up trying to control anxiety while also learning to institute control over engaging in activities that they previously said they could not do because of anxiety.

Although ACT is a relatively recent development in behavior therapy, it has been increasingly demonstrated that it is an efficacious therapeutic approach for alleviating psychological distress across a wide range of behavioral disorders, including anxiety disorders, chronic drug addiction, affective disorders, and parenting disabled children (Strosahl, Hayes, Bergan, & Romano, 1998). In fact, in contrast to the empirically supported treatments designed for specific problems, ACT is a psychological intervention that can be used for persons who have a variety of single or multiple behavioral problems. Perhaps for this reason, ACT often is tested with field effectiveness research methodologies rather than more traditional efficacy-based methodologies that are the norm among second-generation approaches to treatment (e.g., Strosahl et al., 1998).

Case Illustration

To illustrate how an acceptance-based approach to therapy is actually employed, we now return to Steve, our patient who suffers from panic disorder. Similar to the PCT approach to treatment presented in the second-generation section of this chapter, using the ACT therapy approach would involve monitoring of anxiety levels and stressful life events to understand what factors contribute to panic attacks. Further, behavioral techniques, including exposure to bodily sensations and certain exercises such as breathing retraining and relaxation strategies, would still be employed. However, whereas these strategies were formerly employed to control or eliminate anxiety and panic, in ACT, they are employed to shape the patient toward recognizing that panic attacks can be accepted and acknowledged for what they are (e.g., merely inconvenient "false alarms" of the sympathetic nervous system).

As part of the ACT therapeutic process, therapists employ behavioral metaphors to help the patient recognize how efforts to "control" panic sensations actually make the problem worse (Hayes et al., 1996). For example, in the Chinese finger trap metaphor, Steve would be instructed to place his index fingers in an open-ended woven bamboo tube that fits snugly around his index fingers until they touch—the Chinese finger trap! Then he is instructed to discover a method of escape. The device is constructed, however, to constrict more tightly around his fingers, the more he struggles. The solution, of course, is to push his fingers inward, loosening the device and gently twisting it off. The metaphor has great utility in explaining to the patient that the more one struggles trying to control anxiety, the more panic attacks maintain a grip on the patient's life. Similar acceptance-based instructions are used during the selection and assignment of exposure exercises. For instance, during interoceptive exposure, Steve would be encouraged to experience anxiety and try to create a panic attack, rather than try to control it. Paradoxically, these attempts to experience elevated anxiety often reduce anxiety levels and subsequently the probability of having panic attacks. Further, during exteroceptive exposure, Steve would be encouraged to carry out the assigned task, despite his feelings of anxiety. For example, during an exposure assignment to go to a restaurant for 30 minutes, Steve would be encouraged to stay for the specified period of time and also to eat something regardless of how anxious he feels. By giving up previously desperate attempts to eliminate anxiety and panic, Steve would learn to change the function of his previously held belief that panic attacks are "bad" and thereby would be more likely to behave adaptively.

THE FUTURE OF BEHAVIOR THERAPY

Despite the significant growth of behavior therapy as a field and the demonstrated efficacy of behavioral treatments, continued research is warranted on refining existing strategies and developing other interventions. One of the most important unanswered questions pertains to the unknown mechanisms of behavior change and what learning principles are responsible for positive outcomes. Indeed, it is often unclear what exactly leads to behavioral change for even well-studied procedures such as systematic desensitization.

Second, behavior therapists are beginning to examine their strategies without relying solely on the diagnostic nomenclature employed in psychiatry. It has long been known that, despite great efforts to achieve an effective categorization system for psychiatric disturbances, considerable individual differences exist within diagnostic groups. Because this information is crucial in optimizing successful treatment matching of patient problems with strategies, it will be critical to identify which patient and/or therapist characteristics are related to positive outcomes. Additionally, it will be important to investigate whether these predictive relations generalize to patients from various ethnic, gender, and/or socioeconomic groups. Taken together, these efforts will allow a more comprehensive evaluation of pretreatment characteristics that are associated with positive treatment outcome.

Third, although the movement toward empirical validation of psychotherapeutic interventions has looked favorably upon behavior therapy applications, it will be important to monitor carefully how this information will be used and disseminated to the mental health-care system. In many respects, publishing lists of empirically supported treatments has been a commendable effort to communicate to colleagues and consumers that efficacious treatment methods are available to treat many different types of psychological disorders. Additionally, however, direct clinical service issues such as the reimbursement of assessment and/or treatment services have been affected by these changes. Thus, though developing lists of empirically supported therapies has generally been a positive step, at the same time, such changes naturally have led to new questions and concerns that need to be addressed. As one example, published clinical practice guidelines in the form of treatment lists may result in legal proceedings brought against clinicians who do not follow these guidelines (Barlow, 1996). Accordingly, insurance companies may begin to limit reimbursement of services to those psychological disorders for which there are validated treatments. Thus, the regulation of mental health services may involve restricting treatment to those persons who suffer from a disorder for which a standardized treatment exists. Taken together, it is evident that the movement toward empirically supported therapies has been highly influential, at times controversial, and undoubtedly complex. Regardless, behavior therapy has established its role in the mental/behavioral health-care industry as a result of this movement and will certainly continue to evolve and contribute in this arena in clinical, research, and political realms.

Finally, there has been an increasing impetus among behavioral scientists to integrate the important contributions of behavior therapy with other therapeutic orientations, such as psychodynamic and pharmacologic approaches (Bellack & Hersen, 1990), and with other realms of psychological science, including social, developmental, and cognitive psychology (Martin, 1991). These efforts can assure that behavior therapy will continue to expand into new and exciting areas and continue to make important contributions to understanding and treating mental/behavioral problems.

SUMMARY

Behavior therapy has evolved continuously during the past 40 years and has grown from early investigations of conditioning strategies to its present application for virtually every diagnostic mental/behavioral presentation. This evolution has paralleled the changes observed during the same period of time in the field of psychological assessment and diagnosis. For the most part, outcome findings have been impressive and in some cases (e.g., specific phobia, obsessive–compulsive disorder, posttraumatic stress disorder, sexual dysfunction) behavioral therapeutic applications are the treatments of choice. In contrast to other theoretical approaches that have impacted social science during the same period, behavior therapy has progressively evolved, carefully building on the success of previous therapeutic applications. In this regard, although these approaches have evolved over the decades, the importance of operant and classical conditioning phenomena in acquiring and maintaining mental/behavioral problems continues to play a critical role.

Because of the dynamic nature of the field, patients like Steve, depicted in this chapter, would be treated somewhat differently if they sought help from a behavior therapist in each of the past several decades. Although early behavioral interventions focused primarily upon exposure to environmental stimuli associated with problematic behavior, later developments aimed to improve the patient's ability to tolerate the emotional arousal that accompanied these exposures either via training in direct control strategies or those based on acceptance. In sum, behavior therapy has made a significant contribution to understanding the onset and maintenance of mental/behavioral problems and has led scientific efforts to apply this knowledge to treat a myriad of behavioral health-care problems.

REFERENCES

Ayllon, T. (1963). Intensive treatment of psychotic behavior by stimulus satiation and food reinforcement. *Behaviour Research and Therapy, 1*, 53–62.

Barlow, D. H. (1996). The effectiveness of psychotherapy: Science and policy. *Clinical Psychology: Science and Practice, 3*, 236–240.

Barlow, D. H., Craske, M. G., Cerny, J. A., & Klosko, J. S. (1989). Behavioral treatment of panic disorder. *Behavior Therapy, 20*, 261–282.

Barlow, D. H., & Craske, M. G. (1994). *Mastery of your anxiety and panic-II.* Albany, NY: Center for Stress and Anxiety Disorders.

Beck, A. T. (1976). *Cognitive therapy and the emotional disorders.* New York: International Universities Press.

Beck, A. T., Rush, A. J., Shaw, B. F., & Emery, G. (1979). *Cognitive therapy of depression.* New York: Guilford.

Bellack, A. S., & Hersen, M. (Eds.). (1990). *Handbook of comparative treatments of adult disorders.* New York: Wiley.

Chambliss, D. L., Baker, M. J., Baucom, D. H., Beutler, L. E., Calhoun, K. S., Crits-Christoph, P., Daiuto, A., DeRubeis, R., Detweiler, J., Haaga, D. A. F., Johnson, S. B., McCurry, S., Mueser, K. T., Pope, K. S., Sanderson, W. C., Shoham, V., Stickle, T., Williams, D. A., & Woody, S. R. (1998). Update on empirically validated therapies, II. *The Clinical Psychologist, 51*, 3–16.

Hayes, S. C., & Wilson, K. G. (1994). Acceptance and commitment therapy: Altering the verbal support for experiential avoidance. *The Behavior Analyst, 17*, 289–303.

Hayes, S. C., Wilson, K. G., Gifford, E. V., Follette, V., & Strosahl, K. (1996). Experiential avoidance and behavioral disorders: A functional dimensional approach to diagnosis and treatment. *Journal of Consulting and Clinical Psychology, 64*, 1–16.

Linehan, M. M. (1994). Acceptance and change: The central dialectic in psychotherapy. In S. C. Hayes, N. S. Jacobson, V. M. Follette, & M. J. Dougher (Eds.), *Acceptance and change: Content and context in psychotherapy* (pp. 73–86). Reno, NV: Context Press.

Marlatt, G. A. (1994). Addiction, mindfulness, and acceptance. In S. C. Hayes, N. S. Jacobson, V. M., Follette, & M. J. Dougher (Eds.), *Acceptance and change: Content and context in psychotherapy* (pp. 175–197). Reno, NV: Context Press.

Martin, P. R. (Ed.). (1991). *Handbook of behavior therapy and psychological science: An integrative approach.* New York: Pergamon Press.

Meichenbaum, D. H. (1977). *Cognitive-behavior modification.* New York: Plenum Press.

Michelson, L., Mavissakalian, M., & Marchione, K. (1988). Cognitive, behavioral, and psychophysiological treatments of agoraphobia: A comparative outcome investigation. *Behavior Therapy, 19*, 97–120.

Nemeroff, C. J., & Karoly, P. (1991). Operant methods. In F. H. Kanfer & A. P. Goldstein (Eds.), *Helping people change: A textbook of methods* (pp. 122–160). New York: Pergamon Press.

Onken, L. S., Blaine, J. D., & Battjes, R. J. (1997). Behavioral therapy research: A conceptualization of a process. In S. W. Henggeler and A. B. Santos (Eds.), *Innovative approaches for difficult to treat populations* (pp. 477–485). Washington DC: American Psychiatric Press.

Paul, G. L. (1969). Outcome of systematic desensitization II. Controlled investigations of individual treatment, technique variations, and current status. In C. M. Franks (Ed.), *Behavior therapy: Appraisal and status.* New York: McGraw-Hill.

Strosahl, K. D., Hayes, S. C., Bergan, J., & Romano, P. (1998). Assessing the field effectiveness of Acceptance and Commitment Therapy: An example of the manipulated training research method. *Behavior Therapy, 29*, 35–64.

Wolpe, J. (1958). *Psychotherapy by reciprocal inhibition.* Stanford, CA: Stanford University Press.

27

Pharmacological Interventions

DANIEL M. HARRIS, WILLIAM H. WILSON,
AND ANN MARIE HAMER

INTRODUCTION

Psychoactive substances have been identified and used medically and nonmedically for centuries, but scientifically based psychopharmacology is only about 50 years old. Almost all of the medications currently used as psychopharmacological interventions were formulated and approved for use within that time period. Many of the most frequently used medications have been introduced within the past 10 to 15 years (Schatzberg & Nemeroff, 1995). In the mid twentieth century, the first generation of antipsychotic, antidepressant, and antianxiety medications emerged that were discovered largely by serendipity. As we enter the twenty-first century, medications have become an essential component in treating mental disorders, and the process of medication development (see Table 1) has become largely rational, guided by marked advances in neuroscience and technology (Stahl, 1996).

The traditional dichotomy of mind and body has been blurred by scientific findings about mental illness. Epidemiological studies indicate a substantial genetic component for many illnesses. Pharmacological studies show specific effects of particular interventions on the molecular level; for example, the blockade of dopamine receptors leads to a decrease in psychosis, but not of depression. Advanced neuroimaging techniques, such as magnetic resonance imaging (MRI), functional magnetic resonance imaging (fMRI), and positron emission tomography (PET) allow studying of living human brain structure and function in ways which would have been unimaginable only a few years ago. Rigid separation of pharmacological and psychological perspectives on mental illness continue to give way to more holistic, integrative, interactive models of experience and behavior. Similarly, treatment is often multifaceted. Interventions designed to address neurobiological, psychological, and social domains are vitally interlinked. Response to treatment is often based on synergistic effects of the various treatment modalities (Wilson, 1997).

DANIEL M. HARRIS • Oregon Health Sciences University, Portland, Oregon 97201.   **WILLIAM H. WILSON** • Department of Psychiatry, Oregon Health Sciences University, Portland, Oregon 97201.   **ANNE MARIE HAMER** • Oregon State University College of Pharmacy, Portland, Oregon 97201.

Advanced Abnormal Psychology, Second Edition, edited by Hersen and Van Hasselt. Kluwer Academic/Plenum Publishers, New York, 2001.

TABLE 1. Commonly Used Psychiatric Medications[a]

Generic name	Brand name	Type
Antipsychotic medications[b]		
Chlorpromazine	Thorazine	Typical, low-potency
Clozapine	Clozaril	Atypical, for treating refractory illness
Droperidol	Inapsine	Typical, injectable only; for emergency treatment of extreme agitation
Fluphenazine	Prolixin	Typical, high-potency
Fluphenazine decanoate	Prolixin decanoate	Long-acting, depot injectable form of fluphenazine
Haloperidol	Haldol	Typical, high-potency
Haloperidol decanoate	Haldol decanoate	Long-acting, depot injectable form of haloperidol
Loxapine	Loxitane	Typical, mid-potency
Mesoridazine	Serentil	Typical, low-potency
Molindone	Moban	Typical, mid-potency
Olanzapine	Zyprexa	Atypical, first-line agent
Pimozide	Orap	Typical, high-potency
Perphenazine	Trilafon	Typical, mid- to high-potency
Quetiapine	Seroquel	Atypical, first-line agent
Risperidone	Risperdal	Atypical, first-line agent
Thioridazine	Mellaril	Typical, low-potency
Thiothixene	Navane	Typical, high-potency
Trifluoperzine	Stelazine	Typical, high-potency
Ziprasidone	Zeldox	Atypical, not yet marketed, likely to be first-line
Antianxiety medications[c]		
Buspirone	Buspar	Unique medication
Chlordiazepoxide	Librium	Benzodiazepine
Clonazepam	Klonopin	Benzodiazepine
Clorazepate	Tranxene	Benzodiazepine
Diazepam	Valium	Benzodiazepine
Flurazepam	Dalmane	Benzodiazepine
Propranolol	Inderal	Beta-blocker
Lorazepam	Ativan	Benzodiazepine
Oxazepam	Serax	Benzodiazepine
Temazepam	Restoril	Benzodiazepine
Triazolam	Halcion	Benzodiazepine
Antidepressant medications		
Amitriptyline	Elavil	Tricyclic antidepressant
Amoxapine	Asendin	Tetracyclic
Bupropion	Wellbutrin	New generation
Citalopram	Celexa	Selective serotonin re-uptake inhibitor
Clomipraime	Anafranil	Tricyclic antidepressant
Desipramine	Norpramin, Pertofrane	Tricyclic antidepressant
Doxepin	Adaptin, Sinequan	Tricyclic antidepressant
Fluoxetine	Prozac	Selective serotonin re-uptake inhibitor
Fluvoxamine	Luvox	Selective serotonin re-uptake inhibitor
Imipramine	Tofranil	Tricyclic antidepressant
Isocarboxazid	Marplan	Monoamine oxidate inhibitor
Maprotiline	Ludiomil	Tetracyclic
Mirtazapine	Remeron	New generation
Nafazodone	Serzone	New generation
Nortriptyline	Aventyl, Pamelor	Tricyclic antidepressant

TABLE 1. (Continued)

Generic name	Brand name	Type
Antidepressant medications (cont.)		
Paroxetine	Paxil	Selective serotonin re-uptake inhibitor
Phenelzine	Nardil	Monoamine oxidate inhibitor
Protriptyline	Vivactil	Tricyclic antidepressant
Sertraline	Zoloft	Selective serotonin re-uptake inhibitor
Tranylcypromine	Parnate	Monoamine oxidate inhibitor
Trazodone	Desyrel	New generation
Trimipramine	Surmontil	Tricyclic antidepressant
Venlafaxine	Effexor	New generation
Mood-stabilizing medications		
Carbamazepine	Tegretol	Anticonvulsant
Divalproex	Depakote	Anticonvulsant
Lamotrigine	Lamictal	Anticonvulsant, newer, less well studied
Gabapentin	Neurotin	Anticonvulsant, newer, less well studied
Lithium (carbonate, citrate)	Cibalith-S, Eskalith, Eskalith CR, Lithan, Lithobid, Lithotabs	Elemental ion
Topiramate	Topamax	Anticonvulsant, newer, less well studied
Valproic acid	Depakene	Anticonvulsant
Additional medications for substance abuse		
Bupropion	Zyban	Reduces tobacco craving
Disulfiram	Antabuse	Causes alcohol to produce unpleasant symptoms
Methadone	Dolophine	Opiate replacement for heroin
Naltrexone	Revia	Reduces reward experience from alcohol
Additional medications used in head injury and dementia		
Amantadine	Symmetrel	Dopamine agonist
Bromocriptine	Parlodel	Dopamine agonist
Dextroamphetamine	Dexedrine	Stimulant
Donepezil	Aricept	Cognitive enhancer
Methylphenidate	Ritalin	Stimulant
Tacrine	Cognex	Cognitive enhancer
Medications used to treat side effects of typical antipsychotics		
Trihexyphenidyl	Artane	Anticholinergic
Procyclidine	Kemadrin	Anticholinergic
Biperiden	Akineton	Anticholinergic
Benztropine	Cogentin	Anticholinergic
Amantadine	Symmetrel	Dopamine agonist
Diphenhydramine	Benadryl	Anticholinergic/antihistamine

[a]Medications are categorized by original use, primary use, or point of discussion in the text. Use may overlap among categories. Medications are listed only once. Generic name refers to the specific chemical name of the medication. Brand names are pharmaceutical trademarks for specific preparations. The brands listed are the most common in the United States. Brand names differ in other countries.

[b]"Typical" antipsychotics are the older agents that have more side effects than the newer agents. Potency refers to the number of milligrams needed for daily dose. At therapeutic doses, all typical antipsychotics have similar efficacy. Side effects vary with potency. See text for discussion. "Atypical" antipsychotics are the newer, preferred agents. "First-line" drugs are those regarded as the primary treatment, and other medications are used when response to "first-line" agents is inadequate or side effects are intolerable. Clozapine is reserved for patients whose symptoms do not respond to other medications because of the risk of decreased white blood cell production.

[c]As discussed, "antidepressants" also play a significant role in treating anxiety.

The role of medication in treating mental disorders is highly variable. At times, medication is the only treatment that an individual requires for optimal benefit. More often, medication treatment is one component of an integrated treatment plan that also includes psychotherapeutic and social interventions. In other instances, psychotherapeutic or social intervention are the preferred treatment, and medication plays a minor role or is not indicated. At times, pharmacological and nonpharmacological treatments are equally appropriate, and the matter is one of individual preference. Clearly, psychopharmacological medications are powerful tools and can provide considerable benefits if used wisely, but they can also be misused. Rigorous clinical research on treatment outcomes is required to evaluate the utility of specific treatments and combinations of treatments. The challenge for practitioners is to use medications rationally and effectively in a comprehensive treatment plan that best meets the needs of the individual (Diamond, 1998).

This chapter explores the pharmacological component of treatment for the major categories of mental disorders and in the process, reviews the major classes of psychiatric medications.

General Considerations

Before discussing pharmacological interventions for particular disorders, some general considerations regarding pharmacological interventions are presented. Medication of mental disorders is carried out similarly to general medical treatments. Informed consent from the individual or a legally authorized surrogate is required for treatment. Laws vary from state to state regarding competency to give informed consent and procedures for legal authorization for treatment without the person's consent. Ideally, the individual and the prescribing professional (who may be a psychiatrist, general physician, nurse practitioner, or physician's assistant) develop a collaborative relationship, and the individual takes an active role in decision making. Nonmedical mental health professionals play a vital role in this process by helping individuals to understand the risks and benefits of treatment, by monitoring response to treatment, and by facilitating effective communication with the prescribing professional.

Accurate diagnosis of a particular illness and symptoms is an essential first step in treatment planning. The use of standard diagnostic criteria (American Psychiatric Association, 1994) allows clinicians to predict response on the basis of scientifically designed outcome studies. "Efficacy studies" determine drug response under highly controlled conditions. Subjects are selected who clearly meet diagnostic criteria for the medication's principal use and are otherwise healthy. Treatment proceeds according to predetermined schedules and procedures. Subjects who cannot follow the protocol are dropped from the study. These studies provide essential information on drug effects by eliminating confounding variables. However, many of these confounds are present in everyday clinical situations. In contrast, "effectiveness studies" examine the medication response under "real-world" conditions of greater diagnostic variability among subjects, frequent occurrences of other concurrent mental and general medical illness, and less strict adherence to treatment recommendations by study subjects. In real-world clinical situations, treatment sometimes must begin before all of the information is available to make a definitive diagnosis. In such cases, treatment is targeted to specific symptoms and proceeds while information is gathered to continue making a more definitive diagnosis. This practice is analogous to a general medical doctor using medication to bring down a fever while proceeding with tests to determine the particular cause of the patient's elevated temperature.

Pharmacological interventions reduce the severity of symptoms and protect against the recurrence of symptoms; however, medications do not "cure" the disorder. In this respect, psychopharmacological treatments are similar to the treatments of diabetes mellitus with insulin or rheumatoid arthritis with anti-inflammatory agents, where the goal is to reduce symptoms and prevent relapse. There are indications, however, that prompt pharmacological interventions may slow the natural progression of schizophrenia and severe mood disorders. Perhaps someday, treatments based on genetic engineering will correct underlying genetic defects, but no such "cures" should be expected in the immediate future.

Some medications have immediate effects on target symptoms (e.g., relief of anxiety within minutes of ingesting a benzodiazepine), but the therapeutic benefits of many medications develop slowly during a period of weeks (e.g., response to antidepressants) and have their therapeutic effects through a process termed "initiation and adaptation." In such instances, the medication's immediate neurochemical effect is to initiate a complex cascade of neurochemical responses that unfold during a period of weeks. The gradual adaptation of the brain to the medication results in gradual changes in experience and behavior. The initial weeks of treatment are often difficult because the person may have side effects with little or more therapeutic effects. Patience, persistence, and psychosocial support are necessary during this period of waiting for a therapeutic response. At times, sequential trials of several medications are required to find the medication that is most helpful to a particular person. The process of transition from one medication to the next must be carefully orchestrated to avoid drug interactions and symptom relapse.

There are a number of instances in which several psychotropic medications should be used concurrently, at times, because of the specificity of action of the particular drugs. For example, an individual who has bipolar affective disorder and has a depressive episode accompanied by persecutory delusions would probably be treated with three drugs: an antidepressant to normalize mood, a mood stabilizer to prevent emergence of mania, and an antipsychotic to reduce the delusions. At times drugs from similar classes are used together to achieve synergistic effects. Problems of excessive side effects and drug interactions are more likely when several drugs are used at the same time. If multiple drugs are used, there should be a clear rationale for each medication, an understanding of potential interactions, and a clear plan for monitoring the effectiveness of each medication and the possible emergence of adverse effects.

Some medications, particularly the older antidepressants and lithium, are highly toxic and potentially lethal in overdose. Care must be taken to assure that a suicidal or cognitively impaired individual does not have access to a potentially lethal supply of medication. Family members may at times help with monitoring access to medication. A few of the psychotropics, such as the benzodiazepines, can be abused. Other medications, such as the antipsychotics, have little abuse potential but are used on the street to moderate the effects of street drugs. Careful monitoring of treatment reduces the risk that therapeutic agents will be used improperly.

Medications are often quite expensive and represent a significant expense to individuals, government agencies, and health plans. Considerations of cost-effectiveness are having an increasing impact on the choice of medications. Estimations of cost need to take into account all of the costs associated with the illness, not just the price of the drug. For example, an expensive, but effective, medication could result in significant overall savings if it reduced the need for hospital care, eliminated crises with the police, and allowed the individual to return to work, and so forth. But, if there are not distinct advantages between medications, the lower priced agent is clearly the better choice.

Medications are named in several ways, and the designations can be confusing. General terms refer to the most common or original therapeutic use (e.g., "an antidepressant"), despite the fact that the drug may also have other uses (e.g., "antidepressants" are the treatment of choice for some anxiety disorders). Medicines may be referred to by their characteristic neurochemical action (e.g., "the norepinephrine and serotonin re-uptake inhibitors"). Medicines may be grouped on the basis of common chemical structures (e.g., "tricyclic" antidepressants). The chemical name for an individual drug is the "generic name" and is written in lower case ("diazepam"). A manufacturer's trademark for its particular preparation of a drug is indicated by an initial capital letter (Valium).

Depression and Other Mood Disorders

Transient feelings of discouragement, low mood, lack of interest in life, as well as transient states of irritability, elation, and increased energy are a part of normal life and usually occur in response to unpleasant events or especially exciting ones. Mood disorders are diagnosed when affective states become sufficiently intense, prolonged, and unresponsive to everyday events so that individuals experience marked suffering or have marked difficulty with their normal social roles and responsibilities (Agency for Health Care Policy and Research, 1999b; Harris, 1999b). Major depressive disorder is characterized by a constellation of symptoms involving mood, cognition, and bodily functions. Persistent feelings of unhappiness and worthlessness and unresponsiveness to good news or happy events are accompanied by lack of interest in activities that are usually enjoyable, lack of energy, disrupted sleep, decreased libido, and increased or decreased appetite. Suicidal thoughts and attempts are not uncommon. Overly pessimistic thoughts may progress to frankly delusional ideals, such as beliefs that one has caused all of the evil and suffering in the world or that one's body is rotting away. Antidepressant medications provide significant symptomatic improvement for more than 70% of individuals who have major depression. In delusional depressions, an antipsyhchotic medication (discussed later) is used concurrently with antidepressants. Dysthymic Disorder, characterized by persistent but less severe depressive symptoms, also responded to these medications. Antidepressants usually have little or no effect on the mood of people who are not depressed.

Medications help with all of the symptoms of depression, not only with mood. Improvement occurs gradually during a period of several weeks. Frequently, vegetative symptoms such as sleep disturbance and decreased energy begin to improve before mood improves. Improvement may be noticed by family members and caregivers before it is apparent to the depressed person. Newer medications allow safer, more comfortable treatment than was available in the past. Continued treatment with antidepressants following the resolution of depression reduces the rate of recurrence in the future. The optimal length of time to continue full antidepressant doses after symptoms are resolved is somewhat controversial. Two to three years of maintenance treatment is often reasonable, and longer periods are advisable for persons who have had recurrent, severe episodes. Antidepressants should be discontinued by gradually decreasing the dose over several weeks to avoid the anxiety and flu-like symptoms that may accompany abrupt discontinuation.

Four classes of antidepressant medications are currently in use: monoamine oxidase inhibitors (MAOIs), tricyclic antidepressants (TCAs), selective serotonin re-uptake inhibitors (SSRIs), and new generation agents. MAOIs and TCAs have been used since the 1950s. The MAOIs and TCAs are effective antidepressants, but they are quite toxic and often lethal in overdose, a serious concern in treating potentially suicidal individuals. In addition, the MAOIs can cause life-threatening reactions to common foods and medications. The SSRIs and new generation antidepressants are equally effective as the older drugs and much less toxic. Overdose with these drugs may be uncomfortable, but they rarely cause serious medical problems or death. For this reason, most people are now treated with SSRIs or new generation medications. The newer medications have fewer side effects than the older ones, but they are far from perfect.

The antidepressant properties of MAOIs and TCAs were discovered by serendipity in the 1950s. At that time, iproniazid, an MAOI, was used to treat tuberculosis. An astute clinician noted that the mood of depression patients improved during iproniazid treatment. The first TCA, imipramine (Tofranil), was developed with the expectation that it would have antipsychotic properties. It had little effect on psychosis but was observed to improve mood. It was later determined that iproniazid and imipramine each increased the availability of the neurotransmitters norepinephrine and serotonin within synapses, although by different mechanisms. Other drugs that have similar structures and functions were quickly developed. In contrast, the SSRIs and new generation antidepressants were not found by chance. Rather they are the product of concerted research efforts by the pharmaceutical industry to construct molecules that increase synaptic norepinephrine and/or serotonin without causing toxicity and side effects. Symptomatic improvement occurs as the brain adapts to these higher levels of neurotransmitters during a period of around 6 weeks. Because of differences among the drugs, a person who does not respond well to one drug may respond to another. About 70% of patients respond at least moderately well to the first medicine. It is not possible to predict response to specific antidepressants in advance. Rather, the initial drug is chosen on the basis of its side-effect profile and individual preferences of the individual and practitioner.

Two MAOIs, phenelzine (Nardil) and tranylcypromine (Parnate), are commonly available in the United States. A third, isocarboxazid (Marplan), is being phased out by the manufacturer but is available in cases of special need. The MAOIs increase synaptic norepinephrine and serotonin by deactivating the enzyme monoamine oxidase (MAO). MAO degrades norepinephrine and serotonin as a part of normal metabolism. Deactivation of the enzyme leads to the desired effect of increased synaptic norepinephrine and serotonin but has problematic effects as well. The enzyme also normally degrades certain drugs and dietary substances (such as tyramine, an amino acid), protecting the body from the elevations in blood pressure caused by these substances. Thus, the concurrent use of MAOIs and common drugs (e.g., over-the-counter cold preparations and nasal sprays) or foods (e.g., ripe cheeses, wines and beers, prepared meats, Italian broad beans) may lead to myocardial infarction, stroke, or death. Lists of problematic drugs and foods are commonly available. Individuals can safely take MAOIs by judiciously avoiding the drugs and foods. Nevertheless, because of the risk of hypertensive crisis and toxicity in overdose, the MAOIs are primarily used as second- or third-line agents for depressed persons whose symptoms have not responded to other classes of antidepressants. A few newer MAOIs that have markedly better safety profiles (e.g., moclobemide [Aurorix]) are widely used in other countries but are not yet approved for use in the United States.

Tricyclic antidepressants (TCAs) take their name from the characteristic three-ringed chemical structure. These drugs increase norepinephrine and serotonin availability in synapses by blocking the molecular pumps that normally recycle these neurotransmitters back into presynaptic neurons for reuse. Seven TCAs are currently in use: desipramine (Norpramin), amitriptyline (Elavil), nortriptyline (Pamelor, Aventil), trimipramine (Surmontil), protriptyline (Vivactil), doxepin (Adapin, Sinequan), and clomipramine (Anafranil). Clomipramine differs from the other agents in that it primarily inhibits re-uptake of serotonin and was approved by the Food and Drug Administration (FDA) for treating obsessive–compulsive disorder. Nonetheless, clomipramine is widely used to treat depression. Two antidepressants, whose chemical structures contain four rings, rather than three, are usually considered to belong to this group: maprotiline (Ludiomil), amoxapine (Asendin). These agents offer no particular advantages over tricyclics.

As previously noted, the primary drawback to TCAs is their toxicity in overdose. A week's worth of medication is usually a lethal dose. The effects are additive to the sedative properties of alcohol and make an overdose with this combination especially lethal. Other side effects are not dangerous but are sufficiently bothersome that many people choose to discontinue treatment in the early weeks before therapeutic benefits are evident. Side effects may also lead to discontinuing maintenance medication and recurrence of depression. These side effects include anticholinergic side effects (side effects due to blockade of receptors for acetylcholine: constipation, dry mouth, urinary retention, decreased sweating), orthostatic hypotension (dizziness after rising to a standing position), weight gain, decreased libido, impotence, and menstrual irregularity. Not everyone taking TCAs will develop all of these problems. The side effects are particularly troublesome for the elderly. The orthostatic hypotension associated with TCAs may lead to confusion or to potentially serious falls in this population. Despite these drawbacks, TCAs are highly useful medicines for many people.

Five selective serotonin re-uptake inhibitors (SSRIs) are approved for clinical use and are among the most widely prescribed medications in the United States. Fluoxetine (Prozac) became available in the late 1980s, and these others have gradually followed: sertraline (Zoloft), paroxetine (Paxil), fluvoxamine (Luvox, approved for obsessive–compulsive disorder but widely used as an antidepressant), citalopram (Celexa). SSRIs share the common trait of inhibiting the re-uptake of serotonin into presynaptic neurons and having much less effect on the re-uptake of norepinephrine and other neurochemicals. Such relative selectivity in comparison to TCAs and MAOIs leads SSRIs to have fewer side effects and considerable less toxicity. Overdoses of SSRIs, even in combination with alcohol, may be uncomfortable but are seldom lethal. Detractors have blamed these drugs for suicide and violence, although these claims are not supported by the data from longitudinal treatment studies or analysis of the specific cases.

Although considerably safer and better tolerated than the older medications, SSRIs are not free from side effects. Weight gain is common, as is mild GI distress and headache. Decreased spontaneity and apathy may occur after months of treatment and are often confused with a recurrence of depression. Sexual side effects, in the form of decreased sexual desire and difficulty in achieving orgasm, are common in both women and men. SSRIs interfere with the liver's ability to metabolize a variety of medications, so the use of SSRIs can increased blood levels of other medications. Usually this can be handled through dosage adjustment. SSRIs at high doses, or in combination with other medications (such as the MAOIs, other SSRIs, and the cough suppressant dextromethorphan) can precipitate a serious systemic reaction termed the "serotonin syndrome." Symptoms include unstable blood pressure, disorientation, agitation, gastrointestinal distress, hyperactive motor reflexes, and fever.

The new generation antidepressants (also called "novel" or "atypical" antidepressants) are grouped together not on the basis of their chemical structure or their mode of action, but because they are relatively new and do not fit into the other categories. These antidepressants include trazodone (Desyrel), nefazodone (Serzone), bupropion (Wellbutrin), venlafaxine (Effexor), and mirtazapine (Remeron). All of these except trazodone are commonly used as initial treatments for depression. None has serious toxicity in overdose. Neurochemical effects are largely through re-uptake inhibition of norepinephrine and serotonin. Each agent is in some way unique, but it is it not possible to give a detailed description of each one within the space allotted to this chapter. Full descriptions appear in works by Diamond (1998) and Schatzberg and Nemeroff (1995). The efficacy of these agents is comparable to those agents in the other classes. Trazodone, however, is so sedating that few patients can take a full therapeutic dose. It is often used at low doses as a nonaddictive sleeping pill. The medications are generally well tolerated and have relatively few side effects. Individual patients, however, may develop uncomfortable side effects from any of the medications. Bupropion, nefazodone, and mirtazapine are particularly free of sexual side effects. Bupropion also reduces cravings for cigarettes and is marketed under a different trade name (Zyban) for smoking cessation. Mirtazapine has antianxiety effects, is mildly sedating, and causes weight gain. Together with SSRIs, these medications are now the mainstay of antidepressant treatment.

Bipolar Affective Disorder and Mood Stabilizers

Bipolar affective disorder is a common, debilitating condition in which depressive episodes alternate with episodes of mania and periods of relatively normal mood. Manic episodes are characterized by greatly increased energy, little need for sleep, euphoria or irritability, and poor judgment. During manic episodes, individuals may spend money wildly, have spontaneous sexual relationships, drive recklessness, and otherwise endanger themselves and their social situations. Depressive episodes are similar to the episodes of major depressive disorder. Mixed episodes that have simultaneous features of depression and mania are possible. Delusions and hallucinations, as well as suicide attempts, may occur in mania or depression. Milder forms of the illness also occur. Pharmacological treatment reduces the intensity of episodes and prolongs the time between episodes. With treatment, many people who have bipolar disorder lead highly productive, stable lives (Frances, Kahn, Carpenter, Docherty, & Donovan, 1998).

Mood-stabilizing medications are used continuously in treating bipolar disorder. Lithium is the prototypic mood stabilizer. Several medications that were initially developed as antiepilepsy medicines are also widely used as mood stabilizers: divalproex (Depakote), valproic acid (Depakene), and carbamazepine (Tegretol). Newer anticonvulsants have been studied less thoroughly but are being used widely for individuals who do not respond well to usual treatment: lamotrigine (Lamictal), gabapentin (Neurontin), and topiramate (Topamax). The antipsychotic medications discussed later also have antimanic properties.

Lithium has been used as a mood stabilizer since the 1950s. It has no effect on the mood of normal individuals. For treatment of bipolar illness, it helps to keep mood within the normal range. It is effective in treating manic episodes and in preventing their recurrence. It has some antidepressant properties and decreases the recurrence of depressions. Lithium is an element in the same family as sodium and potassium. Like those elements, it is found naturally as salts. When used as medicines, lithium salts dissolve readily, and the positively charged lithium ions are absorbed and distributed through the bloodstream in the same manner as sodium and potassium. It is cleared from the body through the kidneys by the same mechanisms that clear sodium and potassium. Lithium has complex actions on the chemical processes within nerve cells, and its exact therapeutic mechanism is unclear. Unlike the antidepressants and antipsychotics, it does not directly effect neurotransmission. In mania, response to lithium is gradual and requires about 10 days for significant improvement. Blood tests for lithium levels are necessary because individuals vary in the oral dose needed to produce a therapeutic blood level and because therapeutic blood levels are only slightly above toxic. Measurement of blood levels allows maintaining the dose within the narrow therapeutic range. At therapeutic levels, common side effects include mild gastrointestinal distress, mild tremor, and weight gain. Because lithium suppresses thyroid function, supplementary thyroid hormone may be necessary. If lithium levels rise above the therapeutic range, initial side effects are nausea and diarrhea, followed by clumsiness and mental clouding. Overdose may result in coma and death. Not everyone who has bipolar disorder responds to lithium.

In recent years, divalproex and the other anticonvulsants have been used increasingly as mood stabilizers. Presently, divalproex is the most commonly prescribed drug for mania and is quite frequently used as a maintenance medication to prevent future episodes. Divalproex has several advantages over lithium. Individuals who respond to lithium are likely to respond to divalproex. Divalproex is more effective than lithium in rapid-cycling bipolar disorder (depression and mania alternation over a few days) and in mixed episodes (irritability, depressed mood coexist with manic symptoms). Blood levels are measured, but less frequently because the therapeutic range is much wider, and high levels are of less concern. At therapeutic doses, side effects include weight gain and occasionally, mental clouding. Excessive doses result in gastrointestinal disturbance, clumsiness, and further cognitive disturbance. Nonetheless, the medication is relatively safe, even in massive overdoses.

The chemical mechanism of divalproex is complex and not fully understood. As with lithium, the actions occur within nerve cells, rather than at the synapse. During absorption in the intestine, divalproex is split into two identical molecules of valproate. It is the valproate ion, not divalproex, which is active in the nervous system. Valproate can be administered directly in the form of valproic acid (Depakene), but it causes more upset stomach. Other anticonvulsants have mood stabilizing properties but have been less well studied. Carbamazepine has been used for many years but has many interactions with other medications. Gabapentin and lamotrigine are newer medications that are being increasingly employed as second-line agents. Topiramate is receiving attention because it tends to cause weight loss rather than weight gain and thus is acceptable as a long-term medication to people who are unwilling to continue divalproex due to weight change. Antipsychotic medications are fairly effective as mood stabilizers, but side effects have limited their utility. Two of the newer atypical antipsychotics are gaining prominence in treating affective disorder. Clozapine (Clozaril) is useful in some cases of poor response. Olanzapine (Zyprexa) may be useful as a first-line agent, but more study is required.

During episodes of depression, improvement is hastened by using antidepressant medications in conjunction with a mood stabilizer. As with major depression, SSRIs and new generation agents are the usual choices. Antidepressants can provoke manic episodes in bipolar illness but are safely used as long as a mood stabilizer is also given. Antidepressants are not continued as maintenance medications in bipolar disorder because they tend to cause more rapid mood cycling.

Mood stabilizers all have adverse effects on fetal development. Women who have bipolar illness must use adequate birth control methods throughout treatment. Normal pregnancies are possible but require careful planning and collaboration of the woman with her physician, so that medications can be stopped during key periods of fetal development.

Other Somatic Treatments

Various preparations of the herb St.-John'-wort (*Hypericum perforatum*) are sold in the United States without prescription. St.-John's-wort is used medically in Germany and several other European nations (Linde, Ramirez, Mulrow, Pauls, Weidenhammer, & Melchart, 1996). Data from several small clinical trials indicate that standardized preparations of hypericum are effective relative to placebo in treating the symptoms of mild to moderate depression. This substance has not been evaluated for approval by the FDA, and its formulation and purity are not regulated. Caution should be exercised in recommending this substance to depressed patients in place of approved antidepressant medications. St.-John's-wort is usually well tolerated, but side effects and interaction with drugs are being reported with increasing frequency. Its use in combination with prescription serotonergic substances may lead to the medically serious serotonin syndrome reaction. Patients should not use antidepressants and hypericum concurrently. S-adenosyl-methionine (SAMe), a substance naturally produced in the human body, is being developed for several uses including antidepressant pharmaco-therapy. SAMe is currently available in several European countries by prescription. It is not FDA-approved or -regulated in the United States, but it is beginning to appear on the shelves of health food stores as a dietary supplement.

Three other somatic treatments for depression are worth discussing as alternatives or adjuncts to pharmacological intervention. Bright light treatment has proven beneficial in seasonal affective disorder. Light treatment affects the production and regulation of melatonin, a hormone that has multiple effects in the brain. Electroconvulsive therapy (ECT), as presently administered, is arguably the single most effective treatment for depression that is currently available. The present procedure is carried out under anesthesia, with complete muscle relaxation in the surgical area of a hospital, and bears little resemblance to the dangerous, outmoded "shock treatments" of the past. Transcranial magnetic stimulation (TMS) is a promising technology that is in the early stages of development and eventually may play a significant role in treating depression.

ANXIETY DISORDERS

A degree of anxiety and fear are part and parcel of everyday life and may help a person adapt to challenging or dangerous situations, but the extreme, chronic, anticipatory, or uncontrollable anxieties that occur in anxiety disorders impair rather than enhance function-ing. The DSM-IV groups a number of somewhat disparate conditions under this general category. The most prominent are generalized anxiety disorder, panic disorder, specific and social phobias, obsessive–compulsive disorder, and posttraumatic and acute stress disorders. The term "antianxiety medication" usually refers to a single class of drugs, the benzodiaze-pines, of which diazepam (Valium) is the prototypic example. However, antidepressants, a unique agent called buspirone (BuSpar), and several types of agents also play a significant role in treating anxiety. Pharmacological treatment depends on the particular disorder and often needs to be carefully coordinated with psychosocial treatments.

Considerable progress has been made in treating anxiety during the past 40 years. Alcohol and opium alkaloids were used for centuries but suffered from the drawbacks of tolerance, abuse, dependence, and withdrawal (frequently accompanied by seizures) from prolonged use and toxicity in high doses. During the nineteenth and early twentieth centuries, bromides, chloral hydrate, paraldehyde, barbiturates, and meprobamate (Miltown) were intro-duced but were subsequently abandoned because of the same drawbacks. Each of these early nonselective CNS depressants exhibits a dose response continuum ranging from anxiety relief to disinhibition, sedation, hypnosis (sleep), coma, and death. Furthermore, the therapeutic dose/toxic dose window for these agents is typically very narrow. When the benzodiazepines were introduced, beginning with chlordiazepoxide (Librium) in the early 1960s, all of these earlier medications were abandoned as antianxiety medications, although some continue to be used for other indications (e.g., opiates for severe pain, barbiturates for induction of general anesthesia).

Benzodiazepines are effective antianxiety agents and have a very rapid onset of action that is sustained during long-term treatment. When used under medical supervision for well-diagnosed anxiety disorders, they are quite safe and effective. Benzodiazepines available in the United States are chlordiazepoxide (Librium), diazepam (Valium), flurazepam (Dalmane), clorazepate (Tranxene), halazepam (Paxipam), prazepam (Centrax), lorazepam (Ativan), oxazepam (Serax), temazepam (Restoril), triazolam (Halcion), and the two triazolobenzodiazepines, alprazolam (Xanax) and clonazepam (Klonopin). Benzodiazepines act by enhancing the effects of γ-aminobutyric acid (GABA), the brain's primary inhibitory neurotransmitter.

All of the current benzodiazepines have similar pharmacodynamics (all enhance GABA and have equivalent efficacy at relieving anxiety) and are distinguished primarily by their pharmacokinetics (absorption, metabolism, half-life, therapeutic dosage, time to onset, and clearance and elimination). Some, like chlordiazepoxide, diazepam, clorazepate, and halazepam, are relatively long acting (their half-lives are on the order of 20 to 60 hours); others, like lorazepam and clonazepam, are intermediate acting (their half-lives are 15 to 30 hours); and still others, like oxazepam, temazepam, triazolam, and alprazolam, are relatively short acting (their half-lives are 2½ to 12 hours). Similarly, some benzodiazepines are rapidly absorbed and have short times to onset (e.g., diazepam, temazepam, and triazolam), whereas other take much longer to act (e.g., clonazepam and oxazepam). Practitioners typically choose a benzodiazepine by matching its pharmacokinetics with the properties desired for a particular patient (e.g., rapid onset for stress-related anxiety or insomnia or short half-life and rapid clearance for elderly patients whose metabolisms are slowed).

Benzodiazepines have marked therapeutic effects, but they also have disadvantages. Benzodiazepines can be abused, particularly by people who have a history of abusing alcohol or street drugs. The body develops tolerance to benzodiazepines within a few weeks of treatment, so that a withdrawal syndrome occurs if the medication is abruptly discontinued. All benzodiazepines cause some sedation, so caution must be used when driving or using machinery. Use by the elderly must be closely monitored to prevent accidental falls due to sedation. Benzodiazepines interfere with memory, and the short acting agents cause most of the problems. At times benzodiazepines disinhibit behavior and interfere with judgment. This is similar to the disinhibition caused by alcohol.

Buspirone (BuSpar) is a relatively new antianxiety agent that is not addictive and does not potentiate the effects of alcohol or other CNS depressants. Buspirone does not adversely affect cognition or coordination and is not sedating. It has no withdrawal syndrome and no particular abuse potential. In clinical trials, its efficacy is similar to that of diazepam in anxious patients after one month. The principal drawback is that the therapeutic effects occur over a period of a few weeks rather than immediately. This delay in action, compared to benzodiazepines, is at times difficult for patients who know that relief would be immediate if they took benzodiazepines. It also has some antidepressant properties. Thus, it is well suited for treating chronic anxiety and may be especially well suited for use by the elderly, medically ill, and substance abusers. In contrast to benzodiazepines, it does not enhance GABA. Rather, buspirone partially stimulates a subclass of serotonin receptors (5-HT1A receptors). Two other groups of medications are often used in treating anxiety disorders. Sedating antihistamines (e.g., diphenhydramine [Benadryl] and hydroxyzine [Vistaril, Atarax]) are sometimes used for their sedative effects for patients who have a history of substance abuse or who have anxiety-related dermatological conditions that may respond to the antihistamine properties of these agents.

Generalized anxiety disorder (GAD) is characterized by excessive, free-floating, chronic anxiety, that causes the individual distress and interferes with daily life. Benzodiazepines are the most common treatment. Buspirone (BuSpar) is an alternative that is probably under-utilized. Antidepressants, including the TCAs and SSRIs, have some efficacy but are not first-line drugs for GAD.

In panic disorder, overwhelming feelings of dread and doom come out of the blue, accompanied by sweating and rapid heartbeat. Individuals may believe that they are having a heart attack and may present to an emergency room. As episodes tend to occur in public places, agoraphobia develops as an adaptive response. The frequency and severity of panic episodes are reduced by treatment with "antidepressant" medications. Antidepressants from all four classes are effective, but SSRIs are the most commonly used agents. Benzodiazepines, discussed later, are secondary agents. Even when panic attacks are well controlled by medica-tion, behavior therapy may be required to overcome an individual's avoidance of situations that triggered panic in the past.

Specific phobias, such as fears of animals, elevators, or flying, are usually treated by behavior therapy. Social phobias, on the other hand, often respond to antidepressants. Again, SSRIs are the most widely used. Performance anxieties, such as fear of public speaking or of playing music in public, are often allayed by using "beta-blockers" such as propranolol (Inderal). Beta-blockers dampen autonomic arousal and allow the individual to proceed confidently through the feared activity without the usual sweaty palms, shaky hands, weak knees, and such.

Obsessive–compulsive disorder is characterized by repetitive unpleasant thoughts (ob-sessions) and repetitive, ritualistic actions that are designed to limit anxiety (compulsions). Antidepressant drugs that have serotonin-enhancing properties are the most effective phar-macological treatments. As previously noted, two such agents, clomipramine and fluvox-amine, are approved by the FDA for treating obsessive–compulsive disorder rather than depression (Expert Consensus Panel on Obsessive–Compulsive Disorder, 1997).

Posttraumatic stress disorder (PTSD) and acute stress disorders occur following partic-ularly stressful events. Posttraumatic stress disorder may be present years after the event, whereas acute stress disorder is the occurrence of the symptom within the first month following the stressor. PTSD was initially recognized in combat veterans, but events also occur in civilian life that are sufficiently stressful to induce the disorder. Common symptoms include vivid recollections of the events, "flashbacks" of being in the event, sleep disturbance, emotional numbing, and a host of related symptoms. Similar symptoms occur in the acute disorder and are likely to predict development of the chronic disorder. Several agents are useful in treating PTSD, and treatment must be tailored to the individual. SSRIs are useful to many. Agents that block autonomic hyperarousal, such as clonidine and propranolol, may be useful. In other instances divalproex, gabapentin, or other mood stabilizers may be helpful. There are few studies of the acute disorder, but benzodiazepines are often prescribed to relieve anxiety acutely. There has been speculation that prompt treatment will limit the chronic effects of the trauma.

SCHIZOPHRENIA AND OTHER PSYCHOTIC DISORDERS

The hallmarks of psychosis are hallucinations, delusions, and thought disorder. There are many causes for psychosis, including medical and neurological conditions, intoxication and withdrawal from medicines and street drugs, and various psychiatric disorders. The "psychotic disorders" are syndromes in which psychosis is the principal symptom. Among the psychotic disorders, schizophrenia is the most prevalent and perhaps the most problematic. Schizophrenia is a lifelong disabling illness that affects just under 1% of the population. It is caused by a poorly characterized interaction of genetic and environmental factors. Psychotic symptoms usually appear first in early adulthood, following a period of decreased social functioning. Numerous structural and functional abnormalities have been noted, but these findings remain pieces of a conceptual puzzle waiting to be solved. Schizophrenia is best treated by a comprehensive program of antipsychotic medication, specific forms of rehabilitation, supportive psychotherapy, and practical social support. Newer medications, introduced within the past few years, represent marked improvements over the older ones. These medicines have engendered a renewed sense of hope among many people with schizophrenia and among their family members (American Psychiatric Association, 1997; Expert Consensus Panel on Schizophrenia, 1996; Harris, 1999a).

The symptoms of schizophrenia are grouped into four overlapping domains that are designated "positive," "negative," "cognitive," and "affective." Positive symptoms are the defining symptoms of psychosis: hallucination, delusions, thought disorder, bizarre behavior, and the like. "Negative" symptoms include flat or blunted affect, blunting of perception, poverty of thought or speech, apathy and lack of motivation, feelings of emptiness and anhedonia, psychomotor retardation and inactivity, and social isolation. The terms "positive" and "negative" symptoms had their origin in neurological theories that are no longer current, but the distinction between the domains remains useful. Cognitive symptoms include deficits in attention, perception, judgment, and similar executive (problem-solving) functions, memory, and learning. Affective symptoms usually are discouragement, demoralization, and depression of varying severity. Over the years, the severity of symptoms fluctuates. Periods of especially severe symptoms are termed "relapses" or "acute episodes." Complete recovery between episodes is rare, even with optimal treatment.

Antipsychotic medications are grouped into two distinct classes: the older "typical" antipsychotics (also termed "conventional" or "first-generation") and the new "atypical" antipsychotics (also termed "nonconventional" or "second-generation"). Typical antipsychotics treat positive symptoms, are of little or no benefit for the other domains, and may even worsen them. The newer agents are at least as effective as the older ones in treating positive symptoms and are often helpful with negative, cognitive, and affective symptoms as well. All of the older antipsychotics cause motor system side effects that many individuals dislike intensely. The atypicals are virtually free of motor system side effects, and, for that reason they are greatly preferred by many people with schizophrenia. Typical and atypical antipsychotics are used to decrease symptoms during acute exacerbations and as maintenance medicines to prevent relapse during periods of relative remission.

The first antipsychotic, chlorpromazine (Thorazine), was developed in France during the early 1950s as a sedative for use in surgical anesthesia. It was later given to patients with schizophrenia with the expectation that it would decrease agitation. Investigators were surprised by their observation that long-standing psychotic symptoms gradually improved in many patients. Thus chlorpromazine represented a great breakthrough in treating what had been an untreatable disorder, despite the fact that it also produced a number of problematic side effects. The other typical antipsychotics that quickly followed were based on the chlorpromazine model. Even with their limited safety, tolerability, and efficacy (as many as 30% of treated patients have little response), these antipsychotics were widely adopted and resulted in significant symptoms reduction for many individuals with schizophrenia.

The therapeutic action of the typical antipsychotics, it is now thought, is due to blockade of the D2 type of dopamine receptors in the limbic area of the brain. Blockade of dopamine receptors in the basal ganglia gives rise to motor symptoms, including drug-induced parkinsonism (stiffness, slow shuffling gait, tremor) and acute dystonia (cramps). Treatment over months or years often causes muscle tics (termed "tardive dyskinesia") and abnormal postures (termed "tardive dystonias") which may not remit, even if medications are discontinued. The dopamine blockade of hypothalamic areas results in overproduction of the pituitary hormone prolactin and growth hormone. High prolactin levels result in menstrual irregularity and breast engorgement in women and sexual dysfunction and breast development in men.

About a dozen typical antipsychotics are in clinical use. These can be ranked with respect to their affinity for D2 receptors. High-potency agents achieve a dopaminergic blockade with doses of around 10 milligrams per day. These drugs are not sedating and have few anticholinergic side effects, but the motor side effects are pronounced. Anticholinergic agents are often given along with these drugs to reduce motor side effects, but this does not lessen the risk of tardive dyskinesia. Examples of high-potency agents are haloperidol (Haldol), fluphenazine (Prolixin), trifluoperazine (Stelazine), and thiothixene (Navane). Low-potency agents require daily doses of several hundred milligrams per day and have more affinity for receptors other than dopamine. A blockade of receptors for histamine, norepinephrine, and acetylcholine can lead to sedation, orthostatic hypotension, and anticholinergic side effects. Acute motor side effects are less severe due to the intrinsic anticholinergic activity. Examples of low-potency agents are chlorpromazine (Thorazine), thioridazine (Mallaril), and mesoridazine (Serentil). Mid-potency agents, such as loxipine (Loxitane) and molindone (Moban) have daily doses and side effects that fall between those of the other groups. Two antipsychotics are available in long-acting depot preparations (haloperidol decanoate and fluphenazine decanoate) that may be given by injection every 2 to 6 weeks. Depot injectable forms ensure continuous treatment for individuals who have difficulty adhering to a schedule of daily oral medication.

In somewhat rare instances, both typical and atypical antipsychotics can lead to the serious and occasionally fatal neuroleptic malignant syndrome (NMS) that is characterized by severe muscle rigidity, elevated temperature, dysphagia, fluctuating blood pressure, elevated creatinine phosphokinase levels, and mental confusion or coma. NMS is a medical emergency best treated in a general hospital.

Clozapine (Clozaril) was the first atypical antipsychotic developed. It has been in clinical use in Europe since the 1970s and was approved for clinical use in the United States in 1990. Rigorous clinical trials have shown that clozapine is an effective treatment for many individuals whose symptoms do not respond to conventional antipsychotics. To this day, it is considered the single most effective antipsychotic, but side effects limit its use to otherwise refractory cases. Once again, serendipity played a role in the discovery. Clozapine was synthesized for use as a typical antipsychotic and was found lacking in motor system side effects. Clozapine is a relatively weak dopamine blocker and a more potent blocker of some serotonin receptors. For unclear reasons, these actions lead to effects in the limbic system while avoiding effects in the basal ganglia and hypothalamus. Thus, there is antipsychotic activity without motor or hormonal side effects. Clozapine causes a life-threatening decrease in white blood cell production (agranulocytosis) in 1% of patients. It has since been determined that weekly blood monitoring can detect agranulocytosis in its early stages. If clozapine is then discontinued, almost all patients recover fully. Weekly blood tests are required for the first 6 months and every 2 weeks thereafter. Clozapine also has a number of other side effects, including occasional seizures, weight gain, sedation, and increased saliva production. Despite these side effects, it has given many people the chance to live much more normal lives.

The success of clozapine led to a search for compounds that would mimic its neurochemical status without causing agranulocytosis. At this time, three additional atypical antipsychotics are available: risperidone (Risperdal), olanzapine (Zyprexa), and quetiapine (Seroquel). Several others are in late stages of development. All of these combine some dopamine blockade with serotonin blockade. None of them causes agranulocytosis. All are effective antipsychotics. Evidence is accumulating that each of these agents is beneficial in treating all four symptom domains. Low doses of risperidone are often sufficient for antipsychotic activity and produce few or no motor side effects. At the higher end of its therapeutic dose range, risperidone begins to behave more like the typical antipsychotics and causes motor system side effects. Risperidone also increases prolactin levels. Olanzapine and quetiapine are virtually free of motor system side effects throughout their therapeutic ranges and do not elevate prolactin. The risk of tardive dyskinesia is considered minimal if there are no acute motor side effects. Quetiapine is somewhat sedating, especially during the early stages of treatment. Quetiapine has been associated with cataracts in dogs, but these have yet to be observed in people. These drugs usually cause mild to moderate weight gain, which is bothersome to patients. Otherwise they are free of common side effects.

Atypical antipsychotics are priced considerably higher than typical agents. Overall treatment costs may not be increased because the increased effectiveness of the newer medications often leads to decreased use of hospitals and other health-care services.

Substance Abuse Disorders

The abuse of alcohol, tobacco, street drugs, and prescription medications is a major public health problem. Pharmacological interventions have an essential role in treating substance abuse (Agency for Health Care Policy and Research, 1999a). Substance "abuse" consists of a maladaptive pattern of substance use that leads to significant social impairment or distress. In many instances, abuse is coupled with drug "dependence." In drug dependence, a person's body has adjusted to the substance so that larger doses are required, and withdrawal symptoms occur if the substance is not taken. Obtaining and using the substance become the single most important activities in a person's life, and substance use may continue despite obvious detrimental effects on emotions, social relationships, and physical health. Abuse and dependence should be differentiated from the physiological tolerance that may develop in the course of legitimate use of medications For example, an individual who has cancerous bone lesions may have a legitimate need for continuous opiate treatment A person who has recurrent depressions may require maintenance treatment with antidepressants. If either the opiate or antidepressant were abruptly discontinued, the individual would have withdrawal symptoms. Yet these are not examples of substance abuse. The substances are used adaptively to enhance the quality of life, and the continued use of the medicines poses no problems. Withdrawal could easily be managed by gradually reducing the medication dose, if necessary. The ways in which pharmacological interventions are helpful in treating substance abuse disorders include (1) managing acute intoxication; (2) allowing safe detoxification by averting uncomfortable and medically dangerous withdrawal symptoms; (3) treating anxiety, depression, and psychosis induced by substances; and (4) promoting abstinence by reducing cravings, mitigating the intensely pleasurable experience of intoxication, or providing a frankly adverse reaction to intoxication.

Acute, severe emotional problems and behavioral problems are common during intoxications with alcohol and street drugs such as amphetamines and hallucinogens. The primary treatment is observation in a safe environment until the intoxication passes and arrangements have been made for safe detoxification, if necessary. Antipsychotics and benzodiazepines may be carefully administered to control agitation and to prevent harm to self and others.

The withdrawal reactions that occur following abrupt abstinence from alcohol, barbiturates, and, at times, benzodiazepines are often severe and are potentially lethal. Detoxification involves using medications that allow the body to adjust safely to the abstinent state. Symptoms of alcohol withdrawal include elevations in pulse and blood pressure, gastrointestinal distress, tremor, epileptic seizures, hallucinations, and in 5% of untreated cases, death. Most of these symptoms are avoided by using a decreasing dose of benzodiazepines given during a period of 2 to 5 days. Heroin and other opiates have uncomfortable but less medically serious withdrawal states. A variety of medications have been used to make these more comfortable.

Chronic substance abuse often leads to symptoms of anxiety, depression, and psychosis. The primary treatment is abstinence from the abused substance, which often leads to resolution of symptoms without other intervention during a period of weeks to months. Treating the symptoms during the initial phases of abstinence may hasten improvement. Medications should be avoided that are potentially abusable or that would be dangerous if substance abuse recurred. For example, the antianxiety drug buspirone is much less likely to be abused than benzodiazepines, and SSRI antidepressants are far safer in combination with alcohol than TCAs. If substance abuse is ongoing, pharmacological treatment of substance-induced anxiety, depression or psychosis is usually futile.

Several treatments are used to facilitate abstinence. The antidepressant bupropion (Wellbutrin) reduces tobacco cravings and therefore is helpful in stopping cigarette smoking. The trade name "Zyban" is used for bupropion marketed expressly for this purpose. Naltrexone (Revia), an opiate receptor antagonist, blocks the pleasurable experience associated with alcohol intoxication, without causing adverse effects. The pleasure of intoxication is a key reinforcer in maintaining substance abuse. Individuals who take naltrexone and continue to drink find that the experience is neutral rather than pleasurable. Drinking decreases in accordance with the extinction paradigm of drinking theory. In contrast, disulfiram (Antabuse) interferes with the metabolism of alcohol, leading to an accumulation of toxic by-products. If disulfiram is taken daily, alcohol consumption will cause physical symptoms, including flushing, sweating, palpitations, nausea, vomiting, and in rare cases, death. Disulfiram is used by alcoholics who desire additional motivation to remain sober. It is primarily effective for alcoholics who are strongly motivated to remain sober. Others are simply noncompliant with disulfiram or endure the discomfort of the reactions, just as they endure so many other negative consequences of continued alcohol abuse. Medication to lesson craving for cocaine, amphetamine, and opiates has been less successful.

Substance abuse often complicates treatment of other disorders, such as depression, bipolar affective disorder, and schizophrenia. In such cases, treatment must be directed to both disorders simultaneously.

SEXUAL DISORDERS

The DSM-IV groups sexual disorders into three categories: gender identification disorder, sexual dysfunction, and paraphilia. There are no specific pharmacological interventions for gender identification disorder. Pharmacological interventions for sexual dysfunctions often involve treating comorbid conditions that result in sexual abnormalities. For example, decreased sexual desire is a common, treatable symptom of depression. At other times, sexual dysfunction is caused by medications taken for other reasons, and alterations in medications treat the sexual dysfunction. For example, SSRIs cause decreased libido and orgasmic delay. Switching to an alternative antidepressant such as nefazodone or bupropion may eliminate the sexual dysfunction. In contrast, low doses of SSRIs often successfully delay orgasm in men who ejaculate prematurely without eliminating sexual desires.

Pharmacological intervention for paraphilias has largely centered on treating sex offenders. Interventions are most successful for offenders who are genuinely motivated but find it difficult to stop the offensive behavior because of recurrent thoughts, intense erotic desires, or poor impulse control. SSRIs may be useful in reducing aberrant sexual desire. SSRIs may also stop repetitive thoughts of offending behaviors, much as they reduce obsessive thoughts in OCD. The antiadrenergic hormone medroxyprogesterone reduces sexual desire in men and may be given in as a long-acting injection (Depo-Provera). Anticonvulsants such as divalproex delay impulsive behavior and often give individuals time to stop and think before they do something harmful. Involuntary treatment of sexual offenders is less successful and fraught with ethical and legal dilemmas (Berlin, 1997).

PERSONALITY DISORDERS

Personality disorders are a heterogeneous group of conditions in which enduring, pervasive patterns of inner experience and behavior lead to significant distress or impairment in social functioning, and these patterns are not accounted for by other disorders. The DSM-IV subcategorizes personality disorders into three clusters: paranoid, schizoid, and schizotypal (Cluster A); antisocial, borderline, histrionic, and narcissistic (Cluster B); and avoidant, dependent, and obsessive–compulsive (Cluster C). A residual category of "personality disorder not otherwise specified" is also recognized for unusual presentations. Further, a person may exhibit traits from different clusters, and more than one cluster may be diagnosed.

Pharmacological interventions are not directed at treating the personality disorder *per se*, but treating specific symptoms is often helpful. Thus, quasi-psychotic symptoms that may accompany paranoid, schizoid, schizotypal, or borderline disorders may be responsive to antipsychotics. Inadequate impulse control may respond to SSRI antidepressants, or anticonvulsants. Depressive symptoms may respond to antidepressants, and anxiety to anxiolytics. Substance abuse is frequently a complicating factor. There is no pharmacotherapy for the criminality and lack of interpersonal concern associated with antisocial personality disorder, but affective lability and poor impulse control may be mitigated by antidepressants or anticonvulsants. Although not well studied, anger and overt aggression may be reduced by mood stabilizers, antidepressants, or antipsychotics (Fava, 1997).

PSYCHOPHYSIOLOGICAL AND ORGANIC MENTAL DISORDERS

Numerous medical and neurological disorders cause emotional, cognitive, and behavioral symptoms, as does destruction of brain tissue from trauma and dementing processes. The list of illnesses and neurological disorders that cause psychological symptoms is seemingly endless. A short list of common examples includes pituitary insufficiency, Cushing's disease, hyper- or hypothyroidism, folic acid deficiency, pernicious anemia, central nervous system infections and neoplasms, multiple sclerosis, pancreatitis, porphyria, systemic lupus erythematosus, and heavy metal poisoning. In addition, numerous medications that are used to treat medical conditions cause psychological symptoms. The primary treatment for all of these disorders involves treating the underlying medical condition or discontinuing the problematic medication. Psychopharmacological interventions may be useful as adjunctive agents. For example, high-dose steroid hormone treatment may be life saving in severe asthma but may cause psychotic symptoms. Adjunctive antipsychotic medication during steroid treatment mitigates the severity of the psychosis.

In the United States, there are more than 2 million traumatic head injuries each year (Silver, Hales, & Yudofsky, 1997). Half of these result from motor vehicle accidents. The remainder are largely from falls, assaults, and sports injuries. Severe injuries are frequently followed by persistent changes in personality, cognition, and mood, including both depression and mania. Mood stabilizers, antidepressants, or antipsychotics may be useful, depending on the particular symptoms. Stimulants, such as dextroamphetamine (Dexedrine) and methyphenidate (Ritalin), and the dopamine stimulating agents bromocriptine (Parlodel) and amantadine (Symmetrel) reportedly improve memory, concentration, and attentiveness.

Progressive decline in cognitive function affects 10% of persons older than age 65, and the prevalence increases dramatically with advancing age (Borson & Pascualy, 1998). Alzheimer's disease is, by far, the most common cause, followed by multi-infarct dementia, and other conditions that cause progressive loss of brain tissue. Medications help to preserve function in person's with Alzheimer's disease but do not alter the process of neuronal degeneration. When used early in the course of the illness, the cholinesterase inhibitors donepezil (Aricept) and tacrine (Cognex) provide modest increases in cognitive function, which result in a meaningful delay in nursing home placement. Donepezil is the preferred agent because it has fewer side effects. Later in the course of Alzheimer's disease, depression, agitation, and psychosis frequently require pharmacological treatment for the person's comfort and to preserve as much independent function as possible. Low medication doses, slow increases in doses, attention to drug interaction, and frequent monitoring are required to avoid falls and other problems from medications in this frail population.

Summary

Psychopharmacology has advanced greatly during the last half of the twentieth century, and it holds even greater promise for the twenty-first. The combined efforts of neuroscience and psychopharmacology are unlocking the physiological secrets of mental disorder and providing specially designed molecules to help relieve them. This chapter has been an overview of current pharmacological interventions for adults who have psychiatric disorders. Only the most salient issues could be addressed. Readers are encouraged to explore the field in more depth by using the referenced works.

Pharmacological interventions play an essential role in treatment and are best used as one component of a comprehensive, individualized treatment plan that may include psychotherapy, rehabilitation, and attention to concrete social needs. The great strides made by psychopharmacology are to be viewed alongside the advances made in psychotherapy and the challenges to health-care delivery that are posed by economic necessity and social reality. The synergistic combination of biological, psychological, and social modalities offers the best hope of addressing the complex needs of individuals who have emotional, cognitive, and behavioral disorders.

References

Agency for Health Care Policy and Research (1999a). *Pharmacology for Alcohol Dependence, Summary, Evidence Report/Technology Assessment: Number 3*. Rockville, MD: Author. Retrieved March 11, 1999 from the World Wide Web: http://www.ahcpr.gov/clinic/alcosumm.htm

Agency for Health Care Policy and Research (1999b). *Treatment for Depression—Newer Pharmacotherapies, Summary, Evidence Report/Technology Assessment: Number 7*. Rockville, MD: Author. Retrieved April 22, 1999 from the World Wide Web: http://www.ahcpr.gov/clinic/deprsumm.htm

American Psychiatric Association (1994). *Diagnostic and statistical manual of mental disorders*, 4th ed. (DSM-IV). Washington, DC: Author.

American Psychiatric Association (1997). Practice guidelines for the treatment of patients with schizophrenia. *American Journal of Psychiatry*, *154*(Supplement 4), 1–23.

Berlin, F. S. (1997). "Chemical castration" for sex offenders. *New England Journal of Medicine*, *336*, 1030.

Borson, S., & Pascualy, M. (1998). Pharmacologic management of Alzheimer's disease. *Psychiatric Clinics of North America*, *5* 231–268.

Diamond, R. J. (1998). *Instant psychopharmacology, a guide for the nonmedical mental health professional*. New York: W. W. Norton.

Expert Consensus Panel for Schizophrenia (1996). Treatment of schizophrenia. *Journal of Clinical Psychiatry*, *57*(Supplement 12B), 11–27.

Expert Consensus Panel on Obsessive–Compulsive Disorder (1997). Treatment of obsessive–compulsive disorder. *Journal of Clinical Psychiatry*, *58*(Supplement 6), 1–75.

Fava, M. F. (1997). Psychopharmacological treatment of pathological aggression. *Psychiatric Clinics of North America*, *20*, 427–451.

Frances, A. J., Kahn, D. A., Carpenter, D., Docherty, J. P., & Donovan, S. L. (1998). The expert consensus guidelines for treating depression in bipolar disorder. *Journal of Clinical Psychiatry*, *59*(Supplement 4), 73–79.

Harris, D. M. (1999a) Medical technology assessment and health resources plan with recommended clinical practice guidelines for anti-psychotic drugs. Salem, OR: Oregon Health Resources Commission.

Harris, D. M. (1999b) Medical technology assessment and health resources plan with recommended clinical practice guidelines for anti-depressant drugs. Salem, OR: Oregon Health Resources Commission.

Linde, K., Ramirez, G. Mulrow, C. D., Pauls, A., Weidenhammer, W., & Melchart D. (1996). St. John's wort for depression—An overview and meta-analysis of randomized clinical trials. *British Medical Journal*, *313*, 253–258.

Schatzberg, A. F., & Nemeroff, C. B. (1995). *The American Psychiatric Press textbook of psychopharmacology*. Washington, DC: American Psychiatric Press.

Silver, J. M., Hales, R. E., & Yudofsky, S. C. (1997). Neuropsychiatric aspects of traumatic brain injury. In S. C. Yudofsky & R. E. Hales (Eds.), *The American Psychiatric Press textbook of neuropsychiatry*, 3rd ed. Washington, DC: American Psychiatric Press.

Stahl, S. M. (1996). *Essential psychopharmacology: Neuroscientific basis and practical applications*. New York: Cambridge University Press.

Wilson, W. H. (1997). Neuroscientific research in mental health. In T. R. Watkins & J. W. Callicut (Eds.), *Mental health policy and practice today*. Thousand Oaks, CA: Sage.

About the Editors

Michel Hersen (Ph.D., State University of New York at Buffalo) is Professor and Dean, School of Professional Psychology, Pacific University, Forest Grove, Oregon. He is Past President of the Association for Advancement of Behavior Therapy. He has written 4 books, coauthored and/or coedited 114 books, and has published more than 220 scientific journal articles; he is coeditor of several psychological journals and is coeditor, with Alan S. Bellack, of the recently published 11-voume work *Comprehensive Clinical Psychology*. Dr. Hersen has been the recipient of numerous grants from the National Institute of Mental Health, the Department of Education, the National Institute of Disabilities and Rehabilitation Research, and the March of Dimes Birth Defects Foundation. He is a Diplomate of the American Board of Professional Psychology, Distinguished Practitioner, Member of the National Academy of Practice in Psychology, and recipient of the Distinguished Career Achievement Award in 1996 from the American Board of Medical Psychotherapists and Psychodiagnosticians. Dr. Hersen has written and edited numerous articles, chapters, and books on clinical assessment.

Vincent B. Van Hasselt (Ph.D., University of Pittsburgh) is Professor of Psychology and Director, Family Violence Program, Nova Southeastern University, Fort Lauderdale, Florida. He has published over 150 journal articles, books, and book chapters including several on the assessment and treatment of family violence, substance abuse, and police issues and is coeditor of the *Journal of Family Violence*, *Journal of Developmental and Physical Disabilities*, *Aggression and Violent Behavior: A Review Journal*, and *Journal of Child and Adolescent Substance Abuse*. Dr. Van Hasselt has been the recipient of grants from the Buhl Foundation, March of Dimes Birth Defects Foundation, National Institute of Disabilities and Rehabilitation Research, National Institute of Mental Health, U.S. Department of Education, and the National Institute of Justice. He is also a certified police officer, a lecturer at the Broward County (Florida) Police Academy and the FBI National Academy, and a consultant to the FBI Behavioral Science and Crisis Negotiation Units. His clinical and research interests are in the areas of police psychology, behavioral criminology, and critical incident stress.

Author Index

Subject Index